The SAGES
of Qualit
and Patient Safety

John R. Romanelli
Jonathan M. Dort
Rebecca B. Kowalski
Prashant Sinha
Editors

The SAGES Manual of Quality, Outcomes and Patient Safety

Second Edition

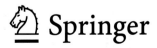 Springer

Editors
John R. Romanelli
Department of Surgery
University of Massachusetts
Chan Medical School - Baystate
Medical Center
Springfield, MA, USA

Rebecca B. Kowalski
Department of Surgery
Lenox Hill Hospital
New York, NY, USA

Jonathan M. Dort
Department of Surgery
Inova Fairfax Medical Campus
Falls Church, VA, USA

Prashant Sinha
Department of Surgery
NYU Langone Medical Center
Brooklyn, NY, USA

ISBN 978-3-030-94609-8   ISBN 978-3-030-94610-4   (eBook)
https://doi.org/10.1007/978-3-030-94610-4

This Springer imprint is published by the registered company Springer Nature Switzerland AG
The registered company address is: Gewerbestrasse 11, 6330 Cham, Switzerland

Preface

The idea that we can continually improve our outcomes in the delivery of healthcare is intrinsic in the nomenclature of calling what we do being in "practice." The concept of improving quality in the practice of medicine dates back to the nineteenth century. From Ignaz Semmelweis' seminal work on handwashing to prevent puerperal sepsis to Florence Nightingale associating high death rates of soldiers in Army hospitals with poor living conditions, physicians and other healthcare providers have often endeavored to find novel ways to improve the delivery of patient care. In surgery, Ernest Codman is credited with the first efforts in quality improvement, recognizing that surgeons could learn from each other and share science to lead to better outcomes for patients, and so he helped found the American College of Surgeons (ACS). Dr. Codman helped to start the Hospital Standardization Program at the ACS, which created and over-saw hospital standards. Today, this is known as the Joint Commission, which is ubiquitous in the healthcare quality arena. He also is the father of implementation of strategies to improve healthcare outcomes. Surgical quality, outcomes, and safety owe a debt of gratitude to this unique surgeon with remarkable foresight over a century ago.

While surgical societies such as ACS or the Society of Thoracic Surgeons (STS) have often led the charge to quality improvement, SAGES, too, has long had a role in this space. SAGES proudly developed the Fundamentals of Laparoscopic Surgery (FLS), the Fundamentals of Endoscopic Surgery (FES), and the Fundamentals of the Use of Safe Energy (FUSE); these programs were borne of the concept of education and accreditation of surgeons as "safe" for their patients; both FLS and FES are requirements for all graduating surgical residents. The SAGES Quality, Outcomes, and Safety (QOS) Committee was formed as a Task Force on Outcomes in 1997, and it eventually led to the creation of the Outcomes Committee in 2003. This committee was expanded into the QOS Committee in 2008, and it leads the society and its 7000+ surgeons and members as more public attention is devoted to healthcare quality. The first edition of the SAGES Quality, Outcomes, and Safety Manual was groundbreaking as it combined didactic study with expert opinion, venturing outside the clinical arena with important writings on topics such as systems improvement, perioperative safety, error analysis, simulation as an educational tool, team training, and an emphasis on the SAGES Fundamentals programs. Published in 2011, this manual edited by David Tichansky, John Morton, and Daniel B. Jones was one of the first scholarly texts to collect these thoughts into one book, and it was well received by the SAGES membership and surgeons around the world.

Much has transpired in the last decade, and the editors of the second edition of the SAGES Quality, Outcomes, and Safety Manual sought to include these topics for discussion. So, while we sought to keep and update some of the fine work of the first edition, we added new sections that are timely and relevant to the surgeon in practice today. We explored areas of enhanced recovery pathways and the avoidance of postoperative opioid use, as the crisis of the abuse of the drugs is widespread and perhaps preventable to some degree. We examined threats to quality, such as healthcare disparities, disruptive behavior, physician wellness and burnout, physicians as second victims of bad outcomes, ergonomics of surgery, and training new surgeons in the era of work hour limitations. We discussed pathways towards quality, such as mentoring, teleproctoring, training to proficiency, and creating procedural benchmarks. We debated controversial issues such as the use of the robot in minimally invasive surgery, prevention of bile duct injury, super-specialization of general surgery and what it means for patients, and non-clinical concerns such as enforced OR attire and consistent operating room teams. And wherever possible, we highlighted the role that SAGES plays in the quality, outcomes, and safety space.

Lastly, it would be remiss of me personally and professionally not to acknowledge the incredible work of Erin Schwarz. Erin is the administrative staff member who ensures that Quality, Outcomes, and Safety continues its important role in SAGES. A textbook project of this magnitude simply would not be possible without her indefatigable efforts to keep the momentum going to complete this project. Erin is a key member of BSC, who are the framework upon which SAGES thrives. My heartfelt gratitude goes to the whole of BSC, but to Erin, I can only humbly say "thank you."

On behalf of my co-editors, Jonathan Dort, Rebecca Kowalski, and Prashant Sinha, I thank you for reading this book and hope it helps you to consider important concepts to improve the care of your surgical patients.

Springfield, MA, USA   John R. Romanelli

Preface

Approximately a decade following the publication of the first edition of this manual, the world of surgery continues to dramatically change. The focus on the quality of care provided by surgeons, the safety of the patients we treat, and the clinical outcomes we see as a result of our care, by both the surgical community and the public, has never been stronger. SAGES remains committed to leading in these areas, and the work and expertise presented in this manual will hopefully serve as a comprehensive resource to all of our SAGES members, as well as to the broader surgical community. This manual covers a wide range of critical topics, from the language and basics of quality, outcomes, and patient safety to education, mentorship, new technologies, and different approaches to care. It is crucial for the care of their patients that surgeons understand all of the elements of how quality is measured, how care outcomes are reviewed, and what the best practices available to them are on how to provide that care. On behalf of the SAGES Quality, Outcomes, and Patient Safety Committee, I am indebted to the time and efforts of the committee members and authors who have helped to create this manual. I also wish to thank my co-editors, John Romanelli, Rebecca Kowalski, and Prashant Sinha, as well as to Erin Schwarz, who has provided all of the administrative support to this endeavor, for all of their hard work in producing this second edition. I hope that you find it to be informative, comprehensive, and useful.

Falls Church, VA, USA   Jonathan M. Dort, MD

Contents

Part III Surgical Safety

Part IV Working Towards Surgical Quality, Outcomes, and Safety

**Part V   Threats to Surgical Quality, Outcomes,
and Safety**

Part VI   Surgical Controversies That Impact Quality

Contributors

Gina Adrales Johns Hopkins University School of Medicine, Baltimore, MD, USA

Thomas A. Aloia University of Texas MD Anderson Cancer Center, Houston, TX, USA

Adnan Alseidi Department of Surgery, University of California San Francisco, San Francisco, CA, USA

Sharon Bachman Department of Surgery, Inova Fairfax Medical Campus, Falls Church, VA, USA

Limaris Barrios Dr. Kiran C. Patel College of Allopathic Medicine (NSU MD), Nova Southeastern University in Florida, Fort Lauderdale, FL, USA

Marylise Boutros Division of Colon and Rectal Surgery, Sir Mortimer B. Davis Jewish General Hospital, Montreal, QC, Canada

L. Michael Brunt Department of Surgery and Section of Minimally Invasive Surgery, Washington University School of Medicine, St. Louis, MO, USA

Stephanie Calcasola Hartford HealthCare, Hartford, CT, USA

Manoj Kumar Choudhury Senior Consultant, GI and MIS, Nemcare Superspecialty Hospital, Assam, India

Nabajit Choudhury The University of Tennessee Health Science Center, Memphis, TN, USA

Freeman Condon Tripler Army Medical Center, Honolulu, HI, USA

Tiffany C. Cox Department of Surgery, Uniformed Services University of Health Sciences & Walter Reed National Military Medical Center, Bethesda, MD, USA

M. Shane Dawson Northwell Health at Lenox Hill Hospital, New York, NY, USA

Peter M. Denk GI Surgical Specialists, Fort Myers, FL, USA

Diana L. Diesen Department of Surgery, University of Texas Southwestern Medical Center, Dallas, TX, USA

Justin B. Dimick Department of Surgery, University of Michigan, Ann Arbor, MI, USA

Jonathan M. Dort Department of Surgery, Inova Fairfax Medical Campus, Falls Church, VA, USA

Christopher G. DuCoin Department of Surgery, University of South Florida Morsani College of Medicine, Tampa, FL, USA

Shaina R. Eckhouse Section of Minimally Invasive Surgery, Department of Surgery, Washington University School of Medicine, Saint Louis, MO, USA

Yasmin Essaji Division of HPB Surgery, Virginia Mason Medical Center, Seattle, WA, USA

Liane S. Feldman Department of Surgery, McGill University, Montreal, QC, Canada

Julio F. Fiore Department of Surgery, McGill University, Montreal, QC, Canada

Benjamin J. Flink Stony Brook University Department of Surgery, Division of Bariatric, Foregut, and Advanced Gastrointestinal Surgery, Stony Brook, NY, USA

Timothy Fokken Department of Surgery, Inova Fairfax Medical Campus, Falls Church, VA, USA

Teresa Fraker Metabolic and Bariatric Surgery Accreditation and Quality Improvement Program (MBSAQIP), Division of Research and Optimal Patient Care (DROPC), American College of Surgeons (ACS), Chicago, IL, USA

Gerald M. Fried Professor of Surgery and Associate Dean for Education Technology and Innovation, Montreal, QC, Canada
Faculty of Medicine and Health Sciences, McGill University, Montreal, QC, Canada
Director, Steinberg Centre for Simulation and Interactive Learning, Faculty of Medicine and Health Sciences, McGill University, Montreal, QC, Canada

Pascal Fuchshuber Sutter East Bay Medical Group, UCSF-East Bay, Oakland, CA, USA

Rebecca Gates Virginia Tech Carilion School of Medicine and Carilion Clinic, Roanoke, VA, USA

Kim Gerling Department of Surgery, Uniformed Services University of Health Sciences & Walter Reed National Military Medical Center, Bethesda, MD, USA

Michael Ghio Tulane University School of Medicine & Tulane Medical Center, New Orleans, LA, USA

William Greif The Permanente Medical Group, Kaiser Walnut Creek Medical Center, Walnut Creek, CA, USA

Anjali A. Gresens Bariatric Surgery, Sentara Medical Group, Norfolk, VA, USA
Department of Surgery, Eastern Virginia Medical School, Norfolk, VA, USA

Rana M. Higgins Medical College of Wisconsin, Milwaukee, WI, USA

Ryan Howard Department of Surgery, University of Michigan, Ann Arbor, MI, USA

Eunice Y. Huang Departments of General and Thoracic Surgery, Monroe Carell Jr. Children's Hospital at Vanderbilt, Nashville, TN, USA

Gretchen Purcell Jackson Departments of General and Thoracic Surgery, Monroe Carell Jr. Children's Hospital at Vanderbilt, Nashville, TN, USA

Intuitive Surgical, Sunnyvale, CA, USA

Daniel B. Jones Department of Surgery, Rutgers New Jersey Medical School, Newark, NJ, USA

Carolyn Judge Department of Surgery, Uniformed Services University of Health Sciences & Walter Reed National Military Medical Center, Bethesda, MD, USA

Michael R. Keating University of Texas Southwestern, Dallas, TX, USA

Deborah S. Keller Division of Colorectal Surgery, Department of Surgery, University of California at Davis, Sacramento, CA, USA

Leena Khaitan University Hospitals, Department of Surgery, Cleveland, OH, USA

James R. Korndorffer Jr Department of Surgery, Stanford University School of Medicine, Stanford, CA, USA

Anai N. Kothari Department of Surgery, Division of Surgical Oncology, Medical College of Wisconsin, Milwaukee, WI, USA

Rebecca B. Kowalski Northwell Health at Lenox Hill Hospital, New York, NY, USA

Danuel Laan Tulane University School of Medicine & Tulane Medical Center, New Orleans, LA, USA

Kathleen Lak Bariatric and Minimally Invasive Gastrointestinal Surgery, Medical College of Wisconsin, Milwaukee, WI, USA

Teresa L. LaMasters Iowa Methodist Medical Center Unity Point Clinic, University of Iowa, Des Moines, IA, USA

James N. Lau Loyola University Medical Center, Department of Surgery, Maywood, IL, USA

Shauna Levy Tulane University School of Medicine & Tulane Medical Center, New Orleans, LA, USA

Anne O. Lidor Department of Surgery, Johns Hopkins University SOM, Baltimore, MD, USA

Cara A. Liebert Department of Surgery, Stanford University School of Medicine, VA Palo Alto Health Care System, Palo Alto, CA, USA

Robert Lim University of Oklahoma School of Medicine Tulsa, Tulsa, OK, USA

Jamie P. Loggins Mission Weight Management Center, Asheville, NC, USA

Matthew Madion Medical College of Wisconsin, Milwaukee, WI, USA

Kelly Mahuron Department of Surgery, University of California San Francisco, San Francisco, CA, USA

John D. Mellinger Southern Illinois University School of Medicine, Department of Surgery, Springfield, IL, USA

Samuel M. Miller Department of Surgery, Yale School of Medicine, New Haven, CT, USA

Jeongyoon Moon Division of Colon and Rectal Surgery, Sir Mortimer B. Davis Jewish General Hospital, Montreal, QC, Canada

Lee Morris Department of Surgery, The Houston Methodist Hospital, Houston, TX, USA

John M. Morton Department of Surgery, Yale School of Medicine, New Haven, CT, USA

Madhuri B. Nagaraj University of Texas Southwestern, Department of Surgery, Dallas, TX, USA

Brian J. Nasca Northwestern University Feinberg School of Medicine, Chicago, IL, USA

Ugoeze J. Nwokedi Department of Surgery, The Houston Methodist Hospital, Houston, TX, USA

Jaisa Olasky Mount Auburn Hospital, Harvard Medical School, Boston, MA, USA

Rocco Orlando III Hartford HealthCare, Hartford, CT, USA

University of Connecticut School of Medicine, Hartford, CT, USA

Charles Paget Virginia Tech Carilion School of Medicine and Carilion Clinic, Roanoke, VA, USA

John T. Paige Department of Surgery, MedicineLouisiana State University (LSU) Health New Orleans School of Medicine, New Orleans, LA, USA

Julio Santiago Perez Valley Health System General Surgery Department, Las Vegas, NV, USA

V. Prasad Poola Southern Illinois University School of Medicine, Department of Surgery, Springfield, IL, USA

Aurora D. Pryor Stony Brook University Department of Surgery, Division of Bariatric, Foregut, and Advanced Gastrointestinal Surgery, Stony Brook, NY, USA

Fateme Rajabiyazdi Department of Systems and Computer Engineering, Carleton University, Ottawa, ON, Canada

Bruce Ramshaw Managing Partner, CQInsights PBC, Knoxville, TN, USA

Stacy M. Ranson Inova Fairfax Medical Campus, Falls Church, VA, USA

Arthur Rawlings General Surgery, University of Missouri, One Hospital Drive, Columbia, MO, USA

Swathi Reddy Johns Hopkins University School of Medicine, Baltimore, MD, USA

Adam Reid Southern Illinois University School of Medicine, Department of Surgery, Springfield, IL, USA

Caroline E. Reinke Department of Surgery, Atrium Health, Charlotte, NC, USA

Amelia T. Collings Department of Surgery, Indiana University School of Medicine, Indianapolis, IN, USA

John R. Romanelli Department of Surgery, University of Massachusetts Chan Medical School - Baystate Medical Center, Springfield, MA, USA

Ingrid S. Schmiederer Department of Surgery, Stanford University School of Medicine, Stanford, CA, USA

New York Presbyterian-Queens, Department of Surgery, Flushing, NY, USA

Benjamin E. Schneider University of Texas Southwestern, Dallas, TX, USA

Erin Schwarz SAGES, Los Angeles, CA, USA

Daniel J. Scott University of Texas Southwestern, Department of Surgery and Simulation Center, Dallas, TX, USA

Marinda Scrushy Department of Surgery, University of Texas Southwestern Medical Center, Dallas, TX, USA

Neal E. Seymour Baystate Medical Center, Department of Surgery, Springfield, MA, USA

Phillip P. Shadduck Duke University, Durham, NC, USA

William C. Sherrill III Department of Surgery and Section of Minimally Invasive Surgery, Washington University School of Medicine, St. Louis, MO, USA

Prashant Sinha Department of Surgery, NYU Langone Medical Center, Brooklyn, NY, USA

Brandon W. Smith Baystate Medical Center, Department of Surgery, Springfield, MA, USA

Eileen R. Smith Section of Minimally Invasive Surgery, Department of Surgery, Washington University School of Medicine, Saint Louis, MO, USA

Dimitrios Stefanidis Department of Surgery, Indiana University School of Medicine, Indianapolis, IN, USA

Jonah J. Stulberg The University of Texas Health Science Center at Houston, Houston, TX, USA

Joseph A. Sujka Department of Surgery, University of South Florida Morsani College of Medicine, Tampa, FL, USA

Dina Tabello Inova Fairfax Medical Campus, Falls Church, VA, USA

Nabil Tariq Department of Surgery, The Houston Methodist Hospital, Houston, TX, USA

Jacob A. Tatum Department of Surgery, Eastern Virginia Medical School, Norfolk, VA, USA

Dana A. Telem National Clinician Scholars Program, University of Michigan, Ann Arbor, MI, USA

Shawn Tsuda Valley Health System General Surgery Department, Las Vegas, NV, USA

Buğra Tugertimur General Surgery Resident, PGY 5, Department of Surgery, Lenox Hill Hospital, Northwell Health, New York City, NY, USA

Sofia Valanci Doctoral student in Experimental Surgery, Education Concentration, McGill University, Montreal, QC, Canada

Valeria S. M. Valbuena University of Michigan, Department of Surgery, Ann Arbor, MI, USA

Sherry M. Wren Department of Surgery, Center for Innovation and Global Health, Stanford University School of Medicine, VA Palo Alto Health Care System, Palo Alto, CA, USA

Tonia M. Young-Fadok Division of Colon and Rectal Surgery, Mayo Clinic, Phoenix, AZ, USA

Joseph Youssef University Hospitals, Department of Surgery, Cleveland, OH, USA

Brenda M. Zosa Department of Surgery, Johns Hopkins University SOM, Baltimore, MD, USA

Part I
Surgical Quality

Chapter 1
Defining Quality in Surgery

Ryan Howard and Justin B. Dimick

Introduction

With recognition of wide variations in surgical performance, demand for information on surgical quality is at an all-time high. Patients and families are turning to their physicians, hospital report cards, and the Internet to identify the safest hospitals for surgery [1]. Payers and purchasers are using efforts to reward high quality (e.g., pay for performance) or steer patients toward the highest quality providers (e.g., selective referral) [2]. In addition to responding to these external demands, providers are becoming more involved in leveraging their own quality measurement platforms to improve surgical care, such as the National Surgical Quality Improvement Program (NSQIP) [3]. Finally, professional organizations are now accrediting hospitals based on their ability to meet certain metrics believed to be associated with better outcomes [4].

Despite the need for good measures of quality in surgery, there is very little agreement about how to best assess surgi-

R. Howard · J. B. Dimick (✉)
Department of Surgery, University of Michigan,
Ann Arbor, MI, USA
e-mail: jdimick@umich.edu

J. R. Romanelli et al. (eds.), *The SAGES Manual of Quality,
Outcomes and Patient Safety*,
https://doi.org/10.1007/978-3-030-94610-4_1

cal performance. According to the widely used Donabedian paradigm, quality can be measured using various aspects of structure, process, or outcome [5]. In addition, many widely recognized quality measurement efforts, such as those by the Leapfrog group, use composite, or "global," measures of quality, which combine one or more elements of structure, process, and outcome [6]. In this chapter, we consider the advantages and disadvantages of each type of quality measure. We close by making recommendations for choosing among these different approaches.

Structure

The structure of surgical care refers to measurable attributes of a hospital (e.g., size and volume) or its providers (e.g., specialty training and years in practice) (Table 1.1). Measures of structure are extensively used in the measurement of surgical quality, owing to their widespread availability. The American College of Surgeons (ACS) and the American Society of Metabolic and Bariatric Surgeons (ASMBS) accredit hospitals for bariatric surgery based largely on measures of structure, including hospital volume, surgeon volume, and other structural elements necessary for providing multidisciplinary care for the morbidly obese [4].

Structural elements have several key strengths as quality measures. First, they are relatively easy to ascertain. Often, structural elements such as volume can be obtained from readily available administrative data. Second, many structural measures are strong predictors of hospital and surgeon outcomes. The most well-known example of this relationship was described by Birkmeyer et al., who observed a fivefold difference in mortality between low- and high-volume hospitals for high-risk surgical procedures [7]. This same relationship holds true for individual surgeon volume as well [8]. Since the early 2000s, the volume-outcome relationship has been demonstrated for dozens of operations [9].

TABLE 1.1 Approaches to measuring the quality of care for aortic surgery with advantages and disadvantages of each approach

Type of measure	Example	Advantages	Disadvantages
Structure	Hospital or surgeon volume	Inexpensive and readily available Good proxy for outcomes	Not actionable for quality improvement Not good for discriminating among individual providers
Process	Prophylactic antibiotics given on time Adherence to venous thromboembolism prevention guidelines	Actionable as targets for improvement Less influenced by patient risk and random errors	Known processes relate to unimportant or rare surgical outcomes Very few "high leverage" processes of care are known
Outcomes	Anastomotic leak rates with bariatric surgery Wound infection with ventral hernia repair	Seen as the bottom line of patient care Enjoy good "buy-in" from surgeons	Sample sizes often too small at individual hospitals Need for detailed data for risk adjustment
Composite	Leapfrog group's "Survival Predictor"	Addresses problems with small sample size Makes sense of multiple conflicting measures	Not granular enough to identify specific clinical areas that need improvement

However, there are certain limitations of using structural quality measures. Most importantly, they are proxies for quality rather than direct measures. As a result, they only hold true on average. For example, while high-volume surgeons are better than low-volume surgeons on average, there are likely to be some high-volume surgeons with bad outcomes and low-volume surgeons with good outcomes [5]. What's more, structural measures are not meaningfully actionable for quality improvement. Hospitals cannot easily change their operative volume, although regionalization of high-risk care may offer a solution to centralize care at more specialized centers and leverage the volume-outcome relationship.

In recent years, structural measures of care have also been found to be lacking when implemented as real-world quality metrics. For example, after certain high-risk cancer operations, there was no mortality difference in hospitals that met the Leapfrog group's minimum volume standards and those that did not [10]. Similarly, even among hospitals designated as bariatric centers of excellence based on volume standards, there is still a 17-fold difference in rates of serious complications [11].

Process

Processes of care are the steps and details of a patient's care that can lead to good (or bad) outcomes. Although processes of care can represent details of care in the preoperative, intraoperative, and postoperative phases, the most familiar process measures focus on details in the immediate preoperative phase of patient care. For example, the Center for Medicare and Medicaid Services (CMS) Surgical Care Improvement Project (SCIP) measures utilization of preoperative antibiotic and venous thromboembolism prophylaxes. Along these lines, one of the most familiar approaches to improving the process of care in surgery is the use of a presurgical checklist, which verifies that a number of best practices (confirming patient name, procedure laterality, administration of antibiotics, etc.) have been performed [12]. This has now become standard practice in the United States.

Process measures have several strengths as quality measures (Table 1.1). First, processes of care are extremely actionable in quality improvement. When hospitals and surgeon are "low outliers" for process compliance (e.g., patients not getting timely antibiotic prophylaxis), they know exactly where to target improvement. Second, in contrast to risk-adjusted outcomes measurement, processes of care do not need to be adjusted for differences in patient risk, which limits the need for data collection from the medical chart and saves valuable time and effort.

However, using processes of care has several significant limitations in surgery. First, most existing process measures are not strongly related to important outcomes. For example, the SCIP measures, which are by far the most widely used process measure in surgery, are not related to surgical mortality, infections, or thromboembolism [13]. Similarly, after implementing the preoperative checklist in 101 hospitals in Ontario, Canada, there was no measurable change in postoperative complications or mortality [14]. The lack of a relationship between process improvement and surgical mortality can be explained by the fact that the complications they aim to prevent are secondary (e.g., superficial wound infection) or extremely rare (e.g., pulmonary embolism). However, there is also a very weak relationship between process measures and the outcome they are supposed to prevent (e.g., timely administration of prophylactic antibiotics and wound infection) [15]. This finding is more difficult to explain. It is possible that there are simply multiple other processes (many unmeasured or unmeasurable) that contribute to good surgical outcomes. As a result, it is likely that adherence to process best practices is necessary but not sufficient for good surgical outcomes.

Outcome

Outcomes represent the end results of care. In surgery, the most commonly evaluated outcomes are mortality, serious complications, and hospital readmissions. For example, the

NSQIP, the largest clinical registry focusing on surgery, reports risk-adjusted morbidity and mortality rates to participating hospitals [3]. While morbidity and mortality have long been the "gold standard" in surgery, patient-reported outcomes such as functional status and quality of life are also critically important.

Direct outcome measures have several strengths (Table 1.1). First, everyone agrees that outcomes are important. Measuring the end results of care makes intuitive sense to surgeons and other stakeholders. For example, the NSQIP has been enthusiastically championed by surgeons and other clinical leaders [16]. Second, outcomes feedback alone may improve quality. This so-called Hawthorne effect is seen whenever outcomes are measured and reported back to providers. For example, the NSQIP in the Veterans Affairs (VA) hospitals and private sector has documented improvements over time that cannot be attributed to any specific efforts to improve outcomes [17].

However, outcome measures have key limitations. First, when the event rate is low (numerator) or the number of cases is small (denominator), outcomes cannot be reliably measured. Small sample size and low event rates conspire to limit the statistical power of hospital outcomes comparisons. For most operations, surgical mortality is too rare to be used as a reliable quality measure [18]. For example, a study examining seven operations for which mortality was advocated as a quality measure by the Agency for Healthcare Research and Quality (AHRQ) found that only one of the seven operations – coronary artery bypass surgery – had high enough caseloads to reliably measure quality with surgical mortality [19].

Accurately measuring and comparing outcomes as a quality improvement instrument is also confounded by many factors. Surgical outcomes are influenced not only by quality of care but also by random variation, sample size, and case mix. Whereas structure and process measure are fixed elements of care, outcomes require additional risk and reliability adjustment to account for these confounders [20]. Acquiring the data necessary to make these adjustments is labor-intensive and expensive. For example, the NSQIP collects more than 80 patient variables from the medical chart for this purpose [17]. Each NSQIP hospital employs a trained nurse clinician to collect this data.

Composite

Composite measures are created by combining one or more structure, process, and outcome measures [21]. Composite measures offer several advantages over the individual measures discussed above (Table 1.1). By combining multiple measures, it is possible to overcome problems with small sample size discussed above. Composite measures also provide a "global" measure of quality. This type of measure has been used for quality for value-based purchasing or other efforts that require an overall or summary measure of quality.

One key limitation with composite measures is that there is no "gold standard" approach for weighting input measures. Perhaps the most common approach is to weight each input measure equally. For example, in the ongoing Premier/CMS pay for performance initiative, individual measures are weighted. However, this approach is also flawed insofar as variation in these composite measures is entirely driven by the process measures [22].

Another limitation with composite measures is that they are not always actionable for quality improvement. By combining information on multiple measures and/or clinical conditions, there is often not enough "granularity" for clinicians to use the information for quality improvement. To target quality improvement efforts, it is often necessary to deconstruct the composite into its component measures and find out where the problem lies (e.g., the specific procedure or complication).

Patient-Reported Outcomes

An important element of surgical quality not captured in the traditional Donabedian paradigm outlined above is patient-reported outcomes. There is now wide recognition of the importance of patient-reported outcomes. These outcomes capture the patient's perspective on their postoperative experience, and common measures include functional status, satisfaction, and quality of life.

CMS now uses the Hospital Consumer Assessment of Healthcare Providers and Systems (HCAHPS) survey as part of its value-based purchasing program. Although it is still unclear how these outcomes can be meaningfully integrated into actionable quality improvement efforts, they are nevertheless a necessary complement to traditional outcome measures [23]. It has been demonstrated that there is a high association between patient satisfaction and traditional objective outcome measures [24]. This suggests that efforts and policies to improve the patient experience can be undertaken without negatively impacting other important outcome measures.

Choosing the Right Measurement Approach

No approach to quality measurement is perfect. Each type of measure – structure, process, and outcome – has its own strengths and limitations. In general, selecting the right approach to measure quality depends on characteristics of the procedure and the specific policy application [5].

Certain characteristics of the surgical procedure should be considered when selecting a quality measure (Fig. 1.1). Specifically, one should consider how risky the procedure is (i.e., how often to complications occur?) and what the volume of the procedure is (i.e., how often is it performed?). For procedures that are both common and relatively high risk (e.g., colectomy and gastric bypass), outcomes are reliable enough to be used as measures of quality (Fig. 1.1, Quadrant I). For

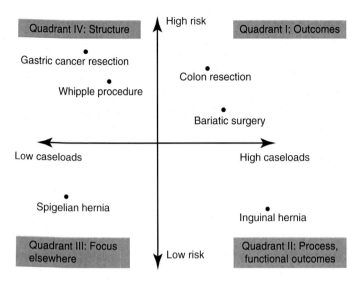

FIGURE 1.1 Choosing among measures of structure, process, and outcomes. For high-risk, high caseload operations (e.g., colectomy and bariatric procedures), outcomes are useful quality measures. For low-risk, common procedures (e.g., inguinal hernia repair), processes of care or functional outcomes are appropriate measures. For high-risk, uncommon operations (e.g., gastric and pancreatic cancer resection), measures of structure, such as hospital volume, are most appropriate. For low-risk, low caseload operations (e.g., spigelian hernia repair), it would be best to focus measurement efforts elsewhere. (Figure modified by Birkmeyer et al. [5])

procedures that are common but low risk (e.g., inguinal hernia repair), measures of the process of care or patient-reported outcomes are the best approach (Fig. 1.1, Quadrant II). For procedures that are high risk but uncommon (e.g., pancreatic and esophageal resection), structural measures such as hospital volume are likely the best approach (Fig. 1.1, Quadrant IV). In fact, empirical data suggests that structural measures such as hospital volume are better predictors of future performance than direct outcome measures for these uncommon, high-risk operations [25]. Finally, for operations that are both uncommon and low risk (e.g., Spigelian hernia repair), it is probably best to focus quality measurement efforts on other, more high leverage procedures.

When choosing an approach to quality measurement, the specific policy application should also be considered. In particular, it is important to distinguish between policy efforts aimed at selective referral and quality improvement. For selective referral, the main goal is to redirect patients to the highest quality providers. Structural measures, such as hospital volume, are particularly good for this purpose. Hospital volume tends to be strongly related to outcomes, and large gains in outcomes could be achieved by concentrating patients in high-volume hospitals. In contrast, structural measures are not directly actionable and, therefore, do not make good measures for quality improvement. For improving quality, process and outcome measures are better because they provide actionable targets. Surgeons and hospitals can improve by addressing problems with process compliance or focus on clinical areas with high rates of adverse outcomes. For example, the NSQIP reports risk-adjusted morbidity and mortality rates to every hospital. Surgeon champions and quality improvement personnel will target improvement efforts to areas where performance is statistically worse than expected.

Improving Quality Measurement

Although the science of surgical quality measurement has come a long way in the past two decades, the methodology is still developing. Here we outline important improvements to quality measurement that address the problems with the process of care and outcome measures discussed above.

A central element of meaningful outcomes reporting and comparison is the use of appropriate risk-adjustment techniques [26]. This process helps account for variation in case mix across hospitals, since a hospital that has a higher proportion of comorbid, complex patients would be reasonably expected to have a higher raw number of complications than a hospital that has younger, less sick patients. The importance of risk adjustment is powerfully illustrated by a study comparing outcomes after emergency colectomy between rural and urban hospitals [27]. Before adjusting for factors such as patient age, gender, race, and comorbidity profile, rural hospitals had a much lower unadjusted 30-day mortality at 10.9% versus 16.3%. However, after adjusting for this difference in patient factors, the difference narrows substantially to 14.3% versus 16.2%, reflecting the fact that rural hospitals tend to have less complex patients.

At present, most clinical registries collect a large number of clinical data elements from the medical record for risk adjustment. This "kitchen sink" approach to risk adjustment is largely based on the assumption that each additional variable improves our ability to make fair hospital comparisons. However, empiric data suggests that only the most important variables contribute meaningfully to risk-adjustment models. For example, Tu and colleagues demonstrated that a 5-variable model provides nearly identical results to a 12-variable model for comparing hospital outcomes with cardiac surgery [28]. Using data from the NSQIP, we have demonstrated similar results for both general surgical procedures [26]. These results should be used to streamline the collection of data for risk adjustment, which will decrease the costs of data collection and lower the bar for participation in these important clinical registries.

Advanced statistical techniques are also needed to address the problem of "noisy" outcome measures [29]. As discussed above, imprecision from small sample size is the Achilles heel of outcomes measurement. Analytic techniques that rely on empirical Bayes theory to adjust hospital outcomes for reliability help mitigate this problem. In this approach, the statistical "noise" is explicitly measured and removed by shrinking the observed outcome rate back toward the average rate. For example, Fig. 1.2 shows risk-adjusted hospital morbidity rates across quintiles for ventral hernia repair, before and after adjusting for reliability. Before adjusting for reliability, rates of morbidity varied eightfold (2.3–17.5%) from the "best" to

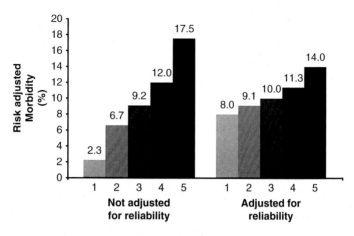

Figure 1.2 Comparison of ventral hernia repair morbidity rates across hospital quintiles (1 = "best hospitals" and 5 = "worst hospitals") before and after adjusting for statistical reliability. After adjusting for reliability, the apparent variation across hospitals is greatly diminished

"worst" quintile. However, after removing chance variation (i.e., "noise") by adjusting for reliability, rates of morbidity varied less than twofold (8.0–14.0%) from the "best" to "worst" quintile.

While this approach has many advantages, reliability adjustment makes the assumption that small hospitals have average performance. Although this approach gives small hospitals, the benefit of the doubt (i.e., they are innocent until proven guilty), under certain circumstances it could bias hospital rankings. For instance, given the well-known relationship between volume and outcome in surgery, these small hospitals may actually have performance below average. Incorporating information about hospital volume could address this bias. We have developed a novel technique for performing reliability adjustment by shrinking to a conditional average (i.e., the outcome expected given hospital volume) to address this problem [6]. This approach is considered a composite measure as it includes two inputs (mortality and volume).

This general approach can also be used to create more sophisticated composite measures of quality. As discussed above, most current approaches for combining measures are flawed. To address this problem, we have developed a method for empirically weighting input measures [30]. Briefly, we first identify a gold standard quality measure, such as mortality or serious morbidity. We then determine the relationship between each candidate measure and this gold standard measure. Finally, each input measure is given a weight based on (1) the reliability with which it is measured and (2) how correlated it is with the gold standard measure. These empirically weighted composite measures have been shown to be better predictors of future performance than individual measures alone.

Measuring Surgeon, Hospital, and Network Quality

Despite continuing uncertainty about how best to methodologically measure performance, value-based payments, surgeon report cards, and national rankings are now a reality of surgical practice. Here we present examples of instruments currently used to compare quality at the surgeon, hospital, and network level and offer strategies for how best to incorporate the above approaches into these measurements.

One example of how surgeon quality is currently measured and presented to patients is via ProPublica's "Surgeon Scorecard," which claims to report risk-adjusted individual surgeon outcomes. Currently, the scorecard attempts to rate surgeons for eight common elective procedures. However, recent studies have shown that this mechanism is underpowered to detect any meaningful difference – to detect a statistically significant difference in outcomes after laparoscopic cholecystectomy, surgeons would need to perform at least 170 of these cases. However, no individual surgeon in the ProPublica scorecard comes close to that volume [31]. An emerging and likely more meaningful approach to individual surgeon rating is the use of intraoperative video assessment, where surgeon skill is evaluated by peer reviewers using standardized instruments. Recent data suggest that surgeon technical skill assessed via video review is directly related to complication rates and mortality [32]. Quality improvement efforts directed at individual surgeon performance are increasingly utilizing video review [33].

Measuring quality at the hospital level requires taking into account the multiple teams, providers, and processes that affect a patient's overall surgical episode. Only once we have an understanding of the root causes that explain outcomes differences between hospitals can best practices be promoted. One such example is the notion of "failure to rescue," which sheds light on the mechanisms underlying variations in surgical mortality rates between hospitals. In a study by Ghaferi et al. using clinically rich data from the NSQIP, hospitals were ranked according to risk-adjusted mortality [34]. When comparing the "best" to "worst" hospitals, they found no significant differences in overall (24.6% vs. 26.9%) or major (18.2% vs. 16.2%) complication rates. However, the so-called failure to rescue (death following major complications) was almost twice as high in hospitals with very high mortality as in those with very low mortality (21.4% vs. 12.5%, $p < 0.001$). This study highlights the need to focus on processes of care related to the timely recognition and management of complications – aimed at eliminating "failure to rescue" – to reduce variations in surgical mortality.

Lastly, measuring the quality of hospitals networks as opposed to individual hospitals is becoming increasingly common. Over the last decade, hospitals have been consolidated into large multicenter networks under the premise that this move would improve the quality of care. Currently, the US News and World Report ranks hospitals networks as opposed to individual hospitals to reflect this. Measuring the quality of these networks largely relies upon traditional structure measures such as volume. By participating in a hospital network, small rural hospitals can refer complex surgical cases to be performed at a high-volume center. We have already discussed that evidence is emerging that such "volume pledge" measures may fall short [10]. Conversely, networks can also be evaluated on how well they decentralize knowledge and best practices, so that care across the network, regardless of hospital size, can be standardized according to accepted guidelines [35]. Future efforts to measure surgical quality may focus on how well guideline-concordant care is delivered across a network of hospitals.

Conclusions

Each type of quality measure – structure, process, and outcome – has its unique strengths and limitations. Structural measures are strongly related to outcomes but do not discriminate among individual providers. Process measures offer actionable steps for improvement but often have a tenuous association with outcomes. Outcomes are the bottom line in surgery, but sampling and adjustment methods are needed to meaningfully compare them between hospitals and surgeons. Other measures such as patient-reported outcomes offer critical information, but their incorporation into quality improvement efforts is less clear. Ultimately, when choosing among the various approaches to define surgical quality, surgeons need to be flexible and consider the specific policy application prior to selecting a single measure.

References

1. Osborne NH, Nicholas LH, Ghaferi AA, Upchurch GR Jr, Dimick JB. Do popular media and internet-based hospital quality ratings identify hospitals with better cardiovascular surgery outcomes? J Am Coll Surg. 2010;210(1):87–92.
2. Rosenthal MB, Dudley RA. Pay-for-performance: will the latest payment trend improve care? JAMA. 2007;297(7):740–4.
3. Birkmeyer JD, Shahian DM, Dimick JB, et al. Blueprint for a new American College of Surgeons: National Surgical Quality Improvement Program. J Am Coll Surg. 2008;207(5):777–82.

4. Dimick JB, Osborne NH, Nicholas L, Birkmeyer JD. Identifying high-quality bariatric surgery centers: hospital volume or risk-adjusted outcomes? J Am Coll Surg. 2009;209(6):702–6.

5. Birkmeyer JD, Dimick JB, Birkmeyer NJ. Measuring the quality of surgical care: structure, process, or outcomes? J Am Coll Surg. 2004;198(4):626–32.

6. Dimick JB, Staiger DO, Baser O, Birkmeyer JD. Composite measures for predicting surgical mortality in the hospital. Health Aff (Millwood). 2009;28(4):1189–98.

7. Birkmeyer JD, Siewers AE, Finlayson EV, et al. Hospital volume and surgical mortality in the United States. N Engl J Med. 2002;346(15):1128–37.

8. Birkmeyer JD, Stukel TA, Siewers AE, Goodney PP, Wennberg DE, Lucas FL. Surgeon volume and operative mortality in the United States. N Engl J Med. 2003;349(22):2117–27.

9. Morche J, Mathes T, Pieper D. Relationship between surgeon volume and outcomes: a systematic review of systematic reviews. Syst Rev. 2016;5(1):204.

10. Sheetz KH, Chhabra KR, Smith ME, Dimick JB, Nathan H. Association of discretionary hospital volume standards for high-risk cancer surgery with patient outcomes and access, 2005–2016. JAMA Surg. 2019;154(11):1005–12.

11. Ibrahim AM, Ghaferi AA, Thumma JR, Dimick JB. Variation in outcomes at bariatric surgery centers of excellence. JAMA Surg. 2017;152(7):629–36.

12. Haynes AB, Weiser TG, Berry WR, et al. A surgical safety checklist to reduce morbidity and mortality in a global population. N Engl J Med. 2009;360(5):491–9.

13. Hawn MT. Surgical care improvement: should performance measures have performance measures. JAMA. 2010;303(24):2527–8.

14. Urbach DR, Govindarajan A, Saskin R, Wilton AS, Baxter NN. Introduction of surgical safety checklists in Ontario, Canada. N Engl J Med. 2014;370(11):1029–38.

15. Stulberg JJ, Delaney CP, Neuhauser DV, Aron DC, Fu P, Koroukian SM. Adherence to surgical care improvement project measures and the association with postoperative infections. JAMA. 2010;303(24):2479–85.

16. Neuman HB, Michelassi F, Turner JW, Bass BL. Surrounded by quality metrics: what do surgeons think of ACS-NSQIP? Surgery. 2009;145(1):27–33.

17. Khuri SF, Daley J, Henderson WG. The comparative assessment and improvement of quality of surgical care in the Department of Veterans Affairs. Arch Surg. 2002;137(1):20–7.

18. Dimick JB, Welch HG. The zero mortality paradox in surgery. J Am Coll Surg. 2008;206(1):13–6.

19. Dimick JB, Welch HG, Birkmeyer JD. Surgical mortality as an indicator of hospital quality: the problem with small sample size. JAMA. 2004;292(7):847–51.

20. Dimick JB, Ghaferi AA, Osborne NH, Ko CY, Hall BL. Reliability adjustment for reporting hospital outcomes with surgery. Ann Surg. 2012;255(4):703–7.

21. Dimick JB, Staiger DO, Hall BL, Ko CY, Birkmeyer JD. Composite measures for profiling hospitals on surgical morbidity. Ann Surg. 2013;257(1):67–72.

22. O'Brien SM, DeLong ER, Dokholyan RS, Edwards FH, Peterson ED. Exploring the behavior of hospital composite performance measures: an example from coronary artery bypass surgery. Circulation. 2007;116(25):2969–75.

23. Bilimoria KY, Cella D, Butt Z. Current challenges in using patient-reported outcomes for surgical care and performance measurement: everybody wants to hear from the patient, but are we ready to listen? JAMA Surg. 2014;149(6):505–6.

24. Sacks GD, Lawson EH, Dawes AJ, et al. Relationship between hospital performance on a patient satisfaction survey and surgical quality. JAMA Surg. 2015;150(9):858–64.

25. Birkmeyer JD, Dimick JB, Staiger DO. Operative mortality and procedure volume as predictors of subsequent hospital performance. Ann Surg. 2006;243(3):411–7.

26. Dimick JB, Osborne NH, Hall BL, Ko CY, Birkmeyer JD. Risk adjustment for comparing hospital quality with surgery: how many variables are needed? J Am Coll Surg. 2010;210(4):503–8.

27. Ibrahim AM, Regenbogen SE, Thumma JR, Dimick JB. Emergency surgery for medicare beneficiaries admitted to critical access hospitals. Ann Surg. 2018;267(3):473–7.

28. Tu JV, Sykora K, Naylor CD. Assessing the outcomes of coronary artery bypass graft surgery: how many risk factors are enough? Steering Committee of the Cardiac Care Network of Ontario. J Am Coll Cardiol. 1997;30(5):1317–23.

29. Dimick JB, Staiger DO, Birkmeyer JD. Ranking hospitals on surgical mortality: the importance of reliability adjustment. Health Serv Res. 2010;45(6 Pt 1):1614–29.

30. Staiger DO, Dimick JB, Baser O, Fan Z, Birkmeyer JD. Empirically derived composite measures of surgical performance. Med Care. 2009;47(2):226–33.
31. Jaffe TA, Hasday SJ, Dimick JB. Power outage-inadequate surgeon performance measures leave patients in the dark. JAMA Surg. 2016;151(7):599–600.
32. Stulberg JJ, Huang R, Kreutzer L, et al. Association between surgeon technical skills and patient outcomes. JAMA Surg. 2020;155:960–8.
33. Dimick JB, Varban OA. Surgical video analysis: an emerging tool for improving surgeon performance. BMJ Qual Saf. 2015;24(8):490–1.
34. Ghaferi AA, Birkmeyer JD, Dimick JB. Variation in hospital mortality associated with inpatient surgery. N Engl J Med. 2009;361(14):1368–75.
35. Ibrahim AM, Dimick JB. Redesigning the delivery of specialty care within newly formed hospital networks. N Engl J Med Catalyst. Mar 30, 2017. http://catalyst.nejm.org/redesigning-specialty-care-delivery. Accessed 26 Aug 2020.

Chapter 2
Never Events in Surgery

Anjali A. Gresens and Jacob A. Tatum

Introduction

"Never events" were first introduced in 2001 by Dr. Ken Kizer, former CEO of the National Quality Forum (NQF) organization that promotes patient safety and quality healthcare [1]. The term refers to medical errors and events that are so egregious that they should be avoidable, preventable, and never occur, such as wrong-site surgery or surgery performed on the wrong patient [2]. Though these might seem shocking, serious preventable surgical errors occur every year despite considerable patient safety initiatives. Overall, medical errors are suspected to contribute to over 251,000 deaths per year in the United States, with an estimated 4000 surgical never

A. A. Gresens (✉)
Bariatric Surgery, Sentara Medical Group, Norfolk, VA, USA

Department of Surgery, Eastern Virginia Medical School, Norfolk, VA, USA
e-mail: AAGresen@sentara.com

J. A. Tatum
Department of Surgery, Eastern Virginia Medical School, Norfolk, VA, USA
e-mail: TatumJA@evms.edu

© The Author(s), under exclusive license to Springer Nature Switzerland AG 2022
J. R. Romanelli et al. (eds.), *The SAGES Manual of Quality, Outcomes and Patient Safety*,
https://doi.org/10.1007/978-3-030-94610-4_2

events occurring yearly [3]. Globally, Haynes et al. estimate a rate of serious incidents occurring in 1/10,000 patients, with up to one million deaths per year [4, 5]. While an individual hospital may only see a wrong-site surgery every 5–10 years, other serious errors may occur more frequently causing undue harm to many patients. From 2007 to 2019, 71% of never events reported to the Joint Commission resulted in fatality [1].

Medical errors and adverse events in healthcare impose a costly toll not only on the patient involved but also to the providers and the institution. The burden is mental as well as financial and can be devastating. In 2011, data from the NQF estimated that serious reportable errors lead to $5.7 billion in additional healthcare costs. When including healthcare expenses, lost productivity, lost income, and disability, costs may exceed $29 billion per year in the United States [6].

Understanding What Events Are Classified by the NQF as "Never Events" in Surgery

Never events should be preventable, and no patient should die from these types of medical errors. In 2002, Dr. Kizer and the NQF proposed a list of serious reportable events to increase accountability and consumer access to critical information and healthcare performance. The goal was to advance the delivery of safe and high-quality healthcare through research, investigation, and collaboration. NQF aimed to facilitate standardized reporting that was uniform across systems, leading to systematic nationwide improvements in patient safety. To be categorized as a "serious reportable event" (SRE) or "never event" according to the NQF, an event must be [7]:

- Unambiguous—clearly identifiable and measurable and thus feasible to include in a reporting system
- Usually preventable—recognizing that some events are not always avoidable, given the complexity of healthcare
- Serious—resulting in death or loss of a body part, disability, or more than transient loss of a body function

Additionally, events included on the list are any of the following:

- Adverse
- Indicative of a problem in a healthcare facility's safety systems
- Important for public credibility or public accountability

Some of these events should absolutely never occur. Others are largely preventable with increased education and improved prevention programs and should trend near zero. The objective of identifying these SREs and never events was not to penalize hospitals and programs but to promote patient safety and advance quality improvement efforts. Reporting is voluntary, but every healthcare organization should be in favor of pursuing research efforts that would identify vulnerabilities. Only by identification can issues be addressed and improved. All organizations are held accountable by their patients, providers, staff, and community in terms of the quality of care they provide, and every organization should strive for the highest-quality care and patient safety measures.

The original list of SREs has evolved into 29 serious reportable events grouped into 7 categories:

- Surgical or procedural events
- Product or device events
- Patient protection events
- Care management events
- Environmental events
- Radiologic events
- Criminal events

A complete list of NQF serious reportable events/never events is found in Table 2.1 [8]. Twenty-six states and the District of Columbia have mandated reporting of SREs [9]. Because each state has a variable approach to reporting SREs, a nationwide effort to learn from these events and enact change is limited.

TABLE 2.1 National Quality Forum serious reportable events/never events [8]

Surgical events

Surgery or other invasive procedure performed on the wrong site

Surgery or other invasive procedure performed on the wrong patient

Wrong surgical or other invasive procedure performed on a patient

Unintended retention of a foreign object in a patient after surgery or other invasive procedure

Intraoperative or immediately postoperative/postprocedure death in an ASA Class 1 patient

Product of device events

Patient death or serious injury associated with the use of contaminated drugs, devices, or biologics provided by the healthcare setting

Patient death or serious injury associated with the use or function of a device in patient care, in which the device is used or functions other than as intended

Patient death or serious injury associated with intravascular air embolism that occurs while being cared for in a healthcare setting

Patient protection events

Discharge or release of a patient/resident of any age, who is unable to make decisions, to other than an authorized person

Patient death or serious injury associated with patient elopement (disappearance)

Patient suicide, attempted suicide, or self-harm that results in serious injury while being cared for in a healthcare setting

Care management events

Patient death or serious injury associated with a medication error (e.g., errors involving the wrong drug, wrong dose, wrong patient, wrong time, wrong rate, wrong preparation, or wrong route of administration)

TABLE 2.1 (continued)

Patient death or serious injury associated with unsafe administration of blood products

Maternal death or serious injury associated with labor or delivery in a low-risk pregnancy while being cared for in a healthcare setting

Death or serious injury of a neonate associated with labor or delivery in a low-risk pregnancy

Patient death or serious injury associated with a fall while being cared for in a healthcare setting

Any Stage 3, Stage 4, and unstageable pressure ulcers acquired after admission/presentation to a healthcare setting

Artificial insemination with the wrong donor sperm or wrong egg

Patient death or serious injury resulting from the irretrievable loss of an irreplaceable biological specimen

Patient death or serious injury resulting from failure to follow up or communicate laboratory, pathology, or radiology test results

Environmental events

Patient or staff death or serious injury associated with an electric shock in the course of a patient care process in a healthcare setting

Any incident in which systems designated for oxygen or other gas to be delivered to a patient contain no gas, the wrong gas, or are contaminated by toxic substances

Patient or staff death or serious injury associated with a burn incurred from any source in the course of a patient care process in a healthcare setting

Patient death or serious injury associated with the use of physical restraints or bedrails while being cared for in a healthcare setting

Radiologic events

Death or serious injury of a patient or staff associated with the introduction of a metallic object into the MRI area

(continued)

TABLE 2.1 (continued)

Potential criminal events
Any instance of care ordered by or provided by someone impersonating a physician, nurse, pharmacist, or other licensed healthcare provider
Abduction of a patient/resident of any age
Sexual abuse/assault on a patient or staff member within or on the grounds of a healthcare setting
Death or serious injury of a patient or staff member resulting from a physical assault (i.e., battery) that occurs within or on the grounds of a healthcare setting

Understanding What Events Are Classified by CMS as "Never Events" in Surgery

The Centers for Medicare and Medicaid Services (CMS) have placed increasing pressure on healthcare institutions to eliminate never events and SREs. In August 2007, CMS announced a "nonreimbursable" policy in which they would no longer pay for costs associated with certain SREs and medical complications. These events are also referred to as hospital-acquired conditions (HACs) or even "no pay" events. Following the lead of CMS, several states and private insurance companies enacted similar policies for their reimbursements. CMS hoped that this new directive would stimulate patient safety protocols to be implemented on an accelerated timeline, therefore reducing the incidence of these complications and their subsequent payouts.

While the CMS list of never events and nonreimbursable HACs is very similar to the SREs defined by the NQF, the lists do differ. Indisputable never events as defined by CMS include surgery performed on the wrong body part, surgery performed on the wrong patient, and performing the wrong surgical procedure on a patient. However, the list of CMS never events and "nonreimbursable"/"no pay" events is expanded to include additional serious adverse events that may not be entirely preventable [10]. Table 2.2 shows the

TABLE 2.2 Comparison of "never events: defined by the NQF ("serious reportable events") versus CMS ("nonreimbursable serious hospital-acquired conditions") [8, 11, 12]

"Never" and "no pay"

Events which overlap between NQF and CMS definitions of "never events"

Surgery on the wrong body part

Surgery on the wrong patient

Wrong surgery on a patient

Foreign body left in patient after surgery

Death/disability associated with intravascular air embolism

Death/disability associated with incompatible blood

Stage 3 or 4 pressure ulcers after admission

Death/disability associated with electric shock

Death/disability associated with a burn incurred within facility

Death/disability associated with a fall within facility

"Never"

Events which should never happen according to the NQF SRE list but are not listed on the CMS HAC list

Postoperative death in a healthy patient

Implantation of wrong egg

Death/disability associated with the use of contaminated drugs, devices, or biologics

Death/disability associated with use of device other than as intended

Patient of any age discharged to the wrong person

Death/disability due to patient elopement

Patient suicide or attempted suicide resulting in disability

(continued)

TABLE 2.2 (continued)

Death/disability associated with medication error

Maternal death/disability with low-risk delivery

Incident due to wrong oxygen or other gas

Death/disability associated with the use of restraints within facility

Impersonating a healthcare provider (i.e., physician or nurse)

Abduction of a patient

Sexual assault of a patient within or on facility grounds

Death/disability resulting from physical assault within/on facility grounds

"No pay"

Adverse events which are classified by the CMS as nonreimbursable HACs but lack the according definition of SRE by the NQF

Death/disability associated with poor glycemic control (diabetic ketoacidosis, nonketotic hyperosmolar coma, hypoglycemic coma, secondary diabetes with ketoacidosis, secondary diabetes with hyperosmolarity)

Catheter-associated urinary tract infection

Vascular catheter-associated infection

Surgical site infection following coronary artery bypass graft (CABG), mediastinitis

Surgical site infection following bariatric surgery (laparoscopic gastric bypass, gastroenterostomy, laparoscopic gastric restrictive surgery)

Surgical site infection following orthopedic procedures (spine, neck, shoulder, and elbow)

Deep vein thrombosis (DVT)/pulmonary embolism (PE) in total knee replacement and hip replacement

Iatrogenic pneumothorax with venous catheterization

complete list of CMS never events and nonreimbursable HACs, highlighting the overlap with the NQF list.

Discussing the Ramifications of "No Pay" After the Occurrence of a Never Event

The CMS "no pay" initiative went into effect in 2008. Payments were withheld from hospitals for designated HACs as laid out in Table 2.2. For true never events like wrong surgeries, if CMS deemed that these events were unreasonable or unnecessary, they would not pay for the corresponding hospital or physician services. The other HACs are a bit more complex. In the past, sicker patients with more comorbidities would be placed in a higher-paying diagnosis-related group (DRG) that would increase the reimbursement to the hospital. When this "no pay" initiative went into effect, the CMS designated HACs would no longer trigger entrance into a higher-paying DRG unless these conditions were present on hospital admission [13]. The amount of money being paid out for these events was relatively small, only $20 million, but the real driving force for CMS was to make hospitals safer for patients. As a result of this policy, hospitals were forced to implement quality improvement projects and reexamine how care was provided. Unquestionably, a focus on patient safety was a positive development. Hospitals created patient safety committees and developed checklists, and administrators began to examine patient care. However, as new protocols were put into place, it was evident that there is no such thing as a true "never event." Quality improved and SREs decreased in frequency, but despite all heroic efforts adverse events still happen [2].

In regard to hospital-acquired patient falls, Fehlberg et al. found that the CMS "no pay" initiative significantly increased the utilization of fall prevention strategies without significantly decreasing the incidence of falls. Fall prevention protocols, such as bed alarms and sitters, were increasingly implemented by nurses as they reported significant pressure from their administrators to prevent falls, taking on increasing personal responsibility. Despite these increased measures, in-hospital falls were not significantly reduced or eliminated. The system-wide policy only seemed to increase resource utilization and employee stress without much evidence that these measures lead to their intended outcome [14]. Even with the best possible care, falls and injuries can occur due to medication impairments, dementia, and other disease impairments.

This is not to say that CMS efforts have failed to make any difference in patient safety: Tracked HACs have decreased over time as hospitals wish to optimize their reimbursement statuses. From 2010 to 2017, the overall reduction in HACs was estimated to be 4.5% annually [15]. The Agency for Healthcare Research and Quality estimates that 910,000 fewer HACs have occurred since 2014 and up to 2.1 million fewer events since 2011. This translates into nearly a $20 billion cost savings and 87,000 fewer HAC-related inpatient deaths [15].

As progress has been made, the initial CMS "no pay" initiative for never events has evolved over the last decade. Not only is payment withheld for services related to wrong surgeries and HACs not present on admission, but CMS now penalizes hospitals who fail to report these events with reductions in their overall reimbursements. By 2015, the Inpatient Quality Reporting (IQR) program was instituted and required hospitals to meet certain quality reporting measures. Hospitals who failed to submit reports, regardless of their quality, would see a 25% reduction in their annual payment rates [16].

Despite all of these initiatives, never events and HACs have not been eliminated. It is estimated that 9 HACs still occur out of every 100 discharges [17]. To further reduce this rate, the Affordable Care Act developed the Hospital-Acquired Conditions Reduction Program (HACRP), effective in fiscal year 2015. The HACRP identifies the 25% worst-performing hospitals in relation to quality measures and reduces their annual Medicare payments by 1% regardless of condition [18]. Though well-intentioned, the HACRP has failed to meet goals of improving patient outcomes, and hospitals have several concerns about the program overall in terms of fairness. Large, urban, public teaching hospitals are significantly more likely to be penalized than small, rural, private nonteaching hospitals based on HACRP grading criteria [13]. The program does not adequately provide risk adjustment for teaching hospitals or low socioeconomic populations with increased medical comorbidities. From a surgical perspective, surgical site infections under the HACRP are not risk adjusted for preoperative diagnosis, elective versus emergent case status, or patient immunosuppression status [7]. This disproportionally affects academic and tertiary care hospitals who care for the sickest and most vulnerable patients who are the most susceptible to HACs. For another example, if hospitals are being graded based on urinary catheter-based infections and central venous catheter-based infections, one way to improve those outcomes would be to avoid placing these catheters altogether [17]. A small private hospital is more likely to transfer sicker patients to a tertiary care center, thus avoiding being penalized for a potential HAC and causing the accepting hospital to endure the consequences.

Undoubtedly, there is work to be done as these programs continue to evolve. Hospitals must operate within the confines of the established laws and are at the mercy of the CMS guidelines and reimbursement policies of private insurers. Clearer guidelines must be established along with risk adjustment and better auditing so that all hospitals are treated fairly and not disproportionately penalized. The focus must remain on patient safety and providing quality care rather than prioritizing the financial bottom line.

Discussing What Systemic Answers Are for the Purpose of Preventing Never Events

As never events continue to be reported every year, significant effort has been made to study their prevention. Human error and failures in communication are prominent themes behind the causes of these events. Thus, many of the strategies used in preventing never events revolve around standardization, most often by using checklists or establishing protocols. The Joint Commission found that 13% of SREs between 1995 and 2006 were due to wrong-site surgery. In further analysis, 76% were performed on the wrong site, 13% were performed on the wrong patient, and 11% involved the wrong procedure. They made it their goal to eliminate wrong-site surgery and announced the implementation of the Universal Protocol for Preventing Wrong Site, Wrong Procedure, and Wrong Person Surgery™ in 2003, mandating its use in hospitals the following year. This protocol requires preoperative verification of the procedure, a pre-procedural time out, and site marking for the proposed procedure. Several professional organizations, such as the American College of Surgeons, have adopted this protocol and recommend its use to procedures outside of the operating room. In 2008, the World Health Organization (WHO) established a 19-point Surgical Safety Checklist for reducing surgical complications and death. A study of nearly 8000 patients showed a significant decrease in inpatient complications from 11% to 7% after implementation [19].

The pre-procedural time-out, also known as the "surgical pause," is perhaps the most well-known and widely regarded part of the Universal Protocol to be implemented and has proven to be effective in reducing errors [20]. Time-outs have become ubiquitous and are used before every surgery, outpatient procedure, and even small procedures done in the office or at a patient's bedside. Pre-procedural time-outs involve the entire team and are composed of a standardized checklist that reviews the relevant patient data, planned procedure, potential risks, and other factors. As recently as 2020, a study from the United Kingdom showed that no wrong-site operations were performed in over 29,000 surgical cases when using a standardized checklist, as 86 wrong-site list errors were caught and corrected ahead of time [21]. Outside of surgery, anesthesia literature noted a reduction in incidence of wrong-site spinal blockade after instituting their own pre-procedural checklist [22]. In interventional radiology, a review of CT-guided procedures encompassing biopsies and drainages noted that a pre-procedural checklist was able to identify safety concerns in 18% of cases. These errors were then resolved prior to the procedure's start. A follow-up survey also showed improvement in the subjective experience of the team and overall team cohesiveness [23].

Likewise, surgical site marking has become a standard procedure to reduce wrong-site surgery. Because site identification is most important in instances of laterality, multiple structures, or multiple levels, the Canadian Orthopaedic Association recommended "marking the incision with a permanent marker" in 1994. The American Academy of Orthopaedic Surgeons launched their "Sign Your Site" campaign in 1998 before the Universal Protocol mandated surgical site marking in 2004 [19]. Marking allows each member of the team, including the patient, a chance to identify a wrong-site error before it occurs. The importance of marking is well demonstrated by a study of ophthalmologists who were able to correctly identify the intended site for operation in only 76.5% of cases by patient name alone and only 87% after looking at the patient [24]. Appropriate site marking and use of the Universal Protocol have shown to significantly reduce the incidence of wrong-site surgery from 0.16% to 0.02% as shown in the neurosurgical literature [25]. While there have been various case reports of breakdowns in marking, such as ink-transfers between sites and patient tattoos causing confusion, these case reports are largely anecdotal and have been resolved before harm comes to patients [26, 27]. There is little to no downside to marking the patient, and multiple studies have demonstrated that the marking process does not affect the sterility of the procedure [28, 29].

To further prevent instances of wrong-site surgery and wrong implants, technology is being increasingly implemented in the operating room. In spinal surgery, intraoperative X-ray is used to reaffirm the correct level prior to incision [30]. It is also common practice for relevant imaging to be displayed in the room and discussed during the time-out so that every team member is aware of the planned intervention. Orthopedic surgery literature demonstrates a database of components used in hip and knee replacements that will notify the surgical team if their combination of prosthetic components is compatible, thus avoiding potentially disastrous mechanical failures. The implementation of the database reduced the rates of incompatibility from 0.14% to 0.06% across thousands of procedures [31]. While the benefit of this technology can be dramatic, it is important to note that these methods are still subject to user error and require a level of proficiency to be effective.

An even more prominent example of a systemic solution relates to one of the most common never events: retained foreign bodies. Retained foreign bodies, often surgical sponges or needles, almost always cause harm to the patient. The best-case scenario for the patient is a prolonged hospital stay, but retained objects can result in infection, reoperation, damage to other structures, and even death. The introduction of radio-frequency (RF)-tagged sponges and scanners has greatly reduced the incidence of retained foreign bodies after operations. Sponge and instrument counts should be performed at the end of every procedure but are skipped or missed in upwards of 45% of cases. Even when counts are performed, these RF devices have found retained sponges despite the correct human count [32]. A very large study of over 13,000 procedures examined sponge counts before and after implementation of these RF devices. The authors found an almost 70% reduction in unreconciled sponge counts using the device. From a cost-benefit standpoint, the use of RF devices resulted in overall reduced costs from saved operating room time and postoperative radiographs due to incorrect counts. Several events of retained sponges were successfully avoided, thus reducing medical and legal fees [33]. However, these devices are only part of the solution as they require the sponges used in a case to have the associated detection chip and require the present team to use the device in the first place. Postprocedure time-outs and checklists have been implemented in some institutions as a potential response.

While human error contributes significantly to never events, the literature also refers to failures of communication within the team. Indeed, the Joint Commission believes upward of 56% of never events relate to communication breakdowns [34]. Even if all protocols are followed, harm can still ensue if the problems identified by these procedures are not brought to the team's attention. A survey of vascular surgery residents noted that residents often did not feel empowered to voice concerns due to the perceived hierarchy established in the operating room [35]. Even the standardized time-out process becomes fallible if not adhered to correctly. One study noted that in 10% of observed time-outs, at least one team member was actively distracted [36]. Another survey of circulating nurses reported that 94% of participants had, at one time or another, experienced active hostility toward the time-out from other members of the surgical team [37]. Even the best protocols and operations can be rendered useless if there is not appropriate buy-in by all team members, as the problems identified cannot be brought to those able to correct them. An overall culture of safety needs to be established that allows for buy-in by all teams and open communication among them to ensure patients are kept safe. Teams that consistently work together in the same environment are more comfortable raising alarms because they can recognize red flags and are more likely to have camaraderie that values each member's opinion.

Great effort has been made toward eliminating never events in the last two decades which has resulted in much success across the whole of the surgery community. Despite their name, "never events" do still occur and continue to be reported. With ongoing efforts and advancing technology, these numbers will continue to decrease, and we can hope that one day these events are a thing of the past.

References

1. Never events. In: Patient safety primer. Agency for Healthcare Research and Quality, Rockville. 2019. https://psnet.ahrq.gov/primer/never-events. Accessed 4 Nov 2020.
2. Fischer JE. Never events. In: Tichansky DS, Morton J, Jones DB, editors. The SAGES manual of quality, outcomes and patient safety. Boston: Springer; 2012. p. 1–8.

3. Anderson JG, Abrahamson K. Your health care may kill you: medical errors. Stud Health Technol Inform. 2017;234:13–7.
4. Haynes AB, Weiser TG, Berry WR, Lipsitz SR, Breizat AH, Dellinger EP, et al. A surgical safety checklist to reduce morbidity and mortality in a global population. NEJM. 2009;360(5):491–9. https://doi.org/10.1056/NEJMsa0810119.
5. Koleva SI. A literature review exploring common factors contributing to Never Events in surgery. J Perioper Pract. 2020;30(9):256–64. https://doi.org/10.1177/1750458919886182.
6. SRE Fact Sheet. Serious Reportable Events NQF. 2011. www.qualityforum.org. Accessed 4 Nov 2020.
7. National Quality Forum (NQF), Serious Reportable Events In Healthcare—2011 update: a consensus report, Washington, DC: NQF; 2011.
8. List of SREs. National Quality Forum, Washington, DC. 2020. http://www.qualityforum.org/Topics/SREs/List_of_SREs.aspx#sre1. Accessed 18 Oct 2020.
9. Variability of State Reporting of Adverse Events. National Quality Forum, Washington, DC. 2011. http://www.qualityforum.org/Topics/SREs/List_of_SREs.aspx#sre1. Accessed 18 Oct 2020.
10. CMS.gov: CMS improves patient safety for Medicare and Medicaid services by addressing never events. Centers for Medicaid & Medicare Services, Baltimore. 2008. https://www.cms.gov/newsroom/fact-sheets/cms-improves-patient-safety-medicare-and-medicaid-addressing-never-events. Accessed 14 Nov 2020.
11. Lembitz A, Clarke TJ. Clarifying "never events and introducing" always events. Patient Saf Surg. 2009;3:26. https://doi.org/10.1186/1754-9493-3-26.
12. CMS.gov: Hospital-acquired conditions. Centers for Medicaid & Medicare Services, Baltimore. 2020. https://www.cms.gov/medicare/medicare-fee-for-service-payment/hospitalacqcond/hospital-acquired_conditions. Accessed 14 Nov 2020.
13. Cassidy A. Health policy brief: medicare's hospital-acquired condition reduction program. Health Aff 2015. https://www.healthaffairs.org/do/10.1377/hpb20150806.512738/full/healthpolicybrief_142.pdf. Accessed 14 Nov 2020.
14. Fehlberg EA, Lucero RJ, Weaver MT, McDaniel AM, Chandler AM, Richey PA, et al. Impact of the CMS no-pay policy on hospital-acquired fall prevention related practice patterns. Innov Aging. 2018;1(3):1–7. https://doi.org/10.1093/geroni/igx036.

15. AHRQ national scorecard on hospital-acquired conditions updated baseline rates and preliminary results 2014–2017. Agency for Healthcare Research and Quality, Rockville. Accessed 14 Nov 2020. 2019. https://www.ahrq.gov/sites/default/files/wysiwyg/professionals/quality-patient-safety/pfp/hacreport-2019.pdf.

16. CMS.gov: Hospital Inpatient Quality Reporting Program. Centers for Medicaid & Medicare Services, Baltimore. 2017. https://www.cms.gov/Medicare/Quality-Initiatives-Patient-Assessment-Instruments/HospitalQualityInits/HospitalRHQDAPU. Accessed 14 Nov 2020.

17. Lawton EJ, Sheetz KH, Ryan AM. Improving the hospital-acquired condition reduction program through rulemaking. JAMA Health Forum. 2020. https://doi.org/10.1001/jamahealthforum.2020.0416.

18. CMS.gov: Hospital-Acquired Condition Reduction Program. Centers for Medicaid & Medicare Services, Baltimore. 2020. https://www.cms.gov/Medicare/Medicare-Fee-for-Service-Payment/AcuteInpatientPPS/HAC-Reduction-Program. Accessed 14 Nov 2020.

19. WHO Guidelines for Safe Surgery 2009: Safe surgery saves lives. WHO Guidelines Approved by the Guidelines Review Committee. World Health Organization, Geneva. 2009. http://www.ncbi.nlm.nih.gov/books/NBK143243/.

20. The WHO safer surgery checklist time out procedure revisited: strategies to optimise compliance and safety. Int J Surg. 2019;69:19–22. https://doi.org/10.1016/j.ijsu.2019.07.006.

21. Geraghty A, Ferguson L, McIlhenny C, Bowie P. Incidence of wrong-site surgery list errors for a 2-year period in a single national health service board. J Patient Saf. 2020;16:79–83. https://doi.org/10.1097/PTS.0000000000000426.

22. Henshaw DS, Turner JD, Dobson SW, Jaffe JD, Reynolds JW, Edwards CJ, Weller RS. Preprocedural Checklist for Regional Anesthesia: Impact on the Incidence of Wrong Site Nerve Blockade (an 8-Year Perspective). Reg Anesth Pain Med. 2019;44:201–5. https://doi.org/10.1136/rapm-2018-000033.

23. Dommaraju S, Siewert B, O'Bryan B, Swedeen S, Appel E, Nakhaei M, Camacho A, Brook OR. Impact of preprocedure time-out checklist for computed tomography-guided procedures on workflow and patient safety. J Comput Assist Tomogr. 2019;43:892–7. https://doi.org/10.1097/RCT.0000000000000940.

24. Pikkel D, Sharabi-Nov A, Pikkel J. The importance of side marking in preventing surgical site errors. Int Risk Saf Med. 2014;26:133–8. https://doi.org/10.3233/JRS-140621.

25. Vachhani JA, Klopfenstein JD. Incidence of neurosurgical wrong-site surgery before and after implementation of the universal protocol. Neurosurgery. 2013;72(4):590–5. https://doi.org/10.1227/NEU.0b013e318283c9ea.

26. Moseley G, Oborski Y, Mayorchak Y, Yau L-A, Flynn P. Ink transfer in pre-operative marking: a patient safety issue? ANZ J Surg. 2020;90:187–8. https://doi.org/10.1111/ans.15412.

27. Edlin JC, Kanagasabay R. Risk of operating on the wrong site: how to avoid a never event. BMJ Case Reports 2018 (May 7, 2018). https://doi.org/10.1136/bcr-2017-223704.

28. Cullan DB, Wongworawat MD. Sterility of the surgical site marking between the ink and the epidermis. J Am Coll Surg. 2007;205:319–21. https://doi.org/10.1016/j.jamcollsurg.2007.02.029.

29. Rooney J, Khoo OKS, Higgs AR, Small TJ, Bell S. Surgical site marking does not affect sterility. ANZ J Surg. 2008;78:688–9. https://doi.org/10.1111/j.1445-2197.2008.04618.x.d.

30. Odgaard A, Laursen MB, Gromov K, Troelsen A, Kristensen PW, Schrøder H, Madsen F, Overgaard S. Mismatch 'never events' in hip and knee arthroplasty: a cohort and intervention study. Bone Joint J. 2019;101B:960–9.

31. DeVine JG, Chutkan N, Gloystein D, Jackson K. An update on wrong-site spine surgery. Global Spine J. 2020;10:41S–4S. https://doi.org/10.1177/2192568219846911.

32. Steelman VM, Shaw C, Shine L, Hardy-Fairbanks AJ. Retained surgical sponges: a descriptive study of 319 occurrences and contributing factors from 2012 to 2017. Patient Saf Surg. 2018;12:20. https://doi.org/10.1186/s13037-018-0166-0.

33. Steelman VM, Schaapveld AG, Storm HE, Perkhounkova Y, Shane DM. The effect of radiofrequency technology on time spent searching for surgical sponges and associated costs. AORN J. 2019;109:718–27. https://doi.org/10.1002/aorn.12698.

34. Etherington N, Wu M, Cheng-Boivin O, Larrigan S, Boet S. Interprofessional communication in the operating room: a narrative review to advance research and practice. Can J Anesth/J Can Anesth. 2019;66:1251–60. https://doi.org/10.1007/s12630-019-01413-9.

35. Lear R, Godfrey AD, Riga C, Norton C, Vincent C, Bicknell CD. Surgeons' perceptions of the causes of preventable harm in

arterial surgery: a mixed-methods study. Eur J Vasc Endovasc Surg. 2017;54:778–86. https://doi.org/10.1016/j.ejvs.2017.10.003.

36. Freundlich RE, Bulka CM, Wanderer JP, Rothman BS, Sandberg WS, Ehrenfeld JM. Prospective investigation of the operating room time-out process. Anesth Analg. 2020;130:725–9.

37. Jones N. Tune-in and time-out: toward surgeon-led prevention of 'never' Events. J Patient Saf. 2019;15:e36–9. https://doi.org/10.1097/PTS.0000000000000259.

Chapter 3
Creating a Surgical Dashboard for Quality

Samuel M. Miller and John M. Morton

The objectives for this chapter should be:
- To describe the characteristics of a surgical quality dashboard
- To discuss AHRQ patient safety indicators (PSIs) and how they are important to include on dashboards

Introduction

Quality continues to evolve as a focus within the healthcare and surgical communities. With more information at our fingertips than ever before, comparisons between countries, healthcare systems, and individual providers have become an assumed part of patients' research before they choose where to receive care. Complications occur in approximately 15% of surgical cases [1]. Many of these complications are preventable, yet despite numerous interventions designed to limit errors and improve patient safety, these numbers continue to rise. Whether it be a review posted by an established patient

S. M. Miller · J. M. Morton (✉)
Department of Surgery, Yale School of Medicine,
New Haven, CT, USA
e-mail: John.morton@yale.edu

© The Author(s), under exclusive license to Springer Nature   41
Switzerland AG 2022
J. R. Romanelli et al. (eds.), *The SAGES Manual of Quality, Outcomes and Patient Safety*,
https://doi.org/10.1007/978-3-030-94610-4_3

in a public forum online, or a manuscript published in a peer-reviewed journal, there can be comfort in knowing that your surgeon has laudable outcomes.

Healthcare institutions continue to look for strategies employed in other fields that may prove useful in the delivery of medical care. Checklists have become an integral part of the operating room as the "time-out" confirms that the entire team is aware of the patient's identity, pertinent medical history, and unique requirements for the upcoming procedure. Algorithms have been built into disease workup as we decide on imaging for a patient with right lower quadrant pain or when to give steroids after a spinal trauma. Nevertheless, as the ability to obtain quantitative data continues to improve, we have not developed an efficient method of analyzing and implementing practical change in the delivery of care.

The *surgical dashboard* has been proposed as part of the solution to improve surgical quality. This condensed display of pertinent information, much like that in a car or airplane, offers the user insight into the workings of his or her machine at present and in the recent past.

Initially developed in the 1970s, their popularity has risen significantly in the last 50 years. These dashboards were designed to present graphical data that made it easy to recognize trends, whether positive or negative. This insight allowed for the identification of areas that needed improvement and also for the evaluation of previous interventions.

Surgical quality dashboards have become even more common over the past decade. With electronic health records having become an integral part of our healthcare system and the increased collection and distribution of health outcomes data, we have access to more data than ever before. Our increasing ability to collect and disseminate these data quickly allows for real-time feedback and focused adjustments in practice. However, with the available data having increased exponentially, it has become more difficult to parse through the troves of information to find those measures that are clinically relevant. Clinicians are often left wanting for a means to efficiently digest this information so that they can incorporate it into their practice. The most effective dashboards of today allow a surgeon to quickly identify trends in their personal practice as well as draw comparisons to colleagues, whether at the institutional or national level.

Characteristics of a Surgical Quality Dashboard

The ideal surgical quality dashboard will combine several characteristics that allow for its efficient use. First and foremost is simplicity. The user should be able to glance at the dashboard and immediately surmise the general tone of the information that is presented. This can be accomplished in many different ways, including using colors to denote positive (green) and negative (red) results or emoticons like "smiley faces" or "thumbs up." While there may be many pieces of information displayed on this dashboard, it is helpful to have one message that is central on the page. Depending on the day, this focus can be placed on a particular metric in which the user excels or an area which might require attention or improvement. This simple theme serves two purposes: to frame the rest of the information that is to follow on the dashboard and to be the sole takeaway if the user is to navigate away from the dashboard without reading further. The act of choosing the data can become an exercise in prioritization for the hospital or health system.

The surgical dashboard must also filter for data that is relevant. In today's world of the electronic health record and national databases, not all data are created equal. It can be difficult to discern which data are clinically impactful. An effective surgical quality dashboard will do just this. Relevant data will vary between different users, different practice types, and different practice settings. In this way, the dashboard must be customizable by the user. One surgeon may be focused on shortening the length of inpatient stay for his patients, while another may be working to limit those of her patients that are discharged with a prescription for narcotics.

Whatever the concern, the dashboard must be built to reflect accurate and relevant information that is tailored to the user's preference. Additionally, the data should be actionable or contemporary. Finally, if an outcome is rare, perhaps, observation of processes should be emphasized. For example, surgical site infections may occur only 5% of cases, but the process of giving antibiotics preoperatively will occur on every case as appropriate. The key relationship here is that the process must be closely linked to the outcome.

The surgical quality dashboard must effectively display the user's current metrics to allow for easy comparison. Often, these data are presented in a graphical manner to allow for the easy identification of trends and should abide by the same principles mentioned previously – the presentation should be simple and relevant. Options should be available to view chronological comparisons with the user's past data as well as with current data at institutional and national levels. This provides feedback to areas in which the user might be excelling and also those where the user needs to focus attention and improve. It is also worthwhile to provide users with institutional comparisons. This can inspire camaraderie among practitioners and can lay groundwork for quality improvement projects at the departmental and institutional levels. There can be more in-depth presentation via run charts which can graphically represent progress in quality improvement initiatives.

Dashboard Metrics

The ultimate purpose of the surgical quality dashboard is to guide practitioners as they strive to improve the experience of their patients. The principles described above provide the framework for the organization of the dashboard, but without actual data, the dashboard may not be helpful. The more advanced displays will be customizable to include metrics that the user selects individually. Additionally, another key concept is to identify who should access the dashboard. All key stakeholders? Selected stakeholders? None of the clinical providers? Should it be available to the public? The following measures will vary in utility based on practice setting but should be included on the dashboard display:

Productivity

A summary of patient care within a given time period should be among the first data points displayed on the surgical quality dashboard. This should include operative cases performed as well as patients seen in clinic. It may be helpful to separate operative cases into those requiring postoperative hospital admission and those performed as outpatient procedures. Certain providers may find a cumulative report of their relative value units (RVUs) to be of value. Efficiency metrics such as average length of stay or third next available open clinic appointment could be represented here.

Mortality

Patient mortality should be front and center on the surgical quality dashboard. Surgical mortality is generally considered to be any patient death that occurs between the time of surgery and postoperative day 30. These data are easy to collect from hospital administrative records and are generally very accurate. In addition, national mortality rates are readily available for many different procedures, and so comparison to the national standard is simple. Including these metrics on the dashboard allows for surgeons to see where they excel and where they might need to focus attention in relation to their peers. The mortality rate should be risk adjusted, as tertiary care centers are more likely to care for sicker patients with increased comorbid conditions. This can drive the mortality rate up but is not necessarily purely a reflection of the surgeon's care and subsequently should not serve as a potential barrier for these patients to be able to find access to care.

Postoperative Outcomes

Postoperative complications are to be included on all surgical dashboards. Compiling these data is often more complicated than mortality, as there is more room for ambiguity in the way these events are recorded. Patient safety indicators (PSI) were created by the Agency for Healthcare Research and Quality (AHRQ) to establish a standard for reporting these postoperative complications (Fig. 3.1) (see Chap. 25 for a more expansive discussion on PSIs). This classification system allows for comparison between practitioners at different institutions and across the nation. These data serve as markers of surgical quality, and poor results are meant to trigger focused investigation.

This display should be customizable by the individual user. Depending on a surgeon's specialty, certain metrics may be more relevant. For example, vascular surgeons may choose to view rates of postoperative acute kidney injury as this can provide feedback on different patients' abilities to metabolize intravenous contrast. Of particular interest to

PATIENT SAFETY INDICATOR
PSI 02 Death Rate in Low-Mortality Diagnosis Related Groups (DRGs)
PSI 03 Pressure Ulcer Rate
PSI 04 Death Rate among Surgical Inpatients with Serious Treatable Complications
PSI 05 Retained Surgical Item or Unretrieved Device Fragment Count
PSI 06 Iatrogenic Pneumothorax Rate
PSI 07 Central Venous Catheter-Related Blood Stream Infection Rate
PSI 08 In Hospital Fall with Hip Fracture Rate
PSI 09 Perioperative Hemorrhage or Hematoma Rate
PSI 10 Postoperative Acute Kidney Injury Requiring Dialysis
PSI 11 Postoperative Respiratory Failure Rate
PSI 12 Perioperative Pulmonary Embolism or Deep Vein Thrombosis Rate
PSI 13 Postoperative Sepsis Rate
PSI 14 Postoperative Wound Dehiscence Rate
PSI 15 Abdominopelvic Accidental Puncture or Laceration Rate
PSI 17 Birth Trauma Rate-Injury to Neonate
PSI 18 Obstetric Trauma Rate-Vaginal DeliveryWith Instrument
PSI 19 Obstetric Trauma Rate-Vaginal Delivery Without Instrument

Figure 3.1 Patient safety indicators published by AHRQ in 2020

bariatric surgeons might be a report of their patients' post-operative weight loss. A general surgeon may want to see a record of hernia recurrences or a breakdown of laparoscopic, robotic, and open procedures.

Hospital Admissions Data

Hospital admissions data are a vital source of information for the surgical quality dashboard. Hospital length of stay (LOS) and discharge disposition offer insight into the immediate postoperative course of patients who are admitted to the hospital. Extended lengths of stay and unexpected discharges to skilled nursing or rehabilitation facilities are often indicators of postoperative complications. In addition, emergency department (ED) visits and readmission rates are valuable to include. Surgeons may not hear if their patients present to the ED or require admission to a nonsurgical service, and so the surgical dashboard may be the only way for them to receive this feedback.

National Standards and NSQIP

The American College of Surgeons put forth the National Surgical Quality Improvement Program (NSQIP) to improve the quality of surgical care through the accurate and detailed collection of outcomes data. Participating sites employ a Surgical Clinical Reviewer to collect preoperative, intraoperative, and postoperative data on randomly selected patients. These data are collected from medical records and include all complications within the 30 days after surgery, regardless of whether these complications take place in the inpatient or outpatient setting. At present, there are over 700 participating hospitals across the world, including 49 of 50 states and 11 countries [2]. This methodology has allowed for more complete and accurate records and for the establishment of a national and international baseline for a variety of perioperative metrics. The NSQIP provides a semiannual report which is broken down by specialty and delivers performance data compared to de-identified peer institutions in a dashboard format. Institutions are ranked by deciles or quartiles, which allows for identification of areas for improvement, which can then internally drive quality improvement projects.

Connecting to Quality Improvement

The surgical quality dashboard, above all, is an instrument to inspire improvement in the quality of care that surgeons deliver to their patients. It allows for both the identification of areas where focused attention is needed and the ability to track change and quantify improvement. However, the dashboard does not provide a course of action by which quality can be improved. There are a number of national organizations that have formed to fill this need to guide hospitals and clinicians through the process of quality improvement.

SCIP

The Surgical Care Improvement Project (SCIP) was created to provide a framework for surgeons to improve the quality of care they offer to their patients. They believe that a "meaningful reduction in complications requires that surgeons, anesthesiologists, perioperative nurses, pharmacists, infection control professionals and hospital executives work together to make surgical care improvement a priority" [3]. By concentrating on complications that are both frequent and expensive, they hope to reduce surgical complications by 25% while also limiting the extraneous costs that these adverse events incur. These parameters have produced a focus on surgical site infections, venous thromboembolism, and adverse cardiac events by monitoring the measures listed in Fig. 3.2.

Set Measures

Set Measure ID	Measure Short Name
SCIP-Card-2	Surgey Patients on Beta-Blocker Therapy Prior to Admission Who Received a Beta-Blocker During the Perioperative Period
SCIP-Inf-1	Prophylactic Antibiotic Received Within One Hour Prior to Surgical Incision
SCIP-Inf-2	Prophylactic Antibiotic Selection for Surgical Patients
SCIP-Inf-3	Prophylactic Antibiotics Discontinued Within 24 Hours After Surgery End Time
SCIP-Inf-4	Cardiac Surgery Patients with Controlled 6 A.M. Postoperative Blood Glucose
SCIP-Inf-6	Surgery Patients with Appropriate Hair Removal
SCIP-Inf-7	Colorectal Surgery Patients with Immediate Postoperative Normothermia
SCIP-venous-thromboembolism-1	Surgery Patients with Recommended Venous Thromboembolism Prophylaxis Ordered
SCIP-venous-thromboembolism-2	Surgery Patients Who Received Appropriate Venous Thromboembolism Prophylaxis Within 24 Hours Prior to Surgery to 24 Hours After Surgery

FIGURE 3.2 Metrics collected by SCIP

AHRQ Safety Program for Improving Surgical Care and Recovery

The Agency for Healthcare Research and Quality created the Safety Program for Improving Surgical Care and Recovery to improve the quality of surgical care. Their stated aim is to "help hospitals and clinicians use AHRQ's Comprehensive Unit-based Safety Program (CUSP) method to enhance the surgical process and improve patients' recovery after surgery" [4]. Specifically, their focus is on decreasing infections and all postoperative complications as well as length of inpatient hospital stays and unexpected postoperative hospital visits. This is accomplished by empowering leaders in all disciplines of healthcare workers to promote a culture of safety and teamwork among each of the members of the surgical team. At present, they are refining their program with the hopes of opening enrollment to additional hospitals in the next several years.

Empowering the Surgical Team

As we work toward improving the quality of care we offer our patients, the importance of cohesion within surgical teams has become evident. At each step of the surgical process, from preoperative evaluation through the operating room and into postoperative recovery, there are groups of people from a multitude of backgrounds working together to help patients regain their quality of life. The surgical quality dashboard should include metrics related to communication between these team members. Records of multidisciplinary rounds, unnecessary or repeated blood draws, and instances of waking patients can all inform surgical teams of areas where they are excelling and also of those where improvement might be needed.

The surgical quality dashboard can also directly facilitate communication. In certain cases, these team members may not ever work together in the same space, and so opportunities for discussion and feedback do not occur naturally. For example, if a physical therapist notices that several patients have peroneal neuropathy after a procedure where their legs were placed in stirrups, this is important feedback for a surgeon to receive so that a simple adjustment in positioning can be made. In addition, there are times when a particular team member may feel more comfortable offering anonymous feedback. The dashboard can serve this purpose as well. While this information may not be displayed in the most prominent position, its inclusion is important.

Future Directions

The surgical quality dashboard has evolved significantly in the last decade. As our ability to track both individual and national data has improved, so too has our ability to identify and address areas in need of attention. As we continue to move forward, there are ways that our surgical quality dashboards can expand. The future may include data from the operating room not previously available such as an "OR Black Box." Data related to prescription filling and monitoring will need to be included, specifically those related to narcotics. In the context of the ongoing opioid crisis, having real-time information about narcotic usage can help a surgeon to adjust prescribing practices to reflect the needs of the average patient, as has already been done in some states. If a surgeon typically prescribes 20 tablets of 5 mg oxycodone after a laparoscopic cholecystectomy and finds that only 40% of patients fill that prescription, he or she may decide to decrease the number of tablets she is prescribing. In addition, it may be helpful for the surgical quality dashboard to include links to evidence-based methods that have been shown to improve certain aspects of surgical care. For example, if a particular surgeon has a high rate of postoperative venous thromboembolism (VTE), links to guidelines for postoperative VTE prophylaxis should be displayed in the same window.

Conclusion

The surgical quality dashboard has never been more important than it is in today's world. With real-time and international data more accessible than ever before, the opportunity for quality improvement has never been greater. By integrating data from sources such as NSQIP and AHRQ, surgeons can see how they compare to their peers and also how their practice has changed over time. By streamlining the presentation of relevant data in a simple format, adjustments can be made that decrease complications, save healthcare dollars, and, most importantly, save patient lives.

References

1. Scott J, et al. Use of national burden to define operative emergency general surgery. JAMA Surg. 2016;151(6):e160480.
2. https://www.facs.org/quality-programs/acs-nsqip/about/history.
3. Griffin F. Reducing surgical complications. Jt Comm J Qual Patient Saf. 2007;33(11):660–5.
4. https://www.ahrq.gov/hai/tools/enhanced-recovery/index.html.

Chapter 4
Understanding Complex Systems and How It Impacts Quality in Surgery

Buğra Tugertimur and Bruce Ramshaw

Introduction

In 1944, President Roosevelt sent a letter to Vannevar Bush, the director of the Office of Scientific Research and Development, to propose a plan for applying similar research principles used in the recent war (WWII) to the war on disease. The Bush report, *Science, The Endless Frontier: A Report to the President*, led to the development of the National Science Foundation (NSF) and then the National Institute of Health (NIH). The applied model is termed the "linear model of innovation" using tools from reductionist science, like controlled research trials.

In healthcare, controlled studies attempt to determine if a treatment is safe and effective and generates recommenda-

B. Tugertimur
General Surgery Resident, PGY 5, Department of Surgery, Lenox Hill Hospital, Northwell Health, New York City, NY, USA
e-mail: btugertimu@northwell.edu

B. Ramshaw (✉)
Managing Partner, CQInsights PBC, Knoxville, TN, USA

© The Author(s), under exclusive license to Springer Nature Switzerland AG 2022
J. R. Romanelli et al. (eds.), *The SAGES Manual of Quality, Outcomes and Patient Safety*,
https://doi.org/10.1007/978-3-030-94610-4_4

53

tions for the average patient. This one-size-fits-all approach is not ideal for complex biologic systems. With an appropriate data and analytics infrastructure in healthcare based on the principles of systems science, we could identify different patient subpopulations and apply the optimal variety of treatments based on which treatment had the best value for each subpopulation. This is the type of data and analytics infrastructure Netflix uses to present the optimal array of movies and shows to customer viewer subpopulations, for example.

Because we don't have this type of data and analytics infrastructure in healthcare, we have had to suffer the consequences of using management strategies during the COVID-19 pandemic, such as social distancing and quarantines, similar to what we did nearly 400 years ago during the plague. On May 12, 2020, during a senate hearing about the lessons learned from our response to COVID-19, Senator Mitt Romney asked Dr. Robert Redfield, the Centers for Disease Control and Prevention (CDC) director, "How is it possible in this day and age that the CDC has never established a real-time system with accurate data?" Dr. Redfield responded, "The reality is there is an archaic system... This nation needs a modern, highly capable data analytic system that can do predictive analysis. I think it's one of the many shortcomings that have been identified as we went through this outbreak, and I couldn't agree with you more, it's time to get that corrected."

Our sense of discovery is an innate compelling drive that has advanced us as a species since the beginning of human existence. According to some philosophers and scientists alike, our constant search for who we are, where we come from, and where we are going is what defines humanity and perhaps even gives meaning and reason to life. While ever so brief in the grand scheme of the universe and Earth, the eras of human evolution have been propelled through history by the nature of our scientific, artistic, literary, and philosophical curiosity. Among these, in science, the concept of reductionism has been central to developing the scientific method leading to innovation and societal advancement for our world.

While reductionism has existed for centuries, it became particularly important in facilitating the Industrial Revolution.

Descartes described reductionism's basic tenant in the seventeenth century: "divide each difficulty into as many parts as is feasible and necessary to resolve it." Reductionism involves reducing an object, system, or process into its comprehensible components to understand the broader phenomenon, therefore assuming that a complex system is equivalent to the sum of its parts [1]. Applied to science, this method of experimentation and research means that all biological phenomena can be understood by unraveling their fundamental biochemical, molecular, and environmental components [2].

Flaws of Reductionism

In modern clinical medicine, the reductionist learning tool is best exemplified by the prospective, randomized, controlled trial (PRCT). While this has been the gold standard in research for testing hypotheses, new medications, and novel medical devices, one fundamental flaw is the attempt to control all variables. In addition to the fact that all variables could never be truly controlled, a change in any one variable in the real world can potentially lead to a different, unintended outcome despite the same intervention.

Another flaw of reductionism, including the PRCT or any algorithm generated from centralized data, is the assumption of generalizability. The concept of generalizability leads to harm in some subpopulations and waste in others in addition to the intended benefit in yet other subpopulations. There are no one-size-fits-all solutions in the real world. For example, a recent analysis of a population health algorithm used by many hospitals in the United States revealed significant harm had occurred to marginalized subpopulations, particularly African-American minorities [3].

In a world with biologic variability that is continuously changing, another flaw of reductionism is the assumption that nothing changes. Static protocols that result in treatment guidelines are not generalizable to all patients, and they are not designed for continuous improvement as things change. Without accumulating new data and interpreting further analyses through feedback loops, any static treatment guideline or static algorithm will degrade over time and lead to more waste and unintentional harm.

The applicability of reductionist PRCTs is also limited by attempting to determine the statistical significance of isolated factors, assuming causation, instead of generating weighted correlations for all identified factors and factor combinations to assess their impact on outcomes. The use of linear statistical methods to prove statistical significance between a variable and outcome measure is not how these statistical tools were intended to be used. The American Statistical Association published a statement in 2016 about this widespread misuse of statistics in science [4].

Our Current Scientific Paradigm Shift

In contrast to Descartes, Aristotle is credited for his observation that "the whole is more than the sum of its parts," which is a central tenant of systems science. Our world is going through the first major scientific paradigm shift since the Renaissance, when the concepts of reductionism were developed. At that time (around A.D. 1300–1600), and for our world over the next few hundred years, this was a significant advancement. We learned how to use raw materials and make useful products. We learned to harness energy and apply it in ways that led to improved quality of life for many people. But there is a growing realization that we're approaching the law of diminishing returns for our reductionist science paradigm. We are expending tremendous resources and working harder yet achieving less improvement in our health and quality of life.

Thomas Kuhn coined the term "paradigm shift" in his book *The Structure of Scientific Revolutions*, published in 1962. He described the process of scientific evolution. He explained that this is not a linear process as previously thought where we would just continue to gain knowledge and improve as a society. According to Kuhn, the impetus for a shift in a paradigm occurs when there are enough anomalies (things that just don't make sense according to the rules of the current paradigm) for people to realize that the solution isn't to figure out why the anomalies are occurring, rather it's to figure out a new paradigm that better aligns with what is happening in the world. The anomalies are only anomalies because the current scientific rules can't account for what is being observed. Figure 4.1 describes some of the differences between the reductionist science paradigm and the systems science paradigm.

	Reductionist Science	Systems Science
Metaphors	Magic Pill/Quick Fix	Emergence/Network
	Machine	Complex adaptive system
Characteristics	Linear	Non-linear
	Predictable	Probabilistic
	Normalcy	Robustness
	Risk reduction	Adaptation/Plasticity
	Homeostasis	Homeodynamics
	Do things just to be safe	Do things to learn and improve
Principles	Can control our biologic world	Can manage our biologic world
	Lower Brain	Higher Brain
	Fragmentation	Holism
	Certainty	Uncertainty
	Secrecy	Transparency
	Competition	Collaboration
	Blame is common after error	Blame is rare
	Didactic Learning (one right answer)	Ensemble Learning (continuous improvement)
	Authoritative Leadership	Empathic Leadership
	Focus on parts of the system or process/"Silos"	Focus on the whole system or process
	Centralized data	De-centralized data
	Need control groups	Control is an illusion

FIGURE 4.1 Reductionist science paradigm vs. systems science paradigm

The Science of Complex Systems Applied to Healthcare

In contrast to reductionism, systems science is rooted in the concepts of measurement and improvement. Regular feedback loops are performed based on insight gained from a variety of data analytics and visualization tools. Instead of providing a "best practice" guideline with a one-size-fits-all approach, systems science has the potential to provide an optimal variety of preventative and treatment options for each appropriate patient subpopulation.

The systems science paradigm accommodates constant change and uncontrollable biologic variability. Instead of one static hypothesis, there are feedback loops that provide insight to inform clinical teams, including patients, so that process and outcome measurements are improved, and measured outcomes are also improved over time.

Real-World Examples of Reductionism Compared with Systems Science

Vitamin Supplements

In 1977, George L. Engel, MD of the University of Rochester, formulated the biopsychosocial model (BPSM), which described a holistic approach in patient care. His philosophy, which was in stark distinction to reductionism, proposed that the physiology of an illness is inseparable from its psychological, behavioral, and social impacts and that the reciprocal influences of all these elements must be considered in understanding and treating disease. His principle was considered an evolution for medical thinking and was adopted in 2002 as the foundation of the World Health Organization's International Classification of Function (WHO ICF).

Compared with this holistic approach to health, an example of a reductionist approach is exemplified by the supplemental vitamin craze in the 1990s. Nobel Prize recipient Linus Pauling is considered the father of molecular biology. In 1970, he published a best-seller book called *Vitamin C and the Common Cold,* which asserted that high doses of daily ascorbic acid could eventually eradicate the cold and many other diseases, including cancer. Despite refutes of his claims by scientists and clinicians, the concepts in his book were embraced by popular culture and promoted in a 1992 article and on the cover of *Time* magazine that claimed vitamins could "fight cancer, heart disease and ravages of aging."

The basis of Pauling's belief was that antioxidants found in vitamins could prevent damage by neutralizing free radicals, which are linked to aging, heart disease, and dementia. While fruits and vegetables are touted for their antitumorigenic benefits based on antioxidants, later research showed that only the balance of numerous antioxidants found naturally within them provides this benefit by creating a protective buffer against free radicals [5]. Not only does this protective effect disappear when antioxidants are consumed in isolation, such as in vitamin supplements, but worse, they are potentially toxic secondary to their pro-oxidative effect through suppression of the body's antioxidant defense system [6]. Recent articles have described the needed paradigm shift from reductionist to systems science in health and nutrition [7, 8].

Football Injuries

To demonstrate another comparison of the reductionist science paradigm and the systems science paradigm, each paradigm's research tools could be applied to the problem of National Football League (NFL) injuries.

Using the reductionist paradigm, a hypothesis would be defined based on observations of the problem and knowledge of potential solutions. A primary investigator might identify a newly available helmet technology that potentially provides more stable cushioning. A study could be designed to prove or disprove the hypothesis that the new helmet technology would reduce the incidence and severity of concussions.

Because this study method requires human subjects research protection, it must be submitted for review and approval to an institutional review board (IRB). There would also need to be research agreements executed for all NFL teams and consent from all the players. This will take at least one entire season to complete, and so the study would not begin until the next NFL season.

Before this second season, the teams would be randomized so that half would use the standard helmets and half would use the new helmet technology. The data would be collected, and the results at the end of the season might show that the new helmet technology has led to a one-third decrease in the incidence and severity of concussions. However, by this time, almost 2 years after the study was designed, there might be other new helmet technologies available, and there is no way to know if they are better than the helmet technology tested in this study.

On the other hand, applying tools from systems science would not attempt to prove anything – there would be no hypothesis. The goal would be to measure and improve outcomes by identifying and measuring factors that might impact those outcomes. Then, by gaining insight through the use of various analytical tools, attempts could be made to improve the outcomes measured, in this case, all types of injuries.

Because there is no attempt to randomize teams or control variables, there is no requirement for an IRB submission. To determine what data should be collected from observing the games, a small team with diverse expertise and perspectives would be assembled. They would propose how best to measure the incidence and severity of all injuries, and all factors the group thinks are potentially significant and may contribute to the incidence and severity of injuries. The group might suggest measuring the preseason training regimens, the weather during each game, the altitude of the stadium, the type of helmet used by each team, the quarter in which the injury occurred, the position of the injured player, etc.

At the end of the season, an analysis would be performed that generates weighted correlations to determine which factors and combinations of factors are most highly correlated with injuries. Based on this insight, highly correlated factors (potentially modifiable) could be addressed. Changes could be implemented that would likely lessen the incidence and severity of injuries in the next season.

For example, the analysis might reveal that three factors were highly correlated with an increase in the incidence and severity of injuries – high and low extremes of temperature and artificial turf. With that knowledge, the artificial turf could be replaced, and heating and cooling technologies could be developed to be used in the next season. Data would then be collected to measure the impact of these improvement attempts. The analysis of this data might demonstrate a decrease in the incidence and severity of all types of injuries.

This is a simplistic example of the potential application of systems science to improve the health of a subpopulation of people (NFL players). These results were obtained by the senior author (BR) when he did a 7th-grade science fair project by watching and recording data for all televised NFL games in 1975. Over the next 25 years, the NFL did replace artificial turf and developed heating and cooling technologies for games played in extreme temperatures.

The full application of systems science, including nonlinear analytics, would allow for feedback loops during each season so any high-signal factors could be discovered well before the end of the season. Also, the analysis of different subpopulations (like linemen vs. quarterbacks) could generate various ideas for improvement based on those unique, position-specific subpopulations.

Which scientific paradigm results in more knowledge faster and is less costly to apply? What if healthcare applied systems science tools to all patients with all types of diseases to measure and improve the value of care provided in our global healthcare system? How quickly could we achieve a sustainable system where costs are lowered, and outcomes are improved over time?

Hernia Mesh

In a reductionist science paradigm, hernia mesh would be inert in the body or at least have the same biologic interaction (generalizability) for all patients. The interaction between hernia mesh and the human body was the first complex problem the senior author (BR) investigated that led to learning the principles of systems science.

Working with two engineers, a materials characterization lab was developed at the University of Missouri-Columbia to analyze mesh after removing it from patients (usually for symptoms of chronic pain, infection, and/or a recurrent hernia). The material removed from the body often looked different and was sometimes harder and more brittle than the soft and flexible material that comes out of the package. But this type of physical change didn't occur in all mesh explants, and it occurred to different degrees in different patients – it could even be different in other parts of the same mesh.

Although these changes that occur in the mesh after implantation in patients have not been correlated with patient outcomes, they demonstrated a large degree of variability from patient to patient. In mesh hernia repairs, we also see variability in patient outcomes. For most patients who have a hernia repaired with mesh, the mesh performs well, and the patient has a good outcome. But in some patients, the mesh may be a contributing factor that leads to an unintentional complication such as chronic pain or a recurrent hernia.

In a systems science paradigm (our real biologic world), the same hernia mesh, placed with the same technique, may result in different outcomes for different patient subpopulations. Figure 4.2 illustrates the systems science concept that different sets of factors for patients who undergo the same treatment, hernia repair with mesh in this example, will result in a subpopulation of patients with good outcomes (benefit), another subpopulation that does not benefit from the procedure, but suffers no harm (waste), and another subpopulation that is harmed unintentionally from the treatment (harm).

Clinical Quality Improvement: A Systems Science Tool

To develop a sustainable healthcare system, we will need to learn how to better measure the value of care provided in the context of the whole, definable patient care processes. The principles of systems science propose that value-based continuous quality improvement (CQI) tools can be applied to lower costs and improve outcomes simultaneously. CQI initiatives can potentially be focused on improving the value of patient care in the actual clinical environment. Using CQI principles is often more appropriate for developing an understanding of the factors that drive improvements in patient care than randomized controlled trials that aim to prove or disprove a hypothesis [9, 10].

Rather than trying to prove or disprove a hypothesis, value-based CQI is implemented to measure and improve the value for each patient care process in which these principles are applied [11]. Unlike traditional clinical research, CQI is not restricted only to patients with specific clinical characteristics defined by study inclusion and exclusion criteria. Instead, CQI allows for more flexible decisions based on situations that healthcare providers face in their everyday practice. CQI can track many outcome measures over the entire patient care cycle over time, not just during a predefined study period.

Lawmakers have recognized the value of CQI initiatives for improving patient care. For example, the use of CQI, defined as a part of healthcare operations, has been one of the exemptions from the HIPAA law since it was implemented in 1996. Also, the US Department of Health and Human Services recognizes that there is a distinction between most quality improvement efforts and research involving human subjects that requires IRB approval. CQI focuses on local process improvement and real-world clinical data and analytics interpreted by the care team. These CQI efforts applied by a clinical team and secondary data uses, such as for

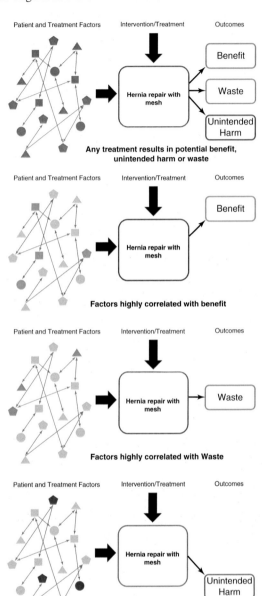

FIGURE 4.2 Illustrations demonstrating the potential outcomes of a treatment, hernia repair with mesh. The outcome that occurs is determined by the state of multiple factors present at the time of the treatment intervention. With the appropriate use of tools from systems science, algorithms can be developed to predict what outcome is most likely to occur and what treatment option may result in the best value-based outcome for any patient or patient subpopulation

academic presentation and publication, do not require submission to an IRB [12].

Analyzing Data

Systems science tools for analyzing data include a variety of data analytics and data visualization methods. Although linear statistics are commonly used in healthcare, various nonlinear analytical tools may be more appropriate when analyzing real-world healthcare data. One group of tools are called principal component analysis (PCA) and factor analysis (FA). Analyses using these tools produce weighted correlations between the factors and combinations of factors with measured outcomes and outcome variations. These weighted correlations can be used to develop predictive algorithms.

There are also many tools and ways to visualize data. The different ways to visualize data depend on the different types of data (discreet, continuous, lists, unstructured, etc.). Data visualizations can help a clinical team drill down into the data to help gain insights that may complement the interpretation of other types of data analyses. Often in healthcare, data is visualized in a static data dashboard where the same data is presented month after month. This minimizes the value of data. Data visualization tools should be interactive and adaptable as each clinical team gains new insights and applies those insights for new ways to visualize and measure their data.

There is no one right way to analyze or visualize data. A clinical team should explore different ways to analyze and visualize a dataset. As clinical teams learn to do this over time, through multiple feedback loops, new insights will be discovered and applied for improvement in measurements and improvement in outcomes. Datasets should be updated with new data that is analyzed and visualized again after new measurements and process improvements are implemented.

The Problem of Suboptimization

Electronic medical records (EMR) systems are designed to document patient care fragments for coding and billing instead of being designed for a whole, definable patient care process. Because of this fragmentation, the opportunity for data collection throughout the entire patient process is lost. A systems science approach would instead provide data collection throughout the whole cycle of care that can be analyzed to measure and improve the outcomes for any definable, whole patient care process.

This care fragmentation leads to the inappropriate application of process improvement tools such as CQI principles (such as Lean and Six Sigma). When improvement tools are applied to a fragment of care (a subprocess) rather than in the context of a whole, definable patient care process, the effort may improve the subprocess, but this will not result in improved outcomes for the whole patient process. The term for optimization of a subprocess without measuring the impact on the entire process is called suboptimization.

Most of the "quality" measures that hospitals are required to report (which might impact their financial reimbursement) are examples of suboptimization: central line infection rate, urinary catheter infection rate, 30-day rehospitalization rate, etc. To make the situation worse, the data from many different types of patient care processes (different contexts) is lumped together at the hospital level, so the data is just noise – it can't be reliably analyzed because of the lack of a definable context.

For example, there are many published reports of process improvement efforts that can result in central line infection rates approaching or even achieving zero infections – which sounds wonderful. But this is not a good outcome if it is isolated to only the subprocess without a measurement of the impact on the outcomes for each whole, definable patient care process. If it's not measured, one can't know the outcomes for each type of patient process in that group of patients who received a central line. One can't know if some patients didn't need a central line. It would be unknown if some patients suffer from other types of complications related to central lines – pneumothorax, bleeding, thromboembolism, etc. Some of these other complications may be more harmful than an infection. By only looking at central line infection, other unintended consequences will occur and might not be identified – a consequence of suboptimization.

Another example of suboptimization is the recent hospital focus on the problem of sepsis. Sepsis, as a diagnosis alone, provides no context. Is it an 80-year-old nursing home patient with sepsis from a urinary tract infection, or is it a 20-year-old motorcycle trauma patient with an open pelvic fracture that has developed sepsis from a necrotizing wound infection? These are two very different patient processes. Developing a treatment for a subprocess like sepsis that is a one-size-fits-all solution can lead to variable outcomes and unintended waste and harm, especially when the outcome of the whole process is not measured. This is what has happened with the effort to implement hospital protocols to treat patients with sepsis. Although these sepsis bundles have led to a decreased short-term (in-hospital) death rate, the unintended long-term harm includes high rates of weakness, cognitive impairment, hospital readmissions, and late death [13].

Systems Science Applied to Healthcare: Implementing a Learning Health System

Noise – Wisdom Continuum
    Data (alone) = Noise
    Data + Context = Information
    Experimentation + Error = Experience
    Information + Experience = Knowledge
    Knowledge + Humility = Wisdom
    – Fergus Connolly
    Noise – Wisdom: The Simplest Note You Need
    fergusconnolly.com April 5, 2019

Systems Science Steps to Implement a Learning Health System

The principles of systems science propose that a learning system in each local clinical environment will be necessary for a sustainable healthcare system. Each local learning system's goal should be to measure and improve the value of care provided in the context of each whole, definable patient care process. The steps to apply a systems science approach include:

1. *Context*: define each whole patient care process. For data to have value, one of the basic rules in systems science applied in a complex system is that data requires "context." That means that the data is generated from a definable, whole process. In healthcare, an example of data not in context is when a surgeon is given their "quality" dashboard. The dashboard typically shows the rate of postsurgical wound infections, for example. But that outcome measure is for all patients that had an operation by that specific surgeon. If the surgeon is a general surgeon, that wound infection rate might include patients who had breast procedures, colon resections, hernia repairs, and maybe even operations for gunshot wounds. Combining an outcome measure from all

these different contexts makes the data confusing, nearly worthless, and may lead to inappropriate interpretations and responses.

2. *Diverse teams*: define the small teams with diverse perspectives who are most involved in caring for the patients in each whole, definable patient process. Over the past few decades, the science of teams has demonstrated how important it is to work in small, diverse teams to optimally manage and improve the outcomes for any complex process. In systems science, it's well known that a small team made up of diverse perspectives focused on any complex problem or process is critical to achieving the best insight and outcomes.

3. *Measure "what matters"*: we collect too much data in healthcare. Most of what we collect for any patient process is just noise and has little or no impact on outcomes that matter the most. A small, diverse team can best identify the patient factors, treatment factors, and outcome measures that matter the most in the context of each whole, definable patient care process.

4. *Value (the most important outcome to measure)*: a basic principle in business and systems science is that you can't improve an outcome if you don't measure it. On the other hand, if you measure something and apply the tools of systems science appropriately, you can improve it. We don't measure the value of care for any whole, definable patient process in healthcare, so we can't lower costs and improve outcomes. This has led to an unsustainable healthcare system globally.

5. *Decentralize the data*: Hospitals, academic medical centers, and large physician practices have centralized data into fragmented silos (EMRs). The current strategy is to centralize the data even more into data lakes or data warehouses, although centralized data limits the ability to learn from it. Centralized data can generate averages but not insights. Averages lead to one-size-fits-all approaches, but individual patients are not well represented by an average. Insights gained to improving patient outcomes while low-

ering cost, maintaining privacy, and maximizing security are only possible through a decentralized data infrastructure.

6. *Analyze the data using a human-computing symbiosis*: a human-computing symbiosis combines the intuition, creativity, and empathy of human team members with computing capabilities to provide various data analysis and visualization outputs. These different strengths are complementary. Figure 4.3 illustrates how the human team can determine what data is most appropriate to program into the computer. The computer provides analyses and data visualizations. The human team will then interpret the analyses and use insights gained to improve measurements and implement process improvements to improve outcomes.

7. *Feedback loops*: one of the essential concepts in systems science is the concept of feedback loops. After data is collected and analyzed, the team interprets the data and generates ideas for improvement. Over time and with the collection of new data, the analysis is done again. Each time the team reviews an analysis of data, they examine the impact of previous process improvement attempts and gain new insights for improvement. The team can use various ways to look at the data and bring in perspectives from outside of the core team to gain insight from new perspectives. For example, obtaining feedback from patients and family members can generate new ideas because of their unique perspective. Another example would be to include an anesthesiologist and a pain specialist in a CQI meeting when considering the implementation of new multimodal surgical pain management strategies to decrease the use of opioids for postoperative pain.

8. *Ensemble model for learning*: applying these systems science concepts in each local clinical environment alone is not adequate for a sustainable healthcare system. Each local team will need to develop a learning network to share knowledge and algorithms with other local clinical teams. This networked learning infrastructure will enable ongoing improvement of value. If we don't collaborate to solve

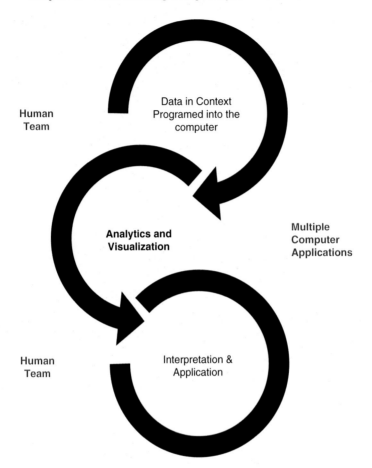

FIGURE 4.3 Human-computer symbiosis applied to healthcare. Small teams made up of people with diverse perspectives relative to each patient process determine what patient and treatment factors are most important to collect and what outcomes measure value in the context of each whole, definable patient care process. Computer programs can perform a variety of data analyses and data visualizations, providing feedback loops for the team to interpret. The team can then apply new insights to suggest improvements in how the data and outcomes are measured and ideas for improvement in the patient process. (Adapted from: Ramshaw [9])

complex problems that we see in healthcare, the goal of a sustainable healthcare system will continue to be elusive. The ensemble learning concepts have been described by the Google AI team as federated learning and federated analytics. There are significant benefits to this model for learning. The complexity is reduced by combining the learning from many small teams and networking that knowledge (ensemble learning). And because the raw data remains in each local environment, the data's privacy and security are maintained. There are examples of ensemble learning in healthcare, used to accurately predict the diagnosis of Type 2 diabetes and maintain privacy [14, 15]. There is even a recent example of an ensemble learning model for diagnosing COVID-19 from routine blood tests [16].

Real-World Application of Systems Science

Starting in 2010, the senior author (BR), working with a small, diverse hernia team, began to apply systems science principles to real patient care as described above. Two examples of using the principles of CQI and nonlinear analytical tools with feedback loops are described below.

Eliminating Drains for Abdominal Wall Reconstruction (AWR)

As a part of our hernia CQI program, we have regularly obtained feedback and input from hernia patients and their family members to get ideas for improvement. Over time, we recognized that many patients had negative experiences with abdominal wall drains. Patients did not like the irritation, discomfort, and hassle of drains, especially when they had to manage them outside of the hospital. We even had one patient who developed an infection at the site where the drain tubing exited the skin, with no problem at the actual incision site.

In an attempt to improve our AWR process, our hernia team did a literature search and found techniques developed by plastic surgeons for abdominoplasty that led to the elimination of abdominal wall drains. These techniques demonstrated better rates of wound complications such as infection, hematoma, and seroma. We were already moving toward techniques to minimize the elevation of skin flaps – first using endoscopic approaches for external oblique component separation and then using the transversus abdominus release (TAR) approach. We added the techniques of wide skin and soft tissue excision, including excision of the umbilicus, and the use of layered quilting (also known as tension reduction) sutures to eliminate the dead space and tension on the skin closure. Although this did increase the operative time (a new improvement opportunity), the rate of wound complications decreased without using a single drain over the next several years [17].

Understanding Chronic Pain After Inguinal Hernia Repair

During one of our hernia team CQI meetings, we were looking at the patients who suffered from chronic pain after inguinal hernia repair and had complications after an operation to relieve their pain. We looked at our operative techniques and the typical patient factors like BMI and smoking, but nothing seemed to explain a pattern for these patients who had bad outcomes. Our patient care manager then spoke up and noted that the patients who had bad outcomes appeared to be the same patients that were more challenging to deal with before surgery.

She described patterns in these patients – some were angry, some had unrealistic expectations (especially those expecting a "quick fix"), and some had high anxiety and/or controlling personalities. We didn't yet know how to measure this, but we thought this might be an important pattern. We needed some sort of measurement tool. Lacking much expertise in this area at the time, we settled on a subjective measure we called "emotional complexity," and we put patients in categories of either high, medium, or low.

As the next 6–9 months went by, we recorded emotional complexity and a few dozen other data points. The subsequent analysis of the data we ran showed that the emotional complexity was the highest modifiable factor predicting our patients' outcomes.

When we found that this was such an important factor, we invited a small group of social science experts to our next CQI meeting to develop a more robust measurement tool [18]. As we learned about the impact of a patient's neurocognitive/emotional state on surgical outcomes from the analysis of data in our patients, we found that this is not that surprising based on recent research in neuroscience and the neurophysiologic impact that traumatic events can have on the brain.

This insight led to the presurgical evaluation of patients' neurocognitive/emotional issues and implementation of cognitive-behavioral therapy (CBT) as part of a "prehabilitation" program for most patients. Since the implementation of this preoperative optimization program, we have seen better outcomes. Some patients were even able to cancel surgery because their pain was improved during this prehabilitation program [19].

Systems Science Applied to Healthcare in Policy and Education

The use of systems science in other industries such as finance, sports, and the military has proven successful. The need to change our reductionist mentality in surgery and medicine is recognized at the national level in the United States, as evidenced by the 21st Century Cures Act, signed into law December 13, 2016. A portion of the law is designed to create a framework for utilizing real-world evidence in the FDA regulatory process for approving drugs and biological products with "data regarding the usage, or the potential benefits or risks… from sources other than traditional clinical trials."

As mentioned by Corrigan-Curry et al. in JAMA Viewpoint on September 4, 2018, an important caveat in the effective practice of guiding national policy will be the need for "shared learning and collaboration across clinicians, patients, health care systems, pharmaceutical companies, and regulators" [20]. While randomized clinical trials currently remain recognized as the gold standard for generating medical and scientific evidence, their limitations in cost, time consumption, and, most importantly, generalizability among populations in a dynamic environment are increasingly becoming recognized.

Lastly, the importance of systems science in healthcare has trickled down to the medical school curriculum for future physicians' early exposure. In 2013, as part of its "Accelerating Change in Medical Education" and "forward-thinking" initiative, the AMA created an initial consortium of 11 medical schools including the Pennsylvania State University College of Medicine and the Warren Alpert Medical School of Brown University, to integrate systems science directly into the medical school curriculum as a "third science." Designed as the third pillar of medical education alongside and equal to basic and clinical science, the goal of this initiative is to promote quality improvement, team science, leadership, socioecological determinants of health, healthcare policy, and economics to prepare the physicians of tomorrow for the evolution of healthcare for a sustainable future based on quality and value. As of 2020, the AMA's consortium consists of 37 medical schools from around the nation [21, 22].

Conclusion

While reductionist science was critical in advancing humanity and healthcare for the past several centuries, using the same anachronistic approach in the era of exponential change and increases in information not only hampers progress but also potentially misguides us despite our good intentions. The reality of the unsustainable nature of our current healthcare system is apparent. The prospect of change is not an easy one, but as human beings, we are a complex species that have, time and time again, proven to be capable of adapting as we gain knowledge and as the world evolves. While our paradigm shift to systems science may be in its infancy, its recognition represents our first steps into the future of evolving healthcare to be centered around the patient through individuality, value, and sustainability.

There are no shortcuts when applying systems science to healthcare or any other industry. If the whole context is not defined, if data is analyzed without understanding the context from which it was obtained, or if process improvements are applied only to a subprocess, the outcome will not be ideal. In other industries, this might lead to an unsatisfied customer, but when the process is a patient care process, the result might include unintended and potentially preventable human suffering. We need to learn to apply systems science principles to measure and improve value in the context of the whole, definable patient processes if we want a sustainable global healthcare system. From reductionist thinking, there is a commonly used saying that "the devil is in the details," but with an understanding of systems science, there is a need to complete the thought: "but an angel can be found in understanding the whole."

References

1. Kricheldorf H. Getting it right in science and medicine: can science progress through errors? Fallacies and facts. Cham: Springer International Publishing; 2016. p. 63. ISBN 978-3-319-30386-4.

2. Montague G. Who am I? Who is she?: a naturalistic, holistic, somatic approach to personal identity. Piscataway: Transaction Books; 2012. p. 308. ISBN 978-3-86838-144-3.

3. Obermeyer Z, Powers B, Vageli C, Mullainathan S. Dissecting racial bias in an algorithm used to manage the health of populations. Science. 2019;366:477–53.

4. Wasserstein R, Lazar N. The ASA statement on p-values: context, process, and purpose. Am Stat. 2016;70(2):129–33.

5. Calabrese V, Cornelius C, Trovato A, et al. The hormetic role of dietary antioxidants in free radical-related diseases. Curr Pharm Des. 2010;16(7):877–83.

6. Bouayed J, Bohn T. Exogenous antioxidants--double-edged swords in cellular redox state: H\health beneficial effects at physiologic doses versus deleterious effects at high doses. Oxid Med Cell Longev. 2010;3(4):228–37.

7. Kaput J, Perozzi G, Radonjic M, Virgill F. Propelling the paradigm shift from reductionism to systems nutrition. Genes Nutr. 2017;12:3.

8. Fardet A, Rock E. From a reductionist to a holistic approach in preventative nutrition to define new and more ethical paradigms. Healthcare. 2015;3:1054–63.

9. Ramshaw B. An introduction to complex systems science and its application to hernia surgery. In: Hope W, editor. Textbook of hernia. Cham: Springer International Publishing; 2017. p. 7–13.

10. Ramshaw B. Applying systems and complexity science to real patient care. J Eval Clin Pract. 2020;26(5):1559–63.

11. Ramshaw B, Forman B, Barker E, Grimsley L. The value proposition for complex abdominal wall reconstruction: how to make it work. Plast Reconstr Surg. 2018;142(3 Suppl):173S–9S.

12. U.S. Department of Health and Human Services. Quality improvement activities FAQs. Available at http://www.hhs.gov/ohrp/policy/faq/quality-improvement-activities/. Accessed 20 Jan 2015.

13. Prescott H, Costa D. Improving long-term outcomes after sepsis. Crit Care Clin. 2018;34(1):175–88.

14. Yang T, Zhang L, Yi L, et al. Ensemble learning models based on noninvasive features for type 2 diabetes screening: model development and validation. JMIR Med Inform. 2020;8(6):e15431.

15. Yao Q, Guo X, Kwok J, et al. Privacy-preserving stacking with application to cross-organizational diabetes prediction. Proceedings of the twenty-eighth joint international conference on artificial intelligence (IJCAI-19):4114–20.

16. AlJame M, Ahmad I, Imtiaz A, Mohammed A. Ensemble learning model for diagnosing COVID-19 from routine blood tests. Info Med Unlocked. 2020;21:100449.

17. Ramshaw B, Dean J, Forman B, et al. Can abdominal wall reconstruction be safely performed without drains? Am Surg. 2016;82(8):707–12.

18. Ramshaw B, Vetrano V, Jagadish M, et al. Laparoscopic approach for the treatment of chronic groin pain after inguinal hernia repair. Surg Endosc. 2017;31(12):5267–74.

19. Landry M, Lewis R, Lew M, et al. Evaluating effectiveness of cognitive behavioral therapy within multimodal treatment for

chronic groin pain after inguinal hernia repair. Surg Endosc. 2020;34(7):3145–52.

20. Corrigan-Curay J, Sacks L, Woodcock J. Real-world evidence and real-world data for evaluating drug safety and effectiveness. JAMA. 2018;320(9):867–8.

21. Just in time for the holidays: AMA's health systems science textbook. American Medical Association. n.d. https://www.ama-assn.org/press-center/press-releases/just-time-holidays-ama-s-health-systems-science-textbook.

22. Member schools of the consortium. American Medical Association. 2020, January 24. https://www.ama-assn.org/education/accelerating-change-medical-education/member-schools-consortium.

Chapter 5
Clinical Care Pathways

Michael R. Keating and Benjamin E. Schneider

What Is a Clinical Care Pathway?

When discussing how clinical pathways may be used in surgery to improve outcomes, it is important to first define "clinical care pathway." This would seem to be a simple question. However, the surgical literature contains many different terms that have been used to define a "clinical pathway," such as critical pathway, care pathway, care map, and integrated care pathway. Though there is no universally accepted definition, Kinsman et al. attempted to create a set of criteria to define a clinical pathway. These include:

1. The intervention is a structured multidisciplinary plan of care.
2. The intervention was used to translate guidelines or evidence into local structures.
3. The intervention detailed the steps in a course of treatment or care in a plan, algorithm, guideline, protocol, or other "inventory of actions."
4. The intervention had timelines or criteria-based progression.

M. R. Keating · B. E. Schneider (✉)
University of Texas Southwestern, Dallas, TX, USA

J. R. Romanelli et al. (eds.), *The SAGES Manual of Quality, Outcomes and Patient Safety*,
https://doi.org/10.1007/978-3-030-94610-4_5

5. The intervention aimed to standardize care for a specific clinical problem, procedure, or episode of healthcare in a specific population.

The authors proposed that if the first criterion was met, then three of the four following criteria being met were sufficient for consideration as a clinical care pathway [1].

The European Pathway Association defines a care pathway as "a complex intervention for the mutual decision making and organization of care processes for a well-defined group of patients during a well-defined period. The aim of a care pathway is to enhance the quality of care across the continuum by improving risk-adjusted patient outcomes, promoting patient safety, increasing patient satisfaction, and optimizing the use of resources" [2].

How Are Clinical Pathways Used in Surgery and How Do They Improve Outcomes?

The intent behind clinical pathways can be broken into two general categories. The first is to improve efficiency of healthcare delivery in order to decrease healthcare costs by, for example, decreasing length of hospital stay. The second is to implement standardized, evidence-based interventions to improve patient outcomes and/or decrease complications (e.g., VTE prophylaxis, multimodal pain therapy). Obviously, there is significant overlap between these two, in that interventions often achieve both decreasing cost of healthcare delivery and improvement of patient outcomes. The most well-known clinical care pathways to surgeons are the enhanced recovery after surgery (ERAS) protocols. The goals of ERAS protocols are preoperative patient optimization, decrease in perioperative stress, maintaining normal postoperative physiologic function, and accelerated recovery time [3]. These protocols were initially developed for cardiac surgery and became much more widespread with their use in colorectal surgery. However, now they are used in many different areas of surgery including bariatric, breast, hepatic, pancreatic, orthopedic, and thoracic surgery. The ERAS Society is an international organization with the mission to "develop perioperative care and to improve recovery through research, education, audit, and implementation of evidence-based practice" [4]. They have published evidence-based guidelines for numerous specialties including colorectal and bariatric surgery with variations for each specialty where appropriate. This section will touch base on general recommendations for each phase of care but not meant to be exhaustive. The general format for these clinical pathways is to break them down into preoperative, intraoperative, and postoperative categories.

Preoperative Recommendations

Preoperative recommendations can be further subcategorized into preadmission and post-admission components. Medical optimization often involves evaluation by other physicians including primary care physicians, cardiologists, pulmonologists, and anesthesiologists. Examples may include identifying patients with obstructive sleep apnea and ensuring that they are being appropriately treated with continuous positive airway pressure (CPAP) devices or ensuring that diabetic patients have adequate glycemic control [5]. Nutritional supplementation may be sought in patients who are malnourished [6]. Smoking cessation (generally for at least 4 weeks) is encouraged in all patients prior to surgery in order to improve respiratory function and decrease wound healing complications. Similarly, alcohol cessation in patients with alcohol abuse is generally recommended for 4 weeks, though in bariatric programs where patients are required to commit to lifelong behavioral changes, preoperative alcohol cessation may be recommended for 1–2 years [7]. Preoperative weight loss, especially in bariatric surgery patients, can make surgery less difficult due to decreased size of the liver but also is associated with decreased complication rates [7]. Another vital (though often overlooked) component of successful clinical pathways is preoperative education and counseling, which aids in decreasing anxiety and improving compliance by setting expectations for patients and their families [7]. One study even found that an ERAS program with staff focused on preoperative stoma education including education on the patient's role in caring for their stoma, routines after surgery, and hands-on practice changing stoma appliances was associated with a significant decrease in hospital length of stay [8].

Post-admission preoperative recommendations include limited fasting, preoperative carbohydrate loading, nausea prophylaxis, and antimicrobial prophylaxis. Despite traditional surgical dogma requiring patients to be nil per os (NPO) after midnight due to concerns for aspiration risk, recent studies have shown that patients may safely have clear liquids up to 2 h before surgery (the current recommendation for solids is 6 h before surgery) with no increase in gastric residual at time of OR, no increase in gastric pH, and no increase in complication rates. Additionally, preoperative fasting leads to decreased liver glycogen stores and increased insulin resistance [9]. Preoperative carbohydrate loading with a low osmolar carbohydrate-rich drink has also been shown to improve insulin resistance, decrease postoperative nausea, and be associated with a decreased hospital length of stay [9–12]. Multimodal nausea prophylaxis is encouraged, including a single dose of dexamethasone given by anesthesia having been shown to be effective and safe in preventing postoperative nausea and vomiting.

Intraoperative Recommendations

Intraoperative protocols largely focus on maintaining homeostasis and controlling pain while minimizing narcotic use. Neuraxial anesthesia and blocks with local anesthetic have been shown to decrease postoperative narcotic use. Transversus abdominus plane (TAP) blocks have been shown to significantly decrease narcotic use on postoperative day 1 as well as significantly decrease time to first bowel movement without differences in postoperative complications [13]. Minimally invasive techniques are well established as safe and have been associated with significantly reduced complications and length of stay [12]. Perioperative fluid overload is associated with postoperative ileus, and restrictive perioperative fluid strategies are associated with reduced complications [12, 14]. Other components of the intraoperative protocols include avoiding hypothermia, strict glycemic control, and decreased use of surgical drains including nasogastric tubes [6].

Postoperative Recommendations

In the postoperative phase of care, the focus is on rapidly returning the patient to a normal state of function and, perhaps even more than pre- or intraoperative phases, highlights the multidisciplinary nature of care pathways. Early mobilization with physical therapy and occupational therapy is essential to ensure the patient maintains strength and functional mobility as well as anticipating discharge needs. Early initiation of PO nutrition has been associated with decreased length of stay, faster time to return of bowel function, and no increase in complication rates including anastomotic leak or pulmonary complications [9]. It can be useful to involve nutritionists postoperatively as well, especially for certain populations, such as bariatric patients, both for inpatient guidance and patient education. Multimodal pain control is another common component of the postoperative protocol and may include acetaminophen, gabapentin, and NSAIDs. The goal of multimodal therapy is to improve pain control while concurrently minimizing narcotics. Minimizing narcotics in turn results in decreased nausea and decreased postoperative ileus. Early involvement of social workers in the postoperative phase can also help with discharge planning to avoid delays in discharge.

Impact of Clinical Pathways in Surgery

Clinical pathways are multidisciplinary care plans that standardize patient care with evidence-based practices and interventions. Their goals are to minimize variability in care deliver, reduce healthcare costs, and improve patient outcomes. Initially, there was some questions as to whether care pathways were safe. One early study by Calligaro et al. in 1995 examined the impact of clinical pathways on hospital costs and outcomes after major vascular surgery. They found that by arranging for much of the preoperative workup (arteriography, cardiac, and anesthesia evaluation) to be done in the outpatient setting rather than during a preoperative admission, and by establishing inpatient clinical pathways, they were able to significantly decrease hospital length of stay and hospital costs with no difference in complications or readmission rates. However, it is worth noting that they did not calculate outpatient costs or costs of skilled nursing facilities. There was also an increased burden on the surgeon and staff in the outpatient setting [15]. A systematic review from 2008 examined indicators used to evaluate clinical pathways, including length of stay, mortality, complication rates, and readmissions. These effects were broken into five categories: financial (length of stay, medical costs), clinical (complication rates, readmission rates), process (number of clinical exams, analysis of deviations), team (team communication/satisfaction), and service (patient satisfaction). The most common domains reported on were financial and clinical, with 87% of controlled studies noting a positive effect in the financial domain and 47% of controlled studies noting a positive effect in the clinical domain; importantly, no studies noted a negative effect of clinical pathways. The authors also commented that "the impact of a clinical pathway will depend on the goals of the project. When a team is only trying to improve the efficiency, we will not find improvements on clinical quality of care or patient safety" [16].

A 2009 prospective cohort study evaluated more granular effects of a clinical pathway in surgery, primarily focused on cost, and found that with a clinical pathway, there was a decrease in unnecessary testing (such as EKGs or lab tests), decreased total nursing time required per patient, decreased hospital length of stay by 23%, and a total cost reduction of 25% with no differences in complications or readmissions [17]. The ERAS compliance group also examined the impact of ERAS protocol compliance on outcomes after elective colorectal surgery. They found that both laparoscopic surgery and ERAS protocol compliance were associated with significantly reduced complications and shorter length of stay. They also found that preoperative carbohydrate loading and totally intravenous anesthesia were associated with shorter hospital stay and that restrictive perioperative fluid use was associated with reduced complications [12]. A systematic review and meta-analysis examining outcomes with ERAS in bariatrics from 2017 found a significant reduction in length of stay. There was also a trend toward decreased readmission and cost reduction, but these were not statistically significant. They found no difference in morbidity, specific complications, or mortality [18]. Similarly, a single-center study comparing outcomes before and after initiating a bariatric ERAS program found significantly decreased length of stay in the ERAS group, with no difference in readmission rate, reoperation rate, 30-day morbidity including bleeding or leak, or mortality [5].

In 2012 a single-center controlled study focusing on effects of clinical pathways for bariatrics on perioperative quality of care found increased rates of timely epidural removal, faster removal of Foley catheters, increased patient mobilization on the day of surgery, faster adoption of oral nutritional supplements, and a decreased length of stay with no impact on morbidity or mortality [19]. A retrospective cohort study from 2020 evaluating the effects of clinical pathways (CPs) on outcomes in patients undergoing a Whipple procedure found that catheters and abdominal drains were removed faster in the CP group, first intake of PO liquids, nutritional support and solids was faster in the CP group, exocrine insufficiency was less common in the CP group, and there was decreased intraoperative transfusion in the CP group. There were no differences in morbidity, mortality, reoperation, or readmission rates [20].

What Are Best Practices That Have Successfully Integrated Clinical Care Pathways?

Implementing a successful ERAS protocol is undeniably challenging, and there are many barriers to success. Some of these include poor communication, resistance to change by staff, lack of institutional support, and additional work imposed by the auditing process, among others. One of the cornerstones of a successful ERAS protocol is its multidisciplinary approach which can involve:

- Surgeons
- Outpatient staff
- Preoperative nurses
- Anesthesiologists
- Operating room nurses
- Recovery room/PACU staff
- Nurses on the surgical floor
- Dieticians
- Pharmacists
- Physical therapists
- Social workers

It can be effective to arrange these pieces into a team structure to divide responsibilities and delineate roles. A 2017 review by Ljunqvist detailed one example of this structure. For clinical pathways in surgery, the surgeon is one of the few members of the team who is present at each step of the patient's care and thus has a more global view of the patient's trajectory. Therefore, a surgeon is often the leader of the team, with close anesthesiologist support. Project managers and coordinators can help organize resources, obtain management approval, and address practical matters such as arranging for education of personnel, creating instructional materials, and auditing the protocol outcomes/adherence. Finally, ancillary services, such as physical therapists and nutritionists, may play specific roles depending on the protocol that has been created. Ljunqvist also recommends scheduling regular meetings, especially at the outset of the program, to evaluate compliance and troubleshoot problems that may arise. Finally, it is important to audit the process, measuring both adherence to the protocol and outcomes. The ERAS Society created the ERAS interactive audit system for this purpose [10]. This allows one to determine:

1. Whether or not the interventions are effective (e.g., time to return to enteral feeding, time to defecate, pain scores)
2. If the protocols are safe (complication rates, number of readmissions, reoperations, ICU admissions, mortality, etc.)
3. Whether results may be skewed by poor adherence to certain parts of the protocol

A recent systematic review evaluating staff experiences with ERAS confirmed the importance of effective multidisciplinary communication, educating staff and patients, and appointing dedicated "champions" to implement an ERAS protocol [21].

Conclusion

Clinical pathways, while a relatively new idea, have a large body of literature from the last several decades which demonstrate that they are safe and can achieve their purpose of reducing healthcare costs while concurrently improving patient outcomes. There are excellent resources to initiate and refine clinical pathways, starting with the ERAS Society guidelines which are evidence based, available for free, and regularly updated. When implementing a clinical pathway, it is important to focus on the multidisciplinary approach, good communication, and being mindful to audit the process in order to ensure adherence and refine it over time.

References

1. Kinsman L, Rotter T, James E, Snow P, Willis J. What is a clinical pathway? Development of a definition to inform the debate. BMC Med. 2010;8:31. https://doi.org/10.1186/1741-7015-8-31.
2. European Pathway Association | CARE PATHWAYS. Accessed 21 Nov 2020. http://e-p-a.org/care-pathways/.
3. Gustafsson UO, Scott MJ, Hubner M, et al. Guidelines for perioperative care in elective colorectal surgery: Enhanced Recovery After Surgery (ERAS®) Society recommendations: 2018. World J Surg. 2019;43(3):659–95. https://doi.org/10.1007/s00268-018-4844-y.
4. List of guidelines. Eras. Accessed 22 Nov 2020. https://erassociety.org/guidelines/list-of-guidelines/.
5. Trotta M, Ferrari C, D'Alessandro G, Sarra G, Piscitelli G, Marinari GM. Enhanced recovery after bariatric surgery (ERABS) in a high-volume bariatric center. Surg Obes Relat Dis Off J Am Soc Bariatr Surg. 2019;15(10):1785–92. https://doi.org/10.1016/j.soard.2019.06.038.
6. Smith TW, Wang X, Singer MA, Godellas CV, Vaince FT. Enhanced recovery after surgery: a clinical review of implementation across multiple surgical subspecialties. Am J Surg. 2020;219(3):530–4. https://doi.org/10.1016/j.amjsurg.2019.11.009.
7. Thorell A, MacCormick AD, Awad S, et al. Guidelines for perioperative care in bariatric surgery: Enhanced Recovery After Surgery (ERAS) Society recommendations. World J Surg. 2016;40(9):2065–83. https://doi.org/10.1007/s00268-016-3492-3.
8. Forsmo HM, Pfeffer F, Rasdal A, Sintonen H, Körner H, Erichsen C. Pre- and postoperative stoma education and guidance within an enhanced recovery after surgery (ERAS) programme reduces length of hospital stay in colorectal surgery. Int J Surg Lond Engl. 2016;36(Pt A):121–6. https://doi.org/10.1016/j.ijsu.2016.10.031.
9. Bisch S, Nelson G, Altman A. Impact of nutrition on enhanced recovery after surgery (ERAS) in gynecologic oncology. Nutrients. 2019;11(5). https://doi.org/10.3390/nu11051088.
10. Ljungqvist O, Scott M, Fearon KC. Enhanced recovery after surgery: a review. JAMA Surg. 2017;152(3):292–8. https://doi.org/10.1001/jamasurg.2016.4952.
11. Yilmaz N, Cekmen N, Bilgin F, Erten E, Ozhan MÖ, Coşar A. Preoperative carbohydrate nutrition reduces postoperative

nausea and vomiting compared to preoperative fasting. J Res Med Sci Off J Isfahan Univ Med Sci. 2013;18(10):827–32.

12. ERAS Compliance Group. The impact of enhanced recovery protocol compliance on elective colorectal cancer resection: results from an international registry. Ann Surg. 2015;261(6):1153–9. https://doi.org/10.1097/SLA.0000000000001029.

13. Hain E, Maggiori L, Prost À la Denise J, Panis Y. Transversus abdominis plane (TAP) block in laparoscopic colorectal surgery improves postoperative pain management: a meta-analysis. Colorectal Dis Off J Assoc Coloproctology G B Irel. 2018;20(4):279–87. https://doi.org/10.1111/codi.14037.

14. Bragg D, El-Sharkawy AM, Psaltis E, Maxwell-Armstrong CA, Lobo DN. Postoperative ileus: recent developments in pathophysiology and management. Clin Nutr Edinb Scotl. 2015;34(3):367–76. https://doi.org/10.1016/j.clnu.2015.01.016.

15. Calligaro KD, Dougherty MJ, Raviola CA, Musser DJ, DeLaurentis DA. Impact of clinical pathways on hospital costs and early outcome after major vascular surgery. J Vasc Surg. 1995;22(6):649–57; discussion 657-660. https://doi.org/10.1016/s0741-5214(95)70055-2.

16. Lemmens L, van Zelm R, Vanhaecht K, Kerkkamp H. Systematic review: indicators to evaluate effectiveness of clinical pathways for gastrointestinal surgery. J Eval Clin Pract. 2008;14(5):880–7. https://doi.org/10.1111/j.1365-2753.2008.01079.x.

17. Müller MK, Dedes KJ, Dindo D, Steiner S, Hahnloser D, Clavien P-A. Impact of clinical pathways in surgery. Langenbecks Arch Surg. 2009;394(1):31–9. https://doi.org/10.1007/s00423-008-0352-0.

18. Małczak P, Pisarska M, Piotr M, Wysocki M, Budzyński A, Pędziwiatr M. Enhanced recovery after bariatric surgery: systematic review and meta-analysis. Obes Surg. 2017;27(1):226–35. https://doi.org/10.1007/s11695-016-2438-z.

19. Ronellenfitsch U, Schwarzbach M, Kring A, Kienle P, Post S, Hasenberg T. The effect of clinical pathways for bariatric surgery on perioperative quality of care. Obes Surg. 2012;22(5):732–9. https://doi.org/10.1007/s11695-012-0605-4.

20. Téoule P, Kunz B, Schwarzbach M, et al. Influence of clinical pathways on treatment and outcome quality for patients undergoing pancreatoduodenectomy? A retrospective cohort study. Asian J Surg. 2020;43(8):799–809. https://doi.org/10.1016/j.asjsur.2019.10.003.

21. Cohen R, Gooberman-Hill R. Staff experiences of enhanced recovery after surgery: systematic review of qualitative studies. BMJ Open. 2019;9(2):e022259. https://doi.org/10.1136/bmjopen-2018-022259.

Chapter 6
Tracking Quality: Data Registries

Brenda M. Zosa and Anne O. Lidor

The methods by which we measure quality surgical care have evolved exponentially over the past 30 years with the growth of technology, demand for accountability, and pursuit to provide the highest-quality care for our patients. However, the framework by which we assess healthcare quality has long been rooted in the Donabedian principles of structure, process, and outcomes [1]. *Structure* represents the physical, technological, and human resources of a healthcare system. These include measures beyond the physical facilities but also include availability of an electronic medical record and data on the provider to patient ratio. While often the easiest to assess, structural measures are the most indirect indicator of quality. *Process* measures are related to the way systems and providers deliver healthcare, such as compliance with evidence-based guidelines and efficiency of delivering care. One of the most familiar process measures is the Surgical Care Improvement Project (SCIP), which, although initially promising, has had some mixed results with regard to how much compliance equates to reductions in postoperative

B. M. Zosa · A. O. Lidor (✉)
Department of Surgery, Johns Hopkins University SOM,
Baltimore, MD, USA
e-mail: lidor@surgery.wisc.edu

© The Author(s), under exclusive license to Springer Nature   91
Switzerland AG 2022
J. R. Romanelli et al. (eds.), *The SAGES Manual of Quality,
Outcomes and Patient Safety*,
https://doi.org/10.1007/978-3-030-94610-4_6

morbidity [2, 3]. *Outcomes* are the metric by which we most closely scrutinize the quality of the care we provide and is arguably the most valuable of measures. It is also the most complex, making "apples to apples" comparisons incredibly challenging across healthcare systems. Multifactorial influences are present at every level, and the success of even the most common procedures is equally affected by the skill of the surgeon, the patient's health status, and the ability of a system to deliver that care and to protect the patient from inadvertent harm.

The emergence of national surgical databases has provided us with platforms to more readily track our outcomes and make meaningful comparisons through the use of statistical modeling that allow us to evaluate data in a risk-adjusted fashion. This enables hospital systems to identify areas of deficiency, enact a plan of action, and assess the effect of that plan on defined quality metrics. This chapter describes the currently existing data registries in surgery and how they have impacted surgical practice.

Society of Thoracic Surgeons (STS)

For better or worse, the incentive to track quality has often been driven by payers, most notably the United States Federal Government. Cardiac surgery was at the heart of the development of national surgical databases. In 1986 the Health Care Financing Administration (HCFA), the predecessor to the Centers for Medicare and Medicaid Services (CMS), released mortality reports on hospitals performing as outliers in cardiac surgery [4]. These reports fueled concern from both the public sector and surgical societies. The validity of these reports was highly criticized for lacking appropriate risk adjustment, in particular when it came to evaluation of outcomes after coronary artery bypass surgery.

The STS recognized the need to better assess quality of care as a surgical specialty and took charge of developing a national database in 1989 [5]. This was among the first surgical databases to include granular clinical data and provide timely risk-adjusted feedback to participating institutions. At the same time, the Department of Veterans Affairs (VA) had begun a nationwide quality improvement project in cardiac surgery, the Continuous Improvement in Cardiac Surgery Program (CICSP). These programs would ultimately lay the foundation for tracking surgical outcomes and promoting data-driven quality initiatives across the country.

National Surgical Quality Improvement Program (NSQIP)

NSQIP was created in response to a federal mandate in 1985 (Public Law 99-166) aimed at improving outcomes for VA hospitals. At the time, the VA was under public scrutiny for high rates of postoperative morbidity and mortality. To address this issue, they first needed to create a system that would allow them to track risk-adjusted outcomes. The National VA Surgical Risk Study was conducted, which collected prospective data at 44 major VA surgical centers. This data established predictive models for risk-adjusted outcomes comparisons that would facilitate assessment of VA hospital performance and the development of the VA NSQIP [6, 7]. Through participation in this program, VA hospitals noted reduction in 30-day mortality after major surgery by 45% and reduction in 30-day mortality by 31% [8]. The federal mandate also required the VA to compare their surgical outcomes to the national average, prompting a pilot study in three academic centers in the private sector which confirmed the predictive models of the VA NSQIP could be applied to other systems. The American College of Surgeons (ACS) then partnered with the VA to conduct the Patient Safety in Surgery (PSS) Study which included 18 non-VA sites and provided further evidence of the validity of NSQIP for hospitals across the nation. Over the study period, participating private sector hospitals noted significant reductions in 30-day postoperative morbidity by 8.7%, surgical site infections

(SSIs) by 9.1%, and renal complications by 23.7% [9]. The culmination of these findings along with positive feedback from the participating sites led to the official establishment of the ACS NSQIP for public enrollment in 2004.

ACS NSQIP became the first nationally validated, risk-adjusted, outcomes-based program for measuring outcomes in a variety of surgical subspecialties, with the ultimate goal of improving the quality of surgical care. Since its creation, ACS NSQIP has become an instrumental tool in quality improvements, outcomes research, and the development of an affective risk calculator. Today over 700 hospitals participate in ACS NSQIP. Preoperative data and 30-day outcomes are recorded for a variety of general and subspecialty surgeries by trained surgical clinical reviewers (SCRs). Hospitals are given semiannual reports on their own risk-adjusted outcomes and offered a blinded comparison to other participating hospitals. This has led to establishment of national benchmarks and various efforts by the ACS to support quality improvement efforts across institutions. Long-term participation in NSQIP has been associated with a reduction in 30-day morbidity and mortality. Studies by both Hall and Cohen found reductions in mortality in 66–69% and reduced morbidity in 79–82% of participating hospitals [10, 11]. However, others have been critical that mere participation in NSQIP is not enough to improve outcomes. Two studies comparing outcomes of NSQIP hospitals to nonparticipating centers found no statistically significant difference in postoperative morbidity over time, suggesting that improved outcomes may be more reflective of regression to the mean over time for certain outliers [12, 13]. In particular, Osbourne et al. [12] found no differences in Medicare payments before and after participation in ACS NSQIP when using nonparticipating hospitals as a control.

It is clear that hospital systems must be committed to improving care and implementing quality improvement projects to make a meaningful impact. There is a wealth of data demonstrating that NSQIP data can serve as a catalyst for change and facilitate monitoring the influence quality improvement initiatives have on targeted outcomes. Examples include a single center initiative at decreasing ventilator time, leading to an eventual zero pneumonia rate, and numerous programs aimed at reducing surgical site infections, in particular after colorectal surgery [14–17]. Beyond local feedback, ACS NSQIP empowers change through the development of collaboratives and best practice guidelines. Currently there are over 65 collaboratives that vary in size and function. These range from health system-wide, regional, to virtual collaboratives. Among the most notable, the Michigan Surgical Quality Collaborative (MSQC) demonstrated improved morbidity in participating hospitals when compared to a non-Michigan ACS NSQIP cohort. This was particularly true when it came to reductions in sepsis, pneumonia, septic shock, cardiac arrest, and need for prolonged mechanical ventilation [18]. The Tennessee Surgical Quality Collaborative also showed significant improvements in surgical site infections (SSIs), decreasing prolonged ventilation, AKI, and wound disruption [19]. Additionally, they estimated a cost savings of over $2,000,000 per 10,000 general and vascular surgery cases.

It is important to note that there is a significant investment incurred by the participating centers. The annual fee ranges from $10,000 to $29,000 a year, but the majority of the cost is in the salary for the SCR, which can range anywhere from $40,000 to $100,000 a year. While NSQIP does not capture cost data, several studies have deduced a cost savings from participating in ACS NSQIP by reducing the incidence of complications [17, 20–23].

Metabolic and Bariatric Surgery Accreditation and Quality Improvement Program (MBSAQIP)

Tracking quality outcomes has become the cornerstone of accreditation for centers of excellence (COE) in bariatric care. In 2012 the ACS Bariatric Surgery Center Network and the American Society for Metabolic and Bariatric Surgery (ASMBS) Bariatric Centers of Excellence combined their respective programs to form MBSAQIP. This now serves as the accreditation body and has created a single bariatric database which over 800 participating institutions currently contribute to. The MBSAQIP database captures high-quality data for the majority of bariatric surgeries that take place in the United States and Canada. An important distinction between NSQIP and MBSAQIP is that while NSQIP randomly samples cases, and thus can miss outliers, MBSAQIP is required to include 100% of bariatric cases at participating centers, thus ensuring a more robust data set.

In addition to bariatric-specific perioperative variables and 30-day outcomes, long-term follow-up data are recorded at 6 months, 1 year, and annually thereafter. The MBSAQIP has recently developed a patient-reported outcome measures (PROMs) program which will send surveys to patients preoperatively, 1-year post-op, and then annually. Semiannual site-specific reports are provided to participating institutions allowing them to benchmark their outcomes to the national average. Accredited sites are required to develop at least one quality improvement initiative per year, and centers who are high outliers for any given measure must address and implement an initiative geared toward reducing that outcome.

MBSAQIP not only stimulates quality improvement initiatives on an individual hospital level, but it has demonstrated that it can facilitate them on a much larger scale. The first national quality improvement collaborative out of the MBSAQIP was aimed at decreasing rates of readmissions. The "Decreasing Readmissions through Opportunities Provided" (DROP) program implemented a bundle at 128 hospitals and demonstrated a 10% reduction in 30-day readmissions overall, with even larger reductions at 32% in centers with the highest rates [24]. Subsequently, the Employing Enhanced Recovery Goals in Bariatric Surgery (ENERGY) study showed successful implementation of an enhanced recovery program across 36 sites with high rates of extended length of stay after bariatric surgery. Adherence to the protocol at targeted centers led to significant decreases in extended length of stay without compromising other outcomes [25].

A recent article by Clapp et al. highlighted the impressive volume of research that has emerged since the release of the first Participant Use Data File (PUF) in 2015, citing 55 published manuscripts and 126 abstracts [26]. It is clear that MBSAQIP has had a resounding impact on surgical research and has proven to be a valuable resource to evaluate outcomes in an evolving field. Over the last 10 years, we have seen a rapid growth in the number of laparoscopic sleeve gastrectomies, becoming the most common bariatric procedure performed. The detailed data captured regarding sleeve gastrectomy has allowed for large-scale analysis of specific technical elements on outcomes. While MBSAQIP data can be utilized to change practice, it is not immune to reporting conflicting results. For example, while one study comparing staple line reinforcement (SLR) to non-reinforced staple lines [27] noted no difference in leak rates after LSG, another study [28] noted a paradoxical increase in leak rates after LSG.

This database like any is not without its limitations. Changes in practice over time have likely led to an element of treatment bias that cannot be accounted for when making comparisons. An evaluation of the 2015 PUF found various data quality issues with data completeness, accuracy, and consistency, which could potentially lead to losing as much as 20% of the entered cases [29]. The majority of these were related to how weight and BMI were recorded, which is clearly an important metric in bariatric surgery.

The aggregate data collected through this robust database has allowed for the creation of a bariatric surgical risk/benefit calculator which provides individualized estimates of postoperative weight loss, resolution of comorbidities, and risk of developing postoperative complications from either sleeve gastrectomy or Roux-en-Y gastric bypass.

Abdominal Core Health Quality Collaborative (ACHQC)

The ACHQC, previously known as the Americas Hernia Society Quality Collaborative, was established in 2013 with the aim of improving the quality of care delivered to patients with ventral hernias. The database formed by this collective is unique in that it provides continuous real-time, risk-adjusted data to participating institutions [30]. It was designed to prospectively collect demographics, granular perioperative details, as well as long-term follow-up data using validated patient-reported outcome measures. It was also intended to facilitate multi-institutional investigations of mesh types and other medical devices in the treatment of hernia disease. A comparison of biosynthetic to polypropylene mesh in clean-contaminated and contaminated wounds using this database elicited some interesting and unexpected results. While there was no significant difference in overall surgical site occurrences between the two types of mesh, biosynthetic mesh was associated with higher rates of major wound complications and unplanned reoperations [31]. By integrating the use of the registry into their routine clinical practice, the Cleveland Clinic Center for Abdominal Core Health has found that the process of conducting a randomized clinical trial was efficient and ensured high-quality data, as the surgeon who was most familiar with the patient's course was the one recording the data. Through these studies [32, 33], the ACHQC has shown one example of how disease-specific databases can be implemented to further surgical science.

Summary

This chapter highlights the history and contributions of some of the most notable surgical databases that are widely used by general surgeons but by no means encompasses the entire spectrum of high-quality surgical registries that exist. There are numerous programs in almost every surgical subspecialty that contribute to advancing global research and quality initiatives. The ACS Trauma Quality Improvement Program (ACS TQIP), Vascular Quality Initiative, Organ Procurement and Transplantation Network, and the National Cancer Data Base (NCDB) are some of the extensive list of quality improvement programs that are currently utilized in surgical practice.

The American Board of Surgery (ABS) recognizes the importance of tracking quality not only on a national level but also for the individual surgeon. As part of the continuous certification process for diplomates, participation in practice improvement is required, either through contributions to one of the national quality improvement registries or by creating an independent practice improvement plan. The goal of the practice improvement requirement is "for diplomates to regularly assess their performance, by reviewing their outcomes, addressing identified areas for improvement, and evaluating the results" [34]. The ABS provides access to the Surgeon Specific Registry (SSR), an online quality improvement tool, where surgeons can track their own individual cases and outcomes independently. This not only facilitates individual practice improvement but has the added potential of meeting certain CMS requirements.

Reliance on databases to measure the quality of surgical care has its own inherent limitations. Despite the robustness of the major surgical databases described, there are no doubt unaccounted risk factors that cannot be adjusted for. True severity of comorbidities, socioeconomic factors, and treatment biases are almost impossible to capture accurately. Outcomes measured are often limited to a 30-day postoperative time frame, when many outcomes of interest may not be evident for a much longer period. This is true for both the NSQIP and MBSAQIP PUF files that are utilized in most published studies. While the SCRs undergo rigorous training and attempts are made to maintain standardized definitions, the way we define certain events, such as ventilator-associated pneumonia, has evolved, making comparisons over time challenging. As practices continue to evolve, there will also be a need to add new variables. We are already seeing this in bariatric surgery where there is not a variable in the MBSAQIP to accurately capture revisions from sleeve to gastric bypass.

Databases have historically lacked quality of life assessments and cost data which are critical for clinicians and interesting to researchers and payers. It is important that surgeons remain engaged with how those measures are recorded and evaluated. The CMS and many other payers have shifted toward pay-for-performance and use performance data to adjust future payments. Both MBSAQIP and ACHQC are approved as qualified clinical data registries in the CMS Merit-based Incentive Payment System (MIPS), which offers surgeons in independent practice opportunities to achieve a higher level of reimbursement that is afforded to larger medical centers that participate in larger programs such as NSQIP. It is important to note that while the benchmarks established by data registries are intended to motivate improvements, oftentimes energy is more focused on "beating" the quality metric than on actually improving the quality of care. We must also be critical of the statistically significant differences we may find when using large data sets that are in reality of minimal clinically significance.

Despite the costs and limitations, we must always remember the overarching goal and purpose of participating in national surgical databases: to continuously strive to provide the highest quality of care to the patients entrusted to us.

Editor's Note

SAGES is and has been interested in data registries for some time. As you have read in this review of registries, many surgical societies have invested time and resources into registry creation. The AHSQC was unique in that it was entirely funded by industry. Mesh manufacturers were keenly interested in product performance and likely were willing to invest in comparative data that showed that their own product performed superiorly to others. While some other product-focused procedures might also benefit from such robust data collection, few other disease-specific registries have yet been developed. One could imagine that an investment into data that showed inferior performance of a product would serve as a disincentive for our industry partners to heavily invest in this concept.

As detailed elsewhere in this textbook, SAGES has been the leader in the prevention of bile duct injuries (BDI), and as such, the concept of a cholecystectomy registry was explored in depth, led by the SAGES Quality, Outcomes, and Safety Committee. This review spanned 2 years and even led to a formal meeting with SAGES leadership and a data company in 2016. The conclusion from this exploration was that there were two major barriers to creating a SAGES data registry: cost and the human cost of data entry. A registry tracking cholecystectomy outcomes (with the aim of prevention of BDI) would require granular data collection, and as such, the surgeons themselves would most likely have to be the inputters of data. Given how ubiquitous cholecystectomy is in the general surgical world, this would impose significant work burden onto surgeons with little tangible benefit (e.g., this would not have been required by CMS for reimbursement). As such, there was concern about how well utilized such a registry would have been, and without a high percentage of usage, there was a likelihood that cases with BDI might not have been entered (with acknowledged concern for inducing medicolegal risk) – thus nullifying the value of such a registry. Again, the AHSQC had initial success because a highly motivated group of academic surgeons with a career focus on hernia surgery committed to the laborious task of data entry, but there was skepticism that surgeons would be similarly motivated with cholecystectomy. Further, the cost of creating the registry would have been between $1.5 and 2 million, which is exorbitant and beyond the realistic ability for a society to fund; data maintenance and storage over time would also have been well over $1 million. As such, the registry plans were abandoned.

Further, SAGES explored the concept – and remains interested in – tracking outcomes of anti-reflux surgery. While this would have been less populated than cholecystectomy in terms of case volumes, we postulated that this would be of high inter-est to the foregut surgeons that comprise a significant percent-age of SAGES' membership. While we pivoted away from a pure data registry due to the aforementioned reasons, a project to conduct video-based assessments of fundoplications is underway and may ultimately serve as a data repository for SAGES members to access. It is the hope of the group conduct-ing this work that we can all learn from one another in terms of technical pearls and that over time this will serve to improve outcomes of the procedure. Much work remains until this is commonplace among SAGES members, but with the ever-increasing computing power and advanced video capture sys-tems and cloud technology, this may become a "twenty-first century" data registry that can be accessed for continual qual-ity improvement.

References

1. Donabedian A. The quality of care. How can it be assessed? JAMA [Internet]. 1988;260(12):1743–8.
2. Chang V, Blackwell RH, Markossian T, Yau RM, Blanco BA, Zapf MAC, et al. Discordance between surgical care improvement project adherence and postoperative outcomes: implications for new Joint Commission standards. J Surg Res. 2017;212:205–13.
3. Altom LK, Deierhoi RJ, Grams J, Richman JS, Vick CC, Henderson WG, et al. Association between Surgical Care Improvement Program venous thromboembolism measures and postoperative events. Am J Surg. 2012;204(5):591–7.
4. Kouchoukos NT, Ebert PA, Grover FL, Lindesmith GG. Report of the Ad Hoc Committee on risk factors for coronary artery bypass surgery. Ann Thorac Surg [Internet]. 1988;45(3):348–9.
5. Clark RE. It is time for a national cardiothoracic surgical data base. Ann Thorac Surg [Internet]. 1989;48(6):755–6.
6. Khuri SF, Daley J, Henderson W, Hur K, Gibbs JO, Barbour G, et al. Risk adjustment of the postoperative mortality rate for the comparative assessment of the quality of surgical care: results of the National Veterans Affairs surgical risk study. J Am Coll Surg. 1997;185(4):325–38.

7. Khuri SF, Daley J, Henderson W, Hur K, Demakis J, Aust JB, et al. The Department of Veterans Affairs' NSQIP: the first national, validated, outcome-based, risk-adjusted, and peer-controlled program for the measurement and enhancement of the quality of surgical care. Ann Surg. 1998;228(4):491–507.

8. Khuri SF. The NSQIP: a new frontier in surgery. Surgery. 2005;138(5):837–43.

9. Khuri SF, Henderson WG, Daley J, Jonasson O, Jones RS, Campbell DA, et al. Successful implementation of the department of Veterans Affairs' national surgical quality improvement program in the private sector: the patient safety in surgery study. Ann Surg. 2008;248(2):329–36.

10. Hall BL, Hamilton BH, Richards K, Bilimoria KY, Cohen ME, Ko CY. Does surgical quality improve in the American College of Surgeons national surgical quality improvement program: an evaluation of all participating hospitals. Ann Surg. 2009;250(3):363–74.

11. Cohen ME, Liu Y, Ko CY, Hall BL. Improved surgical outcomes for ACS NSQIP hospitals over time: evaluation of hospital cohorts with up to 8 years of participation. Ann Surg. 2016;263(2):267–73.

12. Osborne NH, Nicholas LH, Ryan AM, Thumma JR, Dimick JB. Association of hospital participation in a quality reporting program with surgical outcomes and expenditures for medicare beneficiaries. JAMA J Am Med Assoc. 2015;313(5):496–504.

13. Etzioni DA, Wasif N, Dueck AC, Cima RR, Hohmann SF, Naessens JM, et al. Association of hospital participation in a surgical outcomes monitoring program with inpatient complications and mortality. JAMA [Internet]. 2015;313(5):505–11.

14. Fuchshuber PR, Greif W, Tidwell CR, Klemm MS, Frydel C, Wali A, et al. The power of the National Surgical Quality Improvement Program--achieving a zero pneumonia rate in general surgery patients. Perm J. 2012;16(1):39–45.

15. Cima R, Dankbar E, Lovely J, Pendlimari R, Aronhalt K, Nehring S, et al. Colorectal surgery surgical site infection reduction program: a national surgical quality improvement program-driven multidisciplinary single-institution experience. J Am Coll Surg [Internet]. 2013;216(1):23–33.

16. Lutfiyya W, Parsons D, Breen J. A colorectal "care bundle" to reduce surgical site infections in colorectal surgeries: a single-center experience. Perm J. 2012;16(3):10–6.

17. Thanh NX, Baron T, Litvinchuk S. An economic evaluation of the National Surgical Quality Improvement Program (NSQIP) in Alberta, Canada. Ann Surg. 2019;269(5):866–72.
18. Campbell DA, Englesbe MJ, Kubus JJ, Phillips LRS, Shanley CJ, Velanovich V, et al. Accelerating the pace of surgical quality improvement: the power of hospital collaboration. Arch Surg (Chicago, Ill: 1960) [Internet]. 2010;145(10):985–91.
19. Guillamondegui OD, Gunter OL, Hines L, Martin BJ, Gibson W, Clarke PC, et al. Using the national surgical quality improvement program and the Tennessee surgical quality collaborative to improve surgical outcomes. J Am College Surg [Internet]. 2012;214(4):709–14; discussion 714-6.
20. Hollenbeak CS, Boltz MM, Wang L, Schubart J, Ortenzi G, Zhu J, et al. Cost-effectiveness of the national surgical quality improvement program. Ann Surg. 2011;254(4):619–24.
21. McNelis J, Castaldi M. "The National Surgery Quality Improvement Project" (NSQIP): a new tool to increase patient safety and cost efficiency in a surgical intensive care unit. Patient Saf Surg [Internet]. 2014;8:19.
22. van Katwyk S, Thavorn K, Coyle D, Moloo H, Forster AJ, Jackson T, et al. The return of investment of hospital-based surgical quality improvement programs in reducing surgical site infection at a Canadian tertiary-care hospital. Infect Control Hospital Epidemiol [Internet]. 2019;40(2):125–32.
23. Nimeri AA, Bautista J, Philip R. Reducing healthcare costs using ACS NSQIP-driven quality improvement projects: a success story from Sheikh Khalifa Medical City (SKMC). World J Surg [Internet]. 2019;43(2):331–8.
24. Morton J. The first metabolic and bariatric surgery accreditation and quality improvement program quality initiative: decreasing readmissions through opportunities provided. Surg Obes Relat Dis. 2014;10(3):377–8.
25. Brethauer SA, Grieco A, Fraker T, Evans-Labok K, Smith A, McEvoy MD, et al. Employing enhanced recovery goals in bariatric surgery (ENERGY): a national quality improvement project using the metabolic and bariatric surgery accreditation and quality improvement program. Surg Obes Relat Dis [Internet]. 2019;15(11):1977–89.
26. Clapp B, Harper B, Barrientes A, Wicker E, Alvara C, Tyroch A. The MBSAQIP is going viral! 194 hits and still going strong. Surg Obes Relat Dis [Internet]. 2020;16(10):1401–6.

27. Demeusy A, Sill A, Averbach A. Current role of staple line reinforcement in 30-day outcomes of primary laparoscopic sleeve gastrectomy: an analysis of MBSAQIP data, 2015–2016 PUF. Surg Obes Relat Dis [Internet]. 2018;14(10):1454–61.

28. Berger ER, Clements RH, Morton JM, Huffman KM, Wolfe BM, Nguyen NT, et al. The impact of different surgical techniques on outcomes in laparoscopic sleeve gastrectomies: the first report from the metabolic and bariatric surgery accreditation and quality improvement program (MBSAQIP). Ann Surg. 2016;264(3):464–71.

29. Noyes K, Myneni AA, Schwaitzberg SD, Hoffman AB. Quality of MBSAQIP data: bad luck, or lack of QA plan? Surg Endosc. 2020;34(2):973–80.

30. Poulose BK, Roll S, Murphy JW, Matthews BD, Todd Heniford B, Voeller G, et al. Design and implementation of the Americas Hernia Society Quality Collaborative (AHSQC): improving value in hernia care. Hernia. 2016;20(2):177–89.

31. Sahoo S, Haskins IN, Huang LC, Krpata DM, Derwin KA, Poulose BK, et al. Early wound morbidity after open ventral hernia repair with biosynthetic or polypropylene mesh. J Am Coll Surg. 2017;225(4):472–480.e1.

32. Zolin SJ, Petro CC, Prabhu AS, Fafaj A, Thomas JD, Horne CM, et al. Registry-based randomized controlled trials: a new paradigm for surgical research. J Surg Res. 2020;255:428–35.

33. Petro CC, Zolin S, Krpata D, Alkhatib H, Tu C, Rosen MJ, et al. Patient-reported outcomes of robotic vs laparoscopic ventral hernia repair with intraperitoneal mesh. JAMA Surg [Internet]. 2021;156:22–9.

34. ABS practice improvement resources [Internet]. Available from: https://www.absurgery.org/default.jsp?exam-mocpa.

Chapter 7
Accreditation Standards: Bariatric Surgery

Teresa L. LaMasters, Jamie P. Loggins, and Teresa Fraker

Accreditation Standards: Bariatric Surgery

The objectives for this chapter:

1. To describe how accreditation standards were developed and implemented across most of North America with wide acceptance
2. To review current standards for bariatric accreditation
3. To discuss some of the published data as a result of MBSAQIP

T. L. LaMasters (✉)
Iowa Methodist Medical Center Unity Point Clinic,
University of Iowa, Des Moines, IA, USA

J. P. Loggins
Mission Weight Management Center, Asheville, NC, USA

T. Fraker
Metabolic and Bariatric Surgery Accreditation and Quality
Improvement Program (MBSAQIP), Division of Research and
Optimal Patient Care (DROPC), American College of Surgeons
(ACS), Chicago, IL, USA
e-mail: teresa@obesitymedicine.org

© The Author(s), under exclusive license to Springer Nature   107
Switzerland AG 2022
J. R. Romanelli et al. (eds.), *The SAGES Manual of Quality,
Outcomes and Patient Safety*,
https://doi.org/10.1007/978-3-030-94610-4_7

Development of Accreditation Standards

The era of organized bariatric surgery began around 1967 with collaborative meetings and discussion prior to the formation of what would become the American Society for Bariatric Surgery (ASBS). The ASBS was officially founded in 1984 by Dr. Edward Mason at the University of Iowa, and it would later change its name to become what we now know as the American Society for Metabolic and Bariatric Surgery (ASMBS). Even early in the history of bariatric surgery, a need for data collection and evaluation was identified, and therefore the first attempt at a database to better understand outcomes and improve quality was started by Dr. Mason. This registry was housed at the University of Iowa and was called the International Bariatric Surgery Registry. The data collection for this registry began in 1985. It was initially funded by industry support with a planned transition to eventually be supported by member surgeons. This database operated by providing reports to the participating surgeons twice yearly until the database was eventually closed due to a lack of funding [1].

During a similar timeframe, the American College of Surgeons (ACS) with the missions of education and quality had partnered with the surgical specialties of trauma and cancer by forming the Committee on Trauma in 1976 to begin accreditation programs focused on data and improving quality.

There was a period of rapid growth in the number of bariatric procedures performed in the United States with the emergence of laparoscopic techniques of bariatric surgery between 1999 and 2003. The number of gastrointestinal surgeries performed annually for severe obesity increased from about 16,000 in the early 1990s to about 103,000 in 2003 (Fig. 7.1) [2, 3].

During this timeframe, there were many general surgeons looking to transition from open to laparoscopic approaches to procedures inclusive of laparoscopic bariatric surgery. During this period of rapid growth, there were surgeons

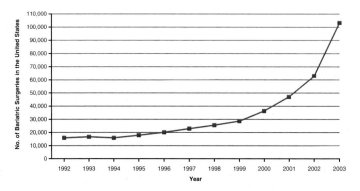

FIGURE 7.1 Historical annual weight loss surgery volume

providing bariatric surgery with limited training in these complex techniques with limited patient education and programmatic support. There was a spotlight on poor bariatric surgery outcomes from many directions including payors, media, malpractice attorneys, and stigmatism from other medical professionals. There were also several reports published during this period demonstrating a high mortality rate of 2–3% and high complication rates, particularly in patients over age 65 years of age [4–6].

A crisis developed when the Centers for Medicare & Medicaid Services (CMS) considered ceasing coverage for all bariatric procedures due to high mortality and complications from bariatric surgery. The Medical Care Advisory Committee for CMS (MEDCAC) committee met on November 4, 2004, to consider the concerning outcomes with bariatric surgery.

The culmination of these reports resulted in a noncoverage proposal for bariatric surgery for patients 65 years or older from Centers for Medicare & Medicaid Services (CMS) on November 23, 2005; however, CMS continued to collect and review safety and outcome data on metabolic and bariatric surgery patients. Fortunately, the rigorous focus from the bariatric surgery community to quality and patient safety did not go unnoticed by CMS. After care review of additional information, CMS granted coverage for all Medicare beneficiaries through a National Coverage Determination (NCD) in 2006 who met certain criteria provided the patient's surgery was performed at a certified Bariatric Surgery Center of Excellence or a Level 1 Bariatric Surgery Center [7].

It was important for the field of bariatric surgery to pivot from unbridled innovation and growth to one of quality outcomes and quality improvement.

Beginning in 2004 and 2005, the first attempt at developing an accreditation program guided by bariatric surgery standards was formed, and as a result, two accreditation programs were developed. One program was under the leadership of the American Society for Metabolic and Bariatric Surgery (ASMBS), and a second was under the leadership of the American College of Surgeons (ACS). Both programs were organized around standards to decrease the variability in care of bariatric surgery patients. There were, however, different philosophies guiding these efforts. The ASMBS program was developed with the creation of a third-party not-for-profit organization to perform the accreditation duties and have the specialty society surgeons at arm's length from the program. The rationale for having a third party involved was to ensure that the data integrity could be protected while simultaneously providing external stakeholders confidence in the process. The ACS program philosophy centered on the expertise of the specialty society determining what constitutes quality in the field without the need for a third-party entity. There was concern from the ACS of a third party having interests that did not align with the mission and goals of the society.

The ASMBS program was called the Bariatric Surgery Centers of Excellence (BSCOE) program, run by the Surgical Review Corporation (SRC). The BSCOE was organized around ten standards, and it provided verification of the surgeon, the practice, and the hospital. The purpose was to create a means for the public and other interested parties to identify bariatric surgery programs that provided standardized and comprehensive care as well as lifelong follow-up care for patients. Data collection and routine reporting of outcomes would allow for evaluation of the true risks and benefits of bariatric surgery while additionally challenging poorly performing programs to evaluate and improve their standards, education, and training [8].

In February 2005, the ACS Board of Regents voted to expand the accreditation programs available with a priority for bariatric surgery. The focus included the need to develop established standards, provide reliable outcomes data, develop a verification process for hospitals and facilities, and to establish credentialing criteria for surgeons. The ACS Bariatric Surgery Center Network (ASC BSCN) convened for planning on March 4, 2005, with 13 bariatric surgeons and outcomes researchers, and the program was formally launched in May 2005.

The initial structure of the ACS BSCN accreditation program (Table 7.1) was modeled off the ACS' trauma verification program with a Level I and Level II designation primarily based around surgical case volumes, services available at facility, and risk profile of patients. It also included a robust data collection platform modeled from the National Surgical Quality Improvement Program (NSQIP) with the notable exception being the increased data capture to 100% data collection (the NSQIP program required a sampling of 25% data collection). Data collection was performed by trained surgical clinical reviewers (SCRs). Bariatric specific endpoints were included as well as long-term follow-up data at 30 days, 6 months, and annually thereafter. The data collection system was developed for quality assessment and quality improvement.

These accreditations became valuable commercially as many insurance payors required participation in one of these two programs. The early results of these accreditation programs resulted in a 1/3 reduction of those (previous) programs who were performing bariatric procedures. There was a sharp and dramatic improvement in mortality and other serious complications in bariatric surgery. These factors led to widespread adoption of the accreditation process because of the significant improvement in patient outcomes.

TABLE 7.1 Initial criteria for Level 1 and Level 2 BSN

Level 1	Level 2 = lower volume and acuity of patients
125 cases per year	25 cases per year
Two surgeons (at least 50 cases per year each)	Surgeon, at least 50 cases every 2 years
Can operate on all patients and risk levels of patients	Cannot operate on high-risk patients including: Age > 60 Significant cardiac or pulmonary issues Male BMI >55, female BMI >60 Nonambulatory patient Elective revisional operations
Full spectrum of services at hospital	
Significant hospital resources criteria	

As time progressed, there were flaws identified in the programs, however. There was a strong emphasis on process and structure but less focus on outcomes. In particular, the ASMBS BSCOE program was exclusionary in nature, based primarily on processes and structure that were not always attributed to improved patient outcomes. It became difficult to determine those programs who were high versus poorly performing based on the data provided for accredited programs. The data collected as a part of the BSCOE in the Bariatric Outcomes Longitudinal Database (BOLD) was extensive but not easily accessible by the participating surgeons and programs. The reporting of the data was not adequate to promote or support quality improvement at the local individual program level.

The flaws in the program and concerns around limitation of access to care for bariatric patients led to the development of a third system, the Michigan Bariatric Surgery Collaborative

(MBSC). This collaborative was focused on high participation, with high-quality data, and sharing of best practices in a collaborative effort. The goal was that all programs in Michigan were expected to participate with the principle of "a rising tide lifts all boats." By encouraging all programs to participate, they were able to improve quality of all programs versus excluding programs. The MBSC was funded by a commercial insurance company – Blue Cross Blue Shield (BCBS) – that served 47% of all patients in Michigan. The collaborative was independent of the insurance company other than receiving funding to operate the collaborative. BCBS also provided insurance coverage for those patients receiving bariatric surgery at participating programs even if the programs did not participate in the ASMBS or ACS accreditation programs. The MBSC was able to demonstrate improved outcomes for the participating bariatric programs, which were similar to, or even better than, programs participating in the other accreditation programs, due to the collaborative focus [9–12].

In response to the MBSC findings, CMS dropped the requirement for its beneficiaries to have bariatric surgery in an accredited facility [13].

During this timeframe, it became clear that the ASMBS BSCOE needed to evolve. There was concern that the third-party organization in charge of the accreditation process may not be aligned with the goals of the ASMBS organization and their leadership. Conflict began to arise, and despite attempts to mitigate the concerns of the organization, it was determined that a new path must be forged to reach the goals of continued quality improvement. The SRC (aka the third party) gave notice to ASMBS that it was not interested in a collaboration of efforts, and the SRC then planned to start their own Centers of Excellence program for bariatric surgery independent of ASMBS. The ASMBS's contract with the SRC was terminated on April 1, 2012 [14].

The combination of these events led to collaboration between the ASMBS and the ACS to create one unified accreditation program and credentialing guidelines. This process began in 2011 and continued through 2012. Initially there were differences between the programs, and a large undertaking to merge the cultures of the program was undertaken. Members of each society came together to create the new accreditation program modeled similarly under the previous ACS BSCN program and other quality programs such as NSQIP. Three working committees were formed which included standards, verification, and data. There was also an oversight committee for governance of the program, called the Committee for Metabolic and Bariatric Surgery. The initial standards were released for public comment in December of 2012. There was a large response from the membership, and these comments were then integrated into the standards. A second draft of the standards was proposed in 2013 with additional comments. The program merged the data collection into the BSCN database with programs beginning to enter new data for the new accreditation program of the Metabolic and Bariatric Surgery Accreditation and Quality Improvement Program (MBSAQIP) on March 1, 2012. The first official set of standards for the new accreditation program MBSAQIP were published on January 28, 2014, in the *Resources for the Optimal Care of the Metabolic and Bariatric Surgery Patient 2014: MBSAQIP Standards and Pathways Manual* [14].

The key aspects of the new program centered around local committees in metabolic and bariatric surgery to evaluate the risk adjusted data and the requirement that the accredited centers use this data for quality improvement. It includes support for integrated health team members to provide education and support within a program structure, data abstraction by independent and trained clinical reviewers, requirement for at least one verified surgeon at the center, and integration of adolescent bariatric surgery standards. The new program provided accreditation for the hospitals and facilities with the requirement that the hospital and facilities demonstrate both the fiscal and administrative support for the program.

The focus of the MBSAQIP is the use of valid, high-quality data provided to individual programs with risk-adjusted reports to allow for individual programs to use the data for continuous quality improvements. Programs are provided reports on individual outcomes as well as comparison data against benchmarks from patients with a similar risk profile. The structure and process of the bariatric programs center around evidence-based and consensus-based standards. Participating programs receive site visits and feedback on compliance with the standards as well as input regarding areas and strategies for quality improvement. MBSAQIP currently has over 839 centers participating in the program, and this number grows each year [15].

The standards are reviewed and updated continuously with new standards published on a triennial cycle. The Standards and Verification committee reviews the standards in lieu of new published evidence, feedback from site reviewers, and feedback from participating programs. Currently, the third edition of the standards in the *Resources for the Optimal Care of the Metabolic and Bariatric Surgery Patient: 2019 Standards* is used to measure programs against one another. This version of the standards is organized under eight separate standards, thereby creating alignment across ACS' entire suite of quality programs in the Division of Research and Optimal Patient Care (DROPC), the ACS' quality division. There are additional qualifications available in Adolescent Bariatric Surgery and Obesity Medicine for programs who meet the additional requirements. The MBSAQIP has remained innovative in response to change and new challenges. In late 2019 and throughout 2020, the United States and the world suffered with a global pandemic of the SARS-CoV-2 coronavirus pandemic with the disease of COVID-19 greatly restricting the ability for in-person site visits and collaboration. Like many organizations during this trying time, the MBSAQIP adapted to this new environment. In collaboration with the other accreditation programs in DROPC, it developed a standardized virtual site visit that was implemented in the summer of 2020. The focus was still on verification of compliance with standards and implementation of continuous quality improvement based on data from the

MBSAQIP risk-adjusted reports. The initial virtual visits were performed with centers applying for renewal of accreditation and subsequently included sites seeking initial accreditation.

Current Standards for Bariatric Accreditation

The current standards allow programs to participate even when the program is new and early in their experience with bariatric surgery. There are different accreditation pathways depending on the volume, experience, and goals of the center. The accreditation pathways available include Data Collection Center, MBSAQIP Comprehensive Center, MBSAQIP Comprehensive Center with Adolescent Qualifications, MBSAQIP Comprehensive Center with Obesity Medicine Qualifications, MBSAQIP Comprehensive Center with Adolescent and Obesity Medicine Qualifications, MBSAQIP Low Acuity Center, MBSAQIP Adolescent Center, and MBSAQIP Ambulatory Surgery Center.

We will give a brief overview of the current standards with a summary of the goal and rationale of the standard (Fig. 7.2) [16].

Standard 1: Institutional Administrative Commitment

- 1.1 Administrative Commitment

This standard is focused on the component of required institutional support for the program. It will not be possible for the metabolic and bariatric program to be successful providing high-quality outcomes with implementation of the standards without strong institutional commitment and support. This support is demonstrated in many ways including infrastructure and cultural support. It requires a signed written commitment from the highest institutional leadership.

8 Optimal Resources for Surgical Quality and Safety

1. Institutional Administrative Commitment
2. Program Scope and Governance
3. Facilities and Equipment Resources
4. Personnel and Services Resources
5. Patient Care: Expectations and Protocols
6. Data Surveillance & Systems
7. Quality Improvement
8. Education: Professional and Community Outreach

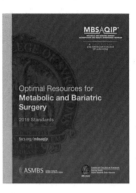

FIGURE 7.2 2019 MBSAQIP Optimal Resources for Surgical Quality and Safety, or "STANDARDS" 15

Rationale: Full support and continuous commitment from institutional leadership is vital to maintaining a MBSAQIP Accredited Center. Resource allocation (such as equipment, personnel, and administrative support), a commitment to patient safety, and an enduring focus on continuous quality improvement are the hallmarks of strong institutional administrative support which help facilitate the success of MBSAQIP centers.

Standard 2: Program Scope and Governance

- 2.1 Volume Criteria
- 2.2 Low Acuity Center Patient and Procedure Selection
- 2.3 Ambulatory Surgery Center Patient and Procedure Selection
- 2.4 Metabolic and Bariatric Surgery (MBS) Committee
- 2.5 Metabolic and Bariatric Surgery (MBS) Director
- 2.6 Metabolic and Bariatric Surgery (MBS) Coordinator

- 2.7 Metabolic and Bariatric Surgery (MBS) Clinical Reviewer
- 2.8 Obesity Medicine Director (OMD)

This standard is the foundation for the accreditation program, speaking to volume, patient selection, governance, and outcome management with high-quality data. It provides minimum procedure volume requirements as well as patient and procedure selection for Low Acuity and Ambulatory Surgery Centers. It also details the composition and responsibilities of the key members for the governance of the accredited programs. This includes the Metabolic and Bariatric Surgery (MBS) Committee, the MBS Director, the MBS Coordinator, the MBS Clinical Reviewer, and the Obesity Medicine Director (OMD) and Pediatric Medical Advisor (PMA), when applicable.

The accreditation and quality improvement are focused on the facility, regardless of how many individual practice locations or surgeons participate at that facility. There is a single unified MBS Committee that consists of, at a minimum, the MBS Director, the MBS Coordinator, the MBS Clinical Reviewer, all surgeons and proceduralists at the center performing procedures for the treatment of metabolic or obesity-related diseases and representatives of the facility administration who are involved in the care or oversight of metabolic and bariatric patients. The cooperation and support of the facility administration is key to the success of a high-quality program with a culture of continuous quality improvement and patient safety.

The MBS Committee is the primary forum for ensuring continuous quality improvement. The MBS Committee is a confidential setting for which the team can share best practices, respond to adverse events, and foster a culture to improve patient care. There must be consensus around care pathways and protocols with a focus on consistency and reliable delivery of intended care. One of the most important aspects of quality improvement is to decrease variability. The consistency of a process is key to supporting continued quality and process improvement.

The MBS Director holds significant responsibility and authority for the leadership of the program. The MBS Director chairs the MBS Committee and is responsible in conjunction with the MBS Committee, to overseeing every aspect of the program. This includes the accreditation process and ensuring continuous compliance with MBSAQIP standards, outcomes and data collection, and development of quality improvement initiatives and quality standards. It also includes education of staff, patient selection and exclusion criteria, the process to safely introduce emerging technologies, institution-wide communication of MBS-related policies, and reporting ethical and quality deviations with plans to remediate or limit privileges. The institution's organizational framework must incorporate the MBS Director position and have a contract or a job description in place that provides the authority and resources to fulfill the required duties. The MBS Director is assisted in their duties by the MBS Coordinator and the MBS Clinical Reviewer.

The center must have a designated MBS Coordinator. The MBS Coordinator works directly with the MBS Director and assists in overseeing all aspects of the program. This includes assistance with program development, managing the accreditation process, maintaining pathways and protocols, patient education, monitoring outcomes data and collection, and education of staff with a focus on patient safety. The MBS Coordinator serves as the liaison between the center and the MBSAQIP and as additionally acts as the liaison between the center and all metabolic and bariatric surgeons, proceduralists, and any general surgeons providing call coverage.

Quality improvement and monitoring of patient safety require timely and accurate data entry and management. This is the responsibility of the MBS Clinical Reviewer (MBSCR). The MBSCR completes specific training on data abstraction and management that includes ongoing recertification. The MBS Clinical Reviewer performs data abstraction on all patients undergoing metabolic and bariatric procedures including the entry of long-term follow-up data for all patients. The MBSAQIP is unique among many accreditation programs in the requirement of 100% data capture rather than a sampling of data. To provide high-quality, prospectively collected clinical data, the data abstraction is performed following objective definitions by an individual who is not providing direct patient care or charting in the patient's medical record. The MBSCR must be integrated with the organizational framework and is a key participant in the quality improvement process with data management and application of the data to specific quality improvement projects.

Rationale: All MBSAQIP-accredited centers must maintain sufficient annual case volume based on their designation level. Additionally, accredited centers must follow any patient and procedure selection criteria specific to their designation level.

Every metabolic and bariatric procedure performed for the treatment of metabolic or obesity-related diseases at a MBSAQIP-accredited center must be entered into the MBSAQIP Registry.

The facility and medical staff provide the structure, process, and personnel to obtain and maintain the quality standards of the MBSAQIP in caring for metabolic and bariatric patients. The administrative and medical staff must commit to broad cooperation to improve the quality of metabolic and bariatric patient care provided at the center.

Standard 3: Facilities and Equipment Resources

- 3.1 Health Care Facility Accreditation
- 3.2 Facilities, Equipment, and Furniture
- 3.3 Designated Bariatric Unit

This standard requires appropriate equipment and facility accommodations for the care of metabolic and bariatric patients. The increased awareness of the needs of the metabolic and bariatric patient population can improve the quality of care for patients of increased size that are encountered throughout a facility in many different departments. This standard also requires a designated area for care of the metabolic and bariatric patient. The designated unit can achieve a higher level of consistency and reliability in care delivery in the program with specific pathways and care protocols. It allows for focused training of staff and more rapid quality and process improvement with a close working relationship with the MBS Director and MBS Coordinator.

Rationale: The center must maintain appropriate facilities and equipment for the care of metabolic and bariatric patients. This includes furniture, wheelchairs, operating room tables, appropriately weight-rated or reinforced toilets, beds, radiology capabilities, surgical instruments, and necessary facility requirements for the safe delivery of care to patients with obesity.

Standard 4: Personnel and Services Resources

- 4.1 Credentialing Guidelines for Metabolic and Bariatric Surgeons
- 4.2 MBSAQIP Surgeon Verification
- 4.3 Metabolic and Bariatric Surgery Call Coverage
- 4.4 Staff Training
- 4.5 Multidisciplinary Team
- 4.6 Advanced Cardiovascular Life Support (ACLS)
- 4.7 Patient Stabilization
- 4.8 Critical Care Unit (CCU)/Intensive Care Unit (ICU) Services
- 4.9 Anesthesia Services
- 4.10 Endoscopy Services
- 4.11 Diagnostic and Interventional Radiology Services
- 4.12 Specialty Services
- 4.13 Pediatric Medical Advisor (PMA)
- 4.14 Pediatric Behavioral Specialist
- 4.15 Children's Hospital Service Requirements

This standard requires centers that are providing metabolic and bariatric procedures to have appropriate personnel, resources, and structure to care for and support those patients throughout the continuum of care. It also provides the unified guidelines for all major organizations for the credentialing of metabolic and bariatric surgeons.

Metabolic and bariatric surgery is one of the greatest success stories in quality improvement. A significant contribution to the improvement of quality over the past 15 years is related to ensuring the initial treating center has the appropriate facility infrastructure, staff training, and multidisciplinary teams in place to avoid adverse outcomes when possible and intervene early should adverse events occur. The center must be prepared for early recognition and intervention for any adverse events in the metabolic and bariatric patient population for both acute and chronic issues that could arise. It is the responsibility of the MBS Director with the MBS Committee to select those patients who are felt to be appropriate for the resources available at the facility with the intention that the accredited center is able to provide for any patient needs. A transfer agreement may be used for unusual events to assist with the care of a patient; however, the transfer agreement is not to be used as a part of standard care pathways for management of common expected or foreseeable adverse events. Specialized staff training around the topics of sensitivity training, safe patient transfer and mobilization, and recognition of signs and symptoms of postoperative complications are key to developing a culture of patient safety. This training provides the team with the necessary educational tools for which to identify those patients who may be experiencing complications and to additionally identify those clinical signs and symptoms which may lead to a failure to rescue.

Rationale: If metabolic and bariatric patients require critical care services, centers and their associated surgeons must ensure that patients receive appropriate care. The facility must maintain various on-site and consultative services required for the care of metabolic and bariatric patients, including the immediate on-site availability of personnel capable of administering advanced cardiovascular life support. Consultants must be available within the specified time as determined by institutional policy.

The responsibility is upon the center, the metabolic and bariatric surgeon, and ultimately the MBS Committee and MBS Director, to appropriately select patients and develop selection criteria for the center relative to the center's available resources and experience. For example, patients who are at risk for specific and predictable complications (renal failure, airway compromise, heart failure, etc.) must be managed in a facility where access to all reasonable medical subspecialty care is available.

All MBSAQIP Comprehensive Center designations must be able to provide CCU and/or ICU services, endoscopy services, and diagnostic and interventional radiology services on-site (some additional specialty services may be provided through a transfer agreement). Centers accredited under less than Comprehensive Center designation levels are eligible to provide these services either on-site or through a transfer agreement.

This standard includes credentialing guidelines for metabolic and bariatric surgeons, criteria for MBSAQIP surgeon verification, outline for metabolic and bariatric surgery call coverage, and requirement for staff training in specific areas on the *topics previously mentioned including sensitivity training, patient transfer and mobilization, and signs and symptoms of postoperative complications. There is an emphasis on early recognition and intervention for adverse events to avoid more severe cascades of complications.* It also includes a requirement for dedicated multidisciplinary teams including consistent operating room teams. The multidisciplinary team is critical for the diverse background of skills and knowledge to best care for patients with the chronic and life-threatening disease of obesity. The consistency these teams contribute to reliability of care delivered is the foundation for high-quality care.

This standard also outlines specialty services to be provided and includes additional criteria for adolescent centers and comprehensive accredited centers with adolescent qualifications.

Standard 5: Patient Care – Expectations and Protocol

- 5.1 Patient Education Pathways
- 5.2 Patient Care Pathways
- 5.3 Written Transfer Agreement
- 5.4 Inpatient Admitting Privileges
- 5.5. Risk Assessment Protocol
- 5.6 Obesity Medicine Services

This standard outlines the requirement of approved pathways and protocols for care of metabolic and bariatric patients at the center. The consistency of the care allows for identification of barriers and areas for which to focus on quality or process improvement. This standard addresses the requirement for surgeons performing metabolic and bariatric procedures at ambulatory surgery centers (ASCs) to have admitting privileges at an inpatient facility to manage the full range of metabolic and bariatric surgery complications to ensure the continuity of care for the patient with the operating surgeon. It also outlines the requirement for ASCs to have a risk assessment protocol that is reviewed annually, which can be applied uniformly for patient selection for treating metabolic and bariatric patients in an outpatient setting.

Rationale: The center must utilize comprehensive clinical pathways that facilitate the standardization of patient care for metabolic and bariatric procedures. Pathways are a sequence of orders and therapies describing the routine care for metabolic and bariatric patients from initial evaluation through long-term follow-up. MBSAQIP requires that patient care pathways be thoroughly documented and followed appropriately by both surgeons and advance practice providers treating metabolic and bariatric patients. Clinical pathways can be documented in a variety of formats, including tables, algorithms, process maps, and paragraph form. All staff caring for metabolic and bariatric patients must be aware of the pathways pertinent to their area of practice.

MBSAQIP Obesity Medicine Qualifications provide an additional designation level for facilities that offer nonprocedural treatment for patients who are overweight and patients with Class I, II, and III obesity. Centers with Obesity Medicine Qualifications employ therapeutic interventions including nutritional intervention, physical activity, behavioral change, and pharmacotherapy. These centers must utilize a comprehensive approach to providing care for patients with obesity as described in the Obesity Medicine Standards (Standards 2.8, 5.6, and 6.4), including the use of additional specialists such as dietitians, exercise specialists, behavioral health professionals, obesity medicine specialists, advance practice providers, and bariatric surgeons to achieve optimal results. Additionally, obesity medicine practitioners function as an effective resource for providing both pre- and postoperative care for metabolic and bariatric patients, while advocating for all patients with obesity.

Standard 6: Data Surveillance and Systems

- 6.1 Data Entry
- 6.2 30-Day and Long-Term Follow-Up
- 6.3 Data Review
- 6.4 Obesity Medicine Data Collection

This standard addresses the data abstraction requirements for short-term and long-term follow-up. It also addresses the requirement for data review with ongoing monitoring of the data specific to the individual center and the individuals performing metabolic and bariatric procedures at the facility. The MBSAQIP requires 100% case capture rather than a sampling of data and provides a high degree of confidence in the data so that quality improvement decisions and projects may be developed from the data. It is important that each center look carefully at the data to understand the story behind the data and how it may be used to guide quality improvement. The MBS Director, MBS Clinical Reviewer, and the MBS Coordinator along with the MBS Committee work closely to monitor outcomes with both risk- adjusted reports as well as non-risk-adjusted reports to best understand the local versus national environment for benchmarking purposes. Access to this data allows for efficient cycles of change and more rapid quality improvement implementation.

For centers seeking Obesity Medicine Qualifications, this standard also includes the requirement for data collection and outcomes monitoring for obesity medicine patients. This requirement is performed independently with local level data management separate from the MBSAQIP data registry. The data management must include reporting and data analysis. Data monitoring can allow for tracking patient outcomes and identification of successful treatment strategies.

Rationale: High-quality data is critical to inform quality improvement and measure the performance of metabolic and bariatric surgery programs.

All metabolic and bariatric procedures performed for the treatment of metabolic or obesity-related diseases must be entered into the MBSAQIP registry, including those performed by nonmetabolic and bariatric surgery credentialed proceduralists and general surgeons.

Data collection is ultimately the responsibility of the MBS Director working collaboratively with the MBS Clinical reviewer, physician offices, and institutional departments to ensure accurate short- and long-term results.

The MBSAQIP Registry collects prospective, risk-adjusted, clinically rich data based on standardized definitions. Data variables to be collected are provided via the MBSAQIP Registry. Data variables are periodically updated, refined, added, or deleted to optimize the information entered into the MBSAQIP Registry while minimizing the data collection burden. Centers are allowed the ability to track additional data elements as desired using custom fields within the MBSAQIP Registry.

Data is validated through multiple mechanisms that are continuously updated to optimize the quality of the data collected. The MBSAQIP Registry was developed to minimize the potential to submit inaccurate data as well as prevent missing data. Centers are required to intermittently submit administrative or other corroborating data as an audit against the data entered. Data are validated in a systematic fashion as part of MBSAQIP site visits. MBS Clinical Reviewers are trained data reviewers who are not directly involved in patient care. Ongoing training and assessment of the MBS Clinical Reviewer's processes and knowledge are monitored as another means to validate data entry. Additional data integrity audits, information, or clarifications may be required by the MBSAQIP.

Data is collected at 30 days, 6 months, 1 year, and annually thereafter. Follow-up data is used to assess morbidity and mortality, as well as the clinical effectiveness concerning changes in weight and weight-related comorbidities. Risk-adjusted metrics have been developed for quality assessment and improvement.

Standard 7: Quality Improvement

- 7.1 Adverse Event Monitoring
- 7.2 Quality Improvement Initiatives
- 7.3 Annual Compliance Reports (ACR)

Patient safety and adverse event monitoring must be implemented through the MBS Committee led by the MBS Director. It includes a protocol to notify surgeons and proceduralists of adverse events and to discuss the patient's care with the MBS Committee when adverse events occur. All mortalities that occur within the first 90 days postoperatively or post-procedurally must be reviewed within 60 days of discovery. All outcomes data must be reviewed on a regular basis.

To deliver safe, effective, and high-quality care to each patient, the accredited center must develop a culture of collaboration and safety among all MBS Committee members. Quality improvement (QI) emphasizes a continuous, multidisciplinary effort to improve the process of care and its outcomes. The Semi-Annual Risk Adjusted Report (SAR) is a risk-adjusted report provided twice annually with comparisons of the individual site level to all MBSAQIP-accredited centers regarding patient complications and outcomes. Each center must use data from the Semi-Annual Risk Adjusted Report (SAR) and other data sources to evaluate areas for improvement. The center must conduct at least one quality improvement initiative each year approved by the MBS Committee with oversight and leadership from the MBS Director. Any center identified as a high outlier on the SAR must develop a QI initiative designed to address the high outlier status.

This standard outlines six basic steps for the basic process for completing a quality improvement initiative. The steps include:

1. Review data – SAR, non-risk-adjusted reports, internal data
2. Identify the problem – high outlier status, or other areas for improvement with a focus on patient safety
3. Propose intervention – discuss contributing factors, root cause analysis
4. Choose quality improvement methodology – may use any consistent methodology that satisfies their unique needs, establish a timeline for review and metrics to track progress
5. Implement intervention and monitor data – consistently implement the intervention, monitor data, and evaluate any missed opportunities of care
6. Present results – gather all documentation and data, review progress, summarize the findings and results of the quality improvement initiative

For MBSAQIP centers renewing their accreditation, they must provide evidence of compliance with the standards each year by submitting the Annual Compliance Report (ACR). Triennially, the program will receive a visit with a surgeon site reviewer in order to ensure compliance with the standards as well as provide guidance and collaboration on best practices.

Rationale: Processes for identifying adverse events and implementing subsequent corrective action plans, measurable through patient outcomes, are inherent cornerstones of continuous quality improvement. Problem resolution, outcomes improvement, and assurances of patient safety ("loop closure") must be readily identifiable through structured quality improvement initiatives.

In support of these efforts, the MBS Director and the MBS Committee at each center must develop a culture of collaboration to report, analyze, and implement strategies based on data to drive improvement in the quality of care offered to metabolic and bariatric patients. While major quality improvement initiatives such as decreasing surgical site infections, leaks, or venous thromboembolism prophylaxis are important, equally important is the examination of pathways of care to maximize the patient experience and effectiveness of metabolic and bariatric procedures. Continuous quality improvement must be reflected in the results of such efforts by the MBS Committee.

Standard 8: Education: Professional and Community Outreach

- 8.1 Support Groups

Obesity is a chronic, progressive, life-threatening disease that requires long-term management and support for successful treatment. Support groups can be an important part of weight maintenance, mental health, provide a community of support, and be a useful tool to control this chronic disease. All accredited centers must provide scheduled, structured, and supervised support groups for metabolic and bariatric patients.

Rationale: Continuous outreach to metabolic and bariatric patients through regularly scheduled, organized, and supervised support groups is critical for maintaining long-term patient engagement and success. Support groups create an environment for both healthcare providers and patients to offer ongoing education and encouragement.

Application of the MBSAQIP Data for Research and Quality Improvement

Thus far, we have explored the history of metabolic and bariatric surgery and reviewed the current standard guidelines for MBSAQIP accreditation. Next, we would like to take a look at what a powerful tool the MBSAQIP is for not only ensuring metabolic and bariatric surgery patients received reliable quality care but also how this robust data registry can be used to further our understanding of metabolic and bariatric surgery while continuously improving the care we deliver.

As was mentioned earlier, one of the most powerful elements of the MBSAQIP data registry is that accreditation standards require 100% data capture. This means that data elements from every metabolic and bariatric surgery performed at every accredited bariatric program must be reported at designated postsurgical milestones including 30 days, 6 months, and annually thereafter. Another exciting element of the MBSAQIP program is that this data is made available at no additional cost, to members of the bariatric team at each MBSAQIP-participating center. This data is shared through the Participant Use Data File (PUF). This file is HIPAA compliant and contains deidentified patient-level aggregate data. The purpose of this file is to facilitate research by providing investigators access to this collective pool of data as a means of improving the quality of care delivered to metabolic and bariatric surgery patients. In 2019 alone, the PUF contains data from 206,570 cases performed at 868 MBSAQIP programs. At the time of this writing in total, the PUF includes data from 967,456 metabolic and bariatric surgery cases performed since 2015 [17]. This makes the MBSAQIP PUF an extremely powerful resource for researchers looking to study trends and answer clinical questions in their efforts to advance the quality and safety of metabolic and bariatric surgery for all patients. To illustrate this, we will explore some of the important published data that was possible as a result of the MBSAQIP program.

As was mentioned earlier, an alarming rise in bariatric surgery morbidity and mortality brought the discipline to a crisis point which was the trigger for the development of the accreditation process. Following implementation of the accreditation process and the focus on laparoscopic techniques and patient selection, there was a tenfold reduction in 30-day mortality in bariatric surgery patients [18]. With this crisis averted, CMS then turned their attention to readmission rates as an important factor escalating medical costs. This led to the first national MBSAQIP quality improvement project: Decreasing Readmissions through Opportunities Provided (DROP). The ambitious goal of this program was to decrease all-cause 30-day readmissions of metabolic and bariatric surgery patients having surgery at accredited programs by 20% in one year. MBSAQIP data indicated most readmissions on bariatric surgery patients stemmed from preventable causes such as dehydration, nausea, medication side effects, and patient expectations [19]. First vetted by a pilot program out of Stanford University, this was to be accomplished through a number of interventions beginning in the presurgical phase and continuing through the perioperative and postoperative periods [18]. Between March 2015 and March 2016, DROP was implemented at 128 MBSAQIP-accredited comprehensive centers. The study followed patients who underwent primary laparoscopic bariatric surgery including adjustable gastric banding, sleeve gastrectomy, and Roux-en-Y gastric bypass. The result was a statistically significant decrease in readmissions by 19% for the laparoscopic sleeve gastrectomy patients, with favorable but not statistically significant reductions in readmission rates for adjustable gastric band and gastric bypass patients [20]. While shy of its ambitious goal, DROP was largely considered a great success and gave a glimpse as to how this comprehensive data registry might be used to improve patient experience and outcomes.

The success of the DROP program quickly gave rise to the second MBSAQIP national quality improvement project. This project, Employing New Enhanced Recovery Goals in Bariatric Surgery (ENERGY), was largely focused on addressing an issue that was becoming a popular across many surgical disciplines, namely, postsurgical length of stay (LOS). The Enhanced Recovery After Surgery (ERAS®) movement had been gaining attention since 2001 largely based on its potential to improve outcomes and decrease cost. In 2016 guidelines specific for the perioperative care of the bariatric surgery patient were published by the ERAS society [21]. Bariatric surgery accreditation has always emphasized the importance of standardized clinical pathways, but the original purpose for these pathways was more to ensure standardization for any given program or hospital. The principals of the ENERGY initiative involved the use of multicenter standardized clinical pathways with the goal improving length of stay for metabolic and bariatric surgery patients. Using the MBSAQIP data, the authors identified accredited metabolic and bariatric surgery programs who were considered statistically significant high outliers for extended length of stay (ELOS) compared to MBSAQIP benchmarks. Secondary outcomes studied included bleeding, readmission, and reoperation, to ensure that patients were not being discharged early only to be subsequently readmitted. Seventy-nine such sites were identified and invited to participate in the program. Participation required adherence to a rigorous protocol that focused on concepts such as opioid-sparing pain management algorithms, goal-directed fluid management, and preoperative nutrition to minimize the effects of insulin resistance. These measures were implemented across various phases of care starting prior to patient's preoperative visit and extended through discharge. Thirty-six programs ended up participating in the program which started in 2016 and included a 1-year preintervention comparison period followed by a

1-year implementation period. In all, 18,048 cases were included in this study. The authors looked at extended length of stay (ELOS) ≥4 days in the pre- and posttreatment groups, which were 8.1% and 4.5%, respectively. This was a significant decrease in ELOS by almost half between the preintervention and implementation groups. In addition, they did not observe any increase in readmission, reoperation, or overall morbidity rates [22]. An interesting finding that was noted was a slight trend toward higher bleeding rates during the implementation phase, which is postulated to be secondary to the opioid-sparing reliance on NSAIDS. This study validated the feasibility and tremendous benefit of decreasing variability of patient care through standardized clinical pathways across multiple centers, with recommendations that such clinical pathways be implemented on a larger scale.

With the lessons learned from the experience of two national quality improvement projects, the MBSC chose to address one of the most serious healthcare epidemics in the United States, the opioid crisis. The experience of the ENERGY project substantiated the feasibility of opioid-sparing protocols in metabolic and bariatric surgery patients, but there was further inquiry needed regarding opioid stewardship. The burning platform, related to opioid overdoses with 72,000 American lives lost in 2017 alone, led to the third nationwide MBSAQIP quality improvement project: Bariatric Surgery Targeting Opioid Prescriptions (BSTOP) [23]. The purpose of this project was to develop and implement protocols for reducing opioid prescriptions in those patients undergoing metabolic and bariatric surgery without sacrificing postoperative analgesia. This project uses clinical pathways centered around patient education and the implementation of opioid-sparing pain management strategies including minimizing perioperative opioid use and regional analgesia. MBSAQIP-accredited centers were invited to participate, and to be included, programs had to agree to follow clinical guidelines for multimodal pain control, provide patient education, and additional elements of data collection to ensure agreement by all stakeholders at both the clinical and administrative levels of each institution. Programs started onboarding for this ambitious program in June 2019. Similar to the ENERGY project, there was a 3-month period of pre-implementation data collection followed by an 18-month period of implementation. At the time of this writing, results from this third national MBSAQIP quality initiative are not yet known, as this study is ongoing with a planned completion date of in June 2020, which may have been delayed by the COVID-19 pandemic. When one considers that regular utilization of prescribed opioids in patients undergoing metabolic and bariatric surgery who were previously opioid naïve is as high as 5.8% at 6 months and 14.2% by 7 years postoperatively, along with a 1.3% mortality rate from new opioid dependence, there is potential for BSTOP to prevent twice as many deaths as the complete elimination of venous thromboembolic events, anastomotic leaks, pneumonia, and bleeding combined [24].

These three national quality initiative projects highlight the power and usefulness of the MBSAQIP data and MBSAQIP-accredited institutions to implement and study change on a national scale. Access to MBSAQIP also makes it a well-built tool to facilitate research at the local/regional level. One such example includes a study examining predictors and outcomes of leak after Roux-en-Y gastric bypass (RYGB) through an analysis of the MBSAQIP data registry. Anastomotic/staple line leak is one of the most dreaded complications of gastric bypass surgery, and fear of leak has led to the continued search of "safer" procedures. Remarkably, however, few studies had been published regarding specific predictors of leak with modern RYGB. Mocanu et al. analyzed all patients who had RYGB surgery at an accredited MBSAQIP center between 2015 and 2016 to identify the prevalence, impact, and predictors of leak in these patients. The study included 77,596 patients. There were 476 leaks with an overall leak rate of 0.6% with a leak-mortality rate of 1.5%. They found an overall total complication rate of 7.5% and a low overall mortality rate of 0.16% in the cohort. Statistically significant risk factors for leak following RYGB included excess BMI, age, operative length, American Society of Anesthesiologist score (ASA) >3, history of a PE, and partially dependent functional status, with the latter two being the most predictive of leak. Interestingly, the investigators found albumin status to be the only protective variable in preventing leak. Clearly, some of these are nonmodifiable risk factors, but the results led the authors to conclude that optimizing preoperative nutrition and preoperative prehabilitation, two achievable goals, may have a role in improving outcomes after gastric bypass surgery [25].

Another group used the MBSAQIP data registry to study a somewhat controversial topic, adolescent bariatric surgery. The World Health Organization defines adolescence being between the ages of 10 and 19 years old, and this is a population that the United States "obesity epidemic" has not spared. With severe obesity (BMI $\geq$120% of the 95th percentile for age and sex) affecting 7.5% of adolescents aged 12–15 and 9.5% for those aged 16–19, the prevalence of the most severe class of obesity has doubled in this population between 1999 and 2012 [26]. These patients are at an elevated risk of developing all the same obesity-related comorbidities as an adult patient, including nonalcoholic fatty liver disease, which is now the leading cause of liver failure in adolescents [27]. Chaar et al. investigated 30-day outcomes from bariatric procedures performed at MBSAQIP centers on all patients $\leq$19 years old from 2015 to 2017. They focused on primary laparoscopic sleeve gastrectomies (LSG) and laparoscopic Roux-en-Y gastric bypass (LRYGB) operations and looked at serious adverse events, organ space infections, and reoperation/reintervention rates. Length of operation, length of stay, and readmissions were measured as secondary outcomes. They identified 1983 adolescent patients that met the profile. Sleeve gastrectomies outnumber gastric bypasses almost 4:1. When compared to 353,726 adult patients undergoing the same procedures during the same timeframe, the authors found no difference in outcomes. They did note a statistically significant difference in the adolescent population favoring sleeve gastrectomy over RYGB in both 30-day serious adverse events (2.9% vs 6.5%) and readmissions (2.6% vs 5.6%). There was a non-statistically significant trend in 30-day reoperation rate again favoring LSG compared to LRYGB (1.1% vs 2.3%) [28]. This led the authors to conclude that adolescents who undergo primary bariatric surgery procedures at MBSAQIP-accredited centers have a safety profile that is similar to adult patients.

In this chapter, we have attempted to provide the reader with a succinct review of the evolution of metabolic and bariatric surgery from a quality standpoint. Metabolic and bariatric surgery is one of the great success stories of modern quality improvement in healthcare, achieving unprecedented safety and improved outcomes for the patients we serve. The key principles of this evolution include the use of high-quality, reliable data organized around evidence-based standards to guide a structured approach to quality and process improvement. These objectives are accomplished by the contributions of multidisciplinary teams under the leadership of the surgeon MBS Director with local MBS Committee guidance and facility administrative support. It is an extraordinary history when one considers that this surgical subspecialty has barely been in existence for 50 years. As a specialty, we have been able to move beyond individual sporadic case outcomes to changes that broadly improve the system of care for patient safety, for which we should all be proud.

Editor's Note

In 2003, the Society of American Gastrointestinal and Endoscopic Surgeons (SAGES) jointly with the ASMBS approved the Guidelines for Institutions Granting Bariatric Privileges Utilizing Laparoscopic Techniques [28]. The guidelines stipulate weight loss surgery should be practiced by appropriately trained surgical teams within programs that provide perioperative and long-term management [28]. In 2003, experts met at the SAGES Appropriateness Conference and established the duodenal switch, banded gastroplasty, laparoscopic adjustable band, and laparoscopic gastric bypass as appropriate operations for weight loss based on current evidence [28]. While other societies such as the ACS, ASMBS, and the Betsy Lehman report use volume criteria (ranging from 25 to 50 procedures annually) to recommend credentialing surgeons, the SAGES guidelines leave the responsibility for privileging on the individual institutions, but recommend input from a committee and the chief of surgery [28].

Minimum Requirements

1. Formal residency training in general surgery within an accredited program with subsequent certification by the American Board of Surgery if required by the institution [28].
2. Documentation that there exists adequate follow-up of patients including nursing care, dietary care, counseling, support groups, exercise training, psychological care if needed, and a method of identifying and managing complications [28].
3. If the surgeon has formal training only in open bariatric surgery, SAGES recommends having a second surgeon who is trained in laparoscopic bariatric surgery and is therefore complementary to their expertise. Alternatively, the surgeon may participate in a proctored experience deemed adequate by the chief of surgery [28].
4. For surgeons without formal training in weight loss surgery (fellowship), preceptorship and/or formal courses are offered as alternatives. Any such courses should meet category 1 continuing medical education requirements and involved both didactics and hands-on experience with inanimate labs or tissue labs [28].
5. If the surgeon has documented formal training in laparoscopic bariatric surgery, SAGES recommends that the volume of open and laparoscopic cases be demonstrated for the type of procedures to be done and that a complementary surgeon experienced in open procedures be available

if needed. The adequacy of case volume/experience is to be determined by the chief of surgery [28].

6. If the surgeon has no documented formal residency training in either laparoscopic open bariatric surgery, they are expected to take a formal course *and* be proctored by a qualified surgeon who is approved by the institution of practice [28].

Institutional Support

Adequate equipment and staff training are expected to be in place prior to starting a bariatric program. Two skilled surgeons are recommended for laparoscopic bariatric procedures or a surgeon and a skilled first assistant [28].

Maintenance of Privileges

SAGES recommends that the chief of surgery or appropriate institutional body should determine the criteria for provisional privileges, monitoring of performance and outcomes, and continuing education requirements such as meetings and courses [28]. The guidelines state that outcome data should be reviewed 6 months after privileges are granted, and regularly thereafter, with comparison of the surgeon's data to national published benchmarks [28]. Any denial of privileges should have an appeal process in place [28].

References

1. Blackstone RP. Chapter 4. The history of the American Society for metabolic and bariatric surgery. In: Nguyen N, Blackstone RP, Morton JM, Ponce J, Rosenthal RJ, editors. ASMBS textbook of bariatric surgery volume I bariatric surgery. New York Heidelberg Dordrecht London: Springer; 2015. p. 47–60.
2. Steinbrook R. Surgery for severe obesity, perspective. NEJM. 2004;350:1076–9. https://www.nejm.org/na101/home/literatum/publisher/mms/journals/content/nejm/2004/nejm_2004.350.

issue-11/nejmp048029/production/images/img_medium/
nejmp048029_f1.jpeg. Accessed 30 Nov 2020.

3. Flum DR, Salem L, Elrod JA, Dellinger EP, Cheadle A, Chan L. Early mortality among Medicare beneficiaries undergoing bariatric surgical procedures. JAMA. 2005;294(15):1903–8. https://doi.org/10.1001/jama.294.15.1903. PMID: 16234496.

4. Flum DR, Dellinger EP. Impact of gastric bypass operation on survival: a population-based analysis. J Am Coll Surg. 2004;199(4):543–51. https://doi.org/10.1016/j.jamcollsurg.2004.06.014.

5. Livingston EH, Langert J. The impact of age and Medicare status on bariatric surgical outcomes. Arch Surg. 2006;141(11):1115–20; discussion 1121. https://doi.org/10.1001/archsurg.141.11.1115. PMID: 17116805.

6. Centers for Medicare and Medicaid Services. Decision memo for bariatric surgery for the treatment of morbid obesity (CAG-00250R). Bariatric surgery in Medicare beneficiaries – reconsideration. Coverage decision memorandum for bariatric surgery for treatment of co-morbidities associated with morbid obesity; Feb 21, 2006.

7. Champion JK, Pories WJ. Centers of excellence for bariatric surgery. Surg Obes Relat Dis. 2005;1(2):148–51.

8. Birkmeyer JD, Shahian DM, Dimick JB, Finlayson SR, Flum DR, Ko CY, Hall BL. Blueprint for a new American College of Surgeons: National Surgical Quality Improvement Program. J Am Coll Surg. 2008;207(5):777–82. https://doi.org/10.1016/j.jamcollsurg.2008.07.018. Epub 2008 Sep 19. PMID: 18954793.

9. Birkmeyer NJ, Dimick JB, Share D, Hawasli A, English WJ, Genaw J, Finks JF, Carlin AM, Birkmeyer JD, Michigan Bariatric Surgery Collaborative. Hospital complication rates with bariatric surgery in Michigan. JAMA. 2010;304(4):435–42. https://doi.org/10.1001/jama.2010.1034. PMID: 20664044.

10. Dimick JB, Nicholas LH, Ryan AM, Thumma JR, Birkmeyer JD. Bariatric surgery complications before vs after implementation of a national policy restricting coverage to centers of excellence. JAMA. 2013;309(8):792–9. https://doi.org/10.1001/jama.2013.755. PMID: 23443442; PMCID: PMC3785293.

11. Nicholas LH, Dimick JB. Bariatric surgery in minority patients before and after implementation of a centers of excellence program. JAMA. 2013;310(13):1399–400. https://doi.org/10.1001/jama.2013.277915. PMID: 24030558; PMCID: PMC3832290.

12. Centers for Medicare and Medicaid Services. National Coverage Determination (NCD) for bariatric surgery for treatment of morbid obesity (100.1). Dec 2012. 100–3(4).
13. Blackstone RP. Chapter 14. Quality in bariatric surgery. In: Nguyen N, Blackstone RP, Morton JM, Ponce J, Rosenthal RJ, editors. ASMBS textbook of bariatric surgery volume I bariatric surgery. Springer; 2015. p. 157–82.
14. American College of Surgeons Website. Accessed 29 Nov 2020. https://www.facs.org/search/bariatric-surgery-centers?allresults=.
15. Optimal resources for metabolic and bariatric surgery 2019 Standards. 2019. American College of Surgeons. Chicago, IL. facs.org/mbsaqip. Accessed 30 Nov 2020.
16. American College of Surgeons Website. Accessed 21 Nov 2020. https://www.facs.org/Quality-Programs/MBSAQIP/participant-use.
17. Nguyen NT, Hohmann S, Nguyen XM, et al. Outcome of laparoscopic adjustable gastric banding and prevalence of band revision and explanation at academic centers: 2007–2009. Surg Obes Relat Dis. 2012;8(6):724–7.
18. Gadaleta D, MD, FACS, FASMBS, Petrick AT, MD, FACS, FASMBS. Raising the standard: DROP—the first national MBSAQIP quality improvement project: decreasing readmissions through opportunities provided. Bariatric Times 2019;16(2):16.
19. Morton JM. The first metabolic and bariatric surgery accreditation and quality improvement program quality initiative: decreasing readmissions through opportunities provided. Surg Obes Relat Dis. 2014;10(3):377–8.
20. Thorell A, MacCormick AD, Awad S, et al. Guidelines for perioperative care in bariatric surgery: Enhanced Recovery After Surgery (ERAS) Society recommendations. World J Surg. 2016;40(9):2065–83.
21. Brethauer SA, M.D., Grieco A, M.P.H., Fraker T, M.S., R.N., Evans-Labok K, B.A., Smith A, Pharm.D., B.C.P.S., McEvoy MD, M.D., Saber AA, M.D., Morton JM, M.D., Petrick A, M.D. Surgery for obesity and related diseases;15(2019):1977–1989.
22. American College of Surgeon Website. Accessed 15 Nov 2020. https://www.facs.org/-/media/files/quality-programs/bariatric/bstop_invitation_letter.ashx.
23. Raebel MA, Newcomer SR, Reifler LM, Boudreau D, Elliott TE, DeBar L, Ahmed A, Pawloski PA, Fisher D, Donahoo WT,

Bayliss EA. Chronic use of opioid medications before and after bariatric surgery. JAMA. 2013;310(13):1369–76.
24. Mocanu V, M.D., Dang J, M.D., Ladak F, M.P.H., M.D., Switzer N, M.P.H., M.D., F.R.C.S.C., Birch DW, M.Sc., M.D., F.R.C.S.C., Karmali S, M.P.H., M.D., F.R.C.S.C. Surgery for obesity and related diseases;15(2019):396–403.
25. Skinner AC, Skelton JA. Prevalence and trends in obesity and severe obesity among children in the United States, 1999–2012. JAMA Pediatr. 2014;168(6):561–6.
26. Welsh JA, Karpen S, Vos MB. Increasing prevalence of non-alcoholic fatty liver disease among United States adolescents, 1988–1994 to 2007–2010. J Pediatr. 2013;162(3):496–500.
27. El Chaar M, King K, Al-Mardini A, Galvez A, Claros L, Stoltzfus J. Thirty-day outcomes of bariatric surgery in adolescents: a first look at the MBSAQIP database. Obes Surg. 2020;25:1–6.
28. Society of American Gastrointestinal and Endoscopic Surgeons Bariatric Surgery Credentialing website. Accessed 27 Mar 2021. https://www.sages.org/wiki/bariatric-surgery-credentialing/.

Chapter 8
Resident Evaluation and Mentorship: Milestones in Surgical Education

Ingrid S. Schmiederer and James N. Lau

Introduction

Residency training is dependent on effective and reliable evaluation. For the purposes of ensuring self-sufficient, competent surgeons with a commitment to patient safety, there is expected to be a consistent framework for both summative and formative assessment of the learner while they are still in training. For program evaluation and accreditation, the Accreditation Council for Graduate Medical Education (ACGME) also sets standards through peer-reviewed processes that ensure generalizable and relevant guidelines for programs and their trainees nationally.

I. S. Schmiederer
Department of Surgery, Stanford University School of Medicine, Stanford, CA, USA

J. N. Lau (✉)
Loyola University Medical Center, Department of Surgery, Maywood, IL, USA
e-mail: James.Lau@lumc.edu

J. R. Romanelli et al. (eds.), *The SAGES Manual of Quality, Outcomes and Patient Safety*,
https://doi.org/10.1007/978-3-030-94610-4_8

Traditionally, evaluation can be broken down into objective measures, such as standardized in-training exam scores, institutional multiple-choice quizzes or verifications of proficiency, and subjective measures, such as observations and end-of-rotation faculty evaluations. On an individual trainee level, a program director might look at the summation of both measures to determine competency or promotion. On an institutional level, the ACGME and institutional officials review these measures to evaluate for program effectiveness and, ultimately, accreditation. There is potential for error at both levels, as individual evaluations are often too subjective or lack consistency comprehensive enough for learners to make necessary changes in their trajectory. The evaluations themselves often ask faculty to rate trainees using numbered scales. Translating resident performance to scales can be difficult because of the loss of detail, introduction of bias, and difficulty in determining cut points. In fact, previous studies have shown that selecting numeric values to characterize subjective competencies is challenging and complex for both the evaluator and the trainee, highlighting the need for a more customizable model of assessment [1]. Furthermore, individual institutions may have unique assessment tools that are not generalizable across other residency programs. At the same time, institutional officials and program directors may focus on "teaching to the test" as they meet program accreditation standards rather than assuring standardized training. This may alter analysis on a national level.

To address some of the potential limitations to resident assessment and evaluation, the ACGME began implementation of the Next Accreditation System (NAS) in 2013 for seven core specialties, including surgery, which ultimately led to the establishment of Milestones [2, 3]. In each specialty, the Milestones resulted from a close collaboration among the ACGME, certifying boards like the American Board of Surgery (ABS), review committees, specialty organizations, program-director associations such as the

Association of Program Directors in Surgery (APDS), and residents in "working groups." The process of establishing Milestones created a national framework for assessment that enables comparison data and enhances resident education with quality and safety [4]. Additionally, the ACGME's requirement to use Milestones to track residents' progress and outcomes has now required further elucidation of these assessment methods so that faculty and program directors might be informed and better trained themselves [5].

This chapter will discuss these Milestones in the context of surgical education – not simply as a perceived obligation or tool for assessment, but also as a means of anchoring and framing mentorship. Surgical faculty often deliver invaluable training based on key educational theory or principles, perhaps without being fully cognizant of the history of these educational ideologies. Certain approaches to surgical skill learning may be more applicable or beneficial for certain trainees, but without the background knowledge, it may be difficult to actually apply the available tools [5]. With focused education about the origins and best practices for Milestones as a developmental tool, as well as elaboration about the development of surgical Entrustable Professional Activities (EPAs), the authors hope to provide an aid and structure for mentors and mentees as they use the evaluation process as an agency for constructive feedback and effective guidance.

Similar to Milestones, Entrustable Professional Activities (EPAs) are a framework around units of work and the assignment of entrustment for the autonomous performance of these work tasks. Created by Olle Ten Cate and colleagues in Utrecht, this framework encapsulates competencies and milestones into discrete, definable and assessable tasks that rely on content experts to determine when supervision levels are attained. EPAs may provide a more manageable way to assess residents' Core Competencies as outlined by ACGME and are presented in a Milestones format to ensure quality healthcare to patients [6].

How Did the ACGME and Its Working Groups Come Up with Milestones?

As described by the ACGME, Milestones are made up of agreed-upon attributes adapted from the ACGME's six Core Competencies (Patient Care and Procedural Skills, Medical Knowledge, Practice-Based Learning and Improvement, Interpersonal Communication Skills, Professionalism, Systems-Based Practice) that were then divided into sub-competencies and organized into a developmental framework of levels using the Dreyfus model of skill acquisition. Developed in 1980 by Hubert and Stuart Dreyfus, the Dreyfus model of skill acquisition proposes a framework of five levels: novice, advanced beginner, competent, proficient, and expert [7]. In general surgery, the levels are briefly broken down into (1) meets expectations of an incoming resident; (2) demonstrates sufficiency at a mid-residency level; (3) demonstrates the majority of the Milestones in the sub-competency; (4) able to substantially demonstrate the Milestones targeted for residency graduation; and (5) an expert resident whose achievements in a sub-competency are greater than the expectation [5]. Students objectively "pass" these levels, along a developmental scale, as they acquire competency in specific skills. With this, residents are considered ready for training completion when they have met the requirements of Level 4. At the completion of training, then, the Milestones are meant to provide data about graduates' performances before entering unsupervised practice [4].

This continuum framework lends itself well to the notion that learning and potential skill level are not finite or bound by time. Therefore, education and expectations might be better suited for learners when the learners are approached by evaluators or mentors based on their competency levels, rather than postgraduate year (PGY) or even age. This concept of competency-based education may prove challenging for a clinical competency committee (CCC) at a residency program that is expected to complete evaluations, to select the Milestone levels and to graduate residents within the traditional 5–7-year timeframe. Still, competency-based education arguably enhances feedback and guidance for surgeons at different levels.

What Is Competency-Based Medical Education and How Does It Apply Here?

Competency-based medical education (CBME) has been called "an approach to preparing physicians for practice that is fundamentally oriented to graduate outcome abilities and [it is] organized around competencies derived from an analysis of societal and patient needs. It de-emphasizes time-based training and promises a greater accountability, flexibility, and learner-centeredness…" [8]

The acquisition of competencies and integrating knowledge, skills, and attitudes in practice should be affirmed in the workplace in a timely manner and in such a way that the learner might self-reflect and adjust their approaches before habits are formed. This competency-based approach requires that trainees are accurately certified for specific competencies after they have demonstrated proficiency or have passed a specific threshold that allows for limited supervision or unsupervised practice [9]. CBME requires frequent and accurate assessments that should represent the full range of ACGME Core Competencies. This is a benefit of having Milestones framework, as it lists these most crucial (and officially-designated) skills needed for graduation. In addition, CBME, along with Milestones, focuses on performance outcomes of the trainees while providing transparency and holding everyone in the education process accountable. Ultimately, a competency-based framework provides a measurable goal and visible educational outcomes which can be utilized for future decision-making [10].

More broadly, as Tekian et al. explain in a comprehensive and constructive review of the Milestones, Milestones also provide an excellent way to guide the process of education with curriculum development, assessment, feedback, and learner self-assessment. Still, Milestones by themselves are not sufficient. Completing the Milestone checklist or scaled system does not capture overall competency every time. This process also requires integration of training experiences, assessments, and holistic feedback [10]. Competency, from this perspective, remains subjective, as it must be constructed and reconstructed to enhance assessment tools that are designed for objective measures. Measurement instruments like the Milestones quantify a construct, but they can also shape how we think about and teach the construct itself [11].

Other studies have demonstrated the utility of narrative evaluations or descriptive comments for a resident's behavior within evaluations, to enhance scale-based evaluations. Observations by multiple raters in multiple situations are known to enhance reliability and validity evidence for assessment tools, in order to obtain the "true" score that properly represents the individual [11]. Despite the perceived ease of a straightforward checklist, a meaningful narrative is more useful in describing the student's progress. Comments and narrative provide a more powerful way to justify one's judgments of a trainee's progress along the road to competence. Not only that, but evaluators can also defend their assessments of trainees' competency and provide specific feedback to improve [10].

This is perhaps where mentorship between faculty and residents plays a crucial role in trainee development and evaluation. There is a wealth of literature in support of the benefit of mentorship for career advancement. Surgical training itself, through Halsted's residency system, uses a mentorship/apprenticeship model to "produce not only surgeons, but surgeons of the highest type...[surgeons] who will stimulate the first youths of our country to study surgery and to devote their energies and their lives to raising the standard of surgical science" [12].

Milestones might guide mentoring conversations at checkpoints throughout training – around evaluators' and trainees' experiences – within a developmental framework. The true challenge is guidance within context-based experience and situational awareness in the real world. The live workplace environment has less controllable social or environmental factors. As a result, the oft-implied workplace curriculum with both direct mentorship guidance and indirect environmental guidance. Becomes the framework in a real-world setting to foster the acquisition of competencies that are necessary for varying stages of accountability. This requires direct observation by evaluators in real time to gain a sense of actual skills of the trainee and this may not be fully captured in the checklist of Milestones or in end-of-rotation meetings, as previously mentioned. Misalignment between observed skills versus expected skills or between expected level of supervision versus actual level of supervision required may place a patient's safety at risk. This also puts the learner in a position to make a potentially preventable medical error [13].

There is no room for veiled language or a reduced checklist approach when protecting patient safety. This is where the "true" resident must be evaluated both within themselves and by their evaluators with clear and observed evidence – to prevent that misalignment of actual versus expected skills. A mentor or teacher must be specific in their feedback. The use of observed examples in real time, as described in the mutually beneficial construct of "entrustment," is proven to be effective. *Can I trust this trainee to care for our patients? Have they given me any reason or situation to doubt their competence? What is the evidence behind my entrustment of this individual in caring for my patient?* The concept of entrustment, then, is essential to our assessment culture. In traditional models, entrustment was an implicit judgment that faculty made on a day-to-day basis. With CBME, it can be explicitly and more objectively expressed by rating trainees using entrustment anchors/scales: through Entrustable Professional Activities (EPAs).

What Are EPAs? How Do They Work for Surgical Training?

Residency is on-the-job training, and therefore, Entrustable Professional Activities (EPAs) are job duties that are measurable units of observable work. EPAs are units of professional practice (tasks) that may be entrusted to a learner to execute unsupervised, once they have demonstrated the required competency. This shifts and broadens the focus from individual competencies to the work that must be performed as a whole. EPAs are important routine activities of a discipline that encompass the ACGME Core Competencies and Milestones within them, for safe and effective performance [13]. Assessing and deciding how much autonomy can be given for this unit of duty requires the integration of multiple competencies. In other words, these units of work add more practical and tangible elements to the developmental framework of Milestones. An EPAs-based workplace curriculum can individually map out a route for individual trainees with summative entrustment decisions at significant moments in their training that lead to acknowledged permission to act in patient care [9].

Surgery allows for workplace assessments to be compartmentalized into discrete duties, since this is essentially how we already work with residents. Ad hoc decisions of entrustment are executed every day with residents and students on surgery rotations. Ten Cate defines competency in the clinical setting as the level at which a professional activity is "mastered": a threshold level that permits trust and where the trainee can act unsupervised [9]. Prior to determining formal duties or EPAs, however, a program must define the operational definition of competence/entrustment. Competency is but a stage in a developmental continuum from novice to mastery. The breadth of competencies that surgeons must assume is large, but the concrete EPAs for a specialty or service are well recognized by the specialty and are manageable by number and category. It is through these stages that Hirschl reinforces that a gradation of responsibility significantly enhances competency-based assessments for surgical residents [14]. Every specialty would know which EPAs are necessary to care for patients safely to master residency expectations. Assessments of EPAs have not been officially incorporated into evaluations of surgical autonomy, but they start to line up with Milestones by providing valuable benchmarks for skills acquisition and characterizing degrees to which a responsibility may be consigned to a trainee [15].

There is a great deal of interest in formulating EPAs for general surgery training and in residency training in general. The American Board of Surgery has undergone a pilot in assigning and evaluating the use of EPAs in broad categories for general surgery residency. There are also EPA pilots formally being conducted and evaluated in undergraduate medical education [16]. Further, once EPAs and bidirectional feedback evolve into a feedback culture on the continuum of training, then further granular feedback might be accomplished through designated nested EPAs [17]. Nested EPAs break down high complexity tasks into smaller ones. This ensures that all members of an interprofessional team have a defined task that is clear and accessible and it elicits feedback that ensures quality care and patient safety.

Overall, Ten Cate defines five levels of supervision that may be employed with each EPA. As Lindeman clarifies through "Entrustable Professional Activities (EPAs) and Applications to Surgical Training," in Resources In Surgical Education (RISE), these are aligned with progressive responsibility measures, like the Milestones, albeit imperfectly, toward independent practice [18]:

1. Observation but no execution by the trainee, even with direct supervision
2. Execution with direct, proactive supervision
3. Execution with reactive supervision, i.e., on request and quickly available
4. Supervision at a distance and/or post hoc
5. Supervision provided by the trainee to more junior colleagues

Looking forward, clinical competency committees could be the formal entrustment committees that assign supervision levels and Milestone levels for residents. Evaluation data for the EPAs can be supported with a myriad of datapoints, such as observed structured assessment of technical skills (OSATs), clinical encounter assessments, teamwork assessments, multisource feedback, simulation verification of proficiencies, operative assessments (i.e., SIMPL), and others. With this, each EPA would be mapped to several Milestones. Residents would then receive assessment of Milestones as entrustment levels are determined. Specific EPAs with entrustment levels would be the focus of biannual feedback sessions for a definable, timely, and actionable course of action. Once generalizable EPAs are more routinely used, a surgical education framework specific to the implementation of entrustment, might be implemented and provide transparency for both faculty and trainees. Ultimately, through identifying gaps in entrustment and in learning, residency leadership will be able to formulate customized teaching plans for mentored guidance in ensuring surgical quality and patient safety.

Bibliography

1. van Mook WNKA, Gorter SL, O'Sullivan H, Wass V, Schuwirth LW, van der Vleuten CPM. Approaches to professional behaviour assessment: tools in the professionalism toolbox. Eur J Intern Med. 2009;20(8):e153–7. https://doi.org/10.1016/j.ejim.2009.07.012.
2. SurgeryMilestones.pdf. Accessed 4 Sept 2020. https://www.acgme.org/Portals/0/PDFs/Milestones/SurgeryMilestones.pdf.
3. Cogbill TH, Malangoni MA, Potts JR, Valentine RJ. The general surgery milestones project. J Am Coll Surg. 2014;218(5):1056–62. https://doi.org/10.1016/j.jamcollsurg.2014.02.016.
4. Nasca TJ, Philibert I, Brigham T, Flynn TC. The next GME accreditation system — rationale and benefits. N Engl J Med. 2012;366(11):1051–6. https://doi.org/10.1056/NEJMsr1200117.
5. Rawlings A, Knox ADC, Park YS, et al. Development and evaluation of standardized narrative cases depicting the general surgery professionalism milestones. Acad Med. 2015;90(8):1109–15. https://doi.org/10.1097/ACM.0000000000000739.

6. Sadideen H, Plonczak A, Saadeddin M, Kneebone R. How educational theory can inform the training and practice of plastic surgeons. Plast Reconstr Surg Glob Open. 2018;6(12):e2042. https://doi.org/10.1097/GOX.0000000000002042.

7. Peña A. The Dreyfus model of clinical problem-solving skills acquisition: a critical perspective. Medical Education Online. 2010;15(1):1-N.PAG. https://doi.org/10.3402/meo.v15i0.4846.

8. Frank JR, Snell LS, Cate OT, Holmboe ES, Carraccio C, Swing SR, Harris P, Glasgow NJ, Campbell C, Dath D, Harden RM, Iobst W, Long DM, Mungroo R, Richardson DL, Sherbino J, Silver I, Taber S, Talbot M, Harris KA. Competency-based medical education: theory to practice. Med Teach. 2010;32(8):638–45.

9. Ten Cate O, Chen HC, Hoff RG, Peters H, Bok H, van der Schaaf M. Curriculum development for the workplace using Entrustable Professional Activities (EPAs): AMEE Guide No. 99. Med Teach. 2015;37(11):983–1002. https://doi.org/10.3109/01 42159X.2015.1060308.

10. Tekian A, Hodges BD, Roberts TE, Schuwirth L, Norcini J. Assessing competencies using milestones along the way. Med Teach. 2015;37(4):399–402. https://doi.org/10.3109/01421 59X.2014.993954.

11. Regehr G, Ginsburg S, Herold J, Hatala R, Eva K, Oulanova O. Using "Standardized Narratives" to explore new ways to represent faculty opinions of resident performance. Acad Med. 2012;87(4):419–27. https://doi.org/10.1097/ ACM.0b013e31824858a9.

12. Kerr B, O'Leary JP. The training of the surgeon: Dr. Halsted's greatest legacy. The American Surgeon; Atlanta. 1999;65(11):1101–2.

13. Carraccio C, Englander R, Gilhooly J, et al. Building a framework of entrustable professional activities, supported by competencies and milestones, to bridge the educational continuum. Acad Med. 2017;92(3):324–30. https://doi.org/10.1097/ ACM.0000000000001141.

14. Hirschl RB. The making of a surgeon: 10,000 hours? J Pediatr Surg. 2015;50(5):699–706. https://doi.org/10.1016/j. jpedsurg.2015.02.061.

15. Wagner JP, Lewis CE, Tillou A, et al. Use of entrustable professional activities in the assessment of surgical resident competency. JAMA Surg. 2018;153(4):335–43. https://doi. org/10.1001/jamasurg.2017.4547.

16. Loomis K, Amiel JM, Ryan MS, Esposito K, Green M, Stagnaro-Green A, Bull J, Mejicano GC (for the AAMC Core EPAs for Entering Residency Pilot Team). Implementing an entrustable professional activities framework in undergraduate medical education: early lessons from the AAMC core entrustable professional activities for entering residency pilot. Acad Med. 2017;92(6):765–70.
17. Angus S, Moriarty J, Nardino RJ, Chmielewski A, Rosenblum MJ. 'Internal medicine residents' perspectives on receiving feedback in milestone format. J Grad Med Educ. 2015;7(2):220–4. https://doi.org/10.4300/JGME-D-14-00446.1.
18. Lindeman B, Petrusa E Phitayakorn, R. Entrustable Professional Activities (EPAs) and applications to surgical training. 2017 June. Retrieved from https://www.facs.org/education/division-of-education/publications/rise/articles/entrustable.

Chapter 9
Implementing Quality Improvement at Your Institution

Michael Ghio, Danuel Laan, and Shauna Levy

Chapter Objectives

- To describe how to align key stakeholders to implement quality improvement locally
- To discuss clinical areas which might benefit from organized quality improvement initiatives

Introduction

In the last several decades there has been a paradigm shift toward improving quality within healthcare that is at least in part motivated by the growing relationship between reimbursement and patient outcomes. Quality improvement (QI) and patient safety are rightfully gaining momentum as healthcare professionals across the country strive to be leaders in improving and innovating care in their respective fields.

M. Ghio · D. Laan · S. Levy (✉)
Tulane University School of Medicine & Tulane Medical Center,
New Orleans, LA, USA
e-mail: mghio@tulane.edu; dlaan@tulane.edu; slevy10@tulane.edu

© The Author(s), under exclusive license to Springer Nature   155
Switzerland AG 2022
J. R. Romanelli et al. (eds.), *The SAGES Manual of Quality,
Outcomes and Patient Safety*,
https://doi.org/10.1007/978-3-030-94610-4_9

Broadly, QI is a thoughtful, deliberate process designed to improve patient outcomes on the whole, whether they be process or outcome measurements. QI includes identification of factors that impact patient outcomes either positively or negatively, with the objective being to minimize elements of care that lead to poor results and implementing or maximizing processes that lead to improved patient care. Once these components are identified, a team is mobilized to form a plan of action for improving outcomes. Implementation of the plan is followed by monitoring and evaluation of the strategies that were executed to improve patient care.

While institutions and quality improvement teams in different fields may share similar goals and methods of deploying strategies, many specifics of QI are site and field dependent. No two hospital sites or healthcare networks are the same, so tailoring of care and quality improvement, which are dependent on such characteristics as patient population, facilities and equipment, variability in surgical procedures, and composition of staff, is individualized at each site. There are, however, many lessons that can be learned from both the successful and unsuccessful practices implemented by different disciplines and institutions. We hope to help the reader understand the fundamental components of basic quality improvement and provide insight into how the respective parts can be tailored to individual institutions.

In this chapter, we will take a look at the history of QI and discuss implementation of QI programs with emphasis on the important role of institutional stakeholders. We will describe why stakeholders are important, how to identify stakeholders, and share strategies for utilizing their skillsets and interests to maximize success. A review of the ways in which successful and unsuccessful QI attempts can benefit institutions and ultimately patient care will follow. We will end with an examination of clinical areas that are likely to benefit from QI and consideration of patient safety in the new era of COVID-19.

History of Quality Improvement Implementation

One of the first impetuses for quality improvement began in 1998 with the *President's Advisory Commission on Consumer Protection and Quality in the Health Care Industry* [1]. The Commission was created by President Bill Clinton in March 1997 with a goal to "advise the President on changes occurring in the health care system and recommend measures as may be necessary to promote and assure health care quality and value and protect consumers and workers in the health care system." [1] This report provided a clear set of goals, including [1]:

1. Reducing the underlying causes of illness, injury, and disability
2. Expanding research on new treatments and evidence on effectiveness
3. Assuring appropriate use
4. Reducing healthcare errors
5. Addressing oversupply and undersupply of healthcare resources
6. Increasing patients' participation in their care

The Commission not only directed that these goals be implemented, but it had the foresight to stipulate that measurable objectives (such as consumer satisfaction, clinical quality performance, service performance measures like waiting time), which were later recognized as a hallmark of quality improvement, be used to evaluate each of these aims [1]. Another influential part of this report was its recommendation to organizations that they structure their systems to include clear leaders and stakeholders with varying levels of motivation. The report released by the *President's Advisory Commission on Consumer Protection and Quality in Health Care Industry* set the foundation for future efforts in QI.

In response to the initial report by President Clinton, in 1999, the Institute of Medicine (IOM) published its popular, landmark publication, *To Err Is Human: Building a Safer Health System*, which showed that close to 100,000 people in the United States were dying each year due to medical errors [2]. This astounding number was more than car crashes (43,458), breast cancer (42,297), and AIDS (16,516) [2]. The initial report also demanded a 50% reduction in medical errors over the next 5 years [2]. There was widespread attention from both the public media and the healthcare sector. Notably, the federal government set aside 50 million dollars annually for patient safety efforts [3]. The IOM continued its investigation of these concerning statistics, in 2001, publishing *Crossing the Quality Chasm: Health System for the twenty-first Century*, which identified six aims that laid the foundation for improving quality improvement [4]. These six aims were [4]:

1. Safe: not doing harm
2. Effective: using proven therapies to treat, not experimental or personal experiences
3. Patient centered: understanding the individual needs of your patient
4. Timely: trying to reduce wait or delays to care
5. Efficient: reducing unnecessary use of resources
6. Equitable: care that does not vary due to gender, ethnicity, location, or socioeconomic status

Subsequent to the release of *Crossing the Quality Chasm: Health System for the twenty-first Century*, the United States saw an increase in the number of grants to study QI, an increase in publications related to patient safety, and a reduction in medical errors [5]. These six pillars remain the guiding force of healthcare QI in the United States and provide a benchmark to focus for the provision of care in the modern era.

Other initiatives designed to continue improving patient safety arose at about this same time, including the development of "serious reportable events" in 2002 by the National

Quality Forum (NQF) [6]. These broadly fell into the following categories, as determined by the NQF [6]:

1. Surgical or Invasive Procedure Events: such as wrong site surgery
2. Product or Device Events: such as a contaminated device resulting in a death/serious injury
3. Patient Protection Events: such as patient suicide while inpatient
4. Care Management Events: such as a serious event/death due to medication error
5. Environmental Events: injury such as electrical shock or burn while in the hospital or injury secondary to use of physical restraints
6. Radiologic Events: such as death or injury of patient or staff associated with introducing a metallic object in MRI field
7. Potential Criminal Events: such as impersonation of healthcare member, abduction of a patient

In 2004, the Joint Commission published its national patient safety goals, and in December of that same year, in response to the Joint Commission's goals, the Institute of Healthcare Improvement (IHI) launched its "100,000 Lives Campaign" with the intent to improve safety and outcomes. In their initial campaign in 2006, the IHI cited statistics showing that about 100,000 people die annually due to medical injuries and high rates of hospital-acquired infection [7]. Per the Institute's initial report, specific aims were defined, including:

1. Deploy rapid response teams that include a physician, nurse, and a respiratory therapist that respond prior to a code event [7].
2. Deliver reliable, evidence-based care for acute myocardial infection (AMI). This was based on the worrisome fact that every year, 350,000 out of a total 900,000 patients die of AMI in the acute period [8].

3. Prevent adverse drug events that result in over 7000 deaths annually [2].
4. Prevent central line infections by examining five components of care aimed at reducing risk: handwashing, barrier precautions, use of chlorohexidine, site choice, and daily evaluation of need, or the removal of a line no longer indicated [7].
5. Prevent surgical site infections by using preoperative antibiotics when indicated, appropriate hair removal, glucose control, and perioperative normothermia [7].
6. Prevent ventilator-associated pneumonia by elevating the head of bed between 30° and 45°, sedation vacations with daily evaluations for extubation, peptic ulcer prophylaxis, and deep venous thrombosis prophylaxis [7, 9, 10].

IHI's campaign was successful, enrolling about 3100 hospitals (75% of all hospitals in the United States at that time) [11]. Over the following 18 months, IHI's efforts were estimated to result in 122,000 fewer deaths [11]. This effort yielded a number of other spin-off projects across the world and encouraged efforts by individual systems.

The development of checklists accelerated as checklists became a well-known means to improve quality of care in various settings. Notably, in 2007, Dr. Peter Pronovost's use of checklists in the intensive care unit was lauded for its prevention of catheter-associated infections [12]. Similarly, Dr. Atul Gawande expanded the use of surgical checklists in 2008; using Dr. Gawande's checklists, the rate of death significantly declined (from 1.5% to 0.8%), and inpatient complications similarly decreased from 11.0% to 7.0% (both statistically significant) [13]. At about the same time, the World Health Organization developed a Surgical Safety Checklist and conducted a global study that was published in the *New England Journal of Medicine* in 2009 showing that use of checklists is associated with both decreased complications and decreased mortality [13].

In 2010, the Health Information Technology for Economic and Clinical Health (HITECH) Act was passed that provided

30 billion dollars to healthcare systems to incentivize hospitals to use electronic health records. In 2011, the NQF again published an update expanding its list of serious events to be aware of while simultaneously reiterating demand for accountability from healthcare organizations [14]. In this report, the NQF recommended healthcare systems search for gaps in their care and encourage frequent and high-quality reviews specific to departments and categories of patient interventions, followed by incorporation of findings to improve care delivered [14]. In 2015, the Department of Health and Human Services announced a change in Medicare's payment policies, such that payments would be based on quality, instead of purely volume, thus representing a further shift in the paradigm.

While the above examples are not an exhaustive list of all the safety and patient-quality care measures taken in the last several decades, they do illustrate the growing importance placed on QI by governing officials, hospitals, and healthcare systems. Although these government agencies, professional organizations, and leaders in the field make the case for QI and provide guidance, frameworks, and insight, it is most often left to individual healthcare networks and hospitals to implement QI.

Identification of Key Stakeholders

At an institutional level, the first step in QI is identifying an area in which a hospital or department can improve on. This can be done through a variety of methods including observation of trends such as a higher than nationally reported infection rate associated with a procedure, use of the American College of Surgeons National Surgical Quality Improvement Program (NSQIP) data, or by having townhall-style sessions to identify deficiencies seen by frontline workers.

Quality can broadly be measured in terms of the following four aspects [15, 16]:

1. Structure: Easily measurable components of a hospital, such as volume (of hospital, individual surgeons), not as readily amenable to quality improvement processes.
2. Process: The individual steps of a patient's care that lead to outcomes. This can be preoperative, intraoperative, or post-operative. Common postoperative process measures include cessation of prophylactic antibiotics within 24 h, removal of urinary catheters, and ambulation within 6 h of surgery.
3. Outcome: Broadly speaking, morbidity and mortality associated with surgery. Frequently seen as the most important to patients and surgeons, given the severity.
4. Composite: Multiple of the above.

Once an area requiring improvement has been identified, a fundamental first step is the identification of key stakeholders. A stakeholder is any individual who is impacted by a project and/or has an ability to influence its success and failure. Stakeholders are important because they provide a variety of lenses through which to identify and view problems along with a diverse group of approaches to addressing needs or shortcomings. Additionally, either directly or indirectly, stakeholders increase awareness of problems, promote transparency during periods of change, and increase the likelihood of commitment to QI through their participation [17].

It is important to think about the range of departments and individuals who play a role related to the area of need and, with that in mind, identify as many stakeholders as possible, from administrators, to pharmacists, nurses, physicians, housekeeping, basically every level of staff at an institution. It is useful to then sort stakeholders through use of a continuum in regard to their power (ability to contribute) and interest level (Fig. 9.1). Each stakeholder is motivated differently: whether by improvement in patient care, recognition for success, financial success if incentives are involved, or efficiency resulting in increased time to use for other activities.

While there is a tendency to invite staff, who are receptive and have readily apparent motivations for participating, it is important to also include staff who may seem resistant to

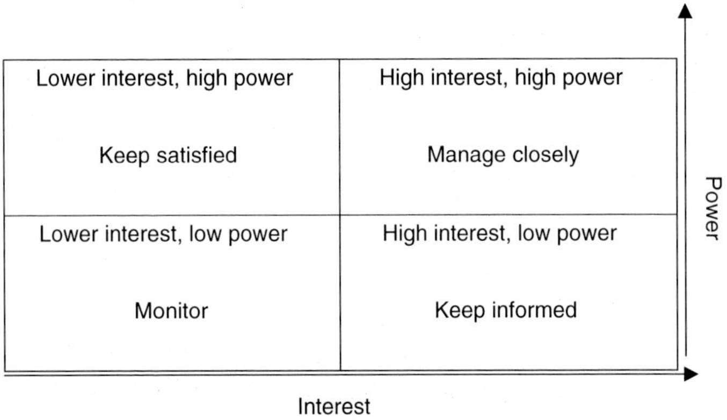

Lower interest, high power	High interest, high power	
Keep satisfied	Manage closely	Power
Lower interest, low power	High interest, low power	
Monitor	Keep informed	

Interest

FIGURE 9.1 Relationship between interest, power, and involvement in quality improvement

change. Missing a stakeholder or failing to identify stakeholders who may resist change can result in inefficient implementation and immediate or delayed failure of a QI project. By targeting naysayers for inclusion on the stakeholder team, their objections can be identified early and ideally be addressed in components of the plan proactively. As a brief example, when thinking about implementing a time out quality improvement project, it is essential to involve all parties in this project. From surgeons, to anesthesiologists, to circulators and scrub techs, each one will have a different opinion on the project's usefulness and the time required for its successful implementation. Failure to engage one of these parties can result in frustration or missing a crucial part of the process.

Analysis of the various stakeholders should be a multidisciplinary effort to ensure every area of the institution that impacts or is impacted by a particular patient outcome is represented. An effective way to approach this is to create a process map – this is a way to identify each action required to complete a task from beginning to completion [18]. A process map should be created for every project and can be accurately created by walking through the desired action, speaking with various staff members, or looking at required documentation [18]. In doing so, one can accurately identify every stakeholder. This is particularly important as the literature has showed the number of steps involved in a surgery or procedure is directly correlated with the numbers of errors and can guide decision-making in a quality improvement project [18].

The identification of each stakeholder is important in and of itself, but each will have a different perspective on the problem and project, and this should be a component of analysis. Stakeholders will often only buy into the quality improvement project if the expected outcome is identifiable or there is some benefit to their particular department or area of responsibility – whether it be financial, improved patient care, or saved time, to name a few. Once a stakeholder's motivation has been identified, evidence must be presented as to how the project will make their specific job more streamlined or meaningful. While not every QI project will make someone's job easier per se, if it improves patient outcomes or makes a seemingly meaningless action more meaningful and purpose driven, its likelihood of being successful is greater. While the inclusion of a diverse group of stakeholders encourages a view of the problem and possible responses, it is natural that the broader the list of stakeholders, the greater the risk for potential conflict as systems are potentially redesigned [17, 19]. Not all stakeholders are flexible or readily adaptable to change. This is where transparency is essential, with a clear focus of the project with an identifiable, visible deficiency that the team is attempting to correct. Examples may include data showing a higher-than expected rate of infections, patient feedback noting an area of deficiency, or reports showing rates of "never events" at your hospital.

Once stakeholders have been identified, the leadership team should be assembled. In our experience, this should include the following members [20]:

1. Project Leader: This individual is primarily in charge of organizing the daily activities and has a vested interest in its success. Ideally, one person takes the lead on an activity.
2. Subject Leaders: These members of the team are those that have leadership roles in the area that you are attempting to improve. For example, if attempting to improve hand hygiene on a surgical floor, this would include the nursing leaders on that floor and the housekeeping leader, in addition to a surgical leader. It is important to identify every level of leadership within a system of change. There will be several people who compose this facet of the team.
3. Project Mentor: Ideally, a QI director or someone else at the institution with experience in implementing projects.
4. Project Mentees: Every project should involve learners (residents, medical students, nursing students, etc.) with an interest in QI who can get involved and learn side by side with the team.
5. Support Members: This can include other physicians, pharmacists, students, or any member who has the time and ability to help with implementation and studying the effects of the project.
6. Patients: Including patients in the team incorporates a perspective often forgotten about, that of likely the biggest stakeholder. Ultimately, these changes should benefit their care, and understanding their perspective is important and educational.

The designation of a leadership team and delineation of responsibilities among members gives the group structure and increases efficiency and opportunity for success [17]. However, for the team to accomplish its goals, there must be a sense of camaraderie with little emphasis on hierarchy. Excitement about the prospect of identifying a common goal to address the problem or area of need is essential, and a thirst for achieving this outcome is important. It is also important the team be receptive to feedback and motivated.

Following selection of the team, the team must articulate what it is trying to accomplish in measurable terms, develop a method for measuring the aim, and articulate how it will evaluate outcomes and project overall. There is excellent support for this "model for improvement" which asks three fundamental questions [21]:

1. What are we trying to accomplish?
2. How will we know a change is an improvement?
3. What change can we make that will result in improvement?

Once the team has established what it is trying to accomplish and how they will measure it, they can develop an initial "PDSA" cycle – standing for "plan, do, study, act." During the plan portion, the team attempts to set a specific goal with a focus on details. For example, returning to our hand hygiene case, the team would need to identify a specific goal (i.e., the percentage, or number of people, etc.) instead of just saying "We will improve handwashing rates." Another part of setting the goal is the need to set a goal timeframe, such as "in 2 weeks." The next step is to then study improvement and act on its changes. These can be either positive or negative results, and it is important to recognize that many quality improvement and patient safety projects can be implemented in a several-week timeframe, not necessarily months to years. The IHI has a project charter sheet that we recommend using for organizing QI plans [22]. When thinking about outcomes, these are broadly classified into three types [20]:

1. Outcome Measures: These are the primary outcomes, e.g., the number of people washing their hands or the number of catheter-associated urinary tract infections, to name a few. These are the outcomes relevant to the patients.
2. Process Measures: These involve looking at the individual steps of the QI project and how they are being implemented, e.g., how many people are being audited for handwashing.

3. Balancing Measures: These refer to an unintentional consequence that the QI project had, e.g., studying if while improving ambulation, the number of patient falls during the study period increased.

The "RE-AIM" method (reach, effectiveness, adoption, implementation, maintenance), which was originally introduced in 1999, is an effective tool to implement a project while ensuring to assess the project's more long-term implementation into the culture of an institution as opposed to a temporary change [23, 24]. One can assess outcome, process, and balancing measures during the implementation phase and use them to guide the team's reaction and/or maintenance phase of the project.

The most important takeaway is that a team's PDSA cycle must be quick to adapt and use lessons learned from prior cycles. If the first implementation cycle of a QI project does not result in improvement of outcome or process measures, or if the balancing measures are too great, the team should not abandon the project but should analyze the process to identify reasons why success was not attained and then develop and implement a second plan. Several cycles of planning and implementation may be necessary to achieve desired outcomes or minimize balancing measures. Rapid cycle methodology requires the use of run charts, which can be used to identify certain trends and guide the next potential change required [19, 25].

We will share a project we are implementing at Tulane Medical Center that we will use moving forward as an example. We recognized that the rate of ambulation was extremely low in our surgical patient population: a dismal 10% were ambulating at least daily. We set a goal of improving the ambulation rate by 25% over 2 weeks by using text message reminders as an inpatient. Our team was led by a resident leader, with general surgery staff surgeons, nursing leadership, and patients also involved. We tested our change by sending two text messages a day to these patients and saw a greater than 50% improvement in ambulation rates among our patients. Our balancing measure was the number of falls in the unit; there was no increase in rate of falls in our population. Because of its simplicity, ease of implementation, and success, this has now evolved into a hospital-wide program aimed at using text messaging to improve various aspects of patient care.

How to Prevent Quality Improvement Fatigue

Frequently in quality improvement and patient safety areas, there is either initial success or failure that is then met with inconsistent follow-up on the project, sometimes with a decline in implementation. It is important that projects are not seen as temporary measures or as isolated projects but as the new norm and standard of care at a hospital. The project's success is frequently determined by its resource requirement, i.e., can it be implemented without constant oversight, a significant monetary inflow, or other factors that may be difficult to maintain longitudinally?

The strongest projects are those that create a culture of change, require few new resources, and have proven, transparent results. On a basic level, the importance of constantly reassessing the PDSA cannot be overstated – quality improvement is defined by the ability to constantly reassess QI measures, from every day to week to month, and redesign the PDSA cycle [22]. True QI can be evaluated on a weekly basis to see if improvements happen then less frequently but still regularly.

It is estimated that up to 70% of change through QI is not sustained, and efforts seen in the United Kingdom showed that 33% of QI projects were not continued 1 year after completion [26, 27]. The National Health Service in the United Kingdom identified ten factors related to process implementation that if scored could predict sustainability [27]. These factors include [27]:

1. Are there benefits beyond helping patients (are jobs easier)?
2. Is there credibility of the benefits? Does evidence support the change and are the benefits visible?
3. Is there adaptability of the improved process? Does the change rely on a specific individual or group?
4. Is there effectiveness of the system to monitor progress? Are there monitoring systems in place?
5. Is staff involved in the change and was new staff hired?
6. Are staff encouraged to express ideas?
7. Is senior leadership engaged and supportive?
8. Is clinical leadership engagement and support?
9. Is there alignment with strategic aim and culture?
10. Is there space and equipment to support change/is infrastructure in place?

We agree that these factors are all important in preventing quality improvement fatigue and should be examined prior to implementation. A project is only as useful as its ability to be continued after initial success, so remaining cognizant of these factors when designing a patient safety project may lead to improved implementation.

Once a QI project has proven successful and implemented as the new norm, it is important to identify new leaders who will continue to assess the outcomes and ensure it is being implemented properly. Oftentimes, this involves inviting mentees with an interest in QI to take on a more substantial role and tasking them with evaluating the project quarterly or at some regular interval. Engaging residents and students is crucial in learning how to develop collaborative initiatives with nursing. Helping mentees understand the goal of quality improvement projects, the fundamental components of designing a project, how their role as a resident is valuable, and the time commitment have all been shown to improve resident involvement [28]. IHI modules provide an introduction to the fundamental topics of quality improvement and patient safety and are a good stepping stone to helping students and residents understand the basics of designing a project. There is a great focus on QI education of residents by the American College of Surgeons through their development of the Quality In-Training Initiative (QITI) that aims to create a culture of change and prioritization of patient safety [25].

Collaboration and networking between hospitals are another strategy to minimizing QI fatigue. Hearing from colleagues at other hospitals about how they created a culture change, implemented projects, and sought to identify stakeholders can ignite passion for QI while providing ideas for further innovation. It also is advantageous for young surgeons and learners as a way to network with experts in the field.

Clinical Areas That Have Established Quality Improvement

Every single surgical field can benefit from QI. Within each surgical department, there are limitless opportunities – from preoperative interventions, intraoperative, postoperative, it is crucial to think about every step of day activity when considering and evaluating areas that would benefit from QI. These exist on a local and national level and require collaboration among providers, whether residents, nurses, attendings, or others. There are certain QI programs that we want to highlight that track patient safety information.

First, the American College of Surgery National Surgical Quality Improvement Program (NSQIP) is a nationally validated, risk-adjusted program that allows hospitals to compare themselves with one another in regard to their complications and is an effective way to gather valuable information about hospital performance. The NSQIP generates semiannual reports showing hospitals' risk-adjusted

30-day morbidity and mortality outcomes along with an odds ratio (1.0 is as expected, >1.0 worse than expected, <1.0 better than expected). This information can provide real-time feedback to hospitals and help identify specific areas for improvement. NSQIP has helped improve the risk-adjusted mortality and risk-adjusted complication rates, preventing between 250 and 500 complications per year [29].

There are a number of quality improvement programs that are specialty specific: Transplant Quality Institute through United Network for Organ Sharing, Metabolic and Bariatric Surgery Accreditation and Quality Improvement Program (MBSAQIP), Trauma Quality Improvement Program (TQIP), Vascular Quality Initiative (VQI), NSQIP Pediatric, and others that we encourage involvement in as these provide useful ways to compare efforts to others.

Within a hospital or healthcare system, frequent review of outcomes in regard to particular departments is a great first step to identifying areas for improvement as is being aware of outcomes achieved at other institutions. In these discussions, it is worthwhile to involve every level of provider and staff to help identify deficiencies. Polling frontline workers about potentially weak sections of their departments as they impact patient outcomes can help delineate areas that need improvement and may identify key stakeholders for a QI project. Institutional administrators and financial directors can help discover financially beneficial projects that will provide additional funding to leverage toward other components of patient care. Whatever the goal may be, a multidisciplinary committee is essential to making meaningful change. Networking between hospitals can provide additional resources for identifying areas to monitor and types of improvement to strive for. Openly and candidly discussing results in regard to individual departments opens the door for dialogue and identification of either deficiencies or areas of success that others would benefit from learning from.

COVID and Quality Improvement: Synchrony in a Dyssynchronous Medical System

In this new COVID-19 world, the importance of QI has intensified. Finding ways to deliver high-quality care is even more important than ever so that repetitive exposure to potentially positive or confirmed positive COVID patients is avoided. There has been an explosion of quality improvement efforts, with high-functioning institutions understanding that efforts must be amplified. Meetings among QI groups should focus on educating frontline workers with useful skills and expertise needed to improve the care they are providing, whether COVID-related or not, to minimize exposure to any patient or to staff. A focus on designing COVID response teams, to manage airway, personal protective equipment, and medications is especially important [30].

There is a growing need for QI and patient safety in the COVID-19 era, with the Federal Communications Commission (FCC) recognizing that telehealth programs, some of which are QI in nature, are essential. In April of 2020, the FCC released a 200-million-dollar budget dedicated to promoting telehealth programs that would provide care for people while reducing exposure of providers to patients [31]. This was an extremely valuable resource that a number of providers took advantage of across the country.

In this environment, it is important to have frequent virtual meetings, leverage support staff, and attempt to maximize the value of in-person interaction with patients when they do take place. We should be careful not to have frivolous interactions that put patients, coworkers, family members, and staff at risk for exposure.

Conclusion

In conclusion, we have stressed the importance of identifying stakeholders and have provided a guide for implementing a QI program. The first step is to draw up a comprehensive list of stakeholders, focusing on how the project will impact stakeholder jobs on a day-to-day basis (i.e., will it eliminate or add new responsibilities) and how the project will ultimately benefit them (whether financially, improved patient outcomes, or other motivation). After bringing the team together, make sure to identify and involve future QI leaders (residents, nursing, medical students, and others) and implement the plan-do-study-act cycle. Of critical importance is the need to respond to both failures and successes – in the case of failures, it is important to attempt to identify what went wrong and implement an updated PDSA cycle that addresses this failure. If a plan resulted in success, the team can move forward with planning for how implementation will continue with less oversight. Awareness and prevention of QI fatigue are essential to sustain long-term results.

Prior to COVID-19, there was a thirst for quality improvement and patient safety projects – now, more so than ever, there is a need for creative methods to impact meaningful patient care given the limitations of current patient care given the ongoing pandemic. Developing projects that improve patient outcomes and motivate them to be active participants in their care is crucial.

References

1. The President's Advisory Commission on Consumer Protection and Quality in the Health Care Industry: report synopsis - PubMed. https://pubmed.ncbi.nlm.nih.gov/10179021/. Accessed 2 Oct 2020.
2. Kohn LT, Corrigan JM, Donaldson MS. To err is human. Building a safer health system, volume 6, vol. 2; 1999. https://doi.org/10.17226/9728.
3. Mission and Budget. Agency for health research and quality. https://www.ahrq.gov/cpi/about/mission/index.html. Accessed 25 Sept 2020.
4. Institute of Medicine (US) Committee on Quality of Health Care in America. Shaping the future; crossing the quality chasm: a new health system for the 21th century. 2001. https://doi.org/10.17226/10027

5. Stelfox HT, Palmisani S, Scurlock C, Orav EJ, Bates DW. The "To Err is Human" report and the patient safety literature. BMJ Qual Saf. 2006;15(3):174–8. https://doi.org/10.1136/qshc.2006.017947.

6. NQF: List of SREs. http://www.qualityforum.org/Topics/SREs/List_of_SREs.aspx. Accessed 2 Oct 2020.

7. Gold JA. The 100,000 lives campaign. WMJ. 2005;104(8):81–2. https://doi.org/10.1001/jama.295.3.324.

8. Outcome Measures. CMS. https://www.cms.gov/Medicare/Quality-Initiatives-Patient-Assessment-Instruments/HospitalQualityInits/OutcomeMeasures. Accessed 2 Oct 2020.

9. Tablan OC, Anderson LJ, Besser R, et al. Guidelines for preventing health-care--associated pneumonia, 2003: recommendations of CDC and the Healthcare Infection Control Practices Advisory Committee. MMWR Recomm Rep. 2004;53(RR-3):1–36. http://www.ncbi.nlm.nih.gov/pubmed/15048056.

10. American Thoracic Society; Infectious Diseases Society of America. Guidelines for the management of adults with hospital-acquired, ventilator-associated, and healthcare-associated pneumonia. Am J Respir Crit Care Med. 2005;171(4):388–416. https://doi.org/10.1164/rccm.200405-644ST.

11. Baehrend J. 100,000 lives campaign: ten years later. http://www.ihi.org/communities/blogs/100000-lives-campaign-ten-years-later. Published 2016.

12. McKee C, Berkowitz I, Cosgrove SE, et al. Reduction of catheter-associated bloodstream infections in pediatric patients: experimentation and reality. Pediatr Crit Care Med. 2008;9(1):40–6. https://doi.org/10.1097/01.PCC.0000299821.46193.A3.

13. Haynes AB, Weiser TG, Berry WR, et al. A surgical safety checklist to reduce morbidity and mortality in a global population. N Engl J Med. 2009;360(5):491–9. https://doi.org/10.1056/NEJMsa0810119.

14. National Quality Forum (NQF). Serious reportable events in healthcare—2011 update: a consensus report. Washington, DC: National Quality Forum (NQF); 2011.

15. Birkmeyer JD, Dimick JB, Birkmeyer NJO. Measuring the quality of surgical care: structure, process, or outcomes? J Am Coll Surg. 2004;198(4):626–32. https://doi.org/10.1016/j.jamcollsurg.2003.11.017.

16. Tichansky DS, Morton J, Jones DB, editors. The SAGES manual of quality, outcomes and patient safety. New York: Springer; 2012. https://doi.org/10.1007/978-1-4419-7901-8.

17. Engaging stakeholders to improve the quality of children's health care. Agency for Health Research and Quality. https://www.ahrq.gov/policymakers/chipra/demoeval/what-we-learned/implementation-guides/implementation-guide1/index.html#about. Accessed 2 Oct 2020.

18. Rosen DH, Johnson S, Kebaabetswe P, Thigpen M, Smith DK. Process maps in clinical trial quality assurance. Clin Trials. 2009;6(4):373–7. https://doi.org/10.1177/1740774509338429.

19. Silver SA, McQuillan R, Harel Z, et al. How to sustain change and support continuous quality improvement. Clin J Am Soc Nephrol. 2016;11(5):916–24. https://doi.org/10.2215/CJN.11501015.

20. Silver SA, Harel Z, McQuillan R, et al. How to begin a quality improvement project. Clin J Am Soc Nephrol. 2016;11(5):893–900. https://doi.org/10.2215/CJN.11491015.

21. Langley GL, Moen R, Nolan KM, Nolan TW, Norman CLPL. The improvement guide: a practical approach to enhancing organizational performance. 2nd ed. San Francisco: Jossey-Bass Publishers; 2009.

22. Plan-Do-Study-Act (PDSA) Worksheet. IHI - Institute for Healthcare Improvement. http://www.ihi.org/resources/Pages/Tools/PlanDoStudyActWorksheet.aspx. Accessed 2 Oct 2020.

23. Glasgow RE, Vogt TM, Boles SM. Evaluating the public health impact of health promotion interventions: the RE-AIM framework. Am J Public Health. 1999;89(9):1322–7. https://doi.org/10.2105/AJPH.89.9.1322.

24. Gaglio B, Shoup JA, Glasgow RE. The RE-AIM framework: a systematic review of use over time. Am J Public Health. 2013;103(6). https://doi.org/10.2105/AJPH.2013.301299.

25. (No Title). https://qiti.acsnsqip.org/ACS_NSQIP_2017_QITI_Curriculum.pdf. Accessed 2 Oct 2020.

26. Beer M, Nohria N. Cracking the code of change. Harv Bus Rev. 2000;78(3):133–41, 216. http://www.ncbi.nlm.nih.gov/pubmed/11183975.

27. Lennox L, Maher L, Reed J. Navigating the sustainability landscape: a systematic review of sustainability approaches in healthcare. Implement Sci. 2018;13(1):1–17. https://doi.org/10.1186/s13012-017-0707-4.

28. Butler JM, Anderson KA, Supiano MA, Weir CR. "It feels like a lot of extra work": resident attitudes about quality improvement and implications for an effective learning health care

system. Acad Med. 2017;92(7):984–90. https://doi.org/10.1097/ACM.0000000000001474.

29. Hall BL, Hamilton BH, Richards K, Bilimoria KY, Cohen ME, Ko CY. Does surgical quality improve in the American College of Surgeons National Surgical Quality Improvement Program: an evaluation of all participating hospitals. Ann Surg. 2009;250(3):363–74. https://doi.org/10.1097/SLA.0b013e3181b4148f.

30. Oesterreich S, Cywinski JB, Elo B, Geube M, Mathur P. Quality improvement during the COVID-19 pandemic. Cleve Clin J Med. 2020. https://doi.org/10.3949/ccjm.87a.ccc041.

31. COVID-19 Telehealth Program. Federal Communications Commission. https://www.fcc.gov/covid-19-telehealth-program. Accessed 2 Oct 2020.

Chapter 10
Creating and Defining Quality Metrics That Matter in Surgery

Anai N. Kothari and Thomas A. Aloia

Creating and Defining Quality Metrics That Matter in Surgery

In March of 2013, Kirk Goldsberry and Eric Weiss introduced "The Dwight Effect" at the MIT Sports Analytics Conference. At that point, the NBA lagged behind other professional sports leagues in the adoption of advanced analytic techniques to evaluate in-game performance [1]. This was especially true for defensive performance, which was difficult to measure and effectively characterize. Since basketball has two key objectives – scoring points and preventing points –

A. N. Kothari
Department of Surgery, Division of Surgical Oncology, Medical College of Wisconsin, Milwaukee, WI, USA
e-mail: akothari@mcw.edu

T. A. Aloia (✉)
University of Texas MD Anderson Cancer Center, Houston, TX, USA
e-mail: thomas.aloia@ascension.org

© The Author(s), under exclusive license to Springer Nature Switzerland AG 2022
J. R. Romanelli et al. (eds.), *The SAGES Manual of Quality, Outcomes and Patient Safety*,
https://doi.org/10.1007/978-3-030-94610-4_10

177

not being able to assess the latter was a significant shortcoming. By combining optical tracking data with visual and spatial analytics, Goldsberry and Weiss were able to reframe how defense in the NBA could be measured [2, 3].

"The Dwight Effect" was the foundation for a new set of advanced defensive metrics that have since led to a transformation in the way basketball is played in the NBA [4]. However, it was not simply creating new metrics that led to this impact – the NBA was already awash in static measures of performance. Instead, insights were obtained by using a deeper understanding of the interaction of the players to identify novel independent variables that better correlated to performance outcomes. Creating and defining quality metrics "that matter" in surgery should have similar focus.

In healthcare, quality metrics are used in multiple ways. From benchmarking to quality improvement efforts to public reporting to reimbursement, quality measures are crucial to support assessment and improvement at the provider, hospital, system, and societal level. Particularly relevant to surgeons, the measurement movement has motivated hospitals and regulatory bodies to transparently report metrics that attempt to measure high-quality surgery. However, attempts to simply apply existing healthcare quality metrics to surgery are limited by inadequate adjustment of risk and incomplete consideration of the unique aspects of perioperative care. As a result, there is a strong incentive for surgeons to move from the sidelines to the playing field when it comes to quality measure design [5].

In this chapter, we introduce aspects of surgical care that can be measured and what data are available to create metrics. We then describe a framework for identifying quality metrics in surgery that matter to patients and providers and the key steps for creating/defining these metrics. Finally, we provide a design tool to create new metrics for surgical application.

From Measuring Surgical Care to Designing Metrics

Approaching metric construction from a design-thinking perspective, the end goal of all measures is quantifying value to achieve the "quadruple aim" (improving patient experience, improving health of populations, reducing the per capita cost of healthcare, and improving the well-being of healthcare providers) [6, 7]. The traditional value equation accounts for outcomes and cost. We propose a modified value equation that further specifies the numerator by accounting for both quality (achieving a positive outcome) and safety (avoidance of harm) (Fig. 10.1) [5]. This can provide a foundation for identifying the inputs necessary to develop new surgical metrics.

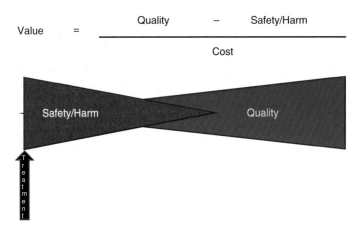

FIGURE 10.1 A framework for developing metrics for surgeons and surgical patients that emphasizes the pursuit of high value care by accounting for quality, safety/harm, and cost. (Aloia et al. [5])

Quality

In 1966, Donabedian introduced a conceptual model for the assessment of quality. Donabedian proposed three major criteria of quality in medical care – structure, process, and outcomes. Each Donabedian component interacts with and influences the next, where structure is defined as the setting where care occurs, process refers to how care is delivered, and outcomes refer to the impact of care [8]. Of these, outcomes are seemingly the most important. However, while some outcomes like mortality are unmistakable, others can be less clear, making them challenging to specify. This has led to a reliance on using structural and process measures to define surgical quality metrics [9].

Existing surgical quality metrics can be grouped based on the Donabedian framework. Postoperative mortality, complications, length of stay, and readmission are outcome indicators. Adherence to components of enhanced recovery after surgery programs and surgical care improvement project (SCIP) measures are examples of commonly used process indicators. Hospital and surgeon volume, nursing ratios, and external designations/accreditations are each structural indicators [10]. In the design of new metrics, using the Donabedian model can provide a template to organize these efforts. Balancing metric value with the work required to obtain data, it is recommended that measure sets contain a balanced portfolio of structure, process, and outcomes measures.

Data that can be used to define quality metrics are available through multiple existing internal and external sources. While impossible to detail all possible data sources, we highlight four major resources: clinical records, registries, billing data/claims, and federal agencies/programs.

Donabedian recognized the important role clinical records play in the assessment of quality. Specifically, patient records provide a narrative summary of how structure, process, and outcomes come together to impact individual patients. However, concerns surrounded their use due to incompleteness and inaccuracy. Many of these concerns have amplified with the transition to the routine use of electronic clinical records [11]. While the electronic health record (EHR) comes with significant promise in the ability to obtain relevant quality improvement data given the availability of electronic documentation, prescription and test information, diagnostics, and many other elements, it is subject to inaccuracies during data entry [12]. Still, electronic health data are an important input to the design of quality metrics.

Clinical registries and databases provide important data for surgeons to use for designing quality metrics. These include institutional databases, local and regional collaborative data-sharing programs, and national datasets that aggregate outcome, process, and structural data [13]. Examples such as the American College of Surgeon's NSQIP program, the Michigan Bariatric Collaborative, and the ACS/NCI's National Care Database provide aggregated data that can be used to measure quality.

Several federal agencies and programs have been established to measure and report on the quality of care, including surgical quality [14]. The Center for Medicare and Medicaid Services (CMS) has several quality programs. These include CAHPS (Consumer Assessment of Healthcare Providers and Systems), Hospital Compare, and the Hospital Inpatient Quality Reporting Program (IQR). Another is the Agency of Health Quality and Research (AHRQ) that has developed several quality indicators, including prevention quality indicators (PQI), inpatient quality indicators (IQI), and patient safety indicators (PSI) [15]. While these are all established quality metrics in their own right, they can also provide a source of data to develop new metrics and adapt for local use.

Safety

Quality is not the only aspect of care that contributes to the numerator of the value equation. Quality closely interacts with safety – together, determining an outcome. Unlike more well-defined models for measuring health quality, no universal approach exists for measuring patient safety. Instead, the focus is on "zero harm" or the avoidance of a negative outcome [16]. Interestingly, most measures that are labeled as surgical quality metrics are better defined as harm metrics. In fact, 95% of publicly reportable metrics in healthcare are harm metrics. For example, postoperative wound infections, deep vein thrombosis, pneumonia, and others are all harm events. Preventing these occurrences, when viewed in the context of the modified value equation, incompletely achieves the aim of high-value care, since they do directly incentivize surgeons to strive for higher-quality/positive outcomes.

There are other collateral damages that can arise from focusing solely on harm metrics including impaired patient access, arrested innovation, challenges in training, and surgeon burnout [17]. Harm metrics can lead to perceived high-risk patients not receiving the same care as their lower-risk counterparts. This is seen across multiple specialties where publicly reported metrics appear to influence decisions for offering surgical treatment [18]. Similarly, in an attempt to avoid harm and promote safety, the process for developing, testing, and implementing new techniques can be slowed [19]. For surgeons that are primarily being measured using harm metrics, there is a potential disincentive to educate and provide trainees the necessary autonomy to help them develop toward their own future independent practice. Finally, the emphasis on harm metrics can contribute to surgeon burnout – few enter surgical practice motivated to avoid harm but instead are intrinsically driven to achieve high quality. Therefore, creating metrics centered on achieving quality might have advantage over those focused on preventing harm [17]. Optimally, metrics that strive to improve quality while also mitigating harm should be prioritized. Ultimately, developing a balanced portfolio of harm and quality measures is more likely to achieve higher levels of value realization.

Cost

The third element and the denominator of the value equation is cost. Measurement of cost quantifies the financial burden associated with rendering a healthcare service, usually in a single episode of care. The challenge in measurement of cost is that it is an opaque term and can describe several items including patient out-of-pocket payments, charges, prices, provision of care costs, indirect costs, and acquisition costs. We propose a framework that focuses on three "real-dollar" domains: [1] patient-borne cost, [2] third-party payors, and [3] institutional cost [20].

Patient-borne cost summarizes the direct and indirect expenses taken on by patients for the care they receive. For example, out-of-pocket costs can be estimated by using copays and deductibles. These direct expenses can be assessed using patient-level billing data. Another type of cost incurred by the patient is indirect and more difficult to assess. Examples of indirect patient costs include lost wages and travel costs. Third-party payor costs focus on reimbursement contributions from insurance companies or governmental health plans. Characterizing and measuring these can be complex, particularly before the initiation of treatment due to lack of transparency into, plan maximums, charge to reimbursement ratios, stop loss provisions, and other differences in third-party contracts. However, post-therapy accounting has become more transparent as penetration of electronic billing platforms embedded in electronic health records has increased access to precise payor funds flow data. Institutional cost includes all of the procurement and production expenses to provision care, such as equipment, pharmacy, staff, services, time, infrastructure, information technology, and many other inputs, both direct and indirect.

Checklist for Creating Surgical Metrics

As described, the volume of data available to surgeons continues to grow at an exponential pace and comes from multiple sources. Data alone, however, do not lead to actual insight, change, and improvement. Instead, data must be translated into usable metrics. This process can be facilitated using a consistent framework. This level of standardization has the advantage of avoiding the temptation to create unneeded and redundant metrics – which is a common practice when faced with increasing available data streams [6].

Several national groups including the National Quality Forum (NQF), CMS, and Physician Consortium for Performance Enhancement (PCPI) have developed guiding principles for developing new measures. Leveraging the expertise of these regulatory organizations can help ensure the creation of high-quality surgical metrics. CMS has formulated a standardized approach that is used across all of the agency's quality programs and initiatives [21]. This blueprint can be broken down into five stages: conceptualization, specification, testing, implementation, and evaluation (Fig. 10.2).

Conceptualization

The initial step to developing a new surgical metric is considering how it will enhance the healthcare system [22]. High-quality metrics should be meaningful to multiple stakeholders including providers, administrators, and patients. To accomplish this, focusing on high-impact areas with real opportunity for improvement is essential. Other considerations include minimizing the burden on providers to both use and collect the measure, prioritizing electronic data to specify the metric, reducing care delivery disparities, and aligning the metric with other quality improvement programs (both local and national) [23].

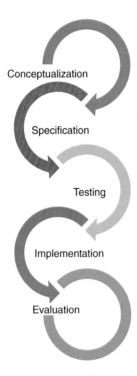

Conceptualization

Specification

Testing

Implementation

Evaluation

Figure 10.2 A checklist for developing surgical quality metrics that matter

The conceptualization phase includes information gathering, engaging subject and content experts, and a public comment process. Information gathering is arguably the most important step of the entire process and focuses on obtaining data that will eventually be used to justify the metric's implementation. This requires a comprehensive literature search and understanding what existing clinical guidelines are already in place. The focus should be on creating a metric that leads to better population health, better care, and/or more affordable care [24].

Specification

Following conceptualization, the next step is specifying the measure. This includes detailing the elements of the metric, defining the type of metric, and determining necessary data sources. Both CMS and NQF outline that quality measures should include a title/description, numerator, denominator, exclusions, and rationale [21].

As an example, the NQF-endorsed quality measure "perioperative temperature management" illustrates how to apply these principles to quality metric specification.

The title/description of the perioperative temperature management measure is "Percentage of patients, regardless of age, who undergo surgical or therapeutic procedures under general or neuraxial anesthesia of 60 minutes duration or longer for whom at least one body temperature greater than or equal to 35.5 degrees Celsius (or 95.9 degrees Fahrenheit) was achieved within the 30 minutes immediately before or the 15 minutes immediately after anesthesia end time." Title/descriptions should clearly describe the population of interest and specify the objective [25].

The numerator for perioperative temperature management is "Patients for whom at least one body temperature greater than or equal to 35.5 degrees Celsius (or 95.9 degrees Fahrenheit) was achieved within the 30 minutes immediately before or the 15 minutes immediately after anesthesia end time." Numerators specify what is necessary to achieve compliance with the measure.

The denominator for perioperative temperature management is "All patients, regardless of age, who undergo surgical or therapeutic procedures under general or neuraxial anesthesia of 60 minutes duration or longer." The denominator exclusions are "monitored anesthesia care and peripheral nerve block." Quality measure denominators describe the total population a metric will be applicable to and highlight those excluded from the measure.

Specifying the metric also involves identifying the necessary data sources to calculate the measure. Measures can be based on a single source or multiple sources of data inputs including administrative data, electronic clinical data, standardized patient assessments, medical records, surveys, and registries.

Testing

Prior to launch, a rigorous assessment of the technical and scientific merit of the measure should be conducted [21]. This is based on four general criteria: importance, scientific acceptability, feasibility, and usability. During this stage, exploration of data collection in a real-world setting is reviewed. Can the data actually be collected? Does collecting data for the metric create substantial hardship (financial cost, number of people needed to maintain the data, etc.)? And, most importantly, does the data being collected measure what was intended? The testing phase is often iterative and requires multiple cycles prior to moving on to the next stage.

Implementation

The implementation stage includes endorsement and complete rollout of the new metric. There are multiple consensus groups that can endorse a new metric including national organizations (ACS, NQF), specialty societies, and local/regional groups. The endorsement process can be long and happen in parallel to the actual rollout of a new measure.

Rollout planning includes preparing for audit and validation, provider education, and pilot programs. In fact, the implementation stage is primarily an education phase – where developers ensure end users understand the purpose of the measure and how to use it. Pilot programs offer a gradual rollout and can help provide feedback from stakeholders using the measure to further improve usability/compliance.

Evaluation

The final stage in metric creation includes the actual use of the measure, ensuring a process for evaluation, and continued maintenance. While a tremendous amount of energy and effort are required to place a new surgical metric into practice, that is just the beginning of the process. The most impactful and consistently used metrics are subject to constant scrutiny. This ensures they remain receptive to changes in literature, public feedback, and maintain scientific validity. Above all, the evaluation phase challenges all metrics to remain relevant and promote quality improvement.

Evaluation of new metrics includes active, ongoing information surveillance. This is similar to the information gathering conducted during development. Many surgical metrics are example of this. For instance, the Surgical Care Improvement Project (SCIP) was developed as a national program to help improve surgical care. SCIP developed several performance measures to help reduce surgical site infections, cardiovascular complications, venous thromboembolism, and respiratory complications [26]. Following broad implementation, many of the SCIP measures were studied to understand if they were actually achieving their intended aim [27]. While they may have contributed to improve surgical care, over time the adherence to the metrics was close to 100% making the impact of the measures difficult to interpret. Ultimately, this ongoing evaluation translated to change, and the SCIP measures were retired in 2015.

Other important considerations during the continued evaluation phase include reassessing the data collected (are there better ways or improved data inputs?), comparisons to other similar measures (are there places of overlap?), and maintenance reviews (should the metric be retained, revised, retired, suspended, removed?).

Model for Patient-Centric Surgical Outcome Measure Development

A possible way to facilitate the conceptualization of new metrics is through surgical societies. These groups are preassembled expert panels and include stakeholders with significant domain expertise. To aid in this process, a structured template can be helpful to allow individuals that may not have formal training in measure development an opportunity to actively participate. We developed a novel tool that leverages the components of the modified value equation to inform the discussion (Table 10.1) [5]. This tool separates patient-centered outcomes into the following domains: safety/harm, quality, short-term utility/disutility, long-term utility/disutility. Use of this tool has been shown to rapidly produce focused procedure-specific metric sets that can be refined through fit testing with patients [5].

TABLE 10.1 A tool for the development of new surgical quality metrics

Relevance: Is it a meaningful measure that identifies potential for improvements?
Scientific soundness: Is it a scientifically valid, accurate, and reproducible measure? Is there clinical evidence to support its use? Can it provide a process–outcome link?
Feasibility: Is it fiscally and logistically workable? Can it be precisely specified and conducted within confidentiality parameters? Is it auditable?
Comprehensiveness: How extensive is the information yielded through the measure?
Quality metric: Survival, resolution of symptoms, and/or degree of recovery
1. Select a procedure
2. List the most common diagnoses that indicate that procedure

(continued)

TABLE 10.1 (continued)

3. Symptom burden: Describe the most common symptoms patients with those diagnoses present with

4. Life interference: Of the symptoms in #3, list 2–3 that are the most disabling to the patient (ability to eat, walk, work, care for self, care for others, enjoy life)

5. Circle the symptoms in #4 that improve/resolve with a "technically successful" procedure in more than 50% of cases

6. Write a metric that addresses one of the circled items

7. Define metric failure

Safety metric: Short-term complication (including readmission)

8. List the 3 most common 30-day surgical complications for the procedure	9. List the median complication grade that occurs with each complication: 5 – death; 4 – organ failure, ICU; 3 – rescue procedure (IR or OR); 2 – medical management at bedside; 1 – no specific intervention)	10. Multiply across, then circle the row with the highest number

First most common (5points)

Second most common (3 points)

Third most common (1 point)

11. Write a metric that addresses the circled item

12. Define metric failure

Safety metric: Long-term disutility

13. List the most common surgically induced disability present at 6–12 months postoperatively

14. Write a metric that addresses the item

15. Define metric failure

Aloia et al. [5]

Conclusion

The perfect surgical metric is likely unattainable. However, creating and defining metrics that matter is a worthwhile effort for surgeons to engage in. With ongoing external pressure for transparent reporting, ensuring surgical metrics are meaningful is of paramount importance. Surgical leadership in developing, specifying, and implementing new measures is crucial. As seen in both healthcare and non-healthcare applications, performance metrics have important consequences – they can reshape the game. A systematic and rigorous approach to metric development can provide assurance that any resultant changes are for the better.

References

1. Goldsberry K, Weiss E. The Dwight effect: a new ensemble of interior defense analytics for the NBA. Sports Aptitude, LLC Web 2013;1–11.
2. Franks A, Miller A, Bornn L, Goldsberry K. Counterpoints: advanced defensive metrics for nba basketball [Internet]. In: 9th annual MIT Sloan sports analytics conference, Boston, MA. lukebornn.com; 2015. Available from: http://www.lukebornn.com/papers/franks_ssac_2015.pdf.
3. Sampaio J, McGarry T, Calleja-González J, Jiménez Sáiz S, Schelling I Del Alcázar X, Balciunas M. Exploring game performance in the national basketball association using player tracking data. PLoS One. 2015;10(7):e0132894.
4. Verrier J. You can't stop NBA offenses—and now, you can't even Hope to contain them [Internet]. The Ringer. 2018 [cited 2020 Nov 29]. Available from: https://www.theringer.com/nba/2018/10/30/18038802/nba-defense-offensive-boom.
5. Aloia TA, Jackson T, Ghaferi A, Dort J, Schwarz E, Romanelli J. Developing minimally invasive procedure quality metrics: one step at a time. Surg Endosc. 2019;33(3):679–83.
6. Henry LR, von Holzen UW, Minarich MJ, et al. Quality measurement affecting surgical practice: utility versus utopia. Am J Surg. 2018;215(3):357–66.

7. Bodenheimer T, Sinsky C. From triple to quadruple aim: care of the patient requires care of the provider. Ann Fam Med. 2014;12(6):573–6.

8. Berwick D, Fox DM. "Evaluating the quality of medical care": Donabedian's classic article 50 years later. Milbank Q. 2016;94(2):237.

9. Birkmeyer JD, Dimick JB, Birkmeyer NJO. Measuring the quality of surgical care: structure, process, or outcomes? J Am Coll Surg. 2004;198(4):626–32.

10. Merkow RP, Bilimoria KY, Ko CY. Surgical quality measurement: an evolving science. JAMA Surg. 2013;148(7):586–7.

11. Tang PC, Ralston M, Arrigotti MF, Qureshi L, Graham J. Comparison of methodologies for calculating quality measures based on administrative data versus clinical data from an electronic health record system: implications for performance measures. J Am Med Inform Assoc. 2007;14(1):10–5.

12. Chan KS, Fowles JB, Weiner JP. Electronic health records and the reliability and validity of quality measures: a review of the literature. Med Care Res Rev. 2010;67(5):503–27.

13. Stey AM, Russell MM, Ko CY, Sacks GD, Dawes AJ, Gibbons MM. Clinical registries and quality measurement in surgery: a systematic review. Surgery. 2015;157(2):381–95.

14. Burstin H, Leatherman S, Goldmann D. The evolution of healthcare quality measurement in the United States. J Intern Med. 2016;279(2):154–9.

15. Elixhauser A, Pancholi M, Clancy CM. Using the AHRQ quality indicators to improve health care quality. Jt Comm J Qual Patient Saf. 2005;31(9):533–8.

16. Thomas EJ. The harms of promoting "Zero Harm". BMJ Qual Saf. 2020;29(1):4–6.

17. Aloia TA. Should zero harm be our goal? Ann Surg. 2020;271(1):33.

18. Shahian DM, Jacobs JP, Badhwar V, D'Agostino RS, Bavaria JE, Prager RL. Risk aversion and public reporting. Part 1: observations from cardiac surgery and interventional cardiology. Ann Thorac Surg. 2017;104(6):2093–101.

19. Marcus RK, Lillemoe HA, Caudle AS, et al. Facilitation of surgical innovation: is it possible to speed the introduction of new technology while simultaneously improving patient safety? Ann Surg. 2019;270(6):937–41.

20. Porter ME, Kaplan RS, Frigo ML. Managing healthcare costs and value. Strategic Finance [Internet]; 2017. Available from:

http://search.proquest.com/openview/0147acbebd6fb625f241bcf
9b3a60f77/1?pq-origsite=gscholar&cbl=48426.
21. Centers For Medicare & Medicaid Services. Blueprint for the CMS measures management system. 2017.
22. Conceptualization [Internet]. [cited 2020 Nov 27]. Available from: https://www.cms.gov/Medicare/Quality-Initiatives-Patient-Assessment-Instruments/MMS/MSP-Conceptualization.
23. Krishnan M, Brunelli SM, Maddux FW, et al. Guiding principles and checklist for population-based quality metrics. Clin J Am Soc Nephrol. 2014;9(6):1124–31.
24. McGlynn EA, Adams JL. What makes a good quality measure? JAMA. 2014;312(15):1517–8.
25. National Quality Forum Measure. Perioperative temperature management – national quality strategy domain: patient safety – meaningful measure area: preventable healthcare harm. Quality ID #424 (NQF 2681) [Internet] 2018. Available from: https://qpp.cms.gov/docs/QPP_quality_measure_specifications/CQM-Measures/2019_Measure_424_MIPSCQM.pdf.
26. Stulberg JJ, Delaney CP, Neuhauser DV, Aron DC, Fu P, Koroukian SM. Adherence to surgical care improvement project measures and the association with postoperative infections. JAMA. 2010;303(24):2479–85.
27. Fry DE. Surgical site infections and the surgical care improvement project (SCIP): evolution of national quality measures. Surg Infect. 2008;9(6):579–84.

Chapter 11
The Role of Surgical Societies in Quality

Benjamin J. Flink and Aurora D. Pryor

Surgical societies have a great ability to galvanize change and help ensure quality outcomes for our patients by leveraging both the knowledge of their members and disseminating guidance, education and knowledge to members to assist in reaching quality outcomes on a broader scale. In fact, the mission statement of SAGES directly addresses quality and is to "innovate, educate, and collaborate to improve patient care" [1] . There are four main ways that a surgical society can help to direct changes to improve the quality of care for surgical patients: (1) clinical guidelines for surgeons and medical professions, (2) direct education and/or certification of surgeons, (3) creation and funding of research and/or quality improvement infrastructure, and (4) education and outreach to non-medical professionals and lay people (Fig. 11.1).

For many, the obvious way that a surgical society can contribute to quality is in the form of clinical guidelines. There are a great multitude of guidelines in a vast number of specialties and subspecialties both in surgery and in the medical

B. J. Flink · A. D. Pryor (✉)
Stony Brook University Department of Surgery, Division of
Bariatric, Foregut, and Advanced Gastrointestinal Surgery,
Stony Brook, NY, USA
e-mail: Aurora.Pryor@stonybrookmedicine.edu

© The Author(s), under exclusive license to Springer Nature   195
Switzerland AG 2022
J. R. Romanelli et al. (eds.), *The SAGES Manual of Quality,
Outcomes and Patient Safety*,
https://doi.org/10.1007/978-3-030-94610-4_11

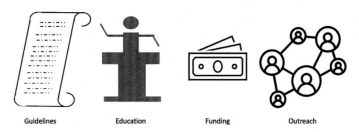

Guidelines   Education   Funding   Outreach

FIGURE 11.1 The roles of surgical societies in quality

realm. It is difficult for the average surgeon in practice to synthesize the broad scope of new literature and appropriately update their practice to deliver the most relevant evidence-based care. Society-based guidelines are an effective way to synthesize surgical literature into the most salient points for clinical practice.

Guidelines play an important role in helping to ensure quality outcomes for our patients through multiple avenues including a synthesis of research, expert opinion when data is limited, as well as providing a template that can be used for reproducing quality care. At their core, guidelines function in discouraging interventions and practices that are ineffective, while simultaneously encouraging those that are either proven or felt to be effective based on best available evidence or, at a minimum, expert opinion [2]. Therefore, guidelines are often an important step in defining what is a standard of care as well as, in some cases, what is a quality outcome.

The importance of society involvement with guidelines is magnified in surgical practice, as there are often many studies that are limited in level of evidence by study design. Often there is a lack of randomized control trials and studies may be retrospective in design or due to relatively rare diseases. In this situation, expert opinions available through a surgical society rise in importance of guideline development. Furthermore, housing the guidelines inside of a large organization such as a surgical society allows for rapid renewal of existing guidelines by utilizing its large group of experts.

While implementation of guidelines can vary, they play an increasingly prominent role in dissemination of best practice guidance from organizations such as SAGES to surgeons around the globe [3, 4]. This process can be expensive, and SAGES is implementing a standard operating procedure for guideline development that will maximize the quality and minimize the production expense of these guidelines [5]. In so doing, SAGES is focusing on a rigorous review of available evidence by volunteer surgeons on a given topic that allows for inclusion of randomized control trials, when available, but also using other sources of data in a regimented way allows for high-quality guidelines that seek to provide the best, unbiased evidence on a particular subject. What allows for the efficient and timely compilation of these guidelines is the connections and expertise that are contained within the SAGES leadership and members. Surgical societies in general are frequently involved with guidelines related to their area of clinical practice, and these play a large role in guiding the practice of surgical subspecialties with regard to what the standard of care is on a given disease process.

Direct education of surgeons and trainees is a very important role for surgical societies. These range from society meetings that help to share the most current research or relevant lectures to members to certifications such as Advanced Trauma Life Support (ATLS) from the American College of Surgeons (ACS) or the Fundamentals of Laparoscopic Surgery (FLS)/Fundamentals of Endoscopic Surgery (FES)/Fundamental Use of Surgical Energy (FUSE) programs that are administered through SAGES. These certifications allow for a formal testing of basic principles of surgical care as they pertain to ensuring mastery of foundational material in laparoscopic and endoscopic surgery. In so doing, they help to maintain a minimum quality standard with regard to the implementation of surgical technologies and skills. These tests also help form the basis of eligibility requirements for taking the American Board of Surgery examinations and are central to achieving and maintaining board certification.

Societies can also contribute to the spectrum of surgical education and certification in other unique ways. SAGES has already been intimately involved with the formation and maintenance of the Fellowship Council which supports fellowship training in several areas of GI surgery. SAGES has led the efforts for training in minimally invasive surgery and surgical endoscopy. SAGES has also recently partnered with the SSAT and ASMBS to lead a new fellowship designation in foregut surgery. These fellowships allow for more standardized training in advanced surgical techniques.

Recently, the American Board of Medical Specialties has recognized that there are distinct areas of clinical specialization beyond an initial certificate. Focused practice designations (FPDs) were first introduced by the American Board of Medical Specialties and "recogniz[e] the value that physicians who focus some or all their practice within a specific area of a specialty and/or subspecialty can provide to improving health care" [6]. FPDs will soon be offered through American Board of Surgery (ABS) for certified surgeons in specific clinical areas, such as bariatric surgery. For surgical FPDs, the ABS is working closely with specialty societies to develop the content and scope of these additional practice areas. These partnerships reinforce to role of societies in assuring quality surgical care.

With continuing education of surgeons outside of certification, society resources and meetings play a key role in allowing access to the most current research in a given field and allow access to the information as well as robust discussion among members and attendees at the given conference. There are also refresher courses and/or mini courses on specific procedures that are offered as part of or in parallel to a given meeting. One such example is the SAGES Master's Program, which is a set of educational programs that may be completed in person at the meeting or online to expand the knowledge and skills of a practicing surgeon. There are 12 domains offered by SAGES, which include acute care, biliary, bariatric, biliary, colorectal, flexible endoscopy, foregut, hernia, leadership and professional development, liver, pancreas, robotic surgery, and solid organ [7, 8]. The SAGES Master's Program is designed to provide a knowledge repository in these specific domains to help deal with the unpredictability that may be experienced in surgical training. This may also be a way to learn about a new approach to a familiar surgical disease or a way to re-familiarize with a procedure and perhaps learn the most recent innovations.

One way being investigated to further ensure surgical skills are verified by an external source that is being developed by SAGES and other surgical societies: video-based assessment (VBA). The essence of this process is to be able to review the operative abilities of a surgeon. VBA reviews have been shown to correlate with complications in a study performed with the Michigan Bariatric Surgery Collaborative [9]. By giving an impartial review of the skills of a surgeon, this can be used to asses competency of surgeons as a form of initial certification as well as allowing for a continuing certification aspect to ensure that a given surgeon is able to perform particular tasks with a certain predetermined proficiency. The VBAs in the Michigan Bariatric Surgery Collaborative also allowed for feedback to surgeons involved that were de-identified and gave each provider ways in which they would be able to further hone their surgical skills. Given that the surgical skills did associate with the outcomes of a given surgeon, such an assessment and concomitant feedback can serve as a powerful tool to help improve quality and safety of operations provided. Robust VBAs are being developed for each of the eight SAGES Master's Programs and will eventually be incorporated into the Master's Program itself as well as eventually becoming part of the educational offerings for residents like the Fundamentals (FLS, FES, FUSE) courses and certificates [10, 11]. VBA is likely also to become a part of the board certification process [12].

Societies may also engage in directed education programs to improve outcomes by producing educational materials for their members to augment the quality of care delivered by practicing surgeons. An example of a program run by SAGES is the Safe Cholecystectomy Program, which focuses on raising awareness and education surrounding avoidance of common bile duct injuries and other complications of laparoscopic cholecystectomy [13]. In focusing on the critical view of safety, discussing the steps needed to obtain it, as well as potential pitfalls and when additional help should be sought, the Safe Cholecystectomy Program directly attempts to tackle a significant comorbidity of a very common procedure performed in the general surgery arena.

Along with the flow of information from a society to its members, societies can create the data infrastructure needed to do research and quality improvement efforts at the society as well as individual investigator level. The most prominent example of data collection inside of a surgical society is the American College of Surgeons (ACS) National Surgical Quality Improvement Program (NSQIP) [14]. There have been thousands of publications that have been made possible through NSQIP data. NSQIP also allows for local use of more extensive data collected by NSQIP data abstractors that are not in the publicly available datasets to help individual hospitals and providers understand and improve their outcomes. In fact, the NSQIP database allows for the development of quality metrics to compare performance across geographic and demographic differences seen among hospitals. Instead of being only judged on meeting a specific metric, this helps to allow for comparison amongst hospitals for them to be able to know what areas could use improvement and ways in which they are already doing well.

There are many additional related databases such as the National Cancer Database and the Metabolic and Bariatric Surgery Accreditation and Quality Improvement Project (MBSAQIP) inside the ACS, the Society of Thoracic Surgeons' National Database, and the Society for Vascular Surgery's Vascular Quality Initiative. Each of these databases, amongst others, has led to the formation of quality metrics and a large body of health services research. These databases require considerable resources, expertise, and coordination that are made possible through partnership with the sponsoring societies. This very important source of quality improvement, risk-adjustment, and overall benchmarking would not be possible without these partnerships. Although the nucleus of this change is housed inside of the surgical society's given database, the information allows for individuals, hospitals, and healthcare organizations to take the lead in pushing and testing for change in the world of surgery. The ability to help individuals and organizations is further augmented through funding that a surgical society can provide to make specific investigations possible.

Even outside of the surgical community, a surgical society can be instrumental with improving surgical care by doing broader outreach to the community. A prime example of this is the Stop the Bleed program sponsored by the ACS. Stop the Bleed training has been shown to be effective in both retention of life-saving skills and knowledge among non-medical personnel around the world [15–17]. Specific societies also gain the power to be able to lobby on behalf of surgeons as a whole, helping to ensure that adequate financial reimbursement to allow for standard treatments to continue is given, as well as to help secure funding for programs that can provide grant funding or education. The collation of voices among the ACS Professional Association Political Action Committee allows for advocacy for surgeons as a whole on the national level. Without overall awareness and momentum outside of a relatively small population of surgeons, it would be difficult to ensure that individual voices would not simply be ignored.

In summary, the resources and knowledge collected by way of the members of a surgical society allow for the gathering of knowledge and resources that would not be available to an individual provider, hospital, or health system. It creates the opportunity to educate members, provide resources for members to improve their own practice, research the status quo, find ways to improve surgical practice as a whole, and define metrics that guide surgical practice. Furthermore, the gathering of surgeons' voices allows for discussion and advocacy for practices that can help to improve the interaction of surgeons within their communities and assist them in reaching their goal of helping their patients. Through the collective work and expertise of a board membership, each surgical society can play a pivotal role in quality improvement.

References

1. SAGES. About the Society of American Gastrointestinal and Endoscopic Surgeons. 2021 [cited 2021]. Available from: https://www.sages.org/about/.
2. Woolf SH, et al. Clinical guidelines: potential benefits, limitations, and harms of clinical guidelines. BMJ. 1999;318(7182):527–30.
3. Grimshaw JM, et al. Effectiveness and efficiency of guideline dissemination and implementation strategies. Health Technol Assess. 2004;8(6):iii–iv, 1–72.
4. Dirks RC, Walsh D, Haggerty S, Kohn GP, Pryor A, Stefanidis D. SAGES guidelines: an appraisal of their quality and value by SAGES members. Surg Endosc. 2021;35(4):1493–9.
5. Rogers AT, et al. Society of American Gastrointestinal and Endoscopic Surgeons (SAGES) guidelines development: standard operating procedure. Surg Endosc. 2021;35(6):2417–27.
6. Specialties, A.B.o.M. Focused practice designation. 2021 [cited 2021]. Available from: https://www.abms.org/board-certification/board-certification-requirements/focused-practice-designation/.
7. Jones DB, et al. SAGES University MASTERS program: a structured curriculum for deliberate, lifelong learning. Surg Endosc. 2017;31(8):3061–71.
8. SAGES. Masters program. 2021 [cited 2021]. Available from: https://www.sages.org/masters-program/.
9. Birkmeyer JD, et al. Surgical skill and complication rates after bariatric surgery. N Engl J Med. 2013;369(15):1434–42.
10. Feldman LS, et al. SAGES Video-Based Assessment (VBA) program: a vision for life-long learning for surgeons. Surg Endosc. 2020;34(8):3285–8.
11. Ritter EM, et al. Video-based assessment for laparoscopic fundoplication: initial development of a robust tool for operative performance assessment. Surg Endosc. 2020;34(7):3176–83.
12. https://www.absurgery.org/default.jsp?news_vba04.21. Accessed 15 Apr 2021.

13. SAGES. The SAGES safe cholecystectomy program. 2021 [cited 2021]. Available from: https://www.sages.org/safe-cholecystectomy-program/.
14. Surgeons, A.C.o. ACS national surgical quality improvement project. 2021 [cited 2021]. Available from: https://www.facs.org/Quality-Programs/ACS-NSQIP.
15. Pasley AM, et al. Stop the bleed: does the training work one month out? Am Surg. 2018;84(10):1635–8.
16. Valsecchi D, et al. The rise of the stop the bleed campaign in Italy. J Spec Oper Med. 2019;19(4):95–9.
17. Villegas CV, et al. Stop the bleed: effective training in need of improvement. J Surg Res. 2020;255:627–31.

Part II
Surgical Outcomes

Chapter 12
Perioperative Risk Assessment

Gina Adrales and Swathi Reddy

Introduction

A careful multidisciplinary approach to preoperative preparation is essential to ensure optimal patient outcomes. Determination of perioperative risk informs shared decision-making regarding the selection and timing of the surgical procedure and postoperative management. In this chapter, we will explore standards of care for preoperative testing and consultation and discuss methods of assessment of perioperative risk.

Delivery of High-Value Preoperative Care

Within the confines of a complex healthcare system, healthcare providers must seek equipoise between testing to identify risk and reduction of unnecessary studies to minimize cost and potential harm. An estimated $18 billion is spent annually in the USA on preoperative testing [1]. While some

G. Adrales (✉) · S. Reddy
Johns Hopkins University School of Medicine,
Baltimore, MD, USA
e-mail: gadrale1@jhmi.edu

© The Author(s), under exclusive license to Springer Nature   207
Switzerland AG 2022
J. R. Romanelli et al. (eds.), *The SAGES Manual of Quality,
Outcomes and Patient Safety*,
https://doi.org/10.1007/978-3-030-94610-4_12

of this expenditure undoubtedly prevents perioperative complications, a portion is wasted on studies that have no impact on surgical management or outcomes. The rate of unnecessary preoperative testing is reported to be 32–45% in various studies [2, 3]. There is a growing recognition that the enormity of healthcare costs in the USA is unsustainable. This has fueled a shift to eliminate low-value care, including a decrease in preoperative medical evaluation and testing.

Choosing Wisely is an initiative of the ABIM Foundation whose mission is to stimulate patient-clinician communication about healthcare that is evidence-based, necessary, and free from harm. This health education campaign is supported by numerous medical and surgical societies, including SAGES, to prevent overuse of treatment and eliminate nonessential or duplicative care. Included in this effort are recommendations to eliminate routine preoperative testing before low-risk surgical procedures, carotid artery disease screening prior to cardiac surgery in the absence of symptoms or comorbidities, and diagnostic cardiac testing in asymptomatic patients before low- to moderate-risk surgery. Such testing may not alter management but could result in delayed care, avoidable healthcare costs, and harm from additional testing.

A potential unforeseen consequence of a reduction of preoperative assessment is a lack of patient and family preparedness. Preoperative assessment entails more than laboratory, radiologic, and cardiac tests. Preoperative evaluation promotes patient education, collaborative anesthesiology and surgical intraoperative care, postoperative and home care plans, and assurance of perioperative tools to deliver individualized care such as management of the difficult airway. While efforts to reduce low-value preoperative testing may be successful, there may be unintended consequences such as surgical no-shows or cancellations due to lack of compliance with preanesthetic eating restrictions or medication cessation [4]. These factors must be considered, particularly in caring for socioeconomically disadvantaged or less educated patient groups.

Who Is at Risk? Methods of Assessment of Perioperative Risk

Evaluation of perioperative risk begins with a history and physical exam. Basic lab testing may be added to determine patients at risk for complications through validated scoring systems.

Preoperative Evaluation and Physical Exam

All surgery patients should first undergo a thorough history and physical exam. The history is essential in stratifying risk and uncovering barriers to care. This discussion should include a detailed history of comorbidities, particularly serious cardiac and pulmonary conditions and anesthetic complications. A history of chronic pain or addiction will guide the intraoperative anesthetic plan and postoperative multimodal pain management. Prior surgical procedures, both minimally invasive and open surgeries, as well as implants including mesh and orthopedic hardware will affect surgical planning, positioning, and assessment of intraoperative procedural risk. Relevant surgical operative notes should be obtained. Prior anesthetic records should be reviewed to determine if there is a history of difficult airway or prior intraoperative cardiopulmonary event. A thorough review of the patient's medication list is crucial and should include anticoagulants and antiplatelet agents, immunosuppressive drugs, and glycemic control agents. Special consideration and advisement should be given regarding cessation of sodium glucose cotransporter-2 inhibitors starting 3–4 days prior to surgery. Medication review often overlooks the use of herbal or vitamin supplements, which can be underreported by patients. Some supplements, such as omega-3 fish oil and ginger, can increase the risk for bleeding due to antiplatelet or thrombotic inhibition effects [5]. Medication modification should be discussed with the patient prior to scheduling surgery, and plans for anticoagulation bridging and postoperative resumption of medications should be formulated in partnership with the primary care provider.

The physical exam should begin with an assessment of overall well-being and collection of vital signs. Uncontrolled hypertension, tachycardia, or bradycardia should prompt evaluation by the patient's primary physician for medical optimization. The general appearance of a patient can be informative with regard to screening for frailty, mobility, and ability to participate in perioperative care. A standard exam should include auscultation of the heart and lungs as well as identification of prior surgical incisions, existing hernias, and skin infection that may affect abdominal surgery and surgical outcomes. Examination concerns specific to anesthesia would be an airway and neck assessment, which is used to ascertain intubation difficulty and risk of cardiopulmonary complication due to sleep apnea or acid reflux. Brief dental exam or history of poor dentition may indicate elevated risk at intubation and risk for infection, particularly after planned prosthetic mesh implants.

For the elective surgical patient, the preoperative evaluation should ideally occur early enough to allow for involvement of a multidisciplinary team including the anesthesiologist, primary care physician, and other subspecialists such as the patient's cardiologist and pulmonologist as needed. A dietician should be involved preoperatively in the case of malnourished, frail, or obese patients. All candidates should be initially evaluated by the primary care provider or a perioperative medical specialist, who will be involved in preoperative optimization of comorbidities as well as postoperative management [6].

Biochemical, Hematologic, and Nutritional Evaluation

Laboratory tests are indicated prior to procedures with higher risk for perioperative complications and in high-risk patients, including morbidly obese and diabetic patients.

Routine hemoglobin and hematocrit levels are recommended by the American Society of Anesthesiologists for patients of advanced age and those preparing for surgery associated with high risk of blood loss [7]. All geriatric patients should have a preoperative creatinine [8]. The need for additional studies, such as liver function panel and coagulation studies, should be directed by the history and physical findings and concern for comorbidities, such as cirrhosis.

We recommend obtaining a hemoglobin A1c in patients with a preexisting diagnosis of diabetes or prediabetes. Fasting glucose level is not recommended for asymptomatic patients [9]. Glycemic control in the diabetic patient is indicated to minimize the risks of infection and wound healing complications. Preoperative protein deficiency is associated with an increased risk of complications, including poor wound healing, and is present in up to 32% of bariatric surgery patients [10]. As such, a nutritional profile including albumin, iron, folate, ferritin, and a fasting lipid panel should be obtained [11]. However, for asymptomatic non-geriatric patients, routine nutrition laboratory testing is not recommended [9].

Surgery-Specific Factors

Surgical urgency is a major determinant of perioperative risk. Urgent or emergent status elevates the risk of complications compared to elective procedures [12]. The American College of Cardiology and American Heart Association define the following: (1) emergency surgery as threatened life or limb without intervention within 6 h, (2) urgent surgery as threatened life or limb without intervention within 24 h, (3) time-sensitive surgery as necessary within 1–6 weeks, and (4) elective surgery as a procedure that can be deferred for up to 1 year [13]. A thoughtful assessment of the risk of blood loss, hemodynamic effect and stress response, fluid requirements, and length of the surgical procedure is important in determining the risk of cardiac events. Surgical risk stratification is based on urgency and surgical type [14]. Breast and ophthalmology procedures are considered low-risk, whereas adrenalectomy and complex bowel surgery are considered high-risk surgeries that warrant assessment of patient functional capacity.

Pulmonary Complications

Postoperative pulmonary complications are a significant contributor to postoperative mortality and morbidity. Even a single mild pulmonary complication is associated with early mortality, ICU admission, and longer hospitalization among patients with American Society of Anesthesiologists (ASA) 3 status [15].

Procedural and patient factors influence the risk of pulmonary complications. Upper abdominal and thoracic procedures impart a decrease in functional residual capacity which can lead to atelectasis and pneumonia. The establishment of pneumoperitoneum is associated with increased peak airway pressures, hypercarbia, and acidosis. Age is an independent predictor of pulmonary complications [16]. All patients should be screened for smoking, as smokers are 1.7 times more likely than nonsmokers to have pulmonary complications and are at greater risk for postoperative general morbidity, wound complications, critical care admission, and neurologic complications [17]. Obstructive lung disease, pulmonary hypertension, and congestive heart failure increase the risk of pulmonary complications [18, 19]. The prevalence of obstructive sleep apnea (OSA) ranges from 35% to 60% in the morbidly obese. Severe undiagnosed obstructive sleep apnea is an independent risk factor for surgical complications [20]. Patients with uncontrolled or suspected obstructive sleep apnea should undergo sleep medicine evaluation with sleep study.

Cardiac Considerations

The American College of Cardiology and American Heart Association outlined an algorithm to assess the risk of a major cardiac adverse event in its 2014 guideline [21]. This includes a determination of the urgency of the surgery and clinical evaluation for acute coronary syndrome. A validated instrument to determine cardiac complication risk, such as the Revised Cardiac Risk Index (Table 12.1), is then applied. Alternatively, the surgical risk calculator by the American College of Surgeons (ACS) National Surgical Quality Improvement Program (NSQIP) is utilized. Patients at low risk (<1%) for a major cardiac adverse event do not need further diagnostic testing. Patients at increased risk with poor functional capacity (<4 Measurement of Exercise Tolerance Before Surgery METs) should undergo pharmacologic stress testing if it is expected that the results would change management. Additional cardiac testing is pursued based on the number of clinical risk factors present. Noninvasive cardiac testing is indicated for patients with one to two risk factors

TABLE 12.1 Revised cardiac risk index [21]

Clinical parameter	RCRI points
History of cerebrovascular disease	1
Diabetes mellitus requiring insulin	1
Serum creatinine >2 mg/dL	1
History of ischemic heart disease	1
High-risk surgery	1
Points	**Risk**
0	0.4%
1	0.9%
2	6.6%

who are undergoing intermediate risk procedures (1–5% risk of cardiac event) such as intraabdominal surgery [14]. Patients with functional capacity greater than 4 METs do not need additional testing.

The Canadian Cardiovascular Society Guidelines on perioperative cardiac risk assessment include the following strong recommendations [22]:

1. Measurement of brain natriuretic peptide (BNP) or N-terminal fragment of proBNP (NT-proBNP) in patients who are 65 years of age or older, are 45–64 years of age with significant cardiovascular disease, or have a Revised Cardiac Risk Index score ≥1
2. No preoperative resting echocardiography, coronary computed tomography angiography, exercise or cardiopulmonary exercise testing, or pharmacological stress echocardiography or radionuclide imaging to enhance perioperative cardiac risk estimation
3. No initiation or continuation of acetylsalicylic acid for the prevention of perioperative cardiac events, except in patients with a recent coronary artery stent or who will undergo carotid endarterectomy
4. Avoidance of α2 agonist or β-blocker initiation within 24 h before surgery
5. Withholding of angiotensin-converting enzyme inhibitor and angiotensin II receptor blocker starting 24 h before surgery
6. Smoking cessation before surgery
7. Daily measurement of troponin for 48–72 h after surgery in patients with an elevated NT-proBNP/BNP before surgery or if there is no NT-proBNP/BNP measurement before surgery, in those who have a Revised Cardiac Risk Index score ≥1, and in those aged 45–64 years with significant cardiovascular disease or aged 65 years or older
8. Initiation of long-term acetylsalicylic acid and statin therapy in patients who suffer myocardial injury/infarction after surgery

The management and timing of surgery in patients with cardiac stents is a frequently encountered issue. Elective surgery is contraindicated in patients with recent coronary stent placements within 6 months of placement due to the elevated risk of stent thrombosis. Timing of elective noncardiac surgery is partially dependent on the type of stent placed (bare metal versus drug-eluting stent) and whether cessation of antiplatelet agents is needed.

Special Considerations in Obese Patients

Obesity is an independent risk factor for cardiovascular disease, and as such, a routine electrocardiogram (ECG) and chest radiograph are recommended as well as a preoperative consultation with the anesthesiologist [6]. Obesity is a known risk factor for coronary artery disease, heart failure, cardiomyopathy, and arrhythmias. In fact, the mortality risk from heart disease is two to three times greater in a patient with a BMI greater than 35 kg/m^2 compared with a person of normal or lean BMI [23]. BMI >35 kg/m^2 is an independent risk factor for postoperative pneumonia, respiratory failure, and surgical site infection [24]. Although intraabdominal surgery is considered an intermediate risk procedure by the American Heart Association, all patients should initially be evaluated by ECG and a chest radiograph. This should be followed by stress testing in indicated patients. Traditional exercise stress testing may not be feasible in obese patients, and nuclear perfusion studies are similarly limited by body habitus. In most cases, pharmacologic stress echocardiography will be the effective alternative of choice [25].

Chronic Liver Disease

Cirrhosis is associated with an increased risk of perioperative morbidity and mortality [9]. MELD scores should be calculated for all cirrhotic patients to assess perioperative risk.

Patients with MELD score >10 are at higher risk for perioperative morbidity [26]. The risk of complications continues to
rise with rising MELD scores. The postoperative mortality
rate for patients with MELD scores of 15 or greater is substantial at over 50% [26].

Frailty

Frailty refers to a vulnerable subset of patients with diminished physical function and limited physiologic reserve. There
are two aspects of frailty, including phenotypic frailty and
deficit accumulation [27]. Phenotypic frailty refers to biologic
decline manifested by weight loss, fatigue, and weakness.
Index frailty or deficit accumulation is determined by an
assessment of comorbidities, weakness, and walking speed.
Frailty assessment tools are designed to identify patients at
risk for postoperative morbidity and mortality, longer hospitalization, and discharge to higher level of care. Preoperative
frailty assessment is recommended for older patients to allow
for more robust discussion with patients and their families
about perioperative risk and postoperative care needs.

Risk Assessment Tools

Over the last decade, multiple perioperative risk assessment
tools have been proposed for surgery patients to assist in risk
stratification. The American Society of Anesthesiologists
(ASA) Status (see Table 12.2) guides planning for intraoperative and postoperative monitoring and is commonly used to
stratify patients in outcomes research. The Revised Cardiac
Risk Index and Caprini Risk Assessment Model for venous
thromboembolism are utilized frequently to assess cardiovascular complication risk and to guide testing and prophylaxis
measures.

In 2013, the ACS published a surgical risk calculator
derived from the NSQIP data, the most robust surgical

TABLE 12.2 American Society of Anesthesiologists (ASA) classification

ASA I	Normal, healthy
ASA II	Mild systemic disease
ASA III	Severe systemic disease
ASA IV	Severe systemic disease that is constant threat to life
ASA V	Moribund patient not expected to survive without the operation
ASA VI	Brain-dead patient whose organs are being removed for donor purposes

outcomes program to date. This calculator estimates the risk of multiple complications within the 30-day postoperative period using 21 predictive variables (https://riskcalculator.facs.org) [28]. This risk calculator has been validated in multiple populations including geriatric patients, various cancer populations, and procedure-specific studies. Limitations of the ACS NSQIP Risk Calculator include that the model is derived from a limited set of 393 participating hospitals, which perform only about 30% of all surgeries in the USA. As such, it may not account for the variation in outcomes seen across all US hospitals. The accuracy of the tool is further dependent on coding and reporting accuracy at the individual institution level [29].

Current Standards of Care: Which Asymptomatic Patients Should Undergo Preoperative Testing and Consultation?

Pulmonary Assessment

In general, routine chest X-rays are not required for asymptomatic patients. Chest radiograph is recommended for patients with known cardiovascular and pulmonary disease; patients more than 50 years old who will have upper abdominal, thoracic, or abdominal aortic surgery; and patients with Class 3 obesity (BMI $\geq$ 40 kg/m^2) [16, 30]. Routine pulmonary function testing is not recommended.

Pulmonary and preoperative anesthesiology evaluation can be considered for patients with severe obesity, history of difficult intubation, elevated Mallampati score, and positive sleep apnea screening questionnaires. The STOP-Bang Questionnaire (see Table 12.3) and Berlin Questionnaire are commonly used [31, 32]. The Berlin Questionnaire calculates risk for sleep apnea based on snoring frequency and intensity, observed apnea during sleep, fatigue after sleep and during waking time, history of falling asleep while driving, and hypertension [32].

Cardiovascular Assessment

Electrocardiogram is recommended for patients with known cardiovascular disease or for patients to undergo higher-risk

TABLE 12.3 STOP-Bang Questionnaire for obstructive sleep apnea [31]

	No	Yes
Snore loudly?		1
Daytime fatigue?		1
Has anyone observed you stop breathing?		1
High blood pressure?		1
BMI $\geq$ 35 kg/m^2		1
Age > 50		1
Neck circumference (>43 cm in males, 41 cm in females)		1
Male sex		1

Low risk 0–2, intermediate 3–4, high risk 5–8 (or >2 and male or BMI > 35 kg/m^2)

surgical procedures, regardless of symptoms. Routine ECG or echocardiogram is not indicated for asymptomatic patients preparing for low-risk surgeries. Stress testing is reserved for higher-risk patients with poor functional capacity (<4 METs).

Conclusion

Identification of patients at risk for perioperative cardiopulmonary complications through careful history and examination and validated risk indices is imperative in the delivery of high-value care. Adherence to standards for selective preoperative testing and consultations reduces cost without the expense of increased mortality or morbidity. For certain patient populations, preoperative evaluation by primary care or anesthesiology providers remains a vital means to deliver patient education, manage expectations, and optimize modifiable perioperative risk factors. This may be particularly important in safety-net hospitals and for frail and socioeconomically disadvantaged patients.

References

1. Benarroch-Gampel J, Sheffield KM, Duncan CB, et al. Preoperative laboratory testing in patients undergoing elective, low-risk ambulatory surgery. Ann Surg. 2012;256:518–28.
2. Beloeil H, Richard D, Drewniak N, Molliex S. Overuse of preoperative laboratory coagulation testing and ABO blood typing: a French national study. Br J Anesth. 2017;119(6):1186–93.
3. Matulis J, Lui S, Mecchella J, North F, Holmes A. Choosing wisely: a quality improvement initiative to decrease unnecessary preoperative testing. BMJ Qual Improv Rep. 2017;6(1):1–5.
4. Mafi JN, Godoy-Travieso P, Wei E, Anders M, Amaya R, Carrillo CA, Berry JL, Sarff L, Daskivich L, Vanala S, Ladapo J, Keeler E, Damberg CL, Sarkisian C. Evaluation of an intervention to reduce low-value preoperative care for patients undergoing cataract surgery at a safety-net health system. JAMA Intern Med. 2019;179(5):648–57.

5. Levy I, Attias S, Ben-Arye E, Goldstein L, Matter I, Somri M, Schiff E. Perioperative risks of dietary and herbal supplements. World J Surg. 2017;41(4):927–34.

6. Eldar S, Heneghan HM, Brethauer S, Schauer PR. A focus on surgical preoperative evaluation of the bariatric patient--the Cleveland Clinic protocol and review of the literature. Surgeon. 2011;9(5):273–7.

7. Apfelbaum JL, Connis RT, Nickinovich DG, et al. Practice advisory for preanesthesia evaluation: an updated report by the American Society of Anesthesiologists Task Force on Preanesthesia Evaluation. Anesthesiology. 2012;116(3):522–38.

8. Chow WB, Rosenthal RA, Merkow RP, et al. Optimal preoperative assessment of the geriatric surgical patient: a best practices guideline from the American College of Surgeons National Surgical Quality Improvement Program and the American Geriatrics Society. J Am Coll Surg. 2012;215(4):453–66.

9. Bierle DM, Raslau D, Regan DW, Sundsted KK, Mauck KF. Preoperative evaluation before non cardiac surgery. Mayo Clin Proc. 2020;95(4):807–22.

10. Major P, Malczak P, Wysocki M, Torbicz G, Gajewska N, Pedziwiatr M, et al. Bariatric patients' nutritional status as a risk factor for postoperative complications, prolonged length of hospital stay and hospital readmission: a retrospective cohort study. Int J Surg. 2018;56:210–4.

11. Parrott J, Frank L, Rabena R, Craggs-Dino L, Isom KA, Greiman L. American Society for Metabolic and Bariatric Surgery integrated health nutritional guidelines for the surgical weight loss patient 2016 update: micronutrients. Surg Obes Relat Dis. 2017;13(5):727–41.

12. Bilimoria KY, Liu Y, Paruch JL, et al. Development and evaluation of the universal ACS NSQIP surgical risk calculator: a decision aid and informed consent tool for patients and surgeons. J Am Coll Surg. 2013;217(5):833–42.e1–e3.

13. Fleisher LA, Fleischmann KE, Auerbach AD, et al. 2014 ACC/AHA guideline on perioperative cardiovascular evaluation and management of patients undergoing noncardiac surgery: executive summary: a report of the American College of Cardiology/American Heart Association Task Force on Practice Guidelines. Circulation. 2014;130(24):2215–45.

14. Raslau D, Bierle DM, Stephenson CR, Mikhail MA, Kebede EB, Mauck KF. Preoperative cardiac risk assessment. Mayo Clin Proc. 2020;95(5):1064–79.

15. Fernandez-Bustamante A, Frendl G, Sprung J, Kor DJ, Subramaniam B, Martinez Ruiz R, Lee JW, Henderson WG, Moss A, Mehdiratta N, Colwell MM, Bartels K, Kolodzie K, Giquel J, Vidal Melo MF. Postoperative pulmonary complications, early mortality, and hospital stay following noncardiothoracic surgery: a multicenter study by the perioperative research network investigators. JAMA Surg. 2017;152(2):157.

16. Smetana GW, Lawrence VA, Cornell JE, American College of Physicians. Preoperative pulmonary risk stratification for noncardiothoracic surgery: systematic review for the American College of Physicians. Ann Intern Med. 2006;144(8):581.

17. Grønkjær M, Eliasen M, Skov-Ettrup LS, Tolstrup JS, Christiansen AH, Mikkelsen SS, Becker U, Flensborg-Madsen T. Preoperative smoking status and postoperative complications: a systematic review and meta-analysis. Ann Surg. 2014;259(1):52–71.

18. Gupta H, Ramanan B, Gupta PK, Fang X, Polich A, Modrykamien A, Schuller D, Morrow LE. Impact of COPD on postoperative outcomes: results from a national database. Chest. 2013;143(6):1599–606.

19. Meyer S, McLaughlin VV, Seyfarth HJ, Bull TM, Vizza CD, Gomberg-Maitland M, Preston IR, Barberà JA, Hassoun PM, Halank M, Jaïs X, Nickel N, Hoeper MM, Humbert M. Outcomes of noncardiac, nonobstetric surgery in patients with PAH: an international prospective survey. Eur Respir J. 2013;41(6):1302–7.

20. Abdelsattar ZM, Hendren S, Wong SL, Campbell DA Jr, Ramachandran SK. The impact of untreated obstructive sleep apnea on cardiopulmonary complications in general and vascular surgery: a cohort study. Sleep. 2015;38(8):1205.

21. Lee TH, Marcantonio ER, Mangione CM, Thomas EJ, Polanczyk CA, Cook EF, et al. Derivation and prospective validation of a simple index for prediction of cardiac risk of major noncardiac surgery. Circulation. 1999;100(10):1043–9.

22. Duceppe E, Parlow J, MacDonald P, Lyons K, McMullen M, Srinatan S, Graham M, Tandon V, Styles K, Bessissow A, Sessler DI, Bryson G, Devereaux PJ. Canadian cardiovascular society guidelines on perioperative cardiac risk assessment and management for patients who undergo noncardiac. Surg Can J Cardiol. 2017;33(1):17–32.

23. Zalesin KC, Franklin BA, Miller WM, Peterson ED, McCullough PA. Impact of obesity on cardiovascular disease. Med Clin North Am. 2011;95(5):919–37.

24. Valentijn TM, Galal W, Hoeks SE, van Gestel YR, Verhagen HJ, Stolker RJ. Impact of obesity on postoperative and long-term outcomes in a general surgery population: a retrospective cohort study. World J Surg. 2013;37(11):2561–8.

25. Supariwala A, Makani H, Kahan J, Pierce M, Bajwa F, Dukkipati SS, Teixeira J, Chaudhry FA. Feasibility and prognostic value of stress echocardiography in obese, morbidly obese, and super obese patients referred for bariatric surgery. Echocardiography. 2014;31(7):879–85.

26. Hanje AJ, Patel T. Preoperative evaluation of patients with liver disease. Nat Clin Pract Gastroenterol Hepatol. 2007;4(5):266–76.

27. Darrell JN, Gregorevic KJ, Story DA, Hubbard RE, Lim WK. Frailty indexes in perioperative and critical care: a systematic review. Arch Gerontol Geriatr. 2018;79:88–96.

28. Bilimoria KY, Liu Y, Paruch JL, Zhou L, Kmiecik TE, Ko CY, et al. Development and evaluation of the universal ACS NSQIP surgical risk calculator: a decision aid and informed consent tool for patients and surgeons. J Am Coll Surg. 2013;217(5):833–42. e1–3.

29. Keller DS, Ho JW, Mercadel AJ, Ogola GO, Steele SR. Are we taking a risk with risk assessment tools? Evaluating the relationship between NSQIP and the ACS risk calculator in colorectal surgery. Am J Surg. 2018;216(4):645–51.

30. Poirier P, Alpert MA, Fleisher L, et al. Cardiovascular evaluation and management of severely obese patients undergoing surgery: a science advisory from the American Heart Association. Circulation. 2009;120(1):86–95.

31. Chung F, Abdullah HR, Liao P. STOP-bang questionnaire: a practical approach to screen for obstructive sleep apnea. Chest. 2016;149:631.

32. Netzer NC, Stoohs RA, Netzer CM, Clark K, Strohl KP. Using the Berlin Questionnaire to identify patients at risk for the sleep apnea syndrome. Ann Intern Med. 1999;131(7):485–91.

Chapter 13
The Current State of Surgical Outcome Measurement

Brian J. Nasca, Jonah J. Stulberg, Marylise Boutros, and Jeongyoon Moon

The Objectives for This Chapter Are as Follows

1. Review the current tools utilized to measure surgical outcomes.
2. How should surgeons interpret current surgical outcome measures?

B. J. Nasca
Northwestern University Feinberg School of Medicine,
Chicago, IL, USA
e-mail: brian.nasca@northwestern.edu

J. J. Stulberg
The University of Texas Health Science Center at Houston,
Houston, TX, USA

M. Boutros (✉) · J. Moon
Division of Colon and Rectal Surgery, Sir Mortimer B. Davis Jewish
General Hospital, Montreal, QC, Canada
e-mail: marylise.boutros@mcgill.ca;
jeongyoon.moon@mail.mcgill.ca

© The Author(s), under exclusive license to Springer Nature   223
Switzerland AG 2022
J. R. Romanelli et al. (eds.), *The SAGES Manual of Quality,
Outcomes and Patient Safety*,
https://doi.org/10.1007/978-3-030-94610-4_13

Introduction

Health services research has rapidly expanded in the past decade, particularly in surgery, with increasing focus on providing high-quality, cost-effective care aimed to improve patients' satisfaction and quality of life (QoL). Health services research in the field of surgery is referred to as surgical outcomes research. The following definition provides a clear description of the nature and purpose of health services research: "Health services research examines how people get access to health care, how much care costs, and what happens to patients as a result of this care. The main goals of health services research are to identify the most effective ways to organize, manage, finance, and deliver high quality care, reduce medical errors, and improve patient safety" [1].

Codman's unrelenting focus on the "end results" of a surgical episode was a call to surgical accountability that has grown into a vast field of surgical outcome measurement [2]. We now have a diverse set of methods and mechanisms for collecting and analyzing surgical outcomes and surgical quality of care. The collective effort to improve drives us to achieve better outcomes for patients, and it is critical that we understand the potential as well as the potential pitfalls of the available data sources. In today's world of "big data," patient outcomes are more accessible to researchers, and when used correctly several new options now exist to study patient outcomes across large databases to determine what factors or techniques produce better outcomes. The ever-enlarging body of literature has great potential, and we will explore the benefits and downfalls of large databases, how those databases are created, how to interpret the findings when they are used, and what to expect in the future from outcomes research. The ultimate goal is to improve overall knowledge to achieve better patient care.

Measuring Surgical Outcomes for Improvement

Federal initiatives driven by the Patient Protection and Affordable Care Act of 2010 require hospitals to demonstrate that they provide high-quality care in order to receive proper compensation, reflecting a shift from quantity- to quality-driven care. In 2012, the Center for Medicare and Medicaid Services (CMMS) launched the Hospital Readmission Reduction Program that incurs reimbursement penalties to hospitals for having higher than expected readmission rates, specifically focusing on Medicare beneficiaries who are over 65 years of age with specific medical conditions and those who underwent coronary artery bypass graft surgery, elective primary total hip arthroplasty, or total knee arthroplasty [3]. Such policy changes at the national level have spurred growing interest in strategies that optimize quality of care, with a special focus on decreasing readmissions and complications among surgical patients.

The ultimate goal of surgical outcomes research is to identify areas in need of improvement and implement specific changes that lead to better quality of care for patients. In order to successfully plan and adopt such change, it is essential to be able to critically evaluate the current care that is being provided, as "we cannot improve what we cannot measure." Donabedian provided a framework for health services research in a landmark paper in 1966, which defined three different elements used to measure quality of care: structure, process, and outcomes [4].

First, *structure* refers to the setting and workforce that compose the healthcare delivery system. Examples relevant to surgical care include fellowship training of surgeons, nurse-to-patient ratio, and case volume. Information on structural components is easily accessible and measurable. However, it is not an accurate proxy for quality and is often fixed and therefore difficult for healthcare providers to act upon.

Second, *process* refers to how care is delivered and, more specifically, care pathways that apply to a large number of patients. Examples include postoperative enhanced recovery protocols and adherence to cancer screening guidelines. Many process measures in surgery are reported and monitored at the national level by the Surgical Care Improvement Project, which was created to reduce important perioperative morbidities, such as surgical site infection, adverse cardiac events, and venous thromboembolism, by setting national standards of best practices in surgery. Process measures reflect the care that patients actually receive and therefore are great targets for quality improvement initiatives. Measuring and reporting of process measures has been associated with significant decrease in perioperative complications among surgical patients [5, 6]. A major limitation is that many of the known processes relate to surgical outcomes that are rare or may not carry significant importance from the patient's perspective.

Third, *outcome* measures reflect the totality of care provided by the healthcare system on the patient. Given that outcome measures focus on the experience of the patient and represents the bottom line of patient care, it is ultimately the most important measure to improve. Traditionally, outcome measures that were the main focus of surgical research were objective measures such as perioperative mortality, morbidity, length of stay, readmission and complication rates, and cost of hospitalization. More recently, there has been a growing interest in subjective outcome measures such as patient satisfaction, as well as patient-reported QoL and functional status.

A major challenge in interpreting and utilizing outcome measures lies in identifying which component(s) of care is (are) most responsible for a poor outcome and how it can be targeted for change. Often, causes of poor outcomes are complex and multifactorial and therefore require multidisciplinary action. Another important challenge is that many surgical outcomes are rare, including adverse events such as postoperative mortality and major morbidity. At a single institution level, insufficient event rates or number of total cases can preclude reliable representation of outcomes or robust analyses to identify possible predictors of this poor outcome [7, 8]. Large scale data collection involving multiple institutions to aggregate and compare outcomes could overcome this important limitation. However, to perform adequate risk adjustments between different care providers, it is important to collect detailed clinical data, which requires significant resources [9]. The American College of Surgeons (ACS)-National Surgical Quality Improvement Project (NSQIP), which is the largest ongoing, national-level initiative aimed at measuring and reporting surgical outcomes, collects more than 80 patient variables for this purpose [10].

Large Nationwide Standardized Databases

Since its founding in 1913, the American College of Surgeons (ACS) has strived to improve surgical quality of care. They formed the Hospital Standardization Program which is now known as the Joint Commission [11]. This program developed a "minimum standard" for accreditation of hospitals. Eventually they improved standards to be an "optimal achievable" level of care [11]. Along the journey of the ACS, they formed the Commission on Cancer (CoC) in 1922 and the Committee on Trauma in 1950 (Quality Programs). The basis of the Veteran's Affairs Surgical Quality Improvement Program (VASQIP) came into being as part of a 1986 mandate by Congress [12]. The Veterans Health Administration completed the National VA Surgical Risk Study from 1991 to 1993 with the aim of developing and validating risk adjustment models for surgical outcomes. With the success and validation of those methods, the Veterans Affairs National Surgical Quality Improvement Program (VASQIP) was founded in 1994 [13].

VASQIP examines 30-day postoperative mortality and morbidity of VA patients collected by examining CPT codes and entered by trained staff. VASQIP does collect unique hospital identifying information that can be used by VA Research and Quality Improvement staff. Key variables examined are mortality, reoperation within 30 days, readmission, and length of stay. Patient outcomes are collected using a systematic sampling of the cases performed at each institution to represent hospital quality. One limitation in the generalizability of VASQIP data is that while the VA Health System serves over 19 million veterans at nearly 2000 facilities, only 10% of veterans are female [12]. This leads to an unbalanced demographic which may limit the generalizability of findings outside of the VA [14].

More recently, the ACS brought the Veteran's Affairs (VA) Surgical Quality Improvement Program (VASQIP) to the private side of healthcare forming the National Surgical Quality Improvement Program (NSQIP) [13]. The ACS has also started credentialing programs for specific disease management like the National Accreditation Program for Breast Cancers (NAPBC) and the Metabolic and Bariatric Surgery Accreditation and Quality Improvement Program (MBSAQIP).

The ACS-NSQIP database began as an effort initiated by the VA health system researchers and clinicians in the late 1980s in response to reports of high complication rates in VA hospitals [15]. Following demonstration of feasibility and potential benefit of collecting and reporting surgical outcomes and associated clinical variables through pilot trials in the VAs and interested non-VA hospitals, the ACS took the lead to expand the initiative to a broader group of hospitals in the USA in 2004 [16, 17]. As of the time of publication of this chapter, there are approximately 700 hospitals participating in and contributing to the ACS-NSQIP database. The ACS-NSQIP is a nationally validated, risk-adjusted, outcome-based clinical registry designed to measure and improve the quality of surgical care. It uses a prospective, peer-controlled, validated database to quantify 30-day, risk-adjusted surgical outcomes, which provide a valid comparison of outcomes among all hospitals in the program [18]. ACS-NSQIP features regular feedback to participating sites, where a semiannual report of the hospital's actual versus risk-adjusted expected mortality and various morbidities is presented by procedure type. Site performance is graded as being worse than expected or better than expected, taking into account various confounding factors, such as hospital structure and surgical case complexity, through risk adjustment modeling [19]. ACS-NSQIP uses trained personnel to collect clinical data, but not administrative billing data. These individuals receive extensive training on the data collection process, have clinical backgrounds (typically nursing), and are regularly audited to assure a very high level of consistency to data reporting. Data are available for analysis by researchers, but hospital identifiers are removed to allow for anonymity across hospitals. ACS-NSQIP developed a risk calculator in 2013 in order to help assess and support surgeon and patient decisions on operations based on empirical data derived from their database.

Another important set of clinical registries are those that focus on cancer outcomes, which take a more longitudinal and comprehensive approach to their data collection methodology. The ACS CoC is a consortium of over 1500 programs with the goal of improving survival and quality of life for cancer patients. They release guidelines and standards to ensure quality care and conduct surveys to assess compliance with their standards. Standardized data collection from CoC-accredited healthcare centers is used to measure quality, outcomes, and treatment patterns. That data is fed into the National Cancer Database (NCDB), which compiles clinical data into quarterly reports for all CoC facilities and has hospital benchmark reports and a Cancer Quality Improvement Program (CQIP) database that includes short-term and longitudinal data released annually. Access to the NCDB, CoC, and CQIP can be applied for, but you must be affiliated with an institution that is a member of a CoC-accredited program to be eligible for access.

Use of a Large National Database for Continuous Evaluation of Quality in Surgical Care

Numerous studies have shown that participation in the ACS-NSQIP is associated with longitudinal improvement in postoperative mortality and morbidity, even without specific efforts taken to improve outcome (so called "Hawthorne effect") [20–22]. However, high-quality studies comparing results for ACS-NSQIP participant and nonparticipant hospitals revealed no significant difference in mortality and complication rates [23, 24]. Although all hospitals demonstrated significant improvement in measured surgical outcomes across time, there was no specific difference in the rate of improvement between ACS-NSQIP participating and nonparticipating sites after rigorous matching of two groups and robust risk adjustment measures [24].

The most important limitation of any outcome-based quality improvement program is that measuring the end results does not necessarily provide answers to improving outcomes. Equivalent or even greater effort is required to identify and implement changes to components of the healthcare system that could potentially improve outcomes. Going back to the more upstream elements of the Donabedian framework, changes may need to happen at multiple levels of structure and process to improve a particular outcome. For example, what could be done to address surgical site infections (SSI)? Perhaps we need to evaluate the existing preoperative, intraoperative, and postoperative care for surgical patients. Are patients managed with evidence-based practices perioperatively in order to effectively reduce SSI (Process)? Would a preoperative SSI checklist help to mitigate SSI (Structure)? Surgical care bundles that include evidence-based, multidisciplinary interventions effectively reduced the rate of SSIs across multiple settings and patient populations [25, 26]. While specific interventions vary between bundles, the bundle approach itself, implementing changes at both the process and structure level with continuous monitoring of outcomes, is believed to drive the improvement in quality of care [25]. Furthermore, in order to implement and sustain these changes in practice, responsible stakeholders including surgeons, allied healthcare professionals, and policy makers must be engaged at multiple levels.

Clinical Registries

Clinical registries are the bedrock of surgical outcomes research and make up the single greatest resource for quality improvement and surgical outcomes researchers in the USA [27]. This category encompasses everything from individual surgeon repositories where surgeons collect and record their own surgical outcomes in a personalized database all the way up to large nationally representative registries that use complex sampling methodology and certified external chart reviewers to estimate quality of care at the hospital level. There are two critical components that determine our confidence in findings derived from clinical registries: blinded (versus unblinded) data collection and objective (versus subjective) standardization of outcomes. When a surgeon is collecting her/his own outcomes, there is an inherent desire to underreport unwanted outcomes (e.g., surgical site infection) [28]. The degree to which this affects the outcome of interest will vary by surgeon, by outcome, and over time, but it is inherent to self-reported datasets and should be a consideration when interpreting any results published from self-reported data. Blinding the data collection process from the surgeon/researcher is a critical element of overcoming our own inherent biases and should be considered whenever possible in the design of quality improvement and research efforts focused on improving surgical outcomes. The second critical element is how a dataset defines a given outcome. As an example, several nicely designed research studies have demonstrated disagreement among surgeons on the definition of a surgical site infection when presented with subjective measures in case scenarios. Therefore, the objective components and strict cutoffs for a given outcome definition are critical to assuring comparison across studies or even across groups within a study when data collection is not centralized. For example, if one institution decides that all patients who require the removal of at least one skin staple to allow for drainage constitutes an infection and another institution requires positive cultures, the dataset will have markedly different surgical site infection rates that do not necessarily reflect differences in the underlying patient outcomes. Therefore, uniform definitions which rely entirely on objective criteria (e.g., white blood cell count, positive cultures, temperature cutoffs) will yield the most consistent results across study populations and are a core principle of most large, national patient registries.

Administrative Registries

Administrative registries compile the administrative and billing records across multiple hospitals and then make the data available for assessment of patient outcomes. The largest administrative registries are the Center for Medicare and Medicaid Services (CMS) administrative claims databases. These are composed of healthcare utilization data derived from reimbursement/claims data and enrollment data from either Medicare- or Medicaid-eligible patients across the USA. CMS data includes demographic information, admission/discharge date, diagnoses, and procedure data as collected for administrative and billing purposes of the hospitals. While this offers enormous potential for surgical outcomes researchers, it is important to recognize the data was collected for operational purposes and not specifically for outcome measurement. Many researchers have therefore demonstrated the systematic underreporting of adverse outcomes such as surgical site infections or deep vein thromboses [29]. Additionally, risk adjustment methods based on comorbidities will be at the mercy of accurate comorbidity documentation within the billing records. Therefore, comorbidities directly linked to increased reimbursement are likely to be much more reliably recorded than those that are not tied to increased reimbursement. This is a critical point to consider when interpreting the results of studies based on administrative databases, as certain research questions will be profoundly affected while others will have this effect normalized across groups. With 98% of persons over 65 enrolled in Medicare, CMS administrative records are a rich dataset with significant value despite their limitations.

Patient Safety Indicators

In 1989 the Agency for Healthcare Research and Quality (AHRQ) was founded as part of the US government's Department of Health and Human Services. Its goal was to improve healthcare through funding and facilitation of research. Following the seminal publication of the Institute of Medicine's "To Err is Human," the AHRQ was given a three-fold task:

1. Identify the causes of preventable healthcare errors and patient injury in healthcare delivery.
2. Develop, demonstrate, and evaluate strategies for reducing errors and improving patient safety.
3. Disseminate such effective strategies throughout the healthcare industry.

From the research funded by over 200 grants awarded by the AHRQ to investigate improving patient safety, AHRQ developed measures to identify patient safety issues to target quality improvement efforts at the institutional level. CMS currently uses 27 indicators developed by AHRQ in order to create an institutional and provider level score for outcomes. Collectively, these are referred to as the Patient Safety Indicators (PSIs).

The reports show the calculated rates of potential in-hospital complications and adverse events following surgeries, procedures, and childbirth utilizing administrative data. As discussed above, administrative data is significantly influenced by the quality and thoroughness of clinical documentation, and this has led to debates over the nuances of better documentation versus the phenomenon of upcoding. Administrative records also do not account for technical considerations of a surgical case and therefore underrepresent issues of case complexity.

Survey Instruments for Outcomes Assessment

Patient-Reported Outcomes

The FDA defines patient-reported outcomes (PROs) as "any aspect of a patient's health status that comes directly from the patient (i.e., without the interpretation of the patient's responses by a physician or anyone else) [30, 31]." PROs were first developed in 1963 with the advent of Health-Related Quality of Life (HRQL) measures, but they played a limited role in medical care until more recently. PROs have become increasingly popular, and they contribute significantly to the approval process for pharmaceutical drugs, and almost 30% of clinical trials between 2007 and 2013 included PROs [32]. As PROs become more standardized, they will likely continue to increase in significance in the future [32]. One limitation of PROs is that they have issues with standardization and generalization across diseases and interventions [30, 31, 33], and this in part has limited their routine integration into surgical care.

Patient-Reported Outcome Measurement System

In an attempt to standardize patient-reported outcomes, US scientists from multiple institutions and representatives from the National Institutes of Health (NIH) formed a group with the goal to "develop and evaluate, for the clinical research community, a set of publicly available, efficient, and flexible measurements of PROs, including HRQL" [30, 31]. They produced Patient-Reported Outcome Measurement System (PROMIS), which established a national resource for measurement of patient-reported function, symptoms, and HRQL in a precise and efficient manner that could be applied to a broad disease and condition set. This made PROs much easier to measure for researchers. PROMIS has five main domains: pain, fatigue, emotional distress, physical function, and social function. These domains were developed through a large study of 11 databases to evaluate how each domain fit with already-published patient-reported data [30, 31]. Each domain is tied to a questionnaire with strong correlation to well-established questionnaires like the SF-36, and they have long and short forms [30, 31].

Press Ganey Surveys

In 1984, Drs. Press and Ganey created a validated survey with the goal of improving quality, safety, and cost of care. The survey integrates Hospital Consumer Assessment of Healthcare Providers (HCAHP) survey questions with their questions. The Press Ganey and HCAHP questions rely heavily on patient satisfaction for things like nursing care and have led to changes to improve patient satisfaction [34]. Their impact on the quality of medical care has been called into question because some practitioners believe hospitals are spending a greater time increasing patient satisfaction instead of increasing quality of care [34]. The hospital-level indicators are not necessarily indicative of hospital outcomes.

Use of Patient-Reported Outcome Measures (PROMs) to Evaluate Surgical Outcomes

The majority of past surgical outcomes research focused on quantifiable measures, such as mortality, complication rates, and length of stay [35]. However, these outcomes may not be the most meaningful to patients and may not be aligned with their priorities. Recovery after surgery is a dynamic and multifactorial process, with the patient as the primary stakeholder [36]. Therefore, it is essential to incorporate patients' perspective and subjective experience into surgical outcomes research [37]. Advantages of PROMs include assessment of various aspects of health, including physical and psychosocial domains, from the patients' perspective [36]; the ability to track the recovery process in the short- and long-term period; and empowering patients to manage their own health and make well-informed treatment decisions that align with their values [38]. Disadvantages of PROMs are that they are hard to measure, are largely subjective and thus hard to make meaningful statistical analysis on their results, and are needed to be kept in databases that are both costly to maintain and labor intensive.

There is important discordance between traditional objective measures of surgical outcomes and patients' lived experience following surgery, as measured by PROMs. For instance, avoiding severe breast symptoms following breast cancer surgery was a more important indicator of quality of care over increased disease-free survival, especially for older age groups [39]. Enhanced recovery after surgery (ERAS) protocols, which have been associated with better objective outcomes like shorter length of stay and decreased complication rates, have not been associated with similar improvement in patient-reported QoL, with report of increased emotional distress among ERAS patients [40, 41]. To evaluate patients' experience following surgery, surgical clinical trials have increasingly adopted PROMs as primary outcomes in addition to standard, clinically oriented outcomes [42].

The field of PROMs has further evolved with recent publication of official guidance regarding their use in evaluating and labeling of medical products by the US Food and Drug Administration (FDA) and the European Medicines Agency (EMA) [43, 44]. Development of PROMs is a rigorous and protocol-driven process, where measures are evaluated for essential properties that include the following [45]:

1. *Reliability*: the degree to which instrument is free of measurement error, as reflected by its ability to produce the same result on repeated measurement for the same outcome level [46].
2. *Validity*: how well the instrument measures the outcome it is intended to measure [47]. There are different measures of validity, including *content validity* (extent to which items of PROM questionnaire reflect the most important aspects of outcome of interest in a given setting) [48], *construct validity* (degree to which PROM relates to other existing measures in a way that is consistent with a priori theoretical hypotheses) [47], and *criterion validity* (how adequately the PROM reflects the existing gold standard) [49].
3. *Responsiveness* (i.e., sensitivity to change): degree to which PROM can detect changes in outcome being measured over time [50].
4. *Practicality*: time, cost, and effort required to administer, score, and interpret PROMs [51].
5. *Interpretability of scores*: ability to assign relevant and understandable meaning to PROM score [46].

Systematic reviews of existing PROMs on recovery following thoracic and abdominal surgery demonstrated a lack of PROMs with sound measurement properties, signaling the need for the development of higher-quality PROMs [37, 42, 52]. Psychometrically robust PROMs should be used in conjunction with clinical outcomes to further drive patient-centered research and improvement in quality of surgical care.

The following PROM-cycle framework (see Fig. 13.1) can be used to support selection, implementation, and evaluation of PROMs by end users, such as clinicians, quality managers, patient representatives, and other experts [53]. The framework has been developed using existing national and international tools for selection and use of PROMs with input from end users who deemed the framework to be relevant and feasible for implementation [53].

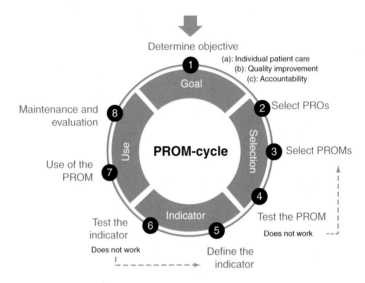

FIGURE 13.1 PROM-cycle framework. (Used with permission courtesy of van der Wees et al. [53])

Phase 1: Goal

First, it is important to determine the objective that the PROM is intended to achieve. The objective of using PROMs in clinical practice is threefold: (a) to guide individual patient care and shared decision-making, (b) to evaluate outcomes in a group of patients to guide quality improvement initiatives, and (c) to increase transparency by reporting outcomes to the public and stakeholders [53, 54]. For instance, using PROMs to evaluate QoL outcomes in patients who undergo pulmonary resection for suspected malignant tumors can assist individual patients in selecting the most appropriate treatment, advocate for change in practice, and compare quality of care across institutions.

Phase 2: Selection

A PROM that best addresses the predetermined objective should then be selected. When selecting an appropriate QoL scale to evaluate postoperative recovery, the PROM should be assessed for its psychometric properties and ability to detect clinically meaningful difference across treatment groups and time. There are two main types of QoL measures: generic scales and condition-specific scales.

Generic scales assess a wide range of health-related QoL issues and can therefore be applicable to a broad population, including the general population. Thus, generic scales can compare a target population to other populations. However, given the broad nature of questions, generic scales may not be specific enough to detect subtle changes in QoL. A common example of a generic QoL scale is the EuroQol-5 dimensions (EQ-5D), which is widely used to describe and value health across numerous health conditions across five dimensions: mobility, self-care, usual function status, pain/discomfort, and anxiety/depression [55]. When tested for its validity and responsiveness among patients undergoing pulmonary resection for cancer, the EQ-5D was limited in detecting changes in QoL across time as predicted by a priori hypothesis (poor responsiveness) and between patient groups (poor discriminant validity) [56].

Specialized scales are developed to assess QoL associated with a particular health condition. As such, their questions are generally more targeted and responsive to change. An example of a specialized scale designed for lung cancer is the European Organization for Research and Treatment of Cancer Quality of Life Questionnaire-Lung Cancer 29 (EORTC QLQ-LC29), which contains five multi-item scales relevant to lung cancer patients, including surgery-related symptoms [57]. Recently, an international, cross-cultural, multicenter phase IV study reported on psychometric properties of EORTC QLQ-LC29, demonstrating excellent internal consistency, reliability, responsiveness to change over time, and group differences when comparing patients with low vs. high performance status [58]. Thus, the EORTC QLQ-LC29 may be a more appropriate and sensitive measure to achieve the goal of assessing postoperative recovery trajectory and QoL in the target population.

Phase 3: Define the Indicator

After selecting an appropriate PROM, the outcome should then be interpreted in relation to the quality of healthcare delivered [53]. The utility of a quality indicator is in its ability to monitor outcomes and provide actionable data [59]. For QoL measures, "minimal clinically meaningful difference," which refers to the smallest difference in QoL score that is considered to be clinically important, is generally used to indicate significant findings used to guide treatment recommendation and/or changes in practice [60].

Phase 4: Use

The PROM and associated quality indicator should be periodically evaluated, verifying that it remains relevant and sensitive to the target population and outcome(s) of interest as practice guidelines change [53]. In fact, the conception of EORTC QLQ-LC29 stemmed from the need to add new items to the existing PROM (EORTC QLQ-LC13) in order to assess effects and side effects of novel therapeutic options that were recently made available for lung cancer patients [61].

Interpreting Outcome Measures

Effective outcome measurement studies can change clinical practice, but accurate interpretation requires that we know the data limitations. Although participation in large multi-institutional databases attempts to reduce bias, the act of self-reporting in and of itself can lead to bias for the voluntary programs. Surgeons already desire to do their best, and the reported outcomes are collected by trained database staff, not the surgeons.

In addition, patients who undergo operations have a great variation in comorbidities. The quality of data collected significantly impacts whether the complexity of the patients is captured in the databases. Despite the NSQIP risk calculator's attempt to account for these comorbidities and associated risks, it cannot account for everything and is certainly not infallible. The operation ultimately lies in the hands of the surgeon on the individual patient. Each operation has its own technical challenges, some much greater than others, and it is not possible to accurately reflect this in large databases. Given the various sources and quality of data in the large databases, their data may be inconsistent.

Mull et al. performed an analysis between VASQIP, SCIP, and PSI measures for 67 VA hospitals and found at most a very weak correlation or agreement between measures for rating hospitals as high- or low-performing [27]. They make the case for not using any one outcome measure but looking at a range of outcome measures and understanding the use for each one.

Evaluating Surgical Innovation: Using the IDEAL Framework (Table 13.1)

Outcomes research also plays a significant role in the field of surgical innovation. In recent decades, surgical techniques have evolved tremendously, from open to minimally invasive surgery and further development of novel surgical approaches, with constant focus on improving patient outcomes. Recent innovations in surgical procedures have not been subject to the same degree of rigorous regulation as for drug development. The process of surgical innovation has been largely unstructured and unregulated and is met with unique

TABLE 13.1 Characteristics of each stage of IDEAL framework

	Idea	Development	Exploration	Assessment	Long-term
Surgeons	Surgical innovators	Early adopters	Larger surgical community with variable training and expertise	Surgeons formally trained and assessed to perform novel technique	Surgeons formally trained and assessed to perform novel technique
Patient population	Highly select group of patients	Select, but larger group of patients	International group of patients	Recruited patients assigned to treatment group	Enumerated patients who are followed long-term
Type of study	Case reports	Prospective case series from single center	Prospective multicenter cohort study	Randomized controlled trials	Long-term population-based observational studies using clinical registry/administrative data

Objectives				
Inform surgeons of safety +/− benefits of innovation Report on recurrent errors requiring further refinement	Develop technical aspects of procedure Collaborative approach to collect patient outcome data and standardize procedure	Define correct indication Clarify potential harms and benefits Plan for future RCTs Establish optimal method of training and assessment	Study relative benefit of innovation compared to conventional approaches	Assess long-term oncologic and functional outcomes and associated quality of life

challenges, including a high degree of technical complexity and significant individual variability among surgeons. To ensure safety and efficacy, surgical innovation should undergo robust evaluation that is guided by evidence-based principles. The IDEAL framework is composed of five stages of evaluating and reporting surgical innovations: Idea, Development, Exploration, Assessment, and Long-term [62]. It was developed by the IDEAL collaborative, composed of surgeons, methodologists, clinical trialists, ethicists, journal editors, and health technology assessment professionals, with the aim of developing an integrated and thorough evaluation pathway for surgical and other complex interventions [63]. IDEAL also promotes high-quality, prospective research design to rigorously test new procedures, with the intention of preventing widespread implementation before proper assessment has taken place.

A good example of how the IDEAL framework has guided implementation of novel surgical technique can be found in the development of transanal total mesorectal excision (TaTME) for rectal cancer. The transanal component of the procedure aims to overcome the limitations of transabdominal approach where dissection of the mid- and distal rectum is often challenged by poor visualization of planes, especially in the narrow and deep pelvis. While this innovative approach may offer technical advantages, it is essential to evaluate whether this novel procedure can also offer adequate oncologic results, risk of complications, and QoL for patients undergoing the procedure.

Idea The first clinical phase consists of a "proof of concept," where a group of surgeon innovators perform the novel surgical procedure on a small number of select patients. This phase is often preceded by a preclinical phase, where a technique is first attempted and practiced on animal models and human cadavers. Whiteford was the first surgeon to describe the use of natural orifice transluminal endoscopic surgery (NOTES) in colorectal surgery, which was later tested in pigs and cadavers and achieved successful excision of intact mesorectum, as well as reduced operative times [64–66]. The first clinical cases of TaTME were performed between 2010 and 2012 by Sylla and Lacy on low-risk rectal cancer patients and reported complete TME specimens with negative margins and uneventful postoperative course [65, 66].

Development Following proof of safety and potential benefit of TaTME as demonstrated in early case series, surgeons who are "early adopters" in the field started to take up the procedure and gain personal experience, leading to the Development phase. In this second phase, the procedure is still performed on select but larger groups of patients, following institutional review board approval, and their outcomes are collected and reported in a prospective manner [62]. Various technical modifications and equipment changes are made while troubleshooting to further refine the procedure. The key aspect of this phase is the collaboration among surgeons across different centers and countries, as well as collaboration with industry, to refine technical aspects of the procedure, maximize the understanding of available devices, and foster technical innovation to make the procedure easier to perform.

Exploration After achieving technical improvement and standardization, attention is shifted to understanding the benefits and potential harms of surgical innovation. Prospective, observational studies involving a larger number of patients from single or multiple practices are performed. A clinical registry of cases is critical in collecting data during the exploration and future stages and should be established if possible to track and learn from early outcomes and provide longer-term data. In this example of TaTME, the international TaTME Registry was launched in 2014 and involved data input from surgeons across the world with varying levels of expertise [67]. Another essential aspect of the exploration phase is establishing an optimal method of teaching and evaluating surgeons who will be adopting the technique with its widespread implementation. In this example of TaTME, a consensus recommendation was proposed by Francis and colleagues, which describes a formal curriculum that involves online modules, simulated training, and formative assessment of competency that is led by a surgeon trained in laparoscopic colorectal surgery with prior experience in transanal surgery [68].

Assessment Does this new surgical procedure with promising early results in terms of safety and patient outcomes also offer advantage over existing, conventional procedures? The Assessment phase aims to answer this question using properly conducted randomized controlled trials (RCT) as the preferred method of study [62]. Again using the TaTME example, three RCTs are currently underway. The overall goal of these trials is to validate the safety and efficacy of TaTME in comparison with conventional procedures for rectal cancer treatment [69].

Long-term studies The focus of the last stage is evaluation of long-term outcomes related to patient QoL, function, and oncological status. The major advantage of setting up a registry early on in evaluation of innovative surgical procedures is that registered patients can be followed long term to assess for outcomes of interest. The international TaTME registry, in conjunction with ongoing trials mentioned above, could be used to track oncological outcomes as well as bowel, sexual, and urinary function and associated QoL, which are of utmost interest among rectal cancer patients.

Although evaluation of TaTME followed steps to adhere to IDEAL framework, a major deviation occurred when surgeons who did not undergo formative training and assessment rapidly adopted this complex procedure, in the absence of robust evidence of safety and efficacy obtained through

RCTs [70]. One can only harken back to the rapid adoption of laparoscopic cholecystectomy and the sharp increase in bile duct injuries as an example of this phenomenon. A recent Delphi consensus reflecting collaborative input from 14 international colorectal societies provided guidance on safe adoption and practice of TaTME [71]. Continuous monitoring and critical evaluation by an international body of expert surgeons and stakeholders are essential in the process of surgical innovation.

Future Methods

Multiple new methods for surgical outcome measurement are on the horizon. Patient-generated outcomes using wearable technology like the single use Zio Patch for 14-day continuous ECG monitoring using an adhesive patch [72] have great promise. Technologies like these bring measures that are more objective to clinicians and researchers and make data capture more convenient for patients. The technology is expanding to allow for data tracking and clinical intervention in real time, and our data storage capacity is growing to enable large warehousing of population-level statistics.

In addition to clinical data capture, several smartphone applications are currently being used to collect patient-generated health data in real time and improve clinical care. The GetWell Loop system allows for automated check-ins and reminders to patients, which has already increased knowledge about postoperative opioid use and disposal [73]. There are challenges to analyzing and validating such data that are unique to interrupted time series and go beyond the scope of this chapter, but the data capture technology holds significant promise for enhanced surgical outcome data research in the future.

As discussed above, definitions of clinical outcomes can vary and diminish the value of using a given outcome such as surgical site infection. With greater technological integration, documentation of incisions and wounds can now be taken by smartphones and uploaded directly to the medical record either remotely or in a clinical setting. Reliance on more objective documentation like photos can push the medical community toward a greater standardization. Simply integrating more image capture capabilities can allow for more consistent assessment of wound changes over time, remote assessment of wounds, and possibly verification of surgical site infections in databases and clinical trials or by quality oversight committees. This would remove the subjectivity inherent in individual assessment.

In addition to static images, video capture of laparoscopic surgeries has become commonplace, as well as video monitoring of operating rooms. "Black box" systems, similar to those in airplanes, have been proposed and implemented at some institutions. Their ultimate goal is to reduce adverse events and improve outcomes. Jung et al. evaluated a black box system with over 100 cases reviewed by trained analysts and found a median of 20 errors and 8 events in each case [74]. Clearly there are many unanswered questions regarding the ethics, potential positives, and potential negatives of video capture in the surgical setting, but this technology is poised to fundamentally change surgical outcomes research.

Finally, many technology experts and researchers agree artificial intelligence (AI) will become a significant contributor to medical and surgical care [75]. Currently machine learning, or "deep learning," is being developed in order to assist with recognition of skin cancer [76]. These same concepts can be applied to many other aspects of surgery including diagnosis, monitoring, reporting of outcomes, or even predicting outcomes. The exact role that AI will play in surgical outcomes assessment and review is yet to be determined, but it is easy to see how these advancements in machine learning may increase the speed at which we recognize adverse outcomes and potentially help us to prevent them.

Conclusion

Health services research is an important driver of value-based and patient-centered care. Out of the three quality indicators, outcomes are the most reflective of the impact of healthcare on patients and therefore are the best target for quality improvement efforts. Surgical outcomes research has grown tremendously in the past two decades through national-level reporting and feedback of procedure-specific outcome data across increasing numbers of collaborating sites. However, in order to lead to meaningful changes, outcome measurements must further be translated to changes in practice and culture at multiple levels. Furthermore, clinical outcomes should be used in conjunction with PROMs that reflect patients' values and needs, to drive patient-centered research and improvement in quality of surgical care. Evaluation of surgical innovation through the IDEAL framework provides an example of how outcomes research could effectively drive a change in practice to improve patient care. Outcomes specific to each stage of development serve as checkpoints to ensure safety and efficacy of surgical innovation. Therefore, surgical outcomes are not only the final results but also measures that are most useful when complemented by attempts to improve care while undergoing constant and critical evaluation. As outcome measurements improve and advance, outcomes researchers and quality improvement specialists have greater opportunities to analyze high-quality data. This data will continue increasing in quality with EMR integration, machine learning techniques, and video/image capture integration.

References

1. What is health services research? Agency for Healthcare Research and Quality. 2002. https://archive.ahrq.gov/about/whatis.pdf.
2. Hicks CW, Makary MA. A prophet to modern medicine: Ernest Amory Codman. BMJ. 2013;347:f7368.

3. Gai Y, Pachamanova D. Impact of the Medicare hospital read-missions reduction program on vulnerable populations. BMC Health Serv Res. 2019;19(1):837.

4. Donabedian A. Evaluating the quality of medical care. 1966. Milbank Q. 2005;83(4):691–729.

5. Munday GS, et al. Impact of implementation of the Surgical Care Improvement Project and future strategies for improving quality in surgery. Am J Surg. 2014;208(5):835–40.

6. Wu AK, Auerbach AD, Aaronson DS. National incidence and outcomes of postoperative urinary retention in the Surgical Care Improvement Project. Am J Surg. 2012;204(2):167–71.

7. Dimick JB, Welch HG. The zero mortality paradox in surgery. J Am Coll Surg. 2008;206(1):13–6.

8. Dimick JB, Welch HG, Birkmeyer JD. Surgical mortality as an indicator of hospital quality: the problem with small sample size. JAMA. 2004;292(7):847–51.

9. Iezzoni LI. The risks of risk adjustment. JAMA. 1997;278(19):1600–7.

10. Khuri SF, Daley J, Henderson WG. The comparative assessment and improvement of quality of surgical care in the Department of Veterans Affairs. Arch Surg. 2002;137(1):20–7.

11. Roberts JS, Coale JG, Redman RR. A history of the joint commission on accreditation of hospitals. JAMA. 1987;258(7):936–40.

12. Khuri SF, Daley J, Henderson W, Hur K, Demakis J, Aust JB, Chong V, Fabri PJ, Gibbs JO, Grover F, Hammermeister K, Irvin G, Mcdonald G, Passaro E, Phillips L, Scamman F, Spencer J, Stremple JF. The Department of Veterans Affairs' NSQIP. Ann Surg. 1998;228:491–507.

13. Ingraham AM, et al. Quality improvement in surgery: the American College of Surgeons national surgical quality improvement program approach. Adv Surg. 2010;44(1):251–67.

14. Massarweh NN, Kaji AH, Itani KM. Practical guide to surgical data sets: Veterans Affairs Surgical Quality Improvement Program (VASQIP). JAMA Surg. 2018;153(8):768–9.

15. Khuri SF, et al. Risk adjustment of the postoperative mortality rate for the comparative assessment of the quality of surgical care: results of the National Veterans Affairs Surgical Risk Study. J Am Coll Surg. 1997;185(4):315–27.

16. Fink AS, et al. The National Surgical Quality Improvement Program in non-veterans administration hospitals: initial demonstration of feasibility. Ann Surg. 2002;236(3):344–53; discussion 353-4.

17. Khuri SF, et al. Successful implementation of the Department of Veterans Affairs' National Surgical Quality Improvement Program in the private sector: the patient safety in surgery study. Ann Surg. 2008;248(2):329–36.
18. Bilimoria KY, Liu Y, Paruch JL, Zhou L, Kmiecik TE, Ko CY, Cohen ME. Development and evaluation of the universal ACS NSQIP surgical risk calculator: a decision aid and informed consent tool for patients and surgeons. J Am Coll Surg. 2013;217(5):833–42.
19. Cohen ME, et al. Optimizing ACS NSQIP modeling for evaluation of surgical quality and risk: patient risk adjustment, procedure mix adjustment, shrinkage adjustment, and surgical focus. J Am Coll Surg. 2013;217(2):336–46.e1.
20. Maggard-Gibbons M. The use of report cards and outcome measurements to improve the safety of surgical care: the American College of Surgeons National Surgical Quality Improvement Program. BMJ Qual Saf. 2014;23(7):589–99.
21. Hall BL, et al. Does surgical quality improve in the American College of Surgeons National Surgical Quality Improvement Program: an evaluation of all participating hospitals. Ann Surg. 2009;250(3):363–76.
22. Ingraham AM, et al. Quality improvement in surgery: the American College of Surgeons National Surgical Quality Improvement Program approach. Adv Surg. 2010;44:251–67.
23. Etzioni DA, et al. Association of hospital participation in a surgical outcomes monitoring program with inpatient complications and mortality. JAMA. 2015;313(5):505–11.
24. Osborne NH, et al. Association of hospital participation in a quality reporting program with surgical outcomes and expenditures for medicare beneficiaries. JAMA. 2015;313(5):496–504.
25. Tanner J, et al. Do surgical care bundles reduce the risk of surgical site infections in patients undergoing colorectal surgery? A systematic review and cohort meta-analysis of 8,515 patients. Surgery. 2015;158(1):66–77.
26. Carter EB, et al. Evidence-based bundles and cesarean delivery surgical site infections: a systematic review and meta-analysis. Obstet Gynecol. 2017;130(4):735–46.
27. Mull HJ, Chen Q, Shwartz M, Itani KM, Rosen AK. Measuring surgical quality: which measure should we trust? JAMA Surg. 2014;149(11):1210–2.

28. Henry LR, von Holzen UW, Minarich MJ, Hardy AN, Beachy WA, Franger MS, Schwarz RE. Quality measurement affecting surgical practice: utility versus utopia. Am J Surg. 2018;215(3):357–66.

29. Baser O, Supina D, Sengupta N, Wang L, Kwong L. Clinical and cost outcomes of venous thromboembolism in Medicare patients undergoing total hip replacement or total knee replacement surgery. Curr Med Res Opin. 2011;27(2):423–9.

30. Cella D, Riley W, Stone A, Rothrock N, Reeve B, Yount S, Amtmann D, Bode R, Buysse D, Choi S, Cook K. The Patient-Reported Outcomes Measurement Information System (PROMIS) developed and tested its first wave of adult self-reported health outcome item banks: 2005–2008. J Clin Epidemiol. 2010;63(11):1179–94.

31. Cella D, Yount S, Rothrock N, Gershon R, Cook K, Reeve B, Ader D, Fries JF, Bruce B, Rose M, PROMIS Cooperative Group. The Patient-Reported Outcomes Measurement Information System (PROMIS): progress of an NIH roadmap cooperative group during its first two years. Med Care. 2007;45(5 Suppl 1):S3.

32. Rivera SC, Kyte DG, Aiyegbusi OL, Slade AL, McMullan C, Calvert MJ. The impact of patient-reported outcome (PRO) data from clinical trials: a systematic review and critical analysis. Health Qual Life Outcomes. 2019;17(1):156.

33. Katz S, Ford AB, Moskowitz RW, Jackson BA, Jaffe MW. Studies of illness in the aged: the index of ADL: a standardized measure of biological and psychosocial function. JAMA. 1963;185(12):914–9.

34. Urden LD. Patient satisfaction measurement: current issues and implications. Lippincotts Case Manag. 2002;7(5):194–200.

35. Neville A, et al. Systematic review of outcomes used to evaluate enhanced recovery after surgery. Br J Surg. 2014;101(3):159–70.

36. Lee L, et al. What does it really mean to "recover" from an operation? Surgery. 2014;155(2):211–6.

37. Fiore JF Jr, et al. How do we value postoperative recovery?: a systematic review of the measurement properties of patient-reported outcomes after abdominal surgery. Ann Surg. 2018;267(4):656–69.

38. Griggs CL, et al. Patient-reported outcome measures: a stethoscope for the patient history. Ann Surg. 2017;265(6):1066–7.

39. Kool M, et al. Importance of patient reported outcome measures versus clinical outcomes for breast cancer patients evaluation on quality of care. Breast. 2016;27:62–8.

40. Khan S, et al. Quality of life and patient satisfaction with enhanced recovery protocols. Color Dis. 2010;12(12):1175–82.

41. Delaney CP, et al. Prospective, randomized, controlled trial between a pathway of controlled rehabilitation with early ambulation and diet and traditional postoperative care after laparotomy and intestinal resection. Dis Colon Rectum. 2003;46(7):851–9.

42. Macefield RC, Avery KNL, Blazeby JM. Integration of clinical and patient-reported outcomes in surgical oncology. Br J Surg. 2012;100(1):28–37.

43. Health, U.D.o, et al. Guidance for industry: patient-reported outcome measures: use in medical product development to support labeling claims: draft guidance. Health Qual Life Outcomes. 2006;4:1–20.

44. Venkatesan P. New European guidance on patient-reported outcomes. Lancet Oncol. 2016;17(6):e226.

45. Reeve BB, et al. ISOQOL recommends minimum standards for patient-reported outcome measures used in patient-centered outcomes and comparative effectiveness research. Qual Life Res. 2013;22(8):1889–905.

46. Lohr KN. Assessing health status and quality-of-life instruments: attributes and review criteria. Qual Life Res. 2002;11(3):193–205.

47. Terwee CB, et al. Quality criteria were proposed for measurement properties of health status questionnaires. J Clin Epidemiol. 2007;60(1):34–42.

48. Frost MH, et al. What is sufficient evidence for the reliability and validity of patient-reported outcome measures? Value Health. 2007;10:S94–S105.

49. Mokkink LB, et al. The COSMIN study reached international consensus on taxonomy, terminology, and definitions of measurement properties for health-related patient-reported outcomes. J Clin Epidemiol. 2010;63(7):737–45.

50. Hays R, Hadorn D. Responsiveness to change: an aspect of validity, not a separate dimension. Qual Life Res. 1992;1(1):73–5.

51. Fernandez B, Dore L, Velanovich V. Patient-centered outcomes in surgical research and practice. J Gastrointest Surg. 2017;21(5):892–5.

52. Pompili C, et al. Patients reported outcomes in thoracic surgery. J Thorac Dis. 2018;10(2):703–6.

53. van der Wees PJ, et al. Development of a framework with tools to support the selection and implementation of patient-reported outcome measures. J Patient Rep Outcomes. 2019;3(1):75.

54. Black N. Patient reported outcome measures could help transform healthcare. BMJ. 2013;346:f167.

55. Devlin NJ, Brooks R. EQ-5D and the EuroQol group: past, present and future. Appl Health Econ Health Policy. 2017;15(2):127–37.
56. Bejjani J, et al. Validity of the EuroQol-5 dimensions as a measure of recovery after pulmonary resection. J Surg Res. 2015;194(1):281–8.
57. Koller M, et al. An international study to revise the EORTC questionnaire for assessing quality of life in lung cancer patients. Ann Oncol. 2017;28(11):2874–81.
58. Koller M, et al. Psychometric properties of the updated EORTC module for assessing quality of life in patients with lung cancer (QLQ-LC29): an international, observational field study. Lancet Oncol. 2020;21(5):723–32.
59. Nothacker M, et al. Reporting standards for guideline-based performance measures. Implement Sci. 2016;11:6.
60. Hays RD, Woolley JM. The concept of clinically meaningful difference in health-related quality-of-life research. PharmacoEconomics. 2000;18(5):419–23.
61. Koller M, et al. Use of the lung cancer-specific quality of life questionnaire EORTC QLQ-LC13 in clinical trials: a systematic review of the literature 20 years after its development. Cancer. 2015;121(24):4300–23.
62. McCulloch P, et al. No surgical innovation without evaluation: the IDEAL recommendations. Lancet. 2009;374(9695):1105–12.
63. Hirst A, et al. No surgical innovation without evaluation: evolution and further development of the IDEAL framework and recommendations. Ann Surg. 2019;269(2):211–20.
64. Telem DA, et al. Transanal rectosigmoid resection via natural orifice translumenal endoscopic surgery (NOTES) with total mesorectal excision in a large human cadaver series. Surg Endosc. 2013;27(1):74–80.
65. Whiteford MH, Denk PM, Swanström LL. Feasibility of radical sigmoid colectomy performed as natural orifice translumenal endoscopic surgery (NOTES) using transanal endoscopic microsurgery. Surg Endosc. 2007;21(10):1870–4.
66. Sylla P, et al. Survival study of natural orifice translumenal endoscopic surgery for rectosigmoid resection using transanal endoscopic microsurgery with or without transgastric endoscopic assistance in a swine model. Surg Endosc. 2010;24(8):2022–30.
67. Foundation, U.P.C., International TaTME Registry. 2014.

68. Francis N, et al. Consensus on structured training curriculum for transanal total mesorectal excision (TaTME). Surg Endosc. 2017;31(7):2711–9.
69. Rouanet P, et al. Rectal surgery evaluation trial: protocol for a parallel cohort trial of outcomes using surgical techniques for total mesorectal excision with low anterior resection in high-risk rectal cancer patients. Color Dis. 2019;21(5):516–22.
70. Roodbeen SX, et al. Evolution of transanal total mesorectal excision according to the IDEAL framework. BMJ Surg Interv Health Technol. 2019;1(1):e000004.
71. Hompes R, et al. International expert consensus guidance on indications, implementation and quality measures for Transanal Total Mesorectal Excision (TaTME). Color Dis. 2020;22:749–55.
72. Lobodzinski SS. ECG patch monitors for assessment of cardiac rhythm abnormalities. Prog Cardiovasc Dis. 2013;56(2):224–9.
73. Stulberg J, Huang R, Chao SY, Wickline VN, Schäfer W, Ko CY, Rosner B. Leveraging a digital care platform to drive quality improvement in postoperative opioid medication use. J Am Coll Surg. 2020;231(4):e19.
74. Jung JJ, Jüni P, Lebovic G, Grantcharov T. First-year analysis of the operating room black box study. Ann Surg. 2020;271(1):122–7.
75. Beam AL, Kohane IS. Big data and machine learning in health care. JAMA. 2018;319(13):1317–8.
76. Esteva A, Kuprel B, Novoa R, et al. Dermatologist-level classification of skin cancer with deep neural networks. Nature. 2017;542:115–8. https://doi.org/10.1038/nature21056.

Other Selected Reading

Bernardi MP, et al. Transanal total mesorectal excision: dissection tips using 'O's and 'triangles'. Tech Coloproctol. 2016;20(11):775–8.
Calvert M, Kyte D, Price G, Valderas JM, Hjollund NH. Maximising the impact of patient reported outcome assessment for patients and society. BMJ. 2019;364:k5267.
Chen TY-T, et al. Bowel function 14 years after preoperative short-course radiotherapy and total mesorectal excision for rectal cancer: report of a multicenter randomized trial. Clin Colorectal Cancer. 2015;14(2):106–14.

Chow A, Mayer EK, Darzi AW, Athanasiou T. Patient-reported outcome measures: the importance of patient satisfaction in surgery. Surgery. 2009;146(3):435–43.

Cohen ME, Liu Y, Ko CY, Hall BL. An examination of American College of Surgeons NSQIP surgical risk calculator accuracy. J Am Coll Surg. 2017;224(5):787–95.

Deijen CL, et al. COLOR III: a multicentre randomised clinical trial comparing transanal TME versus laparoscopic TME for mid and low rectal cancer. Surg Endosc. 2016;30(8):3210–5.

Department of Veterans Affairs, Office of Data Governance and Analytics, Veteran Population Projection Model (VetPop). Veterans Benefits Administration; Veterans Health Administration, Office of the Assistant Deputy. Under Secretary for Health for Policy and Planning; 2016.

Dickson EA, et al. Carbon dioxide embolism associated with transanal total mesorectal excision surgery: a report from the international registries. Dis Colon Rectum. 2019;62(7):794–801.

Ferraris VA, Harris JW, Martin JT, Saha SP, Endean ED. Impact of residents on surgical outcomes in high-complexity procedures. J Am Coll Surg. 2016;222(4):545–55.

Fiore JF Jr, Figueiredo S, Balvardi S, Lee L, Nauche B, Landry T, Mayo NE, Feldman LS. How do we value postoperative recovery?: a systematic review of the measurement properties of patient-reported outcomes after abdominal surgery. Ann Surg. 2018;267(4):656–69.

Gadan S, et al. Does a defunctioning stoma impair anorectal function after low anterior resection of the rectum for cancer? A 12-year follow-up of a randomized multicenter trial. Dis Colon Rectum. 2017;60(8):800–6.

Hyer JM, White S, Cloyd J, Dillhoff M, Tsung A, Pawlik TM, Ejaz A. Can we improve prediction of adverse surgical outcomes? Development of a surgical complexity score using a novel machine learning technique. J Am Coll Surg. 2020;230(1):43–52.

Jones RS, Stukenborg GJ. Patient-Reported Outcomes Measurement Information System (PROMIS) use in surgical care: a scoping study. J Am Coll Surg. 2017;224(3):245–54.

Lacy AM, et al. Minilaparoscopy-assisted transrectal low anterior resection (LAR): a preliminary study. Surg Endosc. 2013;27(1):339–46.

Lelong B, et al. A multicentre randomised controlled trial to evaluate the efficacy, morbidity and functional outcome of endoscopic transanal proctectomy versus laparoscopic proctectomy for low-lying rectal cancer (ETAP-GRECCAR 11 TRIAL): rationale and design. BMC Cancer. 2017;17(1):253.

Motson RW, et al. Current status of trans-anal total mesorectal excision (TaTME) following the second international consensus conference. Color Dis. 2016;18(1):13–8.

Nicholson G, et al. Optimal dissection for transanal total mesorectal excision using modified CO_2 insufflation and smoke extraction. Color Dis. 2015;17(11):O265–7.

Penna M, et al. Four anastomotic techniques following transanal total mesorectal excision (TaTME). Tech Coloproctol. 2016;20(3):185–91.

Penna M, et al. Transanal total mesorectal excision: international registry results of the first 720 cases. Ann Surg. 2017;266(1):111–7.

Penna M, et al. Incidence and risk factors for anastomotic failure in 1594 patients treated by transanal total mesorectal excision: results from the international TaTME registry. Ann Surg. 2019;269(4):700–11.

Pieniowski EHA, et al. Low anterior resection syndrome and quality of life after sphincter-sparing rectal cancer surgery: a long-term longitudinal follow-up. Dis Colon Rectum. 2019;62(1):14–20.

Smith AB, Schwarze ML. Translating patient-reported outcomes from surgical research to clinical care. JAMA Surg. 2017;152(9):811–2.

Strengths and Limitations of CMS Administrative Data in Research. (n.d.). Retrieved from https://www.resdac.org/articles/strengths-and-limitations-cms-administrative-data-research.

Sylla P, et al. NOTES transanal rectal cancer resection using transanal endoscopic microsurgery and laparoscopic assistance. Surg Endosc. 2010;24(5):1205–10.

www.ahrq.gov.

www.facs.org/quality-programs.

www.pressganey.com.

www.resdaq.org

Chapter 14
Developing Patient-Centered Outcomes Metrics for Abdominal Surgery

Julio F. Fiore, Fateme Rajabiyazdi, and Liane S. Feldman

Patient-centered care is a practice that emphasizes the active involvement of patients in health decision-making and self-management, supported by research evidence addressing outcomes that matter to patients [1–3]. Previous studies suggest that involving patients in their care has the potential to improve outcomes, enhance patient experience, and decrease healthcare costs [4–6]. As surgery is one of the most frightening, disruptive, and expensive events in a care continuum, surgical care can greatly benefit from a patient-centered approach [7].

In clinical practice, surgeons generally rely on clinician-centered outcome measures to define whether a surgical

J. F. Fiore (✉) · L. S. Feldman
Department of Surgery, McGill University, Montreal, QC, Canada
e-mail: julio.fiorejunior@mcgill.ca; liane.feldman@mcgill.ca

F. Rajabiyazdi
Department of Systems and Computer Engineering, Carleton University, Ottawa, ON, Canada
e-mail: rajabiyazdi@sce.carleton.ca

© The Author(s), under exclusive license to Springer Nature   259
Switzerland AG 2022
J. R. Romanelli et al. (eds.), *The SAGES Manual of Quality, Outcomes and Patient Safety*,
https://doi.org/10.1007/978-3-030-94610-4_14

procedure was "successful." This traditional approach involves ascertaining that the procedure achieved its intended goal (e.g., effective resection, repair or reconstruction of the diseased structure) while avoiding complications (e.g., anastomotic leaks, surgical site infections). Also, clinicians are motivated to avoid prolonged hospital length of stay (LOS) and healthcare reutilization (i.e., emergency department visits and hospital readmissions) as these events lead to increased healthcare costs and, in the USA, may reduce reimbursement for the health service provided [8]. While these traditional metrics are obviously important, they do not capture the full spectrum of surgical outcomes that are meaningful to patients.

When assessing surgical outcomes, it is important to acknowledge that surgery has short-term deleterious effects on patients' health status even in the absence of complications. For patients, major surgery is a major physiologic stressor leading to a rapid health decline postoperatively requiring weeks or months for full recovery (i.e., getting back to "normal") (Fig. 14.1) [9]. This health decline is primarily caused by the surgical stress response, a cascade of metabolic and hormonal events triggered by tissue trauma that is proportional to the intensity of the intervention [10, 11]. When complications occur, patients often experience delays in their recovery, and some may never return to their preoperative

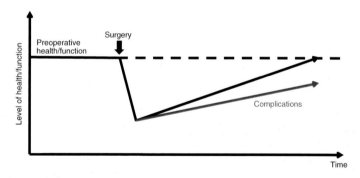

FIGURE 14.1 Trajectory of postoperative recovery and impact of postoperative complications. (Based on information from: Lee et al. [9])

level of health (Fig. 14.1) [12, 13]. While recovering, patients withdraw from household, leisure, and economic activities and often require assistance with activities of daily living [14, 15]. In clinical practice, patients often inquire about the duration of recovery in terms of how long they will need to be away from work, sports, and other activities. This is consistent with research supporting that patients define postoperative recovery as the ability to return to baseline levels of function [16–18]. As such, the ability to quantify the period of recovery after specific procedures would be relevant both in clinical practice and for comparative effectiveness research. However, recovery is a latent construct (i.e., not directly observable or quantifiable [1]) that is difficult to measure [19]. The process of recovery is highly dynamic and comprises multiple dimensions of health (e.g., symptom experiences, functional status, and well-being); therefore, it cannot be easily captured by a single metric [9].

In line with the principles of patient-centered care, recent literature advocates that measurement of recovery needs to include the patients' voice through patient-reported outcome (PRO) measures [9, 20–23]. In comparison with traditional measures of surgical outcomes, PROs have the advantage of allowing a broad assessment of recovery across various patient-centered health domains, engaging patients as the key stakeholders in the recovery process [19]. PROs generally take the form of questionnaires that allow information reported by patients to be translated into objective data that can be more readily analyzed [23]. These questionnaires can be completed at different time points, allowing a better understanding of the recovery trajectory. In this chapter, we will provide an overview about PROs, how they are developed, and summarize current evidence- and consensus-based recommendations for the use of PROs in surgical care. Our primary focus will be on PROs aimed to assess postoperative recovery after abdominal surgery, but the concepts are broadly applicable to the use of PROs to measure surgical outcomes.

What Are Patient-Reported Outcome Measures (PROMs)?

As per the classical definition by the US Food and Drug Administration (FDA), a PRO is "any report of the status of a patient's health condition that comes directly from the patient, without interpretation of the patient's response by a clinician or anyone else." [24] Measurement of PROs is usually conducted via self-reported questionnaires known as PRO measures (or PROMs). As the name suggests, PROMs target aspects of health that are directly relevant to patients, including symptoms, functional status, psychological status, and participation in life activities. A PROM should capture specific domains of health that are relevant to the construct that is being measured (i.e., the underlying theme or subject matter). For example, postoperative "pain" and "physical function" are constructs commonly targeted by PROMs used in surgical research. Each domain is evaluated by one or more items (i.e., close-ended questions with specific response options) that are counted and mathematically combined to produce a summary score. Sometimes, PROMs are multidimensional and contain multiple sub-scores, each representing a different but related health domain. Examples of multidimensional PROMs are generic health status questionnaires, which produce different scores for specific domains such as pain and physical and mental health [25]. These include PROMs such as the Short Form (36) Health Survey (SF-36) [26] and the World Health Organization Disability Assessment Schedule (WHODAS 2.0) [27].

PROMs can be generic or condition-specific. As the name implies, generic PROMs are intended to measure general aspects of health that are not specific to a particular disease or condition [28]. Examples of generic PROMs that have been used to quantify recovery after surgery are the above-mentioned SF-36 [26] and WHODAS 2.0 [27], as well as the Euro Qol Group 5 Dimension Instrument (EQ-5D) [29]. Traditionally, generic PROMs are used to compare self-reported health status across different patient populations and to compare data with population norms. Potential issues related to the use of generic PROMs in the context of surgical research are addressed later in this chapter. Condition-specific PROMs, on the other hand, address aspects of health that are impacted by a specific disease or condition [28]. In other words, they are developed to address issues that are important for a specific patient population. Overall, they are more suited than generic PROMs to detect changes in aspects of health that are condition-specific. Examples of condition-specific PROMs that have been used in surgical outcomes research include the European Organization for Research and Treatment of Cancer QLQ-C30 (EORTC QLQ-C30) questionnaire [30] and the Quality of Recovery measures QOR-9, QOR-15, and QOR-40 [31].

Development of PROMs and Assessment of Measurement Properties

The development of a PROM is a complex and iterative process that requires substantial time, resources, and expertise. For too long, this process was seen as a simple activity that merely required common sense (i.e., creating some questions, intuitively judging their relevance, and attributing subjective scores to responses); however, it is now well understood that there is a great deal of science involved in developing good-quality PROMs and that their measurement properties require careful consideration [32].

Comprehensive guidelines have been published to direct the process of PROM development by researchers [24, 33, 34]. For the purpose of this chapter, this process will be divided in three phases: (1) content validity and item generation, (2) item evaluation and scale formation, and (3) assessment of measurement properties.

The aim of *phase 1* is to establish the PROM's content validity (i.e., the degree to which the content of a PROM is an adequate reflection of the construct to be measured [35]). To many experts, content validity is the most important measurement property of a PROM [36]. It is strongly recommended by guidelines that content validity of a PROM be supported by a conceptual framework, which includes a diagram that explicitly defines the concepts measured by PROM and how they relate to each other [24, 33]. The study by Alam et al. [37], where patients from four different countries were interviewed to elicit concepts relevant to the process of recovery after abdominal surgery, presents a concrete example of conceptual framework development (Fig. 14.2). Once a conceptual framework has been developed, PROM questionnaire items reflecting the essence of the framework should be generated through an iterative process of drafting, evaluation,

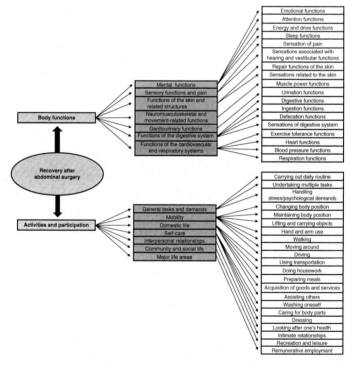

FIGURE 14.2 Conceptual framework of recovery after abdominal surgery. (Based on data from: Alam et al. [37])

and revision [34]. Patients' understanding of the items should be assessed via cognitive interviews [34]. The item pool (i.e., questions) created through this process (i.e., set of candidate items that have not yet been "calibrated") will comprise the preliminary draft of the PROM.

Phase 2 in the process of PROM development includes an assessment of the quality of the items proposed, as well as the development of scoring rules (algorithms). This assessment requires that the PROM preliminary item pool be administered to a large cohort of patients and analyzed psychometrically. In recent years, measurement theory has evolved with the use of modern psychometric techniques for item selection and scoring, such as item-response theory (IRT) and Rasch Measurement Theory (RMT). In brief, these techniques use a range of diagnostic information (error estimates and fit statistics) to determine whether adding the scores from a collection of items is justified [38]. When using RMT, for example, items can be eliminated or modified to "fit" what is expected in a Rasch model (i.e., a statistical model that calibrates items in a unidimensional scale) [39–41]. Traditional methods for PROM development (e.g., classical test theory) use arbitrary ordinal scales with no intrinsic meaning. Thus, response categories like "very good," "good," and "fair" are separated by unknown distances, restricting interpretation, as the distance from one category to the next may not be the same. In contrast, modern psychometric methods provide a nonlinear transformation of ordinal scores into a common interval scale, analogous to a ruler [38]. As a result, this approach facilitates accurate and meaningful interpretation of changes in PROM scores. Modern psychometric approaches also provide a basis for computer adaptive testing (CAT), the next-generation method of administering PROMs [42, 43]. In CAT, PROM items are selected in real time to reflect answers already given, thereby creating measures that are tailored to the patient's level of "ability," resulting in a questionnaire with fewer items and reduced patient burden [44, 45].

In *phase 3*, after content validity and scoring algorithms have been established, it is recommended that the PROM in its final format be administered to a large patient cohort for further assessment of measurement properties using traditional psychometric methods (i.e., classical test theory) [24]. In this phase, analyses using correlations and descriptive statistics evaluate measurement properties such as *internal consistency* (the degree of interrelatedness among items), *reliability* (the proportion of the total variance in scores which is due to "true" differences between patients), *measurement error* (deviations in scores that cannot be attributed to "true" differences), *structural validity* (the degree to which scores are an adequate reflection of the dimensionality of the construct of interest), *construct validity* (the degree to which the scores are consistent with hypotheses based on the assumption that the PROM is actually measuring the construct of interest), and *responsiveness* (the ability of a PROM to detect change over time in the construct of interest) [46]. At this stage, *cross-cultural validity* can also be assessed (the degree to which a translated or culturally adapted PROM is an adequate reflection of the original version) [46]. This analysis provides important information regarding external validity that can be compared against the measurement properties of existing PROMs [24, 46]. Specific standards for the assessment of PROM measurement properties has been proposed by the COSMIN (COnsensus-based Standards for the selection of health status Measurement INstruments) initiative (https://www.cosmin.nl/).

Critical Appraisal of PROMs Used in Abdominal Surgery

The surgical literature is replete with "validated" PROMs, but not all PROMs were created equally. In fact, a recent systematic review by Fiore et al. [32] suggested that there is limited evidence supporting the measurement properties of PROMs currently used in the context of postoperative recovery after abdominal surgery. This review appraised a total of 22

PROMs against quality standards proposed by COSMIN [47] and identified major deficiencies in relation to content validity, internal consistency, reliability, construct validity, and responsiveness, which are considered minimal standards for the selection of PROMs for use in research and clinical practice [48].

One major issue is that patient-centered assessment of postoperative recovery has often relied on generic PROMs. Although these PROMs are helpful for making comparisons with population norms and other patient groups, they miss important domains of health that are relevant for patients undergoing abdominal surgery. For example, items related to gastrointestinal dysfunction (e.g., tolerance of food, constipation) are not covered by generic PROMs frequently used in the surgical literature (e.g., SF-36 and EQ-5D) despite being considered relevant from the perspective of abdominal surgery patients [37]. Due to their questionable content validity, these PROMs have limited ability to detect changes in recovery. Several generic PROMs also have long recall periods (the period of time that patients are asked to consider when responding PRO items, e.g., "last 4 weeks") and, therefore, may have limited ability to capture rapid changes in patients' health condition postoperatively. As mentioned previously, this may potentially be remediated by implementing PROMs specifically focused on postoperative recovery. Although the review by Fiore et al. [32] identified 16 recovery-specific PROMs (11 focused on nonspecific surgical populations and 5 focused on abdominal surgery), most of these PROMs were not developed using modern psychometric methods (IRT or RMT), and evidence supporting their measurement properties in the context of abdominal surgery was limited. A research program initiated at McGill University and supported by SAGES and other funders aims to bridge this major knowledge gap by using state-of-the-art methodology to develop a novel PROM to assess recovery after abdominal surgery [37, 49].

Consensus Recommendations for PROM Use in Abdominal Surgery

While further research on this important topic emerges, consensus recommendations have been proposed to support the implementation of PROMs in surgical research and clinical practice. In 2018, the American Society for Enhanced Recovery (ASER) and the Perioperative Quality Initiative (POQI) proposed a consensus statement on patient-reported outcomes for use within enhanced recovery pathways. The ASER/POQI statement makes relevant remarks regarding the importance of selecting PROMs with an appropriate recall period, suggesting that PROMs with short recall periods (24 h) be administered in the first days after surgery (i.e., during hospital stay) and PROMs with longer recall periods (7 and/or 30 days) be used for assessment of long-term outcomes (i.e., after hospital discharge). The statement emphasizes that PROMs should also be collected at baseline, before surgery. Although ASER/POQI recognizes that, currently, there is limited evidence supporting its measuring properties, the Quality of Recovery 15 (QoR-15 [50]; recall period 24 h) was recommended for use during the early postoperative period. For assessment of long-term outcomes, the WHODAS 2.0 [51] (recall period 30 days) or PROMIS [52] (Patient-Reported Outcomes Measurement Information System, recall period 7 days) were recommended. The latter is a PROM measurement system developed as part of the National Institutes of Health (NIH) Roadmap for Medical Research. This system comprises a set of generic PROMs targeting specific domains of health (e.g., pain intensity, pain interference, fatigue) but also has multidimensional "profiles" targeting multiple domains (PROMIS-29, including physical, mental, and social health). The PROMIS system has the potential advantage of being developed using modern psychometric methods (IRT), accommodating computer adaptive testing, and being calibrated against US population norms. However, the measurement properties of PROMIS measures are yet to be determined in the context of postoperative recovery. Characteristics of the PROMs recommended by the ASER/POQI statement are summarized in Table 14.1.

Other consensus statements covering PROM assessment after surgery include the European Society of Anaesthesiology (ESA) and Intensive Care Medicine (ESICM) outcomes task force [53] and the Standardised Endpoints in Perioperative Medicine (StEP) initiative [54, 55]. Both of these consensuses corroborate the recommendation of QoR-15 as a measure of short-term and WHODAS as a measure of long-term patient-centered postoperative outcomes.

The Future of PROM Assessment in Abdominal Surgery

Tracking postoperative recovery using PROMs is a means to an end, but not the end itself. Achieving scientific and clinical value, the ultimate goal, will occur when PROMs (1) take the center stage in research assessing the comparative effectiveness of interventions aimed to improve recovery after surgery and (2) are used in clinical practice to fill the needs of patients, caregivers, and payers who commonly seek information about recovery expectations (i.e., will the patient resume usual activities after surgery? how long will it take?). The collection of PROM data through electronic platforms [i.e., mobile operating systems (i.e., mobile phones, tablets) and web portals] may empower patients to track their own recovery trajectory in real time and potentially identify complications at a point when they may be more easily treated. Also, electronic data collection may facilitate the use of artificial intelligence (AI) techniques to process PROM data. The use of AI may support patient-centered surgical decision making by identifying patients who are at risk for a slow/eventful postoperative recovery process [56].

Using electronic platforms to collect PROM data is becoming increasingly common. Electronic systems used to store and collect such data are referred to as ePROMs [57]. The main

TABLE 14.1 Characteristics of the patient-reported outcome measures recommended by the American Society for Enhanced Recovery and Perioperative Quality Initiative Joint consensus statement on patient-reported outcomes in an enhanced recovery pathway

Name	Type	Number of items	Rating scale (response options)	Scoring method	Scores produced	Range of scores	Recall period	Available at:
Quality of Recovery-15 (QoR-15)	Condition-specific	15	Numeric rating scale (0–10)	Score sum	Overall score	Total score 0–150 (worst to best)	24 h	https://pubs.asahq.org/anesthesiology/article/118/6/1332/11456/Development-and-Psychometric-Evaluation-of-a
WHO Disability Assessment Schedule 2.0 (WHODAS 2.0)	Generic	12-item version/36-item version	Ordinal scale (5-point)	12-item version: score sum 36-item version: simple scoring (sum) or complex scoring (item-response theory)	12-item version: overall score 36-item version: overall score and subscale scores (cognition, mobility self-care/hygiene, getting along, life activities, participation)	12-item version: 12–60 (best to worst) Total score: 36–180 (worst to best); complex scoring 0–100 (worst to best) Subscale scores: varies	30 days	https://www.who.int/classifications/international-classification-of-functioning-disability-and-health/who-disability-assessment-schedule

| PROMIS measurement system | Generic | Varies | Varies | Item-response theory | Varies | Varies | 7 days | https://www.healthmeasures.net/index.php?option=com_content&view=category&layout=blog&id=147&Itemid=806 |

advantage of ePROMs is that they enable remote data collection and can facilitate data management and assessment by patients, clinicians, and researchers [58]. As discussed earlier, ePROMs also enable the use of computerized adaptive testing (CAT), the next-generation method of administering PROMs via automated selection of (fewer) items to reduce response burden [59]. Research suggests that the use of ePROMs can result in higher patient satisfaction, more accurate and complete data collection, reduced administrative burden, and lower costs [60]. However, ePROMs need to maintain equivalent validity in comparison with paper-based PROMs [61]. Thus, when transforming a paper-based instrument into an ePROM, careful consideration is required to minimize changes in the content and layout [62]. Furthermore, ePROMs' design should be accessible and have an efficient user interface. Such interfaces should be developed using the principles of human-centered design (i.e., with the involvement of patients and healthcare providers) [60, 63].

In the future, we envision that recovery-specific ePROM data will be seamlessly integrated in electronic health records (EHRs). This integration can be done using various approaches, including full-integration, hybrid moderate-integration, or stand-alone low-integration [64]. With a full integration, ePROMs can be incorporated as a part of the secured EHR web platform where patients can view their medical records and answer the ePROM questionnaires. When a moderate hybrid approach is used, the ePROM is presented in a separate platform linked from EHR, and the ePROM data can be viewed in the EHR. Lastly, with the low-integration approach, the ePROM is incorporated in a stand-alone external website where patients enter their responses and data can be viewed only via the external website. Future work is required to study the advantages and disadvantages of these ePROM integration approaches in terms of costs, usability, and patient and provider satisfaction. The integration of PROMs in EHRs is in line with the principles of learning healthcare systems, where data gathered in clinical practice are used in pragmatic studies to inform decision-making, measure performance, and inform quality improvement initiatives [65, 66].

Summary

As surgery enters the era of patient-centered care, it is advocated that postoperative recovery be measured using PROMs as they provide a means to incorporate patients' perspectives and experiences into research and clinical decision-making. In abdominal surgery, this is currently precluded by the lack of PROMs with sound measurement properties. While ongoing studies aim to bridge this gap, guidelines are available to direct the use of PROMs in perioperative care. There is a great deal of research to be done before PROMs are fully embraced by all stakeholders in surgery; however, the integration of PROM data in research and in daily practice has a great potential to transform how we provide care for surgical patients.

References

1. Mayo NE. Dictionary of quality of life and health outcomes measurement. 1st ed. Milwaukee: ISOQOL; 2015.
2. Barry MJ, Edgman-Levitan S. Shared decision making — the pinnacle of patient-centered care. N Engl J Med. 2012;366(9):780–1.
3. Gabriel SE, Normand S-LT. Getting the methods right — the foundation of patient-centered outcomes research. N Engl J Med. 2012;367(9):787–90.
4. Greene J, Hibbard JH. Why does patient activation matter? An examination of the relationships between patient activation and health-related outcomes. J Gen Intern Med. 2012;27(5):520–6.
5. Marshall R, Beach MC, Saha S, et al. Patient activation and improved outcomes in HIV-infected patients. J Gen Intern Med. 2013;28(5):668–74.
6. Munson GW, Wallston KA, Dittus RS, Speroff T, Roumie CL. Activation and perceived expectancies: correlations with health outcomes among veterans with inflammatory bowel disease. J Gen Intern Med. 2009;24(7):809–15.

7. Gray M, Meakins JL. Evidence-based surgical practice and patient-centered care: inevitable. Surg Clin North Am. 2006;86(1):217–20.

8. Borza T, Oerline MK, Skolarus TA, et al. Association of the hospital readmissions reduction program with surgical readmissions. JAMA Surg. 2018;153(3):243–50.

9. Lee L, Tran T, Mayo NE, Carli F, Feldman LS. What does it really mean to "recover" from an operation? Surgery. 2014;155(2):211–6.

10. Desborough JP. The stress response to trauma and surgery. Br J Anaesth. 2000;85(1):109–17.

11. Wilmore DW. From Cuthbertson to fast-track surgery: 70 years of progress in reducing stress in surgical patients. Ann Surg. 2002;236(5):643–8.

12. Zhang LM, Hornor MA, Robinson T, Rosenthal RA, Ko CY, Russell MM. Evaluation of postoperative functional health status decline among older adults. JAMA Surg. 2020;155(10):950–8.

13. Stabenau HF, Becher RD, Gahbauer EA, Leo-Summers L, Allore HG, Gill TM. Functional trajectories before and after major surgery in older adults. Ann Surg. 2018;268(6):911–7.

14. Lawrence VA, Hazuda HP, Cornell JE, et al. Functional independence after major abdominal surgery in the elderly. J Am Coll Surg. 2004;199(5):762–72.

15. Lee L, Mata J, Ghitulescu GA, et al. Cost-effectiveness of enhanced recovery versus conventional perioperative management for colorectal surgery. Ann Surg. 2015;262(6):1026–33.

16. Berg K, Arestedt K, Kjellgren K. Postoperative recovery from the perspective of day surgery patients: a phenomenographic study. Int J Nurs Stud. 2013;50(12):1630–8.

17. Nilsson U, Jaensson M, Hugelius K, Arakelian E, Dahlberg K. A journey to a new stable state—further development of the postoperative recovery concept from day surgical perspective: a qualitative study. BMJ Open. 2020;10(9):e037755.

18. Kleinbeck SVM, Hoffart N. Outpatient recovery after laparoscopic cholecystectomy. AORN J. 1994;60(3):394–8.

19. Lee L, Dumitra T, Fiore J Jr, Mayo N, Feldman L. How well are we measuring postoperative "recovery" after abdominal surgery? Qual Life Res. 2015;24:1–8.

20. Ljungqvist O, Rasmussen LS. Recovery after anaesthesia and surgery. Acta Anaesthesiol Scand. 2014;58(6):639–41.

21. Antonescu I, Mueller CL, Fried GM, Vassiliou MC, Mayo NE, Feldman LS. Outcomes reported in high-impact surgical journals. Br J Surg. 2014;101(5):582–9.

22. Miller T, Mythen M. Successful recovery after major surgery: moving beyond length of stay. Perioper Med. 2014;3(1):4.

23. Davidson GH, Haukoos JS, Feldman LS. Practical guide to assessment of patient-reported outcomes. JAMA Surg. 2020;155(5):432–3.

24. U.S. Department of Health and Human Services Food and Drug Administration. Guidance for Industry. Patient-reported outcome measures: use in medical product development to support labeling claims. http://www.fda.gov/downloads/Drugs/Guidances/UCM193282.pdf. Published 2009. Accessed 23 Sept 2020.

25. Olsen JA, Misajon R. A conceptual map of health-related quality of life dimensions: key lessons for a new instrument. Qual Life Res. 2020;29(3):733–43.

26. Ware JE Jr. SF-36 health survey. In: The use of psychological testing for treatment planning and outcomes assessment. 2nd ed. Mahwah: Lawrence Erlbaum Associates Publishers; 1999. p. 1227–46.

27. Ustün TB, Chatterji S, Kostanjsek N, et al. Developing the World Health Organization disability assessment schedule 2.0. Bull World Health Organ. 2010;88(11):815–23.

28. Black N. Patient reported outcome measures could help transform healthcare. BMJ. 2013;346:f167.

29. Rabin R, Charro F. EQ-5D: a measure of health status from the EuroQol Group. Ann Med. 2001;33(5):337–43.

30. Aaronson NK, Ahmedzai S, Bergman B, et al. The European Organization for Research and Treatment of Cancer QLQ-C30: a quality-of-life instrument for use in international clinical trials in oncology. JNCI. 1993;85(5):365–76.

31. Myles PS. More than just morbidity and mortality – quality of recovery and long-term functional recovery after surgery. Anaesthesia. 2020;75(S1):e143–50.

32. Fiore JF Jr, Figueiredo S, Balvardi S, et al. How do we value postoperative recovery?: a systematic review of the measurement properties of patient-reported outcomes after abdominal surgery. Ann Surg. 2018;267(4):656–69.

33. Patrick DL, Burke LB, Gwaltney CJ, et al. Content validity—establishing and reporting the evidence in newly developed patient-reported outcomes (PRO) instruments for medical product evaluation: ISPOR PRO good research practices task force report: part 1—eliciting concepts for a new PRO instrument. Value Health. 2011;14(8):967–77.

34. Patrick DL, Burke LB, Gwaltney CJ, et al. Content validity—establishing and reporting the evidence in newly developed patient-reported outcomes (PRO) instruments for medical product evaluation: ISPOR PRO good research practices task force report: part 2—assessing respondent understanding. Value Health. 2011;14(8):978–88.

35. Mokkink LB, Terwee CB, Patrick DL, et al. The COSMIN study reached international consensus on taxonomy, terminology, and definitions of measurement properties for health-related patient-reported outcomes. J Clin Epidemiol. 2010;63(7):737–45.

36. Terwee CB, Prinsen CAC, Chiarotto A, et al. COSMIN methodology for evaluating the content validity of patient-reported outcome measures: a Delphi study. Qual Life Res. 2018;27(5):1159–70.

37. Alam R, Montanez J, Law S, et al. Development of a conceptual framework of recovery after abdominal surgery. Surg Endosc. 2020;34(6):2665–74.

38. Petrillo J, Cano SJ, McLeod LD, Coon CD. Using classical test theory, item response theory, and Rasch measurement theory to evaluate patient-reported outcome measures: a comparison of worked examples. Value Health. 2015;18(1):25–34.

39. Pallant JF, Tennant A. An introduction to the Rasch measurement model: an example using the Hospital Anxiety and Depression Scale (HADS). Br J Clin Psychol. 2007;46(1):1–18.

40. Tennant A, Conaghan PG. The Rasch measurement model in rheumatology: what is it and why use it? When should it be applied, and what should one look for in a Rasch paper? Arthritis Care Res. 2007;57(8):1358–62.

41. Hobart JC, Cano SJ, Zajicek JP, Thompson AJ. Rating scales as outcome measures for clinical trials in neurology: problems, solutions, and recommendations. Lancet Neurol. 2007;6(12):1094–105.

42. Hung M, Stuart AR, Higgins TF, Saltzman CL, Kubiak EN. Computerized adaptive testing using the PROMIS physical function item bank reduces test burden with less ceiling effects compared with the short musculoskeletal function assessment in orthopaedic trauma patients. J Orthop Trauma. 2014;28(8):439–43.

43. Gibbons RD, Weiss DJ, Kupfer DJ, et al. Using computerized adaptive testing to reduce the burden of mental health assessment. Psychiatr Serv. 2008;59(4):361–8.

44. Meijer RR, Nering ML. Computerized adaptive testing: overview and introduction. Appl Psychol Meas. 1999;23(3):187–94.

45. Revicki DA, Cella DF. Health status assessment for the twenty-first century: item response theory, item banking and computer adaptive testing. Qual Life Res. 1997;6(6):595–600.

46. Mokkink LB, de Vet HCW, Prinsen CAC, et al. COSMIN risk of bias checklist for systematic reviews of patient-reported outcome measures. Qual Life Res. 2018;27(5):1171–9.

47. Mokkink LB, Terwee CB, Patrick DL, et al. The COSMIN checklist for assessing the methodological quality of studies on measurement properties of health status measurement instruments: an international Delphi study. Qual Life Res. 2010;19(4):539–49.

48. Reeve BB, Wyrwich KW, Wu AW, et al. ISOQOL recommends minimum standards for patient-reported outcome measures used in patient-centered outcomes and comparative effectiveness research. Qual Life Res. 2013;22(8):1889–905.

49. Alam R, Figueiredo SM, Balvardi S, et al. Development of a patient-reported outcome measure of recovery after abdominal surgery: a hypothesized conceptual framework. Surg Endosc. 2018;32(12):4874–85.

50. Stark PA, Myles PS, Burke JA. Development and psychometric evaluation of a postoperative quality of recovery score: the QoR-15. Anesthesiology. 2013;118(6):1332–40.

51. World Health Organization. Measuring health and disability: manual for WHO Disability Assessment Schedule (WHODAS 2.0). Geneva: World Health Organization; 2012.

52. Intro to PROMIS. https://www.healthmeasures.net/explore-measurement-systems/promis/intro-to-promis. Accessed 17 Nov 2020.

53. Jammer I, Wickboldt N, Sander M, et al. Standards for definitions and use of outcome measures for clinical effectiveness research in perioperative medicine: European Perioperative Clinical Outcome (EPCO) definitions: a statement from the ESA-ESICM joint taskforce on perioperative outcome measures. Eur J Anaesthesiol. 2015;32(2):88–105.

54. Myles PS, Boney O, Botti M, et al. Systematic review and consensus definitions for the Standardised Endpoints in Perioperative Medicine (StEP) initiative: patient comfort. Br J Anaesth. 2018;120(4):705–11.

55. Moonesinghe SR, Jackson AIR, Boney O, et al. Systematic review and consensus definitions for the Standardised Endpoints in Perioperative Medicine initiative: patient-centred outcomes. Br J Anaesth. 2019;123(5):664–70.

56. Loftus TJ, Tighe PJ, Filiberto AC, et al. Artificial intelligence and surgical decision-making. JAMA Surg. 2020;155(2):148–58.

57. Coons SJ, Eremenco S, Lundy JJ, O'Donohoe P, O'Gorman H, Malizia W. Capturing patient-reported outcome (PRO) data electronically: the past, present, and promise of ePRO measurement in clinical trials. Patient. 2015;8(4):301–9.

58. Ganser AL, Raymond SA, Pearson JD. Data quality and power in clinical trials: a comparison of ePRO and paper in a randomized trial. In: ePRO: electronic solutions for patient-reporteddata. Surray: Gower; 2010. p. 49–78.

59. Cook KF, O'Malley KJ, Roddey TS. Dynamic assessment of health outcomes: time to let the CAT out of the bag? Health Serv Res. 2005;40(5p2):1694–711.

60. Ross J, Holzbaur E, Wade M, Rothrock T. Patient preferences: pro mixed modes – Epro versus paper. Value Health. 2014;17(7):A515.

61. Coons SJ, Gwaltney CJ, Hays RD, et al. Recommendations on evidence needed to support measurement equivalence between electronic and paper-based patient-reported outcome (PRO) measures: ISPOR ePRO good research practices task force report. Value Health. 2009;12(4):419–29.

62. Gwaltney CJ, Shields AL, Shiffman S. Equivalence of electronic and paper-and-pencil administration of patient-reported outcome measures: a meta-analytic review. Value Health. 2008;11(2):322–33.

63. Harniss M, Amtmann D, Cook D, Johnson K. Considerations for developing interfaces for collecting patient-reported outcomes that allow the inclusion of individuals with disabilities. Med Care. 2007;45(5):S48–54.

64. Wu AW, Kharrazi H, Boulware LE, Snyder CF. Measure once, cut twice—adding patient-reported outcome measures to the electronic health record for comparative effectiveness research. J Clin Epidemiol. 2013;66(8, Supplement):S12–20.

65. Flum DR, Alfonso-Cristancho R, Devine EB, et al. Implementation of a "real-world" learning health care system: Washington state's comparative effectiveness research translation network (CERTAIN). Surgery. 2014;155(5):860–6.

66. Medicine Io. Patients charting the course: citizen engagement and the learning health system: workshop summary. Washington, DC: The National Academies Press; 2011.

Chapter 15
Enhanced Recovery Protocols: A Toolkit for Success

Deborah S. Keller

Introduction

Undergoing surgery is analogous to running a marathon. The marathon runner practices, preparing their body and mind to be in their most fit state for the race. They use all methods available to minimize exertion and optimize their performance and endurance during the physical stress of the race. After the race, they harness their preparation and evidence-based science to avoid injury and expedite recovery. No athlete would go into a marathon without appropriate training, guidance, and support. As surgeons, we should ensure our patients train in the same fashion and receive similar guidance and support for surgery. Major surgery can lead to a variety of physiological stressors including organ dysfunction,

The author received no financial support or funding for this work.

D. S. Keller (✉)
Division of Colorectal Surgery, Department of Surgery, University of California at Davis, Sacramento, CA, USA

© The Author(s), under exclusive license to Springer Nature Switzerland AG 2022
J. R. Romanelli et al. (eds.), *The SAGES Manual of Quality, Outcomes and Patient Safety*,
https://doi.org/10.1007/978-3-030-94610-4_15

physical trauma, and hormonal and neurological disturbances. Without proper preparation and education, the surgical process can lead to morbidity, delayed recovery, and even mortality for the patient, with additional strain on the healthcare system.

Enhanced recovery pathways (ERP) or enhanced recovery after surgery (ERAS) protocols are structured perioperative programs that apply evidence-based interventions coupled with patient engagement to all stages of the surgical process. Enhanced recovery represents a paradigm shift in surgical practice that aims to help patients prepare and recover better and faster than traditional methods. The protocols reexamine traditional perioperative care tenets and replace them with current best practices, when appropriate. In turn, postoperative complications and costs are minimized while improving postoperative recovery and patient outcomes after major surgery.

From personal experience, the success of an ERP is based on four key factors:

- The local applicability of the evidence-based measures applied
- The development of a coordinated multidisciplinary team that can offer patient support along the entire care continuum
- The effective implementation of the program
- The participation of the patient who becomes critical in their own preparation and recovery

As a rule, surgeons are risk-adverse, so implementing change is never a simple task. But presenting the proposed ERP changes as evidence, not just clinical suggestions, in conjunction with a structured framework, can help with acceptance and change management experience. In this chapter, I summarize the history and clinical application of enhanced recovery and highlight the key elements in successfully implementing an ERP into practice in surgery. The implementation here is presented like a "toolkit" and aligned with the SAGES Master's Program framework. The SAGES

Master's Program framework categorizes learning into the three levels of targeted performance: Competency, Proficiency, and Mastery [1]. Competency is defined as what a graduating general surgery chief resident or minimally invasive surgery (MIS) fellow should be able to achieve; in ERP, this is likened to performing the institutional assessment for specific quality improvement targets and defining the multidisciplinary team and protocol that the hospital would like to implement. Proficiency is what a surgeon approximately 3 years out from training should be able to accomplish; from the ERP perspective, this is compatible with developing an action plan for implementing the intervention and a plan for evaluating implementation and devising a program to audit performance and compliance. Mastery is what more experienced surgeons should be able to accomplish after 7 or more years in practice. Mastery is applicable to SAGES surgeons seeking in-depth knowledge in areas of controversy, best practices, and the ability to mentor colleagues. For ERP, this could be developing clinical practice guidelines, implementation models for other surgery service lines, or introducing new technology or progressive topics into study, like same-day discharge and opioid-free surgery (Table 15.1).

Understanding Enhanced Recovery Protocols

Enhanced recovery pathways or protocols (ERP) – also known as enhanced recovery after surgery (ERAS) programs – are evidenced-based pathways designed to standardize surgical care, improve outcomes, and lower healthcare costs. ERPs were first introduced by Danish surgeon Henrik Kehlet in the 1980s. Kehlet studied the impact of the surgical stress response on the recovery process and combined anesthetic, surgical, and postoperative approaches to modify the stress response after surgery [2]. This work developed into multimodal fast-track pathways, which reduced the physiological stress and postoperative organ dysfunction from surgery by optimizing perioperative care and postoperative rehabilitation [3–6].

TABLE 15.1 SAGES Master's Program levels of targeted performance in enhanced recovery

Competency	Proficiency	Mastery
What a graduating general surgery chief resident or MIS fellow should be able to achieve	What a surgeon approximately 3 years out from training should be able to accomplish	What more experienced surgeons should be able to accomplish after 7 or more years in practice
Institutional assessment Change management Define the program/ intervention/ initiative that the hospital would like to implement and devise a plan for evaluating it Understanding the patient has a key role	The second process is to define an action plan for implementing the intervention and a plan for evaluating implementation Implementation science Ensuring compliance	Developing practice guidelines Headlining controversial topics, such as opioid-free pain management, same-day surgery/23-h discharge Best practices for audit methodology Applying new technology to improve outcomes Using mHealth options for post-discharge surveillance Clinical trials to advance the science of enhanced recovery

The specific components of ERP were assembled after rigorous study of mechanisms of how metabolic injury and physical interventions affected recovery, as well as the scientific evaluation of the effectiveness of each measure to enhance the recovery process. Processes for systemic inflammatory and catabolic response of various organ systems to surgery, deranged fluid homeostasis and vascular responsiveness, anemia, and pain pathology were targets for specific interventions [3]. These interventions formed the initial foundation of ERP: standardized preoperative information, reduction of surgical stress responses, optimized dynamic pain relief, and early mobilization and oral nutrition [7]. With the evolution of ERP, traditional perioperative care dogmas such as immobilization, routine drains and nasogastric tubes, and fasting until return of bowel function were eliminated in favor of evidence-based tenets such as normoglycemia and elimination of fasting, carbohydrate loading before surgery, regional anesthetic techniques, maintenance of normothermia and fluid balance during surgery, optimal treatment of postoperative pain, and prophylaxis. These recommendations were broken into interventions for all stages of care in the surgical process – preoperative, intraoperative, postoperative, and post-discharge periods – and published as evidence-based guidelines [8, 9]. These original key principles remain but have evolved to have a greater focus on expanding the use of prehabilitation, minimal invasive surgical techniques, and opioid-sparing pain control [10–16].

The concept of ERP was a paradigm shift from traditional surgical care and recovery. However, this shift provided a major enhancement in surgical care and recovery. ERPs were first initiated in colorectal surgery, and the most robust data remains in these procedures. However, their evidence-based benefits have been proven across nearly all surgery service lines, and guidelines currently exist for management in bariatrics, breast, cytoreductive, cardiac, gastrointestinal, hepato-pancreatic biliary, obstetric, orthopedic, pulmonary, thoracic, neonatal intestinal, gynecologic/oncology, and urologic surgery (https://erassociety.org/guidelines/list-of-guidelines/).

There are multiple controlled trials, systematic reviews and meta-analyses, and cohort studies demonstrating consistently reduced hospital length of stay, postoperative morbidity, and convalescence without increasing readmission rates after surgery [9, 17–33]. The same principles have been proven safe and feasible in special patient populations, such as older adults, Crohn's disease, and stoma patients [27, 34–42]. With the propagation of ERP and earlier hospital discharge, there were concerns of a rebound increase in readmission rates. The initial works showed no significant increases or changes in readmission rates. As ERP experience has matured, readmission rates have actually decreased along with length of stay and complication rates [28, 43]. While there are ongoing studies on the impact of ERAS on patient outcomes, it appears that essentially any surgical specialty, patient population, and age group should be considered for an ERP.

In addition to the clinical benefits, ERPs have consistently improved healthcare utilization and reduced hospital costs [23, 29, 44–53]. The cost savings results primarily from the decrease in hospital length of stay after ERP implementation. The total cost savings in acute hospitalizations after surgery has been estimated as a greater than 15% cost savings per patient [54]. Thus, ERP can help improve healthcare value in the current environment of rising healthcare costs.

Questions initially arose about the safety and acceptability of this shift away from traditional length-of-stay patterns with ERP, where patients are sent home from the hospital after only a few days postsurgery [55, 56]. However, with proper education, established communication lines, and ensuring all patient care needs are met, recovery at home can actually be optimal. Patients are familiar with the surroundings, have access to their belongings and support system, and can control their environment, which promotes a less stressful and less traumatic recovery. Further, in the pandemic environment where hospital visitation by family members may be prohibited or limited, patients have unrestricted family support while recovering at home. Studies have shown patients embraced the protocols, reporting significantly less pain, used fewer opiates, and returned to physical activities faster than patients managed with traditional techniques [57–59].

There are ways to help improve individual outcomes after implementing ERP into practice. Compliance and adherence to the protocol elements matter. Strict adherence is associated with a reduced incidence of postoperative symptoms, complications, and length of stay (LOS) in elective surgery [60–64]. While adherence matters, few studies report on actual adherence rates with their programs [65]. Furthermore, strict adherence to all elements in a multimodal protocol can be a challenge in all patient populations [66]. Studies have tried to identify the relative importance of the individual elements and which are the key components to ensure compliance with [60–64, 67]. However, there are large discrepancies in the elements found to be independent predictors of successful outcomes across all studies, including age, restriction of intravenous fluid, use of a preoperative carbohydrate drink, utilization of minimally invasive surgery, removal of nasogastric tube before extubation, early mobilization, early nonsteroidal anti-inflammatory drug initiation, and early removal of thoracic epidural analgesia. This is not unexpected, as each institution is unique in its patient and provider population, starting point, and quality needs. However, there are categorical demographic and procedural variables the multidisciplinary team can use to recognize which patients will need extra attention adhering to the standardized pathways, including preoperative anxiety, chronic pain, preoperative chemoradiation, and intraoperative conversion [68].

Implementing an Enhanced Recovery Pathway into Practice

While the concept and evidence supporting ERP is well established, few medical centers have been able to embed them seamlessly in their culture. Even among SAGES surgeons, a 2016 survey found less than half regularly used some elements of ERPs (48.7%) and 30% were unfamiliar with the concept [69]. To many in the surgical world, ERP principles remain foreign or unimplemented, to the patients' detriment [70]. Among those reporting ERP use, there was wide variety in the specific elements and discharge used, with a universal need for information on implementation, compliance, and measuring outcomes. With the established benefits, developing a framework for a successful ERP is key to improving a surgical department's quality and outcomes. Here, we describe the steps aligned with the SAGES Master's Program levels of targeted performance: Competency, Proficiency, and Mastery.

Competency

Goals

- Defining the multidisciplinary team and assigning roles
- Literature and evidence review
- Gap analysis and benchmarking
- Institutional assessment for quality improvement targets
- Developing the multimodal protocol

The first step to competency is to assemble a multidisciplinary team and define leaders. There needs to be one overall leader, tasked with coordinating the meetings and ongoing comprehensive details related to the ERP. Under the overall leader are "champions" of enhanced recovery in your organization. They should become subject matter experts in the science of ERP, help change the culture during implementation, and oversee ongoing refinements in the process. It is suggested that the champions be well-known and respected individuals that are mid-career, not too "junior" such that their voice is unknown, yet not too "senior" that their clinical demands are too much to devote the necessary time for this interactive role. For instance, Division Chiefs rather than Department Chairs would be a good appointment. The team should include a representation of every group the patient could interact with during their hospital stay and recovery process. It should be diverse in discipline, including allied health and support services, and experience level, with house staff and attendings all represented. A true multidisciplinary team can help serve as a check and balance system for patient safety and help the implementation of the protocol, by having members that enter, process, approve, and deliver elements of the ERP. It is important to remember that every member of the team has a unique, equal, and important voice in the process. A strong multidisciplinary team with good lines of communication can also help ensure patient engagement and education on the ERP. Suggestions for a multidisciplinary team include administrative officers in patient safety, finance, and quality improvement roles; surgery; nursing (from inpatient, outpatient, and perioperative areas); anesthesia; pharmacy; nutrition; physical therapy; case management; social work; wound ostomy care nurses; data analysts; and unit managers of common postoperative care wards.

In the current landscape, many organizations, departments, and even individual providers have attempted to introduce an ERP or elements of an ERP into practice. When created and implemented without the top-down support and centralization under a primary leader, it is not possible to standardize communications and order sets, rollout the program in an efficient fashion, or use common metrics and time frames for auditing. The program will be carried out in silos, with redundancy and variation across all steps. By definition, this framework will fail to meet the overall goals of a standardized, cost-efficient, and effective ERP. While a major culture change (that could potentially impact the egos of engaged providers), the best thing for the organization as a whole in this situation is to start from scratch. Place a fresh leader in charge over the champions, ensuring higher-level support. Then, include those who previously led stand-alone programs as champions in the multidisciplinary team, respecting their experience and input (Fig. 15.1).

Following establishment of the team, the next step to becoming competent in enhanced recovery is to do your homework – perform a literature search from a search engine

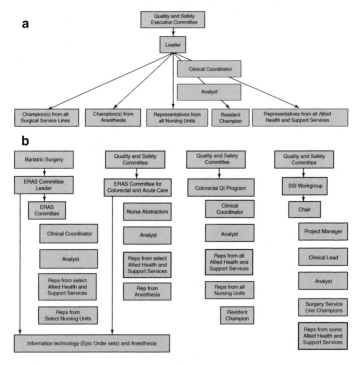

FIGURE 15.1 Enhanced recovery pathway structure in ideal (**a**) and noneffective (**b**) models

such as PubMed® of "enhanced recovery," "enhanced recovery after surgery," "prehabilitation," *and* your specific surgery discipline, such as "colorectal surgery" *or* "bariatric surgery." This will allow you to review the publications on subject matter, from recent clinical trials to classic foundation studies. Reviewing the literature can also help you learn about tools, techniques, and methodology that have been helpful to patients and providers that have already gone through this process. After a broad initial review, your initial search can be refined by adding in process measures (e.g., risk assessment, nutrition, cardiovascular exercise, minimally invasive surgery, early ambulation) and outcome measures (e.g., length of stay, complication rates, readmission rates, costs, patient discharge destination) for work more specific to your institution's interests. Following this literature search, reviewing guidelines and existing protocols for enhanced recovery protocols in your surgery service will help establish a strong understanding of the process, outcomes, and elements in existing protocols, as well as the evidence behind selecting them. Valuable sites for this information are surgical society pages, the ERAS Society, Cochrane Database, and surgical department websites that employ known subject matter leaders. From your review of the literature and evidence, present a sample of key pieces to the administration and multidisciplinary team. These are basics of financial benefits and clinical outcomes, to give the group a sense of urgency and need to implement a protocol. An example of these key papers for colorectal surgery is seen in Table 15.2.

With the team in place, the next step for competency is for the team to perform an assessment of the quality improvement needs at your institution. This information can be derived from a variety of sources, including your institution's divisional morbidity and mortality reports; administrative billing data, nationally validated, risk-adjusted, outcomes-based programs (e.g., ACS NSQIP®); and member-driven healthcare performance analytic agencies (e.g., Vizient, Optum). These data can identify the specific gaps or deficiencies you have in processes that are affecting the overall quality; they can be outcome measures (result of system processes, such as urinary tract infection rate, length of stay, and readmission rates) or process measures (the specific steps in a process that lead to a particular outcome metric, such as routine removal of Foley catheters on day 1 after surgery and patient education sessions on surgical expectations) [71]. While process metrics may ultimately be more important, outcome metrics are more visible and easier to audit change from. In addition, outcome metrics such as readmission are targets for the Centers for Medicare and Medicaid Services (CMS) value-based programs, which can penalize providers for higher-than-expected rates in an effort to reduce excess hospital readmissions, lower healthcare costs,

TABLE 15.2 Suggested key literature on enhanced recovery in colorectal surgery

King PM, Blazeby JM, Ewings P, et al. The influence of an enhanced recovery programme on clinical outcomes, costs and quality of life after surgery for colorectal cancer. Colorectal Dis. 2006;8:506–513	Keller DS, Bankwitz B, Woconish D et al. Predicting who will fail early discharge after laparoscopic colorectal surgery with an established enhanced recovery pathway. Surg Endosc. 2014;28:74–79
Kehlet H, Wilmore DW. Evidence-based surgical care and the evolution of fast-track surgery. Ann Surg. 2008;248:189–198	Thiele, RH, Rea, KM, Turrentine, FE, et al. Standardization of care: impact of an enhanced recovery protocol on length of stay, complications, and direct costs after colorectal surgery. J Am Coll Surg. 2015;220:430–43. https://doi.org/10.1016/j.jamcollsurg.2014.12.042
Spanjersberg WR, Reurings J, Keus F, van Laarhoven CJ. Fast track surgery versus conventional recovery strategies for colorectal surgery. Cochrane Database Syst Rev. 2011;CD007635	West, MA, Loughney, L, Lythgoe, D, et al. Effect of prehabilitation on objectively measured physical fitness after neoadjuvant treatment in preoperative rectal cancer patients: a blinded interventional pilot study. Br J Anaesth. 2015;114:244–51
Lawrence JK, Keller DS, Samia H et al. Discharge within 24 to 72 hours of colorectal surgery is associated with low readmission rates when using enhanced recovery pathways. J Am Coll Surg. 2013;216:390–394	Carmichael, JC, Keller, DS, Baldini, G, et al. Clinical practice guideline for enhanced recovery after colon and rectal surgery from the American Society of Colon and Rectal Surgeons (ASCRS) and Society of American Gastrointestinal and Endoscopic Surgeons (SAGES). Surg Endosc. 2017;31:3412–3436

TABLE 15.2 (continued)

Smart NJ, White P, Allison AS, Ockrim JB, Kennedy RH, Francis NK. Deviation and failure of enhanced recovery after surgery following laparoscopic colorectal surgery: Early prediction model. Colorectal Dis. 2012;14:e727–34	Francis, NK, Walker, T, Carter, F, et al. Consensus on training and implementation of enhanced recovery after surgery: a Delphi study. World J Surg. 2018;42:1919–1928. https://doi.org/10.1007/s00268-017-4436-2
Aarts MA, Okrainec A, Glicksman A, Pearsall E, Victor JC, McLeod RS. Adoption of enhanced recovery after surgery (ERAS) strategies for colorectal surgery at academic teaching hospitals and impact on total length of hospital stay. Surg Endosc. 2012;26:442–450	van Rooijen, S, Carli, F, Dalton, S, et al. Multimodal prehabilitation in colorectal cancer patients to improve functional capacity and reduce postoperative complications: the first international randomized controlled trial for multimodal prehabilitation. BMC Cancer. 2019;19:98
Lee L, Li C, Landry T et al. A systematic review of economic evaluations of enhanced recovery pathways for colorectal surgery. Ann Surg. 2014;259:670–676.	

and improve patient safety and outcomes [72]. The team can compare their internal state with other internal departments, other hospitals, and federal benchmarking levels for each metric. From this benchmarking, they can determine which areas have performance gaps compared to published standards. Selecting one or two measures as the initial focus of the ERP can help keep all parties focused and engaged during the implementation process. It may also make parties resistant to change more likely to "buy in" to the protocol. Common outcome measures selected are readmissions, length of stay, catheter-associated urinary tract infections, and surgical site infections, as these are linked to financial penalties. While not all members of the department may be open to introducing a new ERP and changing their current practice, they need to be open to reducing readmissions, length of stay, catheter-associated urinary tract infections, and surgical site infections. Thus, introducing the ERP as a way to help the bottom line and improve outcomes instead of a process change may help acceptance with colleagues.

The final step in competency is developing the institution's multimodal protocol with the multidisciplinary team. ERP elements are fairly uniform. The availability of specific medications or services may differ across institution, though. Surgery departmental websites with known ERAS programs are an excellent source to reference ERP models. A sample of our department's ERP for colorectal surgery is seen in Fig. 15.2. The Agency for Healthcare Research and Quality (AHRQ) Safety Program for Improving Surgical Care and Recovery (ISCR), a collaborative program with the American College of Surgeons (ACS) and Johns Hopkins Medicine Armstrong Institute for Patient Safety and Quality, also offers a wealth of templates, if needed. The steps of competency are summarized in Fig. 15.3.

Proficiency

Goals

- Education in all patient-facing divisions
- Developing a plan for implementation
- Implementation
- Constructing a plan for evaluating the implementation
- Creating a plan for audit and ensuring ongoing compliance

The proficiency stage is an in-depth planning phase. The specific goals and processes have already been defined. The next step is to define how to put them in place. This is specific for each institution and must take into account local factors. From a broad perspective, the proficiency step is most successful by planning education sessions with all patient-facing

Pre-operative 4-6 Weeks before	
Screen	Anemia, cognition, diabetes, falls, frailty, function
Multimodal prehabilitaton	
Referral	Primary provider, specialist, or anesthesia clinic, as needed
Optimize	Polypharmacy, stop supplements, smoking, and alcohol
Day before	
Oral and mechanical bowel prep	1g Neomycin, 500mg metronidazole at 2, 3, and 9pm Miralax/gatorade at 2pm
Diet	Clear liquids until 4 hours before schedule surgery time (G2/ Water/ smart water/ pedialyte)
Skin cleansing	Shower with antibacterial soap (dial or chlorhexidine liquid)
Immunonutrition	Ensure drink 2× daily (6 days prior to surgery)
Pre-emptive analgesia	Gabapentin 600mg PO at 6pm
Day of surgery	
Carb loading (at home)	− Clear liquids (G2/ water/ smart water/pedialyte) until 4 hours before hospital arrival; If arrival at or before 9:00 am, then NPO from midnight − Ensure/ impact 2 hrs before scheduled start time
Ileus prophylaxis (preop unit)	Alvimopan 12mg PO (1 pre-op dose in all cases)
Pre-emptive analgesia (preop unit)	Celecoxib 200mg, Tylenol 975mg PO
Stoma patients (preop unit)	Notify NP if stoma trial patient
Intraoperative	
Pre-emptive analgesia	TAP block (notify regional anesthesia team and consent) − If using regular local, administer at end of case − If using EXPAREL, administer at start of case
Antibiotics-within 60 mins of incision	Ceftriaxone 1 or 2g and 500mg metronidazole
	If documented PCN allergy, per institution's nomogram
DVT prophylaxis	SubQ Heparin 5,000u
	SCD's
Foley	Insert Foley sterile in OR
PONV prophylaxis	Dexamethasone 8mg at induction
	Zofran 4mg at reversal
Skin prep	Clipping hair
	Chlorhexidine–3 min airdry
Maintain normothermia	Warm air device, fluid warmer, room temp
Maintain euglycemia	Tight glycemic control 80–120
Goal directed fluid therapy	Use crystalloid, avoid salt/water overload / 1.5–2ml/kg/hrs
Wound protectors	Extraction site and laparotomy incisions
Clean closure	Entire team changes gloves and gowns for skin closure
	Clean closure tray opened and used
Multimodal pain management	Anesthesia to use opioids only as needed after induction
	Toradol 30mg at closure (no Toradol in Crohn's disease)

FIGURE 15.2 Sample of an enhanced recovery pathway in colorectal surgery

Postoperative (identify patient as Eras)	
POD #0	
Fluids	Crystalloid @ 1cc/kg/ideal body weight/hr for 6hrs, then 40cc/hr
Diet	Transitional diet POD 0
PONV	Alvimopan 12mg BID while inpatient (7d max) ONLY if open case (STOP in MIS case)
Analgesia	Gabapentin 300mg PO q8hrs or 300mg PO QHS if >70yrs
	Toradol 15mg IV q6hrs (Hold in Crohn's disease patients)
	Acetaminophen 975mg PO q8hrs
PRN and pain adjuncts	− Oxycodone 5mg PO q6hrs prn pain 4–6/10 (moderate) − Oxycodone 10mg PO q6hrs prn pain 7–10/10 (severe) − Dilaudid 0.5mg IV q3 hrs prn pain 8–10/10 ("breakthrough")
	− Selective if persistent pain/ pre-existing opioids: − Add Lidocaine patch to the abdomen − Add Roboxin 750mg PO QID for muscle spasm − PCA-Fentanyl–25-50mcg Q10 min (and stop all other prn meds)
Activity	To chair 3–6 hrs post op, ambulate q6 hrs (goal 2000 steps)
POD #1 onward	
Fluids	DC IVF
Diet	Transitional diet
	Ensure supplement (or diabetic glucerna) at least once per day
POI prophylaxis	Alvimopan 12mg PO BID (open cases)
DVT prophylaxis	40mg Lovenox SC daily
Analgesia	Gabapentin 300mg PO q8hrs or 300mg PO QHS if >70yrs
	Celecoxib 200mg PO BID if CrCl >30 mL/min − Celecoxib 100mg PO BID if older than 70yrs − If renal failure or Crohn's disease, no NSAIDS-> Use prn − medications − If recent MI or stents, no Celecoxib; use Toradol 30mg IV q6hrs
	Acetaminophen 975mg PO q8hrs
PRN and pain adjuncts	− Oxycodone 5mg PO q6hrs prn pain 4–6/10 (moderate) − Oxycodone 10mg PO q6hrs prn pain 7–10/10 (severe) − Dilaudid 0.5mg IV q3 hrs prn pain 8–10/10 ("breakthrough")
PONV prophylaxis	Prn: Zofran 4mg IV q6hrs or Reglan 10mg IV q6hrs
Activity	Out of bed for all meals and at least 6 hours daily
	Ambulate 4× daily; increase distance each day (goal 2000-4000 steps)
Other	DC Foley if not removed in OR (Day 2 for low pelvic cases and pouches)
	Head of bed elevated to 30 degrees at all times
Ancillary services	Enterostomal therapy teaching for all ileostomy and colostomy patients
	Physical therapy as needed for disposition
	Nutrition therapy
DC planning	Follow -up appointment scheduled − Option for PCP for staple removal, Telehealth visit
	Early notification for home care needs to social work/ case management
	Lovenox for DVT prophylaxis X 28 days post discharge for all colorectal cancer and IBD resection cases (not stoma creations, stoma closures)
	Train patient/caregiver to perform injection, start POD 1 (nursing order)

FIGURE 15.2 (continued)

Discharge planning	
Defined discharge criteria:	Walking?
	Passing flatus/ stoma function?
	Pain controlled with PO meds?
	Tolerating PO diet?
	Ready to go home?
	Follow -up appointment scheduled prior to discharge?
Discharge prescriptions:	Gabapentin 300mg PO q8hrs × 2 weeks
	Tylenol 650mg and Motrin/ Advil/ Ibuprofen 600mg PO q8hrs × 2 weeks
	Bowel regimen: Colace and Miralax
	Tramadol 100mg q8hrs prn severe pain × 6–12 tabs prn (depending on medication use in the hospital prior to discharge and case complexity) 6-stoma closure; 10-colectomy, anorectal; 12-proctectomy, pouch, APR
	Lovenox as above

FIGURE 15.2 (continued)

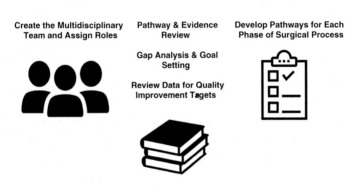

Create the Multidisciplinary Team and Assign Roles

Pathway & Evidence Review

Gap Analysis & Goal Setting

Review Data for Quality Improvement Targets

Develop Pathways for Each Phase of Surgical Process

FIG. 15.3 Competency level steps

groups. These should include the preoperative nurses, postan-esthesia care unit nurses, floor nurses, surgical residents, case management, anesthesia residents/certified registered nurse anesthetists, and your administrative support staff. In these sessions, you should communicate the background, protocol, and particular roles that group will play. It should be noted that these standardized processes are aimed to make their work easier, not create more work by changing what they are used to doing. Seek their input and be open to changes based on their experience. Ask for ongoing feedback so these groups are clear you're partners in this quality improvement goal. Having written communication is also important. Ensure there are patient and provider education booklets or handouts created detailing the ERP elements for the surgery lines and changes from usual practice with their rationale. Advertise the program on the department website and social media platforms and offer to give grand rounds to partnering departments.

After educating all groups, develop an implementation plan to roll out your ERP. Implementation is a set of activities designed to put the program into practice. It requires a coordinated change at the organizational and practice levels; thus, implementation is not easy. It should be thought of as an ongoing process, not a single event on the "rollout day." Having a timeline of the process mapped over a year is advisable (Fig. 15.4). This should be reviewed at all committee meetings. Committee meetings should also be scheduled regularly, such as monthly, with clear roles and action steps for all participating members. The skills of emotional intelligence, leadership, team dynamics, culture, buy-in, motivation, and sustainability are central to a successful ERP implementation and should be demonstrated by the leader and team members. The first step of implementation is the baseline. Baseline occurs before actually trying to put the ERP into practice and serves as a final inventory check phase before the formal implementation. Here, ensure all order sets, checklists, templates, and common phrases have been created by your institutions' information technology (IT) partners and are live in the electronic medical record (EMR) system. Confirm all parties communicating with patients or putting in

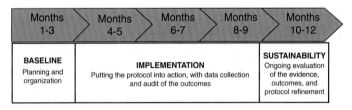

Months 1-3	Months 4-5	Months 6-7	Months 8-9	Months 10-12

BASELINE Planning and organization	**IMPLEMENTATION** Putting the protocol into action, with data collection and audit of the outcomes	**SUSTAINABILITY** Ongoing evaluation of the evidence, outcomes, and protocol refinement

FIGURE 15.4 Timeline for implementation of an enhanced recovery pathway

orders are aware and educated about the ERP. Have a data collection and audit plan in place, as well as an analyst in charge of generating reports for the committee and supporting executives. There are many options for how to accomplish these processes, including developing them manually at the institutional level with variables pulled from the patient records, creating automated reports from your electronic medical record system (NSQIP), or participating claims database or even the ERAS® Interactive Audit System (Encare). Common elements for data collection include patient demographics (e.g., age, physical status, body mass index, gender, frailty, independence level, comorbidities), patient outcome measures (e.g., hospital length of stay, readmissions, reoperation, complications/morbidity, and mortality), benefits and costs per patient in the pathway, patient compliance with the elements (overall and individual ERP elements, as percentage or number of elements chosen), and provider compliance with pathway elements within their specialty (overall and individual ERP elements, as percentage or number of elements chosen). A simple institutional-level report is seen in Fig. 15.5. The audit should provide high-level and detailed documentation, monitoring, and evaluation of variances and outcomes. The audit should be performed regularly, such as monthly at initiation, and then quarterly after well established. Reports should be reviewed by the multidisciplinary committee regularly. Over time, it can determine barriers/obstacles to success and help the committee develop action plans to address. Tools such as six sigma and statistical process control can be applied to evaluate changes over time and reductions in outliers with the ERP [73–82].

The final step in the implementation plan is sustainability. This is an ongoing process where the team can use information from the audit to identify issues in the process or structure of care that impact compliance with the ERP and make necessary changes. Barriers to success can be identified, and facilitators to success put into place. Staffing and organizational barriers include resistance or difficulty adapting to change, consultants or locums, patient coverage, disagree-

Item and phase	Surgeon 1	Surgeon 2	Surgeon 3	Surgeon 4	Total
Preop counseling					
Screen anemia, DM, Frailty, malnutrition					
Prehab 4–6 weeks					
Immunonutriton × 5 days					
Volume loading					
Oral/mechanical bowel prep					
Preop pain management					
Anitbiotic prophylaxis					
DVT prophylaxis					
Tap block					
Minimally invasive approach					
Goal directed fluid					
No abdominal or pelvic drainage					
Intraop opioid sparing regimen					
No routine ng tube					
Post OP iv fluid restriction <100ml/hr					
Limited PACU stay <240					
PONV prophylaxis					
Early diet					
Early ambulation					
Early foley D/C					
Scheduled NSAID/gabapentin/tylenol					
Scheduled (open) or stopped (MIS) ENTEREG					
Avoidance of pca					
Early d/c post op iv fluids					
Opioid free stay					
Mean los					
Number of total patients					
Compliance rate					
Complaince compared to last month					

FIGURE 15.5 Monthly surgeon scorecard compliance report sample

ment with the protocol recommendations, scheduling, and lack of resources to implement the protocol elements. Facilitators included education on the patient and provider benefits and also good communication, strong leadership support, integration of enhanced recovery protocol order sets and computer order entry systems to ease the workload, and feedback of the audit data, and including all staff in celebrating program "wins". Patient-related barriers include characteristics of the population (e.g., high comorbidities, frailness, emergency cases, poor social support, poor health literacy) and concerns about care following discharge. Facilitators include patient engagement and education, early communication, and patient feedback of compliance with ERP elements. It is important to have ongoing committee meetings and continue to address barriers faced. The care process is not static; new procedures, instruments, medications, and evidence are constantly introduced. With this, it is imperative to continually update your ERP and communications with new evidence to ensure the best outcomes are sustained. The elements of proficiency are seen in Fig. 15.6.

Mastery

Goals

- Develop alternative pathways for high-risk patients and procedures.
- Trial and implement new tools to improve compliance.
- Research and clinical trials.

After successfully implementing an ERP with ongoing audit and reassessment, you will essentially enter Mastery level. At this point, an audit will be able to highlight the outliers in a well-implemented protocol. Drilling down on these points may demonstrate specific high-risk patient populations, such as elderly patients, patients on chronic opioid medications, and ileostomy creation or closure cases. Elements

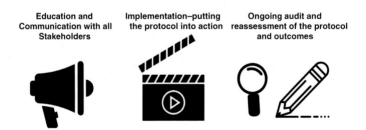

Education and Communication with all Stakeholders

Implementation–putting the protocol into action

Ongoing audit and reassessment of the protocol and outcomes

FIGURE 15.6 Proficiency level steps

in your standardized protocol may be failing to help these patients. There is an opportunity to investigate the outcome variables, and adjust one of more elements in the ERP, as appropriate for that population. Following up the outcomes after tailoring the protocol elements to the specific patient needs can help elevate your enhanced recovery practices for success in all patients.

Using tools, such as wearable devices or mobile health apps, can also help further ERP benefits. Wearable sensors are designed to monitor cardiorespiratory function, which may help early discharge processes, as well as early detection of clinical deterioration after discharge [83]. Activity trackers can be used to monitor ambulation, a major element of ERPs directly associated with early recovery [84, 85]. Finally, mobile apps with education and electronic checklists can help ensure compliance with ERP elements and patient engagement, even after discharge [86–88]. It is beneficial to have accomplished the Mastery level before adding health technologies to an ERP to ensure appropriate patient education, communication, and easy implementation of the additional tool.

Having a well-established ERP also makes evaluating the impact of an individual component in the protocol feasible. At the Mastery level, the committee can look at the benefits of opioid reduction, the impact of adding or removing a specific medication, and cost analyses, among other topics [76, 89–92]. Formal clinical or randomized controlled trials are also possible to increase the evidence base of ERP elements. With Institutional Review Board approval of your ERP, these studies can be published to help guide others looking to improve surgical outcomes. The elements of Mastery are seen in Fig. 15.7.

Develop alternative pathways for high-risk patients and procedures   **New tools to improve compliance**   **Research and Clinical trials**

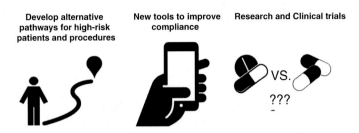

FIGURE 15.7 Mastery level steps

Conclusion

Enhanced recovery pathways are a proven method to improve patient outcomes after surgery. While the benefits are well known, the process of putting an ERP into practice can be daunting. Here, the end-to-end process is presented like a "toolkit" and aligned with the SAGES Master's Program levels of Competency, Proficiency, and Mastery. Details on the activities in each level and checklists documenting completion can help successfully guide users through the enhanced recovery process.

References

1. Jones DB, Stefanidis D, Korndorffer JR, et al. SAGES University MASTERS program: a structured curriculum for deliberate, life-long learning. Surg Endosc. 2017;31:3061–71.
2. Kehlet H. The stress response to surgery: release mechanisms and the modifying effect of pain relief. Acta Chir Scand Suppl. 1989;550:22–8.
3. Kehlet H. Multimodal approach to control postoperative pathophysiology and rehabilitation. Br J Anaesth. 1997;78:606–17.
4. Kehlet H, Wilmore DW. Multimodal strategies to improve surgical outcome. Am J Surg. 2002;183:630–41.
5. Kehlet H, Wilmore DW. Evidence-based surgical care and the evolution of fast-track surgery. Ann Surg. 2008;248:189–98.
6. Kehlet H. Fast-track colorectal surgery. Lancet. 2008;371:791–3.

7. Kehlet H. Fast-track colonic surgery: status and perspectives. Recent Results Cancer Res. 2005;165:8–13.

8. Gustafsson UO, Scott MJ, Hubner M, et al. Guidelines for perioperative care in elective colorectal surgery: Enhanced Recovery After Surgery (ERAS®) Society recommendations: 2018. World J Surg. 2019;43:659–95.

9. Carmichael JC, Keller DS, Baldini G, et al. Clinical practice guidelines for enhanced recovery after colon and rectal surgery from the American Society of Colon and Rectal Surgeons and Society of American Gastrointestinal and Endoscopic Surgeons. Dis Colon Rectum. 2017;60:761–84.

10. Carli F, Zavorsky GS. Optimizing functional exercise capacity in the elderly surgical population. Curr Opin Clin Nutr Metab Care. 2005;8:23–32.

11. Merki-Künzli C, Kerstan-Huber M, Switalla D, et al. Assessing the value of prehabilitation in patients undergoing colorectal surgery according to the enhanced recovery after surgery (ERAS) pathway for the improvement of postoperative outcomes: protocol for a randomized controlled trial. JMIR Res Protoc. 2017;6:e199.

12. King AB, Spann MD, Jablonski P, Wanderer JP, Sandberg WS, McEvoy MD. An enhanced recovery program for bariatric surgical patients significantly reduces perioperative opioid consumption and postoperative nausea. Surg Obes Relat Dis. 2018;14:849–56.

13. Pache B, Hübner M, Jurt J, Demartines N, Grass F. Minimally invasive surgery and enhanced recovery after surgery: the ideal combination. J Surg Oncol. 2017;116:613–6.

14. Spanjersberg WR, van Sambeeck JD, Bremers A, Rosman C, van Laarhoven CJ. Systematic review and meta-analysis for laparoscopic versus open colon surgery with or without an ERAS programme. Surg Endosc. 2015;29:3443–53.

15. Brandal D, Keller MS, Lee C, et al. Impact of enhanced recovery after surgery and opioid-free anesthesia on opioid prescriptions at discharge from the hospital: a historical-prospective study. Anesth Analg. 2017;125:1784–92.

16. Vlug MS, Wind J, Hollmann MW, et al. Laparoscopy in combination with fast track multimodal management is the best perioperative strategy in patients undergoing colonic surgery: a randomized clinical trial (LAFA-study). Ann Surg. 2011;254:868–75.

17. Greco M, Capretti G, Beretta L, Gemma M, Pecorelli N, Braga M. Enhanced recovery program in colorectal surgery: a meta-analysis of randomized controlled trials. World J Surg. 2014;38:1531–41.

18. Miller TE, Thacker JK, White WD, et al. Reduced length of hospital stay in colorectal surgery after implementation of an enhanced recovery protocol. Anesth Analg. 2014;118:1052–61.

19. ERAS CG. The impact of enhanced recovery protocol compliance on elective colorectal cancer resection: results from an international registry. Ann Surg. 2015;261:1153–9.

20. Berian JR, Ban KA, Liu JB, et al. Association of an enhanced recovery pilot with length of stay in the National Surgical Quality Improvement Program. JAMA Surg. 2018;153:358–65.

21. Delaney CP, Brady K, Woconish D, Parmar SP, Champagne BJ. Towards optimizing perioperative colorectal care: outcomes for 1,000 consecutive laparoscopic colon procedures using enhanced recovery pathways. Am J Surg. 2012;203:353–5; discussion 355.

22. Eskicioglu C, Forbes SS, Aarts MA, Okrainec A, McLeod RS. Enhanced recovery after surgery (ERAS) programs for patients having colorectal surgery: a meta-analysis of randomized trials. J Gastrointest Surg. 2009;13:2321–9.

23. King PM, Blazeby JM, Ewings P, et al. The influence of an enhanced recovery programme on clinical outcomes, costs and quality of life after surgery for colorectal cancer. Color Dis. 2006;8:506–13.

24. Larson DW, Lovely JK, Cima RR, et al. Outcomes after implementation of a multimodal standard care pathway for laparoscopic colorectal surgery. Br J Surg. 2014;101:1023–30.

25. Lau CS, Chamberlain RS. Enhanced recovery after surgery programs improve patient outcomes and recovery: a meta-analysis. World J Surg. 2017;41:899–913.

26. Lawrence JK, Keller DS, Samia H, et al. Discharge within 24 to 72 hours of colorectal surgery is associated with low readmission rates when using enhanced recovery pathways. J Am Coll Surg. 2013;216:390–4.

27. Pawa N, Cathcart PL, Arulampalam TH, Tutton MG, Motson RW. Enhanced recovery program following colorectal resection in the elderly patient. World J Surg. 2012;36:415–23.

28. Shah PM, Johnston L, Sarosiek B, et al. Reducing readmissions while shortening length of stay: the positive impact of an

enhanced recovery protocol in colorectal surgery. Dis Colon Rectum. 2017;60:219–27.

29. Thiele RH, Rea KM, Turrentine FE, et al. Standardization of care: impact of an enhanced recovery protocol on length of stay, complications, and direct costs after colorectal surgery. J Am Coll Surg. 2015;220:430–43.

30. Wind J, Polle SW, Fung Kon Jin PH, et al. Systematic review of enhanced recovery programmes in colonic surgery. Br J Surg. 2006;93:800–9.

31. Zhuang CL, Ye XZ, Zhang XD, Chen BC, Yu Z. Enhanced recovery after surgery programs versus traditional care for colorectal surgery: a meta-analysis of randomized controlled trials. Dis Colon Rectum. 2013;56:667–78.

32. Raue W, Haase O, Junghans T, Scharfenberg M, Muller JM, Schwenk W. 'Fast-track' multimodal rehabilitation program improves outcome after laparoscopic sigmoidectomy: a controlled prospective evaluation. Surg Endosc. 2004;18:1463–8.

33. Rawlinson A, Kang P, Evans J, Khanna A. A systematic review of enhanced recovery protocols in colorectal surgery. Ann R Coll Surg Engl. 2011;93:583–8.

34. Tejedor P, Pastor C, Gonzalez-Ayora S, Ortega-Lopez M, Guadalajara H, Garcia-Olmo D. Short-term outcomes and benefits of ERAS program in elderly patients undergoing colorectal surgery: a case-matched study compared to conventional care. Int J Color Dis. 2018;33:1251–8.

35. Gonzalez-Ayora S, Pastor C, Guadalajara H, et al. Enhanced recovery care after colorectal surgery in elderly patients. Compliance and outcomes of a multicenter study from the Spanish working group on ERAS. Int J Color Dis. 2016;31:1625–31.

36. Boon K, Bislenghi G, D'Hoore A, Boon N, Wolthuis AM. Do older patients (>80 years) also benefit from ERAS after colorectal resection? A safety and feasibility study. Aging Clin Exp Res. 2021;33(5):1345–52.

37. Keller DS, Lawrence JK, Nobel T, Delaney CP. Optimizing cost and short-term outcomes for elderly patients in laparoscopic colonic surgery. Surg Endosc. 2013;27:4463–8.

38. Verheijen PM, Vd Ven AW, Davids PH, Vd Wall BJ, Pronk A. Feasibility of enhanced recovery programme in various patient groups. Int J Color Dis. 2012;27:507–11.

39. Spinelli A, Bazzi P, Sacchi M, et al. Short-term outcomes of laparoscopy combined with enhanced recovery pathway after ileocecal resection for Crohn's disease: a case-matched analysis. J Gastrointest Surg. 2013;17:126–32.

40. Hignett S, Parmar CD, Lewis W, Makin CA, Walsh CJ. Ileostomy formation does not prolong hospital length of stay after open anterior resection when performed within an enhanced recovery programme. Color Dis. 2011;13:1180–3.

41. Joh YG, Lindsetmo RO, Stulberg J, Obias V, Champagne B, Delaney CP. Standardized postoperative pathway: accelerating recovery after ileostomy closure. Dis Colon Rectum. 2008;51:1786–9.

42. Ottaviano K, Brookover R, Canete JJ, et al. The impact of an enhanced recovery program on loop ileostomy closure. Am Surg. 2021;87(12):1920–5. https://doi.org/10.1177/0003134820982847.

43. Wood T, Aarts MA, Okrainec A, et al. Emergency room visits and readmissions following implementation of an enhanced recovery after surgery (iERAS) program. J Gastrointest Surg. 2018;22:259–66.

44. Adamina M, Kehlet H, Tomlinson GA, Senagore AJ, Delaney CP. Enhanced recovery pathways optimize health outcomes and resource utilization: a meta-analysis of randomized controlled trials in colorectal surgery. Surgery. 2011;149:830–40.

45. Delaney CP, Chang E, Senagore AJ, Broder M. Clinical outcomes and resource utilization associated with laparoscopic and open colectomy using a large national database. Ann Surg. 2008;247:819–24.

46. Jung AD, Dhar VK, Hoehn RS, et al. Enhanced recovery after colorectal surgery: can we afford not to use it. J Am Coll Surg. 2018;226:586–93.

47. Khanijow AN, Wood LN, Xie R, et al. The impact of an enhanced recovery program (ERP) on the costs of colorectal surgery. Am J Surg. 2021;222(1):186–92.

48. Lee L, Li C, Landry T, et al. A systematic review of economic evaluations of enhanced recovery pathways for colorectal surgery. Ann Surg. 2014;259:670–6.

49. Lee L, Mata J, Ghitulescu GA, et al. Cost-effectiveness of enhanced recovery versus conventional perioperative management for colorectal surgery. Ann Surg. 2015;262:1026–33.

50. Roulin D, Donadini A, Gander S, et al. Cost-effectiveness of the implementation of an enhanced recovery protocol for colorectal surgery. Br J Surg. 2013;100:1108–14.

51. Sammour T, Zargar-Shoshtari K, Bhat A, Kahokehr A, Hill AG. A programme of Enhanced Recovery After Surgery (ERAS) is a cost-effective intervention in elective colonic surgery. N Z Med J. 2010;123:61–70.

52. Stone AB, Grant MC, Pio Roda C, et al. Implementation costs of an enhanced recovery after surgery program in the United States: a financial model and sensitivity analysis based on experiences at a quaternary academic medical center. J Am Coll Surg. 2016;222:219–25.

53. Stowers MD, Lemanu DP, Hill AG. Health economics in enhanced recovery after surgery programs. Can J Anaesth. 2015;62:219–30.

54. Patil S, Cornett EM, Jesunathadas J, et al. Implementing enhanced recovery pathways to improve surgical outcomes. J Anaesthesiol Clin Pharmacol. 2019;35:S24–8.

55. Levy BF, Scott MJ, Fawcett WJ, Rockall TA. 23-hour-stay laparoscopic colectomy. Dis Colon Rectum. 2009;52:1239–43.

56. Delaney CP. Outcome of discharge within 24 to 72 hours after laparoscopic colorectal surgery. Dis Colon Rectum. 2008;51:181–5.

57. Delaney CP, Fazio VW, Senagore AJ, Robinson B, Halverson AL, Remzi FH. 'Fast track' postoperative management protocol for patients with high co-morbidity undergoing complex abdominal and pelvic colorectal surgery. Br J Surg. 2001;88:1533–8.

58. Hughes M, Coolsen MM, Aahlin EK, et al. Attitudes of patients and care providers to enhanced recovery after surgery programs after major abdominal surgery. J Surg Res. 2015;193:102–10.

59. de Paula TR, Nemeth SK, Kurlansky P, Simon HL, Miller LL, Keller DS. A randomized controlled trial examining the impact of an anorectal surgery multimodal enhanced recovery program on opioid use. Ann Surg. 2022;275(1):e22–9; Publish Ahead of Print

60. Cakir H, van Stijn MF, Lopes Cardozo AM, et al. Adherence to enhanced recovery after surgery and length of stay after colonic resection. Color Dis. 2013;15:1019–25.

61. Jurt J, Slieker J, Frauche P, et al. Enhanced recovery after surgery: can we rely on the key factors or do we need the bel ensemble. World J Surg. 2017;41(10):2464–70.

62. Gustafsson UO, Hausel J, Thorell A, Ljungqvist O, Soop M, Nygren J. Adherence to the enhanced recovery after surgery protocol and outcomes after colorectal cancer surgery. Arch Surg. 2011;146:571–7.

63. Pecorelli N, Hershorn O, Baldini G, et al. Impact of adherence to care pathway interventions on recovery following bowel resection within an established enhanced recovery program. Surg Endosc. 2017;31:1760–71.

64. Pedziwiatr M, Kisialeuski M, Wierdak M, et al. Early implementation of Enhanced Recovery After Surgery (ERAS(R)) protocol - compliance improves outcomes: a prospective cohort study. Int J Surg. 2015;21:75–81.

65. Wolk S, Distler M, Mussle B, Sothje S, Weitz J, Welsch T. Adherence to ERAS elements in major visceral surgery-an observational pilot study. Langenbeck's Arch Surg. 2016;401:349–56.

66. Bakker N, Cakir H, Doodeman HJ, Houdijk AP. Eight years of experience with enhanced recovery after surgery in patients with colon cancer: impact of measures to improve adherence. Surgery. 2015;157:1130–6.

67. Lyon A, Payne CJ, Mackay GJ. Enhanced recovery programme in colorectal surgery: does one size fit all? World J Gastroenterol. 2012;18:5661–3.

68. Keller DS, Tantchou I, Flores-Gonzalez JR, Geisler DP. Predicting delayed discharge in a multimodal enhanced recovery pathway. Am J Surg. 2017;214:604–9.

69. Keller DS, Delaney CP, Senagore AJ, Feldman LS, SAGES SMARTTF. Uptake of enhanced recovery practices by SAGES members: a survey. Surg Endosc. 2017;31(9):3519–26.

70. Kehlet H, Joshi GP. Enhanced recovery after surgery: current controversies and concerns. Anesth Analg. 2017;125:2154–5.

71. Lilford RJ, Brown CA, Nicholl J. Use of process measures to monitor the quality of clinical practice. BMJ. 2007;335:648–50.

72. Desai NR, Ross JS, Kwon JY, et al. Association between hospital penalty status under the hospital readmission reduction program and readmission rates for target and nontarget conditions. JAMA. 2016;316:2647–56.

73. Benneyan JC, Lloyd RC, Plsek PE. Statistical process control as a tool for research and healthcare improvement. Qual Saf Health Care. 2003;12:458–64.

74. Chen TT, Chang YJ, Ku SL, Chung KP. Statistical process control as a tool for controlling operating room performance: retrospective analysis and benchmarking. J Eval Clin Pract. 2010;16:905–10.

75. Groom R, Likosky DS, Rutberg H. Understanding variation in cardiopulmonary bypass: statistical process control theory. J Extra Corpor Technol. 2004;36:224–30.

76. Keller DS, Stulberg JJ, Lawrence JK, Delaney CP. Process control to measure process improvement in colorectal surgery: modifications to an established enhanced recovery pathway. Dis Colon Rectum. 2014;57:194–200.

77. Keller DS, Stulberg JJ, Lawrence JK, Samia H, Delaney CP. Initiating statistical process control to improve quality outcomes in colorectal surgery. Surg Endosc. 2015;29(12):3559–64.

78. Keller DS, Reif de Paula T, Yu G, Zhang H, Al-Mazrou A, Kiran RP. Statistical Process Control (SPC) to drive improvement in length of stay after colorectal surgery. Am J Surg. 2020;219:1006–11.

79. Mohammed MA. Using statistical process control to improve the quality of health care. Qual Saf Health Care. 2004;13:243–5.

80. Sedlack JD. The utilization of six sigma and statistical process control techniques in surgical quality improvement. J Healthc Qual. 2010;32:18–26.

81. Thor J, Lundberg J, Ask J, et al. Application of statistical process control in healthcare improvement: systematic review. Qual Saf Health Care. 2007;16:387–99.

82. Vetter TR, Morrice D. Statistical process control: no hits, no runs, no errors. Anesth Analg. 2019;128:374–82.

83. Breteler MJM, Numan L, Ruurda JP, et al. Wireless remote home monitoring of vital signs in patients discharged early after esophagectomy: observational feasibility study. JMIR Perioper Med. 2020;3:e21705.

84. Schwab M, Brindl N, Studier-Fischer A, et al. Postoperative complications and mobilisation following major abdominal surgery with vs. without fitness tracker-based feedback (EXPELLIARMUS): study protocol for a student-led multicentre randomised controlled trial (CHIR-Net SIGMA study group). Trials. 2020;21:293.

85. Hedrick TL, Hassinger TE, Myers E, et al. Wearable technology in the perioperative period: predicting risk of postoperative complications in patients undergoing elective colorectal surgery. Dis Colon Rectum. 2020;63:538–44.

86. Kneuertz PJ, Jagadesh N, Perkins A, et al. Improving patient engagement, adherence, and satisfaction in lung cancer surgery with implementation of a mobile device platform for patient reported outcomes. J Thorac Dis. 2020;12:6883–91.

87. Schlund D, Poirier J, Bhama AR, et al. Value of an interactive phone application in an established enhanced recovery program. Int J Color Dis. 2020;35:1045–8.

88. Mata J, Pecorelli N, Kaneva P, et al. A mobile device application (app) to improve adherence to an enhanced recovery program for colorectal surgery: a randomized controlled trial. Surg Endosc. 2020;34:742–51.

89. Keller DS, Ermlich BO, Schiltz N, et al. The effect of transversus abdominis plane blocks on postoperative pain in laparoscopic colorectal surgery: a prospective, randomized, double-blind trial. Dis Colon Rectum. 2014;57:1290–7.
90. Marcotte JH, Patel KM, Gaughan JP, et al. Oral versus intravenous acetaminophen within an enhanced recovery after surgery protocol in colorectal surgery. Pain Physician. 2020;23:57–64.
91. Rice D, Rodriguez-Restrepo A, Mena G, et al. Matched pairs comparison of an enhanced recovery pathway versus conventional management on opioid exposure and pain control in patients undergoing lung surgery. Ann Surg. 2021;274(6):1099–106.
92. Vincent WR, Huiras P, Empfield J, et al. Controlling postoperative use of i.v. acetaminophen at an academic medical center. Am J Health Syst Pharm. 2018;75:548–55.

Chapter 16
Perioperative Pain Management for Abdominal Operations

Tonia M. Young-Fadok

Introduction

A major role of the surgeon is to be well-versed with a broad range of interventions, both those under the purview of our Anesthesia colleagues and those which we may be best placed to deliver or, in some cases, to request of our colleagues. A patient's age, comorbidities, and allergies, as well as resource availability and provider preference, will all have an effect on the treatments used at individual institutions. Nevertheless, the primary goal is to have a multimodal opioid-sparing analgesic regimen. Combining different classes of analgesics can provide an additive or synergistic effect for pain relief. These multimodal techniques have long been promoted but have gained increased traction recently with the more widespread adoption of enhanced recovery after

T. M. Young-Fadok (✉)
Division of Colon and Rectal Surgery, Mayo Clinic,
Phoenix, AZ, USA
e-mail: youngfadok.tonia@mayo.edu

© The Author(s), under exclusive license to Springer Nature   311
Switzerland AG 2022
J. R. Romanelli et al. (eds.), *The SAGES Manual of Quality,
Outcomes and Patient Safety*,
https://doi.org/10.1007/978-3-030-94610-4_16

surgery (ERAS®) pathways. Perioperative analgesia is just one facet of ERAS® care pathways, which include a set of evidence-based practices to reduce perioperative stress, maintain postoperative physiological function, and accelerate recovery.

In addition to pain management strategies preoperatively and postoperatively which are generally under surgical management, intraoperative pain management strategies include systemic and regional anesthesia techniques. In the past, the latter were solely under the purview of our Anesthesia colleagues. This is true of neuraxial techniques such as epidural and spinal analgesia, and paravertebral and quadratus lumborum blocks, which are unique to anesthesiologists. However, other blocks may be best performed by the surgeon. The type of block is dependent on the nature of the operation and available institutional expertise.

Summary

- The primary goal is to minimize pain while minimizing opioids and their side effects.
- No pain = no patient.
- Learn the anatomy of abdominal wall blocks.
- Become informed regarding systemic and regional pain management modalities.

Preoperative Measures

Patient Education

Setting appropriate expectations regarding postoperative pain lays the foundation for the patient's overall experience. This groundwork discussion begins in the office during the preoperative counseling session. Comprehensive education can help alleviate the patient's fear of the unknown and has been demonstrated to reduce perioperative anxiety and possibly reduce postoperative pain and opioid use in patients undergoing abdominal operations. Such counseling can be performed by the surgeon, anesthesiologist, or nurse educator.

In addition to providing education and setting expectations, the clinician should obtain information about the patient's past history. Important details to consider include the patient's comorbidities, allergies, and whether he or she takes pain medications such as opioids chronically. The planned surgical approach (minimally invasive or open) should also be taken into consideration. The clinician should adjust the analgesic regimen to account for these factors.

Receptor Blockade

Preemptive analgesia describes treatment that is initiated before surgery to reduce sensitization of the peripheral and central pain pathways. The tissue injury that occurs during surgery causes propagation of nociceptive signals, which increase responsiveness in peripheral and central neurons, amplifying pain. Administration of analgesics prior to incision can blunt this response and reduce both postoperative pain and the development of chronic pain.

Acetaminophen, gabapentinoids (gabapentin and pregabalin), and COX-2 inhibitors such as celecoxib have all been used for preemptive analgesia. They are available as oral formulations and are cost-effective. These medications can be used in combination and should be timed appropriately relative to the operation in order to achieve the maximum opioid-sparing effect, in order to decrease opioid-related side effects. Adjustments should be made based on hepatic function (for acetaminophen), renal function, age, and allergies.

Gabapentinoids were initially developed as anticonvulsants and have been used in the treatment of chronic neuropathic pain. Prior studies demonstrating that administration of a single preoperative dose of gabapentin or pregabalin was associated with decreased postoperative pain and opioid consumption were contradicted by studies showing no difference in pain scores and opioid consumption when patients received a single preoperative dose of pregabalin between 100 and 300 mg. Benefits were only seen with multiple continued postoperative doses that can cause dizziness, sedation, visual disturbance, and peripheral edema. Initial advice that gabapentinoids should be given as a single, lowest possible preoperative dose to limit side effects has been replaced with advice to no longer use these agents.

Celecoxib is a selective COX-2 inhibitor that acts by reducing prostaglandin synthesis during inflammation. A recent meta-analysis of randomized controlled trials demonstrated that administration of celecoxib before noncardiac surgery showed modest benefits in terms of postoperative opioid consumption, pain scores, nausea, and vomiting. No significant difference was noted between groups that received 200 mg versus 400 mg and between groups that received a single preoperative dose versus continued postoperative dosing.

Summary: Preoperative Receptor Blockade

- Celecoxib may be considered.
- Gabapentinoids have been removed due to side effects especially in the elderly.
- Acetaminophen may be given preoperatively or in an operation <6 h duration, held and given intravenously at the end of the case.

Intraoperative Measures

Coordination with the anesthesiology team is critical to successful intraoperative pain management. There are several options for pain control, including infusions and blocks. Some can be administered by the anesthesiologist and some can be administered by the surgeon, depending on the institution.

The goal of the anesthetic regimen is to promote rapid awakening with minimal side effects and to minimize the use of opioids. Avoiding long-acting benzodiazepines, using propofol for induction of anesthesia, and using short-acting opioids (fentanyl, sufentanil, remifentanil) help to minimize side effects. To date there is no definitive data to indicate whether use of anesthetic gases versus total intravenous anesthesia (TIVA) offers a superior response regarding pain, although TIVA helps to minimize the risk of postoperative nausea and vomiting (PONV).

Prior to Incision: Anesthesiologist-Controlled

NMDA Antagonists

The N-methyl-D-aspartate (NMDA) glutamate receptors are involved with nociception and the development of chronic pain. NMDA-receptor antagonists provide a nonopioid mechanism of analgesia.

Ketamine, used in subanesthetic doses at 0.1–0.5 mg/kg, can be initiated prior to incision as a preemptive analgesic. It can also be continued postoperatively in the management of severe acute pain, hyperalgesia, and is also particularly useful in patients with opioid tolerance. Side effects include neuropsychiatric effects, but they are typically nil when ketamine is given at extremely low doses <0.1 mg/kg. Ketamine in subanesthetic doses is associated with very little respiratory depression and sedation and thus may be useful in patients with morbid obesity. It is also associated with reduced need for IV patient-controlled analgesia use and reduced postoperative nausea and vomiting.

Magnesium infusion appears to be associated with reduced postoperative pain and opioid consumption. The first randomized trial to address the perioperative use of magnesium occurred in 1996 [1] and showed that a 20% magnesium 15 mL bolus followed by an infusion of 2.5 ml/h for 20 h reduced pain and morphine consumption in patients undergoing total abdominal hysterectomy. A 2013 systematic review [2] demonstrated a reduction in morphine consumption by 24.4% following administration of magnesium, with no statistically significant difference between patients who received bolus only, bolus with infusion, or infusion only. Further meta-analyses and systematic reviews have supported these findings. Common dosing regimens involve a bolus of 30–50 mg/kg and infusions of 8–15 mg/kg/h.

Lidocaine Infusion

Intravenous lidocaine can be given preoperatively as part of a multimodal analgesic regimen. A systematic review indicated that perioperative lidocaine was associated with reduced postoperative pain, opioid requirements, duration of ileus, nausea/vomiting, and length of stay. The effects were most notable in patients undergoing abdominal procedures. Intravenous lidocaine can be used as an alternative to neuraxial or regional anesthesia when those measures are contraindicated or unsuccessful. Longer-acting local anesthetics are not used in intravenous infusion due to risk of toxicity, including cardiac arrest and death. The availability of intravenous lidocaine as a component of the perioperative analgesic regimen may be institution-dependent.

Continuous Epidural Analgesia

Continuous epidural anesthesia has been shown to offer improved postoperative analgesia, decreased pulmonary and cardiac morbidity, and earlier return of gastrointestinal function in patients who undergo open abdominal operations. The benefits in minimally invasive operations are less certain. Local anesthetics such as bupivacaine and ropivacaine are commonly used for epidural anesthesia. Opioids such as fentanyl and hydromorphone can be added as well but may be absorbed systemically and cause opioid-related side effects of nausea, vomiting, pruritus, and respiratory depression.

Anticoagulants should be administered with caution in these patients due to the risk of epidural hematoma. Adverse effects of local anesthetics given via epidural include hypotension, sensory deficits, motor weakness, and urinary retention. In individuals with morbid obesity, the compression on the epidural space can lead to a need for increased doses and precipitate a high block that necessitates airway management. The excess weight can also exacerbate cardiac side effects of the local anesthetic.

Spinal Analgesia

Single-dose administration of epidural or spinal opioids can be associated with reduced pain and reduced requirement for systemic opioids but is also associated with the typical constellation of opioid-induced side effects, including ileus in up to a third of patients. Options include lipophilic opioids (fentanyl and sufentanil), which have a more rapid onset but a shorter duration of action, and hydrophilic opioids (morphine and hydromorphone), which have slower onset but longer duration.

Paravertebral Block

This block involves injection of local anesthetic immediately adjacent to the thoracic vertebra, where the spinal nerve emerges from the intervertebral foramen. It is highly dermatome-dependent and has primarily been utilized for unilateral hernia repair or breast surgery, although the potential uses are being expanded. Inadvertent pleural puncture and iatrogenic pneumothorax are the primary risks; ultrasound has improved the safety and efficacy. However, the use of paravertebral blocks for abdominal operations remains somewhat limited, as the anesthetic coverage for these procedures necessitates bilateral injections at multiple dermatomal levels.

Quadratus Lumborum Block

The quadratus lumborum (QL) block refers to a set of four anatomically defined blocks that are categorized based on where the local anesthetic is injected relative to the QL muscle: lateral (QL1), posterior (QL2), anterior (QL3), and intramuscular (QL IM) (Fig. 16.1). The lateral QL1 block reliably covers T10-L1, and the posterior QL2 and anterior QL3 blocks cover T4 to T12/L1. Thus, the QL2 and QL3 blocks are useful in cases where incisions extend both above and below the umbilicus. Local spread to the paravertebral and epidural area may also account for a portion of their analgesic effect.

While these blocks provide reliable anesthesia, reduce opioid consumption, and improve pain scores, there are a few drawbacks. The blocks are typically performed with the patient in both lateral decubitus positions, are best performed with ultrasound, and require intermediate to advanced skills to perform, adding to procedure time. Lower extremity weakness is a frequent side effect, occurring in 1% of QL1 blocks, 19% of QL2 blocks, and up to 90% of QL3 blocks.

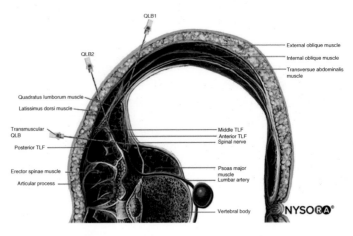

FIGURE 16.1 Quadratus lumborum blocks. (Source: NYSORA.com (https://www.nysora.com))

Summary

- Consider magnesium infusion to block NMDA receptors.
- Consider ketamine infusion or boluses to block NMDA receptors.
- Consider lidocaine infusion.
- Epidural analgesia is effective for open cases but may increase length of stay of laparoscopic cases.
- Long-acting narcotic spinals are effective for pain relief but associated with ileus.
- Quadratus lumborum blocks provide effective pain relief, but there is a trade-off between effectiveness above T10 (umbilicus) and lower extremity weakness.
- Paravertebral blocks are effective but primarily reserved for cases involving limited dermatomes given the need to inject bilaterally at all involved dermatomes.

After Incision

Ultrasound-guided transversus abdominis plane (TAP) blocks may be placed by the anesthesiologist prior to incision, but TAP blocks placed by the surgeon became very popular after popularization of the "two-click" technique. Unfortunately, this was a misguided attempt to simplify the technique and is only applicable to a very specific anatomic approach, in the triangle of Petit. The most accurate – and hence most effective – TAP blocks should be placed using ultrasound to visualize the correct plane *on the surface* of the transversus abdominis muscle, *beneath* the fascia separating this muscle from the internal oblique muscle.

The (TAP) block was first introduced in 2001 by Rafi and was described as a blind anatomy-guided technique aimed at placing a single injection of local anesthetic into the lumbar triangle of Petit, bordered by the external oblique, latissimus dorsi, and iliac crest. Since 2007, ultrasound guidance has been used to direct injection of local anesthetic into the transversus abdominis plane, through which branches from T6-L1 run to innervate the anterior abdominal wall. Anteriorly, this plane lies between the overlap of the lateral rectus abdominis and the transversus abdominis muscles. Posterolaterally, the plane is found beneath the fascial layer between the internal oblique and the transversus abdominis, i.e., the nerves are intimately associated with the *surface* of the transversus abdominis muscle, *beneath* the fascia separating this muscle from the internal oblique. After coursing between the innermost and internal intercostal muscles, the T6-T8 intercostal nerves enter the plane at the level of the costal margin. These nerves then splay out with multiple interconnections, forming the cephalic TAP plexus. The T9-T12 nerves enter the plane posterior to the midaxillary line and similarly form interconnections to form the caudad TAP plexus. The associated lateral cutaneous branches arise before the main nerves enter the TAP plane and supply the lateral abdominal wall between the costal margin and iliac crest.

Because the plane is large and the nerves enter at various points, there are three main approaches to access the transversus abdominis plane, all named according to their point of entry. The *posterior* approach accesses the compartment at the level of the lumbar triangle of Petit or the anterolateral aspect of the quadratus lumborum. Because these landmarks can be difficult to identify in patients who are obese (due to increased depth) or elderly (due to decreased muscle mass), the addition of ultrasound greatly facilitates placement of the block. Ultrasound guidance drastically improves correct placement of the block into the correct plane, compared to both blind and laparoscopic-guided techniques. With the addition of ultrasound, a *lateral* approach between the midaxillary and anterior axillary line may also augment the ability to visualize the layers in the abdominal wall. The *subcostal* approach utilizes ultrasound to inject local anesthetic between the rectus and transversus abdominis muscles near the xiphoid; the needle is then directed inferolaterally to distend the transversus abdominis plane.

Ultrasound has also been used to perform posterior TAP blocks, targeting the intersection of the oblique and transversus abdominis muscles with the quadratus lumborum, just superficial to the transversalis fascia (Fig. 16.2). Volunteer studies have demonstrated that with this approach, the local anesthetic spreads to both the transversus abdominis plan and the paravertebral space. This suggests that posterior TAP blocks may have a dual mechanism of action.

Randomized controlled trials have compared ultrasound-guided posterior, lateral, and subcostal TAP blocks. Four trials demonstrated that subcostal TAP blocks resulted in lower pain scores within the first 24 h following cholecystectomy [3–6], although interestingly one other study showed no difference [7]. Posterior TAP blocks appeared superior to lateral TAP blocks in patients undergoing Caesarian section and

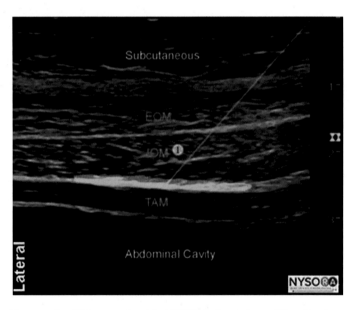

FIGURE 16.2 Ultrasound-guided TAP block anatomy. Visualized are the external oblique muscle (EOM), internal oblique muscle (IOM), and transversus abdominis muscle (TAM). The TAP plane is highlighted – on the surface of the TAM and beneath the fascia separating it from the IOM. (Source: NYSORA.com (https://www.nysora.com))

appeared to anesthetize more dermatomes compared to lateral TAP blocks in patients undergoing laparoscopic gynecologic surgery. Taken together, this suggests that the subcostal and posterior approaches should be considered in place of the lateral approach.

Studies investigating the overall effect of TAP block have yielded somewhat mixed results, possibly due to the relatively short duration of the block. Long-acting liposomal bupivacaine has been approved for TAP blocks as the block does not target a specific nerve, but rather a plane. A recent randomized controlled trial comparing regular bupivacaine to liposomal bupivacaine during TAP blocks in patients undergoing colorectal resection demonstrated no difference between opioid consumption and pain scores within the first 72 h [8]. The block can be performed before the incision or after the procedure is complete, by either the Anesthesiology or the surgical team.

Continuous infusion catheters can be inserted into the TAP space to potentially prolong the duration of the block. In a 2015 study [9], healthy volunteers underwent a TAP block with ropivacaine, followed by continuous catheter infusion of ropivacaine on one side and placebo on the other. There was decreased extension of the block after 4–8 h, and there were notably fewer dermatomes anesthetized on the placebo side at 24 h compared to the ropivacaine side. However, a recent study evaluated single-injection TAP versus TAP injection plus continuous catheter infusion of ropivacaine in patients undergoing laparoscopic live donor nephrectomy [10]. In these surgical patients, there was no difference between the two groups.

Transversalis Fascia Block

The transversalis fascia (TF) block was developed in an effort to provide an efficient, simple, safe, and effective abdominal wall block that did not require any ultrasound expertise. The transversalis fascia courses posteromedially and becomes contiguous with the fascial planes investing the QL muscle. Once the surgeon has gained intraabdominal access, the fascia can be accessed more posteriorly and therefore closer to the nerve root than an ultrasound-guided TAP block. A laparoscopic decompression needle with a beveled tip is connected to a 20-ml syringe with connector tubing. The TF is identified caudad to the costal margin, as laterally as possible, just before it courses behind the retroperitoneal fat at the lateral peritoneal reflection. The needle is guided into this location via an ipsilateral lower abdominal port, with the bevel oriented medially. A single "click" confirms placement under the fascia, and the injectate is administered (Fig. 16.3).

A cadaveric study [11] has confirmed that the TF block has improved longitudinal and posterolateral spread of the injectate, with consistent spread to the intercostal (T8-T12) and ilioinguinal/iliohypogastric nerves (L1). Quality improvement studies have demonstrated a 70% reduction in opioid use with the TF block, compared to a blind laparoscopic TAP block.

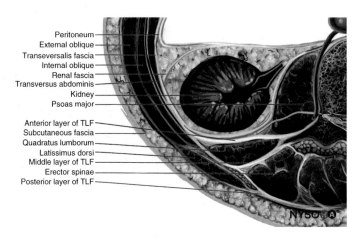

FIGURE 16.3 Anatomy relevant to transversalis fascia (TF) block. (Source: NYSORA.com (https://www.nysora.com))

Rectus Block

The rectus block reliably provides analgesia to the entire midline in the area innervated by the T7-T11 nerves. The TAP block reliably only covers the abdomen below the umbilicus; thus, in cases where an incision is present above the umbilicus, the rectus block is an excellent supplement. The local anesthetic is deposited in the posterior rectus space just below the costal margin. Ultrasound or laparoscopic guidance can be used to ensure correct placement of a single injection. Alternatively, the block can be performed with placement of continuous infusion catheter, following hydrodissection with 20 mL of local anesthetic such as bupivacaine. This approach has been found to be effective at reducing opioid use following laparotomy (Fig. 16.4).

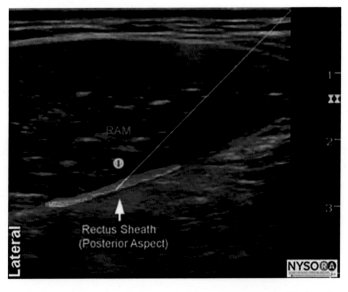

FIGURE 16.4 Relevant ultrasound anatomy for rectus block. The injectate is delivered between the muscle and the posterior sheath, as indicated by the highlighted area. (Source: NYSORA.com (https://www.nysora.com))

Intercostal Block

While traditionally used for thoracic surgery or to treat pain associated with rib fractures, the intercostal block can also be considered for open upper abdominal incisions. The block targets the ventral rami of the sensory nerve within the neurovascular bundle at the inferior aspect of each rib. The chief risk is that of pneumothorax, which may occur in 1–2% of cases. Tube thoracostomy may be required, but this is fairly rare; observation and supplemental oxygen are frequently sufficient.

The relatively short duration of action of the local anesthetic limits the effectiveness of the intercostal block. Catheters inserted into the intercostal space can be used for continuous infusion, which has been shown to reduce analgesic requirements following open cholecystectomy. Use of an extended-release formulation such as liposomal bupivacaine has been shown to have decreased intubation requirements and ICU/hospital length of stay in patients with rib fractures when compared to epidural analgesia [12]. The thoracic surgery literature has also demonstrated that these two techniques have a similar safety profile.

Local Wound Infiltration

The technique of simply infiltrating local anesthetic in the tissues adjacent to the wound should not be dismissed. The surgeon and anesthesiologist should carefully consider the overall dose, the volume of tissue to be anesthetized, as well as the duration of the operation when determining the injectate. Short- and intermediate-duration anesthetics such as lidocaine should be mixed with longer-acting anesthetics such as bupivacaine and ropivacaine if an earlier onset of analgesia is required for a shorter operation. Liposomal bupivacaine could also be used; however, it has a decreased spread compared to standard bupivacaine, so more passes of the needle are required to achieve a better effect.

Intraperitoneal Lidocaine

Administration of intraperitoneal lidocaine has been most frequently studied following either laparoscopic cholecystectomy or gynecologic procedures A 2000 study showed that 15-minute instillation of 200 mL of saline mixed with 200 mg of lidocaine under the right diaphragmatic surface resulted in no pain on deep inspiration in 72% of lidocaine group versus 8% of the control group, as well as reduced analgesic requirements in the immediate 24 h after surgery [13]. A 2017 randomized trial in women undergoing Cesarean section showed a reduction in opioid use following administration of intraperitoneal lidocaine [14]. While the administration of intraperitoneal lidocaine is fairly simple, it has not gained widespread popularity. A 2011 randomized controlled trial showed similar reductions in pain scores and fentanyl use in patients who received either intravenous or intraperitoneal lidocaine with laparoscopic appendectomy [15], indicating that the more readily accessible intravenous route provides similarly effective analgesia.

Postoperative Measures

Some of the interventions discussed in the previous section on intraoperative measures can carry over into the postoperative phase, including anesthetic blocks, ketamine infusion, and lidocaine infusion. These may be initiated prior to incision or may be performed after the procedure is complete.

It is important to continue a multimodal opioid-sparing regimen in the postoperative phase. Multiple enhanced recovery after surgery (ERAS) guidelines recommend using scheduled acetaminophen and nonsteroidal anti-inflammatory drugs (NSAIDs) as the foundation of a multimodal regimen, assuming no medical contraindications. Other nonopioid medications provide a supplemental effect. Opioids should be administered on an as-needed basis as a rescue analgesic.

Acetaminophen can be given as an intravenous or oral form and should be given as a scheduled dose. When combined with opioids, it not only improves analgesia but also promotes an opioid-sparing effect with reduced nausea, vomiting, and sedation. As it is cleared by the liver, acetaminophen should be avoided in cases of renal insufficiency. The maximum daily dose as recommended by the manufacturer of Tylenol is 3 g per day in an adult.

NSAIDs have an additive effect when given with acetaminophen, hence the reason these medications form the backbone of the multimodal regimen as recommended in multiple ERAS guidelines. NSAIDs can be given in an intravenous format (ketorolac) or oral format (ibuprofen, naproxen, or COX-2 inhibitor celecoxib). They have a potent analgesic effect; 600 mg of ibuprofen can be as efficacious as 15 mg of oxycodone. When given with opioids, they have an opioid-sparing effect and a resultant decrease in opioid-related side effects such as nausea and vomiting. They should be administered on a scheduled rather than an as-needed basis if possible. Side effects of NSAIDs include gastrointestinal irritation or bleeding, platelet dysfunction, and renal dysfunction. Nonselective NSAIDs are generally avoided after bariatric operations due to the risk of ulceration and bleeding. COX-2 inhibitors such as celecoxib can be used instead.

Interestingly, a meta-analysis from 2014 found no increased postoperative bleeding between a group of postoperative patients taking ketorolac and a control group [16]. Another study comparing ketorolac to an IV opioid found no increase in gastrointestinal or operative site bleeding except in study participants aged 75 and older [17]. There is some data to suggest an association between postoperative NSAID use and increased anastomotic leak [18, 19]; however, further studies are needed to evaluate this claim.

Transdermal lidocaine, frequently placed as a patch, is generally well-tolerated and has a reasonably low-risk profile, particularly when compared to the other available opioid and nonopioid options. However, its use is contraindicated within

96 h of administration of intraoperative liposomal bupivacaine, so this will be highly dependent on institutional availability of liposomal bupivacaine.

The exact dosing regimen for gabapentinoids postoperatively is unclear, but pregabalin and gabapentin were often used as part of a multimodal regimen. Compared to the other nonopioid options, however, gabapentinoids have more adverse effects that can act synergistically with opioids, including sedation and dizziness, and for this reason have been removed from many ERAS protocols.

Tramadol has a weak opioid-type mechanism, as it targets mu receptors weakly. It also inhibits reuptake of serotonin and norepinephrine as a nonopioid mechanism of action. Overall, tramadol has a lower risk of addiction, constipation, and respiratory depression. The last feature makes it a more attractive option for pain management in patients with morbid obesity, compared to opioids. Tramadol does increase the risk of seizure and so should be used with caution in patients with a history of seizure.

Opioid medications have been central to the management of postoperative pain. However, their side effects of nausea, vomiting, constipation, ileus, sedation, and respiratory depression serve to inhibit a patient's recovery. The majority of enhanced recovery pathways therefore highlight the use of a multimodal pain regimen with scheduled nonopioid analgesics, with opioids reserved for breakthrough pain when the multiple above measures fail. While it is challenging to achieve a completely opioid-free postoperative course in abdominal surgery, the use of a multimodal regimen as part of an ERAS pathway has been shown to consistently reduce opioid requirements.

Non-pharmacologic Measures

A few other non-pharmacologic adjuncts can contribute to a patient's postoperative pain management. Application of ice and/or heat may provide some measure of pain relief.

Additionally, abdominal surgery can often result in ileus, the discomfort which may be relieved by early ambulation. Abdominal binders have been shown to decrease pain and improve mobility following abdominal surgery. Other adjuncts with a potentially positive effect include music therapy, aromatherapy, and acupuncture. These therapies should be used in addition to pharmacologic methods, and their availability certainly varies by institution.

Summary (Table 16.1)

- Acetaminophen 1000 mg q 8 h
- NSAID q 8 h (scheduled at 4-h point between acetaminophen doses)
- Low-dose ketamine infusion
- Transdermal lidocaine patches (if liposomal bupivacaine not used)
- Non-pharmacologic measures
  - Reassurance and education
  - Abdominal binder
  - Ice packs
  - Heating pads
  - Music therapy
  - Aromatherapy
  - Acupuncture

TABLE 16.1 Summary of perioperative pain control measures

Preoperative	Non-pharmacologic	Pharmacologic
	Patient education/ setting expectation	Acetaminophen
		Celecoxib [Gabapentinoids (gabapentin, pregabalin) currently not recommended]

(continued)

TABLE 16.1 (continued)

Intraoperative	**Blocks**	**Medications**
	Continuous epidural anesthesia	NMDA antagonists (ketamine, magnesium)
	Spinal analgesia	Intravenous lidocaine
	Paravertebral block	Intraperitoneal lidocaine
	Quadratus lumborum block	
	TAP block	
	Transversalis fascia block	
	Rectus block	
	Intercostal block	
	Local wound infiltration	
Postoperative	**Non-pharmacologic**	**Pharmacologic**
	Ice/heat	Acetaminophen
	Ambulation	NSAIDs (ketorolac, ibuprofen, naproxen)
	Abdominal binder	[Gabapentin – not recommended]
	Acupuncture	Lidocaine patch
	Aromatherapy	Tramadol
	Music therapy	Opioids

- Short-acting opioid (fentanyl, etc.)
- Weak opioid (tramadol, etc.)
- Opioids for breakthrough

Special Considerations

Chronic Opioid Use

It should be the team's goal to minimize the use of opioids in the management of postoperative pain overall. Patients who take opioids chronically should be considered the major exception to this rule. We have found it helpful to continue the patient's baseline opioid schedule to prevent withdrawal and also use multimodality pain management to avoid escalation of their baseline needs. A ketamine infusion is frequently used in these patients, as it tends to work very well in cases of chronic opioid use. Working with an in-house pain management service and/or coordination with the patient's outpatient pain specialist is essential in these cases.

Morbid Obesity

Obesity causes unpredictability of the pharmacokinetics and pharmacodynamics of the drugs used in a multimodal pain regimen. There are several reasons for this. Due to increased adiposity, the volume of distribution will be significantly altered. Hepatic clearance of drugs is generally unchanged but could become affected if the patient has fatty infiltration, fibrosis, or cirrhosis of the liver. Renal clearance may initially be increased due to higher renal blood flow but may become decreased later on if renal dysfunction sets in. Additionally, obstructive sleep apnea makes patients more susceptible to opioid-induced respiratory depression. It is therefore all the more important to avoid opioids and to carefully utilize a multimodal regimen in these patients.

Disclaimer The field of ERAS incorporates available evidence to optimize recovery of patients undergoing an operation. It is an exciting and rapidly evolving field, as evidenced by the following: Between inception and completion of this chapter, gabapentinoids went from being a part of many pain management protocols to being excluded from them as evidence became available regarding side effects that negated their benefits.

References

1. Tramer MR, Schneider J, Marti RA, Rifat K. Role of magnesium sulfate in analgesia. Anesth. 1996;84(2):340–7.
2. Albrecht E, Kirkham KR, Liu SS, Brull R. Peri-operative intravenous administration of magnesium sulfate and post-operative pain: a meta-analysis. Anaesthesia. 2013;68(1):79–90.
3. Khan KK, Khan RI. Analgesic effect of bilateral subcostal TAP block after laparoscopic cholecystectomy. J Ayub Med Coll Abbottabad. 2018;30(1):12–5.
4. Baral B, Poudel PR. Comparison of analgesic efficacy of ultrasound guided subcostal transversus abdominis plane block with port site infiltration following laparoscopic cholecystectomy. J Nepal Health Res Counc. 2019;16(41):457–61.
5. Ramkiran S, Jacob M, Honwad M, Vivekanad D, Krishnakumar M, Patrikar S. Ultrasound-guided combined fascial plane blocks as an intervention for pain management after laparoscopic cholecystectomy: a randomized control study. Anesth Essays Res. 2018;12(1):16–23.
6. Bhatia N, Arora S, Jyotsna W, Kaur G. Comparison of posterior and subcostal approaches to ultrasound-guided transverse abdominis plane black for postoperative analgesia in laparoscopic cholecystectomy. J Clin Anesth. 2014;26(4):294–9.
7. Houben AM, Moreau AJ, Detry OM, Kaba A, Joris JL. Bilateral subcostal transversus abdominis plane block does not improve the postoperative analgesia provided by multimodal analgesia after laparoscopic cholecystectomy: a randomized placebo-controlled trial. Eur J Anaesthesiol. 2019;36(10):772–7.
8. Guerra L, Philip S, Lax EA, Smithson L, Pearlman R, Damadi A. Transversus abdominis plane blocks in laparoscopic colorectal surgery: better pain control and patient outcomes with liposomal bupivacaine than bupivacaine. Am Surg. 2019;85(9):1013–6.
9. Petersen PL, Hilsted KL, Dahl JB, Mathiesen O. Bilateral transversus abdominis plane (TAP) block with 24 hours ropivacaine

infusion via TAP catheters: a randomized trail in healthy volunteers. BMC Anesthiol. 2013;13(1):30.

10. Yeap YL, Wolfe JW, Kroepfl E, Fridell J, Powelson JA. Transversus abdominis plane (TAP) block for laparoscopic live donor nephrectomy: continuous catheter infusion provides no additional analgesic benefit over single-injection ropivacaine. Clin Transpl. 2020;34(6):e13861.

11. Garbin M, Portela DA, Bertolizio G, Gallastegui A, Otero PE. A novel ultrasound-guided lateral quadratus lumborum block in dogs: a comparative cadaveric study of two approaches. Vet Anaesth Analg. 2020;47(6):810–8.

12. Sheets NW, Davis JW, Dirks RC, Pang AW, Kwok AM, et al. Intercostal nerve block with liposomal bupivacaine vs epidural analgesia for the treatment of traumatic rib fracture. J Am Coll Surg. 2020;231(1):150–4.

13. Elhakim M, Elkott M, Ali NM, Tahoun HM. Intraperitoneal lidocaine for postoperative pain after laparoscopy. Acta Anaesthesiol Scand. 2000;44(3):280–4.

14. Patel R, Carvalho JCA, Downey K, Kanczuk M, Bernstein P, Siddiqui N. Intraperitoneal instillation of lidocaine improves postoperative analgesia at cesarian delivery: a randomized double-blind, placebo-controlled trial. Anesth Analg. 2017;124(2):554–9.

15. Kim TH, Kang H, Hong JH, Park JS, Baek CW, et al. Intraperitoneal and intravenous lidocaine for effective pain relief after laparoscopic appendectomy: a prospective, randomized, double-blind, placebo-controlled study. Surg Endosc. 2011;25(10):3183–90.

16. Gobble RM, Hoang HLT, Kacniarz B, Orgill DP. Ketorolac does not increase perioperative bleeding: a meta-analysis of randomized controlled trials. Plastic Reconstr Surg. 2014;133(3):741–55.

17. Strom BL, Berlin JA, Kinman JL, Spitz PW, Hennessy S, et al. Parenteral ketorolac and the risk of gastrointestinal and operative site bleeding. A postmarketing surveillance study. JAMA. 1996;275(5):376–82.

18. Modasi A, Pace D, Godwin M, Smith C, Curtis B. NSAID administration post colorectal surgery increases anastomotic leak rate: systematic review/meta-analysis. Surg Endosc. 2019;33(3):879–85.

19. Huang Y, Tang SR, Young CJ. Nonsteroidal anti-inflammatory drugs and anastomotic dehiscence after colorectal surgery: a meta-analysis. ANZ J Surg. 2018;88(10):959–65.

Selected Reading and Resources

Gustafsson UO, Scott MJ, Hubner M, Nygren J, Demartines N, Francis N, Rockall TA, Young-Fadok TM, Hill AG, Soop M, de Boer HD, Urman RD, Chang GJ, Fichera A, Kessler H, Grass F, Whang EE, Fawcett WJ, Carli F, Lobo DN, Rollins KE, Balfour A, Baldini G, Riedel B, Ljungqvist O. Guidelines for perioperative care in elective colorectal surgery: enhanced recovery after surgery (ERAS((R))) society recommendations: 2018. World J Surg. 2019;43(3):659–95. PMID: 30426190. https://doi.org/10.1007/s00268-018-4844-y.

https://www.nysora.com: NOTE: This online resource includes highly detailed anatomic illustrations. Its illustrations may be reproduced by any entity acknowledging the source without requiring additional permission. Highly recommended.

Young-Fadok T, Craner RC. Regional anesthesia techniques for abdominal operations. In: Ljungqvist O, Francis NK, Urman RD, editors. Enhanced recovery after surgery (ERAS®), a complete guide to optimizing outcomes. Cham: Springer; 2020. p. 149–62.

Chapter 17
Classification and Analysis of Error

Cara A. Liebert and Sherry M. Wren

Background

The Institute of Medicine estimates that medical errors cause between 44,000 and 98,000 preventable hospital deaths and one million injuries per year in the USA [1]. One study has suggested that 70% of adverse events are preventable, with the most common types being technical errors (44%), diagnostic errors (17%), failure to prevent injury (12%), and medication errors (10%) [1, 2]. Preventable errors result in a total estimated cost of between $17 billion and $29 billion per year in US hospitals [1]. The National Quality Forum (NQF) in 2002 defined "never events" as errors in medical care that are clearly identifiable, preventable, and serious in their consequences for patients and that indicate a real problem in the

C. A. Liebert
Department of Surgery, Stanford University School of Medicine, VA Palo Alto Health Care System, Palo Alto, CA, USA
e-mail: cara.liebert@stanford.edu

S. M. Wren (✉)
Department of Surgery, Center for Innovation and Global Health, Stanford University School of Medicine, VA Palo Alto Health Care System, Palo Alto, CA, USA
e-mail: swren@stanford.edu

© The Author(s), under exclusive license to Springer Nature   335
Switzerland AG 2022
J. R. Romanelli et al. (eds.), *The SAGES Manual of Quality, Outcomes and Patient Safety*,
https://doi.org/10.1007/978-3-030-94610-4_17

safety and credibility of a healthcare facility [3]. In 2011, the NQF updated this list and delineated five specific events for surgery or invasive procedures: (a) surgery or other invasive procedure performed on the wrong site, (b) surgery or other invasive procedure performed on the wrong patient, (c) wrong surgical or other invasive procedure performed on a patient, (d) unintended retention of a foreign object in a patient after surgery or other invasive procedure, and (e) intraoperative or immediately postoperative/post-procedure death in an ASA Class 1 patient [4].

It is estimated that over 4000 surgical "never event" malpractice claims occur each year in the USA, resulting in mortality in 7% of these cases, permanent injury in 33%, and temporary injury in 59% [5]. Since the Institute of Medicine's report *To Err Is Human*, there has been considerable attention to improving patient safety through identification and reduction of potentially avoidable errors across all healthcare delivery systems.

Medical Error

A *medical error* is an unintended act or action that does not achieve its intended outcome and can range from non-consequential to life-threatening [6]. Errors can stem from the failure of a planned action to be completed as intended or the use of a wrong plan to achieve an aim [1]. *Human errors* in medicine are further defined as a flaw in reasoning, understanding, or decision-making of a health problem or execution of a clinical task [7]. Examples in the care of surgical patients include transfusion errors, medication errors, wrong-site surgery, wrong-procedure surgery, retained foreign objects, and iatrogenic injuries. Factors that contribute to errors include individual factors as well as flaws in healthcare systems that fail to prevent errors from occurring. Due to the high acuity and high stress environment, errors with serious consequences are most likely to occur in operating rooms, emergency departments, and intensive care units. Common medical error terms are defined in Table 17.1.

TABLE 17.1 Error definitions and related terms

Term	Definition
Medical error	Unintended act or one that does not achieve its intended outcome and can range from non-consequential to life-threatening [6]
Human error	A flaw in reasoning, understanding, or decision-making of a health problem or execution of a clinical task [7]
Active failure	Unsafe acts committed by providers in the form of slips, lapses, mistakes, and procedural violations [8]
Latent failure	Healthcare system failures that are often hidden and can lead to either error-prone situations or holes in the defense against active failures [7]
Adverse event	An unexpected and undesired incident that harms a patient as a direct result of the care or services provided [7]
Sentinel event	Patient safety event that results in death, permanent harm, or severe temporary harm [9]
Surgical never event	Medical errors associated with serious harm to patients, such as retained foreign bodies, wrong-site surgery, wrong-patient surgery, and wrong-procedure surgery [5]
Near miss	A "close call" or event that had the potential to result in an adverse event but did not [7]
Patient safety	Prevention of healthcare-associated harm caused by errors of commission and omission [10]
Root cause analysis	A formal process of focused review that aims to identify a chain of events and wide variety of contributory factors that lead up to an adverse event or near miss at the systems level [11, 12]

Adverse Events and Near Misses

Errors can lead to *adverse events* or *near misses*. An *adverse event* is an unexpected and undesired incident that harms a patient as a direct result of the care or services provided [7].

In healthcare, the most common root cause of adverse events is poor communication [13]. A *near miss*, or "close call," is an event that had the potential to result in an adverse event but did not [7]. Near misses can occur when a potential or impending error is identified and avoided. Alternatively, a near miss can occur when a provider makes an error, but this error is identified and corrected prior to harm to the patient [1]. Near misses offer a critical opportunity for the providers and healthcare system to perform a root cause analysis and intervene before the error occurs again and leads to an adverse event. Near misses may occur many times before an actual harmful incident and typically outnumber adverse events by a factor of more than 300 [14]. Taking advantage of near misses has the real potential to improve patient safety by analyzing error-prone situations or practices which can be the basis of "error traps" waiting to catch other patients and providers. In addition, there can be less anxiety about blame since no one has been harmed. They serve as key opportunities for process improvement and prevention of future adverse events.

Surgical adverse events and near misses are frequently used as metrics of quality care in healthcare systems and national organizations such as the Joint Commission. Among analysis of errors reported by surgeons at teaching hospitals, 66% were intraoperative errors, 27% preoperative, and 22% postoperative [13]. The most common factors contributing to errors in this study were inexperience/lack of competence in a surgical task, communication breakdown, and fatigue/excessive workload [13]. Eighty-six percent of these adverse events were identified to have cognitive factors contributing to the error, such as error in judgment (63%) and failure of vigilance (49%) [13].

Sentinel Events

Sentinel events are patient safety events which are not primarily related to the patient's underlying condition and result in the death, permanent harm, or severe temporary harm of a patient [9]. The reporting of most sentinel events by a hospital or healthcare system to the Joint Commission is voluntary and therefore represents only a proportion of actual sentinel events [9].

The Joint Commission Sentinel Events [9]

- Surgical
  - Invasive procedure, including surgery, on the wrong patient, at the wrong site, or the wrong procedure
  - Unintended retention of a foreign object in a patient after an invasive procedure or surgery
  - Fire, flame, or unanticipated smoke, heat, or flashes occurring during an episode of patient care or procedure

- Nonsurgical
  - Hemolytic transfusion reaction involving administration of blood or blood products having major blood group incompatibilities
  - Prolonged fluoroscopy with cumulative dose >1500 rads to a single field or any delivery of radiotherapy to the wrong body region or >25% above the planned radiotherapy dose
  - Severe neonatal hyperbilirubinemia (>30 mg/dL)
  - Unanticipated death of a full-term infant
  - Discharge of an infant to the wrong family
  - Any intrapartum maternal death
  - Severe maternal morbidity not primarily related to the natural course of the patient's illness when it results in permanent harm or severe temporary harm
  - Abduction of any patient receiving care, treatment, and services
  - Elopement of a patient from staffed care setting leading to death, permanent harm, or severe temporary harm to the patient
  - Rape, assault, or homicide of any patient receiving care, treatment, and services while on site at the hospital

- Rape, assault, or homicide of a staff member, licensed independent practitioner, visitor, or vendor while on site at the hospital
- Suicide of any patient receiving care, treatment, and services in a staffed care setting or within 72 h of discharge from the hospital or emergency department

Surgical Never Events

Surgical never events represent a subset of sentinel events causing serious harm to patients and include events such as retained foreign bodies, wrong-site surgery, wrong-patient surgery, and wrong-procedure surgery [5]. Of 9744 paid malpractice claims for surgical never events in the USA between 1990 and 2010, retained foreign body was the most common (49.8%), followed by wrong procedure (25.1%), wrong-site surgery (24.8%), and wrong-patient surgery (0.3%) [5]. In multivariable logistic regression, surgeons with clinical privilege disciplinary reports or state licensure disciplinary reports were more likely to have surgical never events (adjusted OR = 1.73, 95% CI, 1.47–2.03) [5]. Based on paid malpractice claims, the estimated annual incidence of surgical never event claims is 4082 in the USA each year [5]; however, the true incidence is likely much higher as many do not reach the legal process. Between 1990 and 2010, malpractice payments for surgical never events totaled $1.3 billion [5].

Based on data published by the Joint Commission, from 2012 to 2018, there were 700 reported retained foreign objects (Fig. 17.1), with the most common retained objects being surgical sponges, guidewires, and instruments [9, 15–17]. The three most frequent locations for retained sponges are the abdomen/pelvis (50%), vagina (24%), and chest (9%) [17]. In general surgery cases of retained sponges, sponge counts were performed in 90% of cases, and 86% of those counts were considered correct at the time of the count [17].

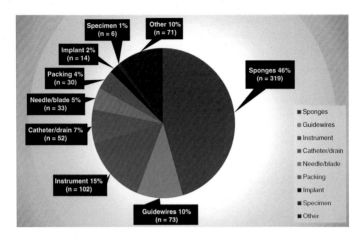

FIGURE 17.1 Retained foreign objects reported to the Joint Commission, 2012–2018. (Adapted from data reported by the Joint Commission and Steelman et al. [9, 15–17])

Error Classification

Active and Latent Failures

Error is commonly classified as *active* versus *latent failure*. *Active failure* is typically a human error that results from a person's inappropriate behavior and can be subclassified into slips, lapses, and mistakes [7, 18]. Slips and lapses are *errors of execution*, with slips defined as a failure to recognize information that the individual would typically identify and lapses defined as moments of attention loss [7]. In these types of error, the provider's intent was correct but due to the slip or lapse, an error occurred. On the other hand, mistakes are *errors of intention* or *errors of planning*, often due to incorrect or inadequate plan [7]. In the case of mistakes, the correct outcome will not occur even with good execution of the plan. Mistakes can be subclassified into *knowledge-based* or *rule-*

based errors. Knowledge-based mistakes occur when a health-care provider makes an error based on inadequate knowledge or expertise, such as iatrogenic injury due to poor under-standing of surgical anatomy [7]. Rule-based errors occur when there is either misapplication or failure to apply a cor-rect protocol [7]. Active failures can also be classified as *errors of commission,* such as administration of an incorrect medication or treatment, versus *errors of omission*, such as failure to order an indicated treatment [1].

Latent failures are healthcare system failures and can lead to either error-prone situations or holes in the defense against active failures [7]. These latent failures include defensive gaps, weaknesses, or absences that can be uniden-tified in a healthcare system for a significant period to time before a combination of active failures exposes them [8]. Types of latent failures include preconditions for unsafe acts such as fatigue, unsafe supervision of trainees, and failures at the organizational level [18]. Examples of organizational level failures include inadequate peer reviews, improper or incomplete credentialing, failure to proactively review high-risk processes for error, inappropriate staffing, and lack of review of adverse events [18]. Poor communication can be classified as a latent failure if it represents an organizational culture that does not promote open and effective communi-cation [18]. When identified and exposed, these latent fail-ures can be addressed, corrected, and eliminated as sources of error.

Types of Errors

One method of classification proposed by Leape et al. orga-nizes errors by diagnosis, treatment, and prevention [2]:

- Diagnostic
    - Error or delay in diagnosis
    - Failure to employ indicated tests
    - Use of outmoded tests or therapy
    - Failure to act on results of monitoring or testing

- Treatment
  - Error in the performance of an operation, procedure, or test
  - Error in administering the treatment
  - Error in the dose or method of using a drug
  - Avoidable delay in treatment or in responding to an abnormal test
  - Inappropriate (not indicated) care

- Preventative
  - Failure to provide prophylactic treatment
  - Inadequate monitoring or follow-up of treatment

- Other
  - Failure of communication
  - Equipment failure
  - Other system failure

Error-Catalyzing Factors

Multiple factors have been identified that can catalyze error in medicine [10]. These catalyzing or contributing factors can be divided into organization- or team-related factors, individual-related factors, and patient-related factors [10]. Examples of organization- or team-related factors include unhealthy patient safety culture, poor communication systems, inadequate resources, system inefficiencies, failure to promote informed shared decision-making, and failure to seek an independent opinion when warranted [10]. Individual-related factors can include knowledge deficits, technical skill deficits, inexperience, poor communication skills, haste, work overload, cognitive biases, cognitive overload, fatigue, and distractions [10]. Patient-related factors include language barriers, compliance, and biases of systems related to a patient's age, gender, race, or socioeconomic status [10]. Although one factor may play a primary role in medical error, most commonly multiple factors coexist.

The Swiss Cheese Model

To a certain degree, slips, lapses, and mistakes by providers are inevitable in every healthcare system. Adverse events are more likely to occur when both active and latent failures coexist or when multiple latent conditions occur simultaneously, which is referred to as the Swiss cheese model of system accidents [8]. In this model, first described by British psychologist James Reason, a systems approach is taken with the premise that humans are fallible and that errors are consequences of systemic factors such as recurrent error traps and flawed organizational processes [8]. This model describes multiple layers of defenses in a healthcare system (slices of cheese) which are safeguards to block errors. Ideally, each of these layers of defense would remain intact, but in reality there are defects in these processes (holes in the cheese) that are continually opening, shutting, and shifting their location [8]. If an error were to occur, a "hole" in any single layer of defense would not normally lead to patient harm. However, when multiple holes in layers of defense momentarily align, errors can lead to patient harm. In the Swiss cheese model of error, holes in defenses typically arise due to a combination of both *active failures* and *latent failures* [8]. Thus, it is imperative that organizational leaders identify and address latent failures in the healthcare system in order to prevent, protect, and mitigate against the effects of active failures. By examining near misses and adverse events using the Swiss cheese model, we can attempt to understand why the error occurred and identify methods to correct these holes.

Stein and Heiss built upon Reason's Swiss cheese model by further defining each layer of defense. In their model (Fig. 17.2), the layers of defense, or "slices," include education, training, institutional policies and procedures, technology, communication, and checklists. Training can include prior experience, simulation, didactic exercises, and ongoing exposure [18]. Institutional policies and procedures can be organization-specific or nationally accepted and are designed to promote safe, standardized care [18]. Examples of technol-

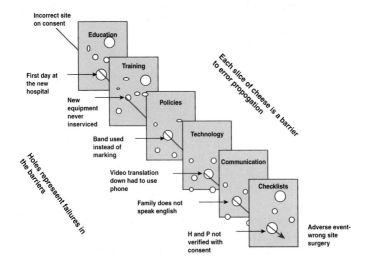

FIGURE 17.2 Swiss cheese model of adverse events. (Visual model portraying the adverse event of wrong-site surgery in a child with right inguinal hernia using a modified Swiss cheese model. Figure originally published in Stein and Heiss, Seminars in Pediatric Surgery, 2015 [18]. Reproduced with permission from Elsevier)

ogy can include electronic medical record pop-ups or best practice alerts, which are vulnerable to alert fatigue [18]. Checklists provide a layer of defense by ensuring confirmation of critical patient information and structured surgical briefings, debriefings, and handoffs [18].

Error Analysis

At the basis of error analysis is the concept that error is not the conclusion but rather the starting point of an investigation [7]. Learning from adverse events and near misses is a cornerstone of patient safety and improvement. There are several methods for investigation and analysis of medical errors, including clinical case review at forums (such as morbidity and mortality conference or peer review), contributory factors, root cause analysis (RCA), failure mode and effects analysis (FMEA), and fishbone diagrams.

Contributory Factors

One method for analyzing medical errors builds off the work of James Reason and classifies error-producing conditions and organizational factors in a single broad framework [19]. This model requires that the user starts by examining the series of events leading to the adverse event or near miss and then further investigates the conditions and organizational context in which the incident occurred [19]. Table 17.2 outlines this framework with examples of common contributory factors to errors.

TABLE 17.2 Framework of factors influencing clinical practice and contributing to adverse events

Framework	Contributory factors	Examples of problems that contribute to errors
Institutional	Regulatory context Medicolegal environment	Insufficient priority given by regulators to safety issues; legal pressures against open discussion, preventing the opportunity to learn from adverse events
Organizational and management	Financial resources and constraints Policy standards and goals Safety culture and priorities	Lack of awareness of safety issues on the part of senior management; policies leading to inadequate staffing levels

TABLE 17.2 (continued)

Framework	Contributory factors	Examples of problems that contribute to errors
Work environment	Staffing levels and mix of skills Patterns in workload and shift Design, availability, and maintenance of equipment Administrative and managerial support	Heavy workloads, leading to fatigue; limited access to essential equipment; inadequate administrative support, leading to reduced time with patients
Team	Verbal communication Written communication Supervision and willingness to seek help Team leadership	Poor supervision of junior staff; poor communication among different professions; unwillingness of junior staff to seek assistance
Individual staff member	Knowledge and skills Motivation and attitude Physical and mental health	Lack of knowledge or experience; long-term fatigue and stress
Task	Availability and use of protocols Availability and accuracy of test results	Unavailability of test results or delay in obtaining them; lack of clear protocols and guidelines
Patient	Complexity and seriousness of condition Language and communication Personality and social factors	Distress; language barriers between patients and caregivers

Adapted from Vincent et al. NEJM 2003 [11]

Root Cause Analysis (RCA)

Root cause analysis, also called systems analysis, is a formal process of focused review that aims to identify a chain of events and wide variety of contributory factors that lead up to an adverse event or near miss at the systems level [11, 12]. The objective of this analysis is to reveal gaps and inadequacies in the healthcare system which can then be addressed in order to prevent future events. Root cause analysis is an event analysis tool that can be applied retrospectively to identify and understand what happened, why it happened, and what should be done to correct it [7]. In comparison with traditional clinical case review, it follows a predefined protocol for identifying specific contributing factors [7]. A formal root cause analysis is typically conducted by an interdisciplinary team of four to five individuals [12]. Five goals of root cause analysis are (1) to determine human and other factors involved in critical incidents, (2) to determine related processes and systems, (3) to analyze underlying causes and effect systems through a series of "why" questions, (4) to identify possible risks and their potential contributions, and (5) to determine a potential improvement in processes and systems [7]. When identifying *root causes* (RC) and *contributing factors* (CF), each human error should have an identified preceding cause and statements should include both cause and effect [12]. A root cause analysis of surgical never events submitted to the Joint Commission between 2004 and 2010 cited lack of leadership and communication as the most common causes of wrong-site surgery and retained foreign bodies. Figure 17.3 outlines common steps in the root cause analysis process.

The Institute for Healthcare Improvement has proposed a modified root cause analysis termed "root cause analysis and actions" or RCA^2 [20]. This process utilizes the basic framework of a root cause analysis with emphasis on a standardized process, action, risk-based prioritization, and understanding that multiple causes usually contribute to an adverse event [20]. RCA^2 focuses on the identification and

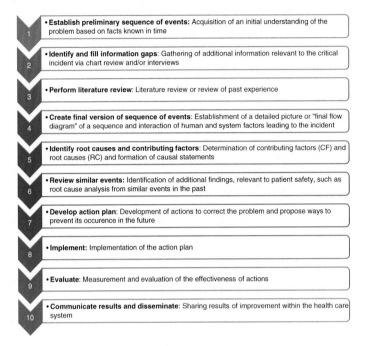

1 • **Establish preliminary sequence of events:** Acquisition of an initial understanding of the problem based on facts known in time

2 • **Identify and fill information gaps:** Gathering of additional information relevant to the critical incident via chart review and/or interviews

3 • **Perform literature review:** Literature review or review of past experience

4 • **Create final version of sequence of events:** Establishment of a detailed picture or "final flow diagram" of a sequence and interaction of human and system factors leading to the incident

5 • **Identify root causes and contributing factors:** Determination of contributing factors (CF) and root causes (RC) and formation of causal statements

6 • **Review similar events:** Identification of additional findings, relevant to patient safety, such as root cause analysis from similar events in the past

7 • **Develop action plan:** Development of actions to correct the problem and propose ways to prevent its occurence in the future

8 • **Implement:** Implementation of the action plan

9 • **Evaluate:** Measurement and evaluation of the effectiveness of actions

10 • **Communicate results and disseminate:** Sharing results of improvement within the health care system

FIGURE 17.3 Steps of root cause analysis (RCA). (Steps adapted from *Medical Error and Harm: Understanding, Prevention, and Control* by Milos Jenicek and VA National Center for Patient Safety *Root Cause Analysis (RCA) Step-By-Step Guide* [7, 12])

implementation of sustainable systems-based improvements to make patient care safer [20].

Failure Mode and Effects Analysis (FMEA)

Failure mode error analysis is a team-based, systematic technique used to prospectively identify potential vulnerabilities or failure points in high-risk systems prior to the occurrence of an adverse event [18, 21]. This process was initially developed in the aerospace and nuclear power industries but is increasingly being applied in healthcare systems. The five primary steps of FMEA are (1) create a flow diagram of the process under evaluation to identify its component steps, (2) identify potential errors or failure modes at each step, (3) score the failure modes numerically to prioritize them according to the risk they pose, (4) identify possible causes for the failures, and (5) generate corrective actions to address these failures [21]. The process of FMEA has been recommended by several national organizations, including the Institute for Safe Medication Practices, the Joint Commission on Accreditation of Healthcare Organizations, and the National Patient Safety Agency in the UK [21].

Fishbone Diagram

A fishbone diagram (Fig. 17.4), also referred to as a cause-and-effect diagram or Ishikawa diagram, is a cause analysis

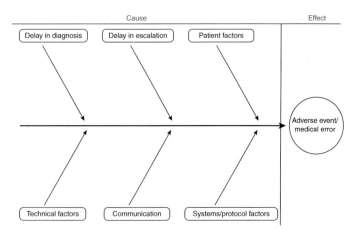

FIGURE 17.4 Fishbone diagram. Example of fishbone diagram to represent contributing factors and causes of an adverse event

tool that can be used to analyze adverse events [22]. These can easily be adapted into morbidity and mortality conference discussions and help educate all attendees and trainees in error analysis and to start thinking broadly about factors that contribute to adverse events.

Prevention of Error in Surgery

Strategies to reduce medical errors in a healthcare system should aim to reduce the frequency of errors by taking human limitations into account, make errors more visible when they occur so their impacts can be mitigated, and provide remedies to rescue patients when errors have occurred [23]. The Joint Commission has created annual National Patient Safety Goals, which inform their sentinel event alerts, standards and survey processes, performance measures, and Joint Commission Center for Transforming Healthcare projects [24]. Additionally, the National Quality Forum has developed safe practice recommendations to prevent never events (Fig. 17.5) [5].

Checklists, such as the World Health Organization Surgical Safety Checklist (WHO SSC) and Surgical Patient Safety System (SURPASS), can improve patient outcomes in surgery and reduce error [26]. A nonrandomized clinical trial has demonstrated that adherence to the postoperative SURPASS checklist is associated with decreased readmission and adherence to both the WHO SSC and preoperative SURPASS checklists is associated with reduced surgical complications and need for reoperation [26].

FIGURE 17.5
National Patient
Safety Foundation
recommendations
for achieving total
systems safety.
(Adapted from:
National Patient
Safety Foundation.
*Free from Harm:
Accelerating Patient
Safety Improvement
Fifteen Years after To
Err Is Human.*
Boston, MA:
National Patient
Safety Foundation;
2015. Available at
ihi.org [25])

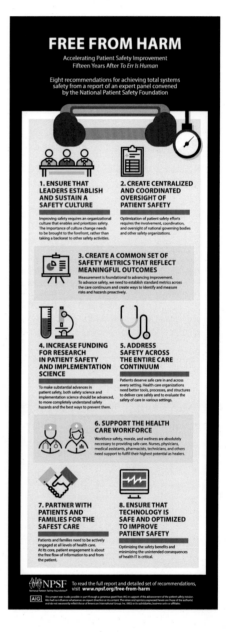

Summary

In all healthcare systems, human error is inevitable. While it is not possible to eliminate medical error completely, strategies can be put in place to design safer healthcare systems to reduce error and mitigate its consequences [23]. Even apparently single error events are typically due to a convergence of multiple contributing factors or latent failures, and prevention requires a systems approach to correct the conditions that contributed to the errors [1].

Errors in healthcare can be classified as near misses and adverse events and can be divided into active failures, such as slips, lapses, and mistakes, or latent failures, such as defensive gaps or weaknesses. Multiple latent failures within a healthcare system increase the likelihood that human error will result in an adverse patient event, as illustrated by the Swiss cheese model. Latent conditions present an opportunity to identify and proactively correct systems-based failures or weaknesses prior to the occurrence of an adverse event. Error and adverse event reporting is key to prompt identification and correction of latent failures. Root cause analysis is a key strategy in the accurate identification of error and modification of latent conditions to prevent future occurrences.

References

1. Institute of Medicine (US) Committee on Quality of Health Care in America. In: Kohn LT, Corrigan JM, Donaldson MS, editors. To err is human: building a safer health system. National Academies Press (US); 2000. http://www.ncbi.nlm.nih.gov/books/NBK225182/. Accessed 11 Nov 2020.
2. Leape LL, Lawthers AG, Brennan TA, Johnson WG. Preventing medical injury. QRB Qual Rev Bull. 1993;19(5):144–9. https://doi.org/10.1016/s0097-5990(16)30608-x.
3. Michaels RK, Makary MA, Dahab Y, et al. Achieving the National Quality Forum's "never events": prevention of wrong site, wrong procedure, and wrong patient operations.

Ann Surg. 2007;245(4):526–32. https://doi.org/10.1097/01.sla.0000251573.52463.d2.

4. NQF: Serious Reportable Events. http://www.qualityforum.org/topics/sres/serious_reportable_events.aspx. Accessed 1 Dec 2020

5. Mehtsun WT, Ibrahim AM, Diener-West M, Pronovost PJ, Makary MA. Surgical never events in the United States. Surgery. 2013;153(4):465–72. https://doi.org/10.1016/j.surg.2012.10.005.

6. Leape LL. Error in medicine. JAMA. 1994;272(23):1851–7.

7. Jenicek M. Medical error and harm: understanding, prevention, and control. Productivity Press; 2010. https://doi.org/10.1201/9781439836958.

8. Reason J. Human error: models and management. BMJ. 2000;320(7237):768–70. https://doi.org/10.1136/bmj.320.7237.768.

9. Sentinel event data - event type by year. https://www.joint-commission.org/resources/patient-safety-topics/sentinel-event/ Sentinel. Event Data - Event Type by Year. Accessed 27 Nov 2020.

10. Seshia SS, Bryan Young G, Makhinson M, Smith PA, Stobart K, Croskerry P. Gating the holes in the Swiss cheese (part I): expanding professor Reason's model for patient safety. J Eval Clin Pract. 2018;24(1):187–97. https://doi.org/10.1111/jep.12847.

11. Vincent C. Understanding and responding to adverse events. N Engl J Med. 2003;348(11):1051–6. https://doi.org/10.1056/NEJMhpr020760.

12. Root Cause Analysis. VA National Center for Patient Safety. https://www.patientsafety.va.gov/media/rca.asp. Accessed 14 Nov 2020.

13. Gawande AA, Zinner MJ, Studdert DM, Brennan TA. Analysis of errors reported by surgeons at three teaching hospitals. Surgery. 2003;133(6):614–21. https://doi.org/10.1067/msy.2003.169.

14. Cuschieri A. Nature of human error. Ann Surg. 2006;244(5):642–8. https://doi.org/10.1097/01.sla.0000243601.36582.18.

15. Steelman VM, Shaw C, Shine L, Hardy-Fairbanks AJ. Unintentionally retained foreign objects: a descriptive study of 308 sentinel events and contributing factors. Jt Comm J Qual Patient Saf. 2019;45(4):249–58. https://doi.org/10.1016/j.jcjq.2018.09.001.

16. Steelman VM, Thenuwara K, Shaw C, Shine L. Unintentionally retained guidewires: a descriptive study of 73 sentinel events. Jt Comm J Qual Patient Saf. 2019;45(2):81–90. https://doi.org/10.1016/j.jcjq.2018.08.003.

17. Steelman VM, Shaw C, Shine L, Hardy-Fairbanks AJ. Retained surgical sponges: a descriptive study of 319 occurrences and contributing factors from 2012 to 2017. Patient Saf Surg. 2018;12:20. https://doi.org/10.1186/s13037-018-0166-0.

18. Stein JE, Heiss K. The Swiss cheese model of adverse event occurrence--closing the holes. Semin Pediatr Surg. 2015;24(6):278–82. https://doi.org/10.1053/j.sempedsurg.2015.08.003.

19. Vincent C, Taylor-Adams S, Chapman EJ, et al. How to investigate and analyse clinical incidents: clinical risk unit and association of litigation and risk management protocol. BMJ. 2000;320(7237):777–81. https://doi.org/10.1136/bmj.320.7237.777.

20. RCA2: improving root cause analyses and actions to prevent harm. Institute for Healthcare Improvement (IHI). http://www.ihi.org:80/resources/Pages/Tools/RCA2-Improving-Root-Cause-Analyses-and-Actions-to-Prevent-Harm.aspx. Accessed 27 Nov 2020.

21. Ashley L, Armitage G. Failure mode and effects analysis: an empirical comparison of failure mode scoring procedures. J Patient Saf. 2010;6(4):210–5. https://doi.org/10.1097/pts.0b013e3181fc98d7.

22. Quality toolbox (2nd ed.) - Knovel. https://app-knovel-com.laneproxy.stanford.edu/web/toc.v/cid:kpQTE00001. Accessed 27 Nov 2020.

23. Makary MA, Daniel M. Medical error-the third leading cause of death in the US. BMJ. 2016;353:i2139. https://doi.org/10.1136/bmj.i2139.

24. National Patient Safety Goals. https://www.jointcommission.org/standards/national-patient-safety-goals. Accessed 27 Nov 2020.

25. Free from harm: accelerating patient safety improvement fifteen years after to err is human. Institute for Healthcare Improvement (IHI). http://www.ihi.org:80/resources/Pages/Publications/Free-from-Harm-Accelerating-Patient-Safety-Improvement.aspx. Accessed 27 Nov 2020.

26. Storesund A, Haugen AS, Flaatten H, et al. Clinical efficacy of combined surgical patient safety system and the world health organization's checklists in surgery: a nonrandomized clinical trial. JAMA Surg. 2020;155(7):562–70. https://doi.org/10.1001/jamasurg.2020.0989.

Chapter 18
Disclosure of Complications and Error

Rocco Orlando III and Stephanie Calcasola

Communication with patients about medical error is one of the most difficult issues that confront surgeons. While surgeons strive to care for patients without mistakes, the complexity of the care process allows for the possibility of surgeon error, system error, or error committed by any member of the care team. Most errors are the result of human rather than technical failures [1]. The current movement to enhance patient safety and improve healthcare quality will certainly reduce error with the goal of error-free care. The introduction of high reliability principles has resulted in dramatic reductions in preventable harm when diligently implemented in a hospital or healthcare system [2]. Human

R. Orlando III (✉)
Hartford HealthCare, Hartford, CT, USA

University of Connecticut School of Medicine, Hartford, CT, USA
e-mail: rocco.orlando@hhchealth.org

S. Calcasola
Hartford HealthCare, Hartford, CT, USA
e-mail: Stephanie.calcasola@hhchealth.org

© The Author(s), under exclusive license to Springer Nature   357
Switzerland AG 2022
J. R. Romanelli et al. (eds.), *The SAGES Manual of Quality,
Outcomes and Patient Safety*,
https://doi.org/10.1007/978-3-030-94610-4_18

fallibility can be limited by robust systems, yet medical error will unfortunately continue to occur and will never be completely eliminated.

In the eyes of the patient and family, there may be confusion between an understanding of complications and error. While adverse events may occur as the result of the underlying disease or unavoidable consequences of a surgical intervention, it is important to be truthful and transparent in discussing these events with patients, families, and members of the care team. While the discussion in this chapter is focused on error, the underlying principles apply equally to disclosure and complications. At times, it may not be clear initially whether or not the source of a poor outcome is the result of medical error or an unavoidable complication. In those cases, diligent evaluation and use of the process of root cause analysis will usually clarify the cause of the adverse event.

The definition of error that was adopted by the Institute of Medicine in the seminal report *To Err Is Human* [3] was proposed by James Reason in 1990: "occasions in which a planned sequence of mental or physical activities fails to achieve its intended outcome" [4]. This definition includes errors that may not result in an adverse event, the concept of the "near miss." The Harvard Medical Practice Study defined adverse events as "an injury that was caused by medical management (and not the disease process) that either prolonged the hospitalization or produced a disability at the time of discharge or both" [5]. This definition is not only precise but also includes significant errors which might not result in disability or prolonged hospital stay. These errors may not result in an adverse event but can still be troubling to patients or the healthcare team. The rise of the high reliability movement in healthcare has emphasized the analysis of near misses – errors that do not result in patient harm but provide the opportunity to improve process and avoid future harm.

Toward a Taxonomy of Error

The traditional taxonomy of error employed by most surgeons is the model of the morbidity and mortality conference. This approach recognizes the time-honored concepts of technical error, judgment error, error of omission, and error of commission [5]. The morbidity and mortality conference analyzes all adverse events on a surgical service – deaths and complications – and the formal structure recognizes that while some adverse events are preventable, others are not. This taxonomy of error is incomplete because it is unduly focused on the actions of the surgeon. While the surgeon may, indeed, commit a technical error or make an error in judgment (such as a delay in diagnosis), this approach does not recognize the myriad of other kinds of medical error: cognitive errors, medication errors, nursing care errors, system errors, and latent errors. Latent error refers to the injury which can result from a complex chain of events in the care process – any one of the events might not result in injury, but taken together, an adverse event occurs. A more inclusive categorization of error is useful because it may provide guidance in changing systems of care to prevent future error (Table 18.1).

Reason's definition of error is more broad and helpful as surgeons consider what to disclose to patients when errors occur. From a pragmatic and ethical standpoint, any error

TABLE 18.1 Taxonomy of error

Traditional surgical paradigm	Practical taxonomy of error
Technical error	Cognitive error
Judgment error	Technical error
Delay in diagnosis	System error
Error in diagnosis	Latent error
Error of omission	Medication error
Error of commission	Device failure

which reaches the threshold of the Harvard Medical Practice Study, resulting in prolonged hospital stay, death, or disability, must be reported to the patient. However, errors recognized by Reason must also be reported at times, specifically those which do not result in injury but may come to the patient's attention. These errors, the "near misses," must be discussed with the patient to avoid a loss in confidence in the caregivers. It is important to explain to patients and families that health-care systems analyze near misses – looking for opportunities to make care safer and to engender more trust in physicians and hospitals.

Regulatory Aspects of Error Disclosure

The climate of healthcare now requires that errors be disclosed. This has resulted from the patient safety movement and recognition that transparency and public accountability are essential to maintaining trust in healthcare. In the past, the culture of medicine was to withhold admission of errors. Physicians commonly withheld the disclosure of errors from patients. Errors were only disclosed when the mistake was obvious or significant injury resulted. At times, adverse events were ascribed to the patient's disease rather than to error. The prevailing wisdom was that admission of error would increase the risk of malpractice litigation. Physicians were embarrassed and unsure of disclosure strategies when confronting error. Patients now expect to be fully informed and involved in their care.

The momentum for the disclosure of error has developed as a result of the patient safety and quality movement. In the USA, the Joint Commission on Accreditation of Healthcare Organizations (the Joint Commission) issued the first nation-wide disclosure standard in 2001 [7]. This standard requires that patients be informed about all outcomes of care including "unanticipated outcomes." The importance of the Joint Commission in the realm of hospital care gave great impetus to the movement to disclose errors. The National Quality

Forum (NQF), an organization that operates at the federal level with strong ties to CMS, has developed standards for the disclosure of unanticipated outcomes [8]. The NQF safe practice standards are used by the Leapfrog Group, a coalition of 29 large healthcare purchasing organizations. A total of 1300 hospitals currently report information about these standards, including disclosure, to the Leapfrog Group.

The Institute for Healthcare Improvement, the Agency for Healthcare Research and Quality (AHRQ), and numerous medical specialty societies have all called for policies of disclosure. AHRQ has published guidelines for the disclosure of error most recently updated in 2019 [9]. Medical society recommendations for transparent disclosure of error have become quite specific in calling for open discussion and disclosure when errors occur. The AMA Code of Ethics had been vague in the past but was updated in 2016. It now recommends not only that physicians be forthcoming when they make an error but also recommends that they encourage colleagues to disclose when they are aware of the error of another physician [10, 11].

Internationally, initiatives in Australia and the UK have been notable. In 2003, Australia initiated an "Open Disclosure Standard" in pilot programs across the country. In the UK, the "Being Open" initiative has been put in place with an extensive educational campaign. These programs have advocated transparent communication and provided tools for enhancing communication with patients. They have been voluntary and have not specifically addressed poor outcomes which have occurred as a result of medical error [10].

As the regulatory agencies have established standards for the disclosure of error, governmental authorities are beginning to mandate disclosure. Although there are no laws requiring disclosure at the national level, in 2005, then Senators Hillary Rodham Clinton and Barack Obama sponsored a bill, the National Medical Error Disclosure and Compensation Act (MEDiC), calling for full disclosure of errors [8]. The bill did not pass, but it linked disclosure, quality, and the medical liability system. The recognition at the federal level that issues of quality, openness, and liability are all closely related is important, yet from a regulatory perspective, these initiatives are more likely to be implemented at the state rather than federal level.

Several states have passed legislation mandating disclosure of serious unanticipated outcomes. Laws are now in effect in ten states including Nevada, Florida, New Jersey, Pennsylvania, Oregon, Vermont, and California [10]. The most stringent law is in place in Pennsylvania which requires that hospitals notify patients in writing within 7 days of a serious event. The Pennsylvania law also prohibits the use of these communications as evidence of liability. These laws share a common approach which requires that hospitals develop mechanisms for disclosure, rather than individual physicians. Forty-five states have enacted "apology laws" which protect certain information transmitted in disclosures, especially expressions of regret or other forms of apology [10]. Enforcement of these laws is only stipulated in the Pennsylvania law. Many of the laws are sufficiently vague that regulation of disclosures seems difficult, at best. Nonetheless, they represent progress because apologies are not admissible in court as part of a malpractice action in most of these states.

Error Disclosure and Risk of Litigation

Physicians have been most concerned that disclosure will increase the likelihood of a malpractice action. These concerns have done much to impede the flow of information to patients and families. Despite this, it is now clear that patients want to know about all errors that cause them harm. A large survey of emergency department patients revealed that 80% wanted to be informed immediately of any medical error. A large majority also supported reporting errors to government agencies, state medical boards, and hospital committees [13]. This study also demonstrated that patients wished to be informed not just about error resulting in injury but also about "near misses." A large survey of health plan members reported increased patient satisfaction and trust when presented scenarios in which full disclosure was advocated. The study also indicated that patients felt that they would be less likely to seek legal advice with full disclosure [14].

American and Canadian physicians appear to embrace the soundness of disclosing errors. These attitudes have changed significantly during the last 20 years. In a 1991 survey of house officers, three out of four said that they had not reported an error to a patient, largely because of concern about litigation [15]. By 2006, in a survey of 2637 physicians, 98% supported disclosing serious medical errors to patients. Seventy-four percent thought that disclosing errors would be difficult, and 58% actually reported disclosing a serious error. Physicians who supported disclosing errors were more likely to believe that disclosure made patients less likely to sue [16]. Physicians were more likely than hospital risk managers to support providing a full apology for error, while the risk managers were more likely to support disclosing error in the first place [17].

The relationship between disclosure and risk of litigation is not at all clear. In 1987, the Veterans Affairs Hospital in Lexington, Kentucky, introduced a disclosure program years before any other. An analysis of the results in 1999 showed that the number of claims during the 12-year period increased, but payments made decreased [18]. Nonetheless, there is a paucity of data which relates the likelihood of a lawsuit to a policy of complete disclosure of error. Despite the lack of solid data, most experts believe that disclosure of error and apology likely reduces the risk of litigation. Based upon the University of Michigan experience, Boothman and Campbell et al. have demonstrated that forthright disclosure and a willingness to apologize are associated with a reduced risk of malpractice actions [19]. In 2014, Mello et al. summarized the outcomes in several states with the same finding [20].

Communication and Resolution Programs (CRPs)

Boothman's work in Michigan along with the work at the Veterans administration led to the establishment of formal programs to facilitate disclosure and early resolution. One of the most important adverse consequences of the tort system is that even in cases where medically induced harm occurs, these cases have often resulted in greater impact to a patient or family that must wait years for financial restitution. To promote communication and patient safety with patients after medical error, healthcare leaders and organizations have developed and implemented formal communication and resolution programs (CRPs) [18, 22–24]. The intent of CRPs is to ensure that patients and families injured by medical error receive prompt "authentic" communication and disclosure of the error. In addition, CRPs are guided by a principled and comprehensive approach with the patient and family engaged throughout the process [18, 22, 24, 25]. Gallagher and team have identified a key success factor for CRPs: the commitment of the healthcare organization to "ensure that patients and families injured by medical care receive prompt attention, honest and empathic explanations, and sincere expressions of reconciliation including financial and non-financial restitution" [25].

The early successes (reduced rate of claims, lawsuits, liability costs, and shorter times to resolution) from the University of Michigan Health System "Early Disclosure and Offer Program" and the Lexington, Kentucky, Veterans Affairs Hospital's program [18, 24, 26] provided the path for others to model [18, 24, 25, 27]. Although interest and momentum are increasing for healthcare organizations to adopt CRPs, there have been challenges with replicating the success of the earlier programs [28–31]. More than 200 hospitals have implemented CRPs [26]. CRPs require a shift in mindset and culture where transparency and engaging patients proactively are the hallmarks of the program. This is in contrast to the traditional "deny and defend" models [18]. Moore and colleagues explored the experiences of patients and families who were injured by medical error and who participated in a CRP program [33]. The CRP experience was positive overall for 60% of the participants. Satisfaction was highest when patients and families reported the communications to be "empathetic and not adversarial." Additionally, patients reported "a strong need to be heard and expected the attending physician to listen without interrupting during the conversations about the event" [33]. Central to all CRPs is the active engagement of the patient and family in the process. Engaging the patient as soon as possible after a medical error is foundational to the program [18, 22–25, 27–30].

Healthcare organizations that have implemented CRPs have been able to improve patient safety across the organizations as a result of implementing the CRP. Mello and colleagues reported the CRP program process gave opportunity to not only identify the patient safety opportunity but actually deploy system changes to improve care design. Some of these best practices include sharing findings with staff to promote transparency, reeducation, policy change, safety alerts, and human factors engineering to name a few [28, 29]. Elements of a principled CRP process start with communication with the patients when the medical error occurs, concurrent investigation to understand why, communicating findings and apologizing, and closing the loop by implementing measures to avoid reoccurrences of the error [34]. Resources are available to guide healthcare leaders in implementing CRPs [23, 29, 34]. In 2017, the Agency for Research and Quality published the CANDOR toolkit (Communication and Optimal Resolution) to aid healthcare organizations in implementing CRPs.

Strategies for Disclosing Error to Patients

Gallagher and his colleagues have observed that surgeons are more inclined to disclose error than their medical colleagues [19]. This may result in part from the fact that surgical errors are often more clear and unambiguous. They documented better ability of surgeons to disclose error using a standard-ized set of patient scenarios [19]. Surgeons are probably bet-ter at disclosing error because of their greater familiarity with transmitting information about complications. Surgeons tend to be direct in describing adverse events and are good at pro-viding details about the consequences of medical error. However, surgeons are reluctant to state that an adverse event was a "mistake" or "error" [19]. Although surgeons may be better than their colleagues in other specialties, until recently there was very little guidance about how to commu-nicate error. The lack of guidance contributes to the tendency of surgeons to avoid the use of the word error or mistake.

When an error occurs, it is necessary to disclose it forth-rightly to the patient. The first decision centers on who should be present when the error is disclosed. This should be dis-cussed prior to meeting with the patient and family. Often, other members of the team should be present to fully address the patient's needs – this may include nursing, hospital administration, risk management, or other physicians. It is often advisable to have a trusted senior surgeon present. When a severe complication or death has occurred, the sur-geon may have concerns that arise from guilt or emotional distress as a result of the poor outcome. The voice of a senior surgeon who does not feel responsible for the complication and who has participated in this kind of meeting in the past may be very helpful. The meeting should take place in a pri-vate setting and all participants should be introduced. The conversation with the patient should take place using clear, simple language, and the tone should be calm and empathic.

The surgeon must provide all of the facts about the event. The source of the error must be identified, paying particular attention to whether it is a technical error, human error, or system failure. It is entirely appropriate to express regret for the adverse outcome and to offer a formal apology if the outcome is the result of system failure or error. These conver-sations should be carried out with empathy and sensitivity. It is very important to accept responsibility for the adverse outcome and to avoid the use of the passive voice. During these conversations, it is important to not attribute blame to others or to claim a lack of understanding of the events. In many cases, all of the facts are not known at the time of initial disclosure. In those cases, the surgeon and team should commit to letting the patient and family know the results of the hospital investigation and analysis. There should be a timely follow-up in in fully informing the patient and family about the outcome of the investigation. Delay in having these discussions can engender a further breakdown in trust.

Following a discussion of the error and resulting injury, the surgeon should review its implications with the patient. The consequences of the error should be reviewed, and the surgeon should explain what will be done to mitigate the problem. The emotional needs of the patient and family should be remembered at this time, and any necessary support should be offered. The patient should also be told what measures will be taken to ensure that a similar error does not occur in the future to another patient.

From an institutional standpoint, the disclosure should be part of a response which includes patient safety and risk management activities – ensuring that a similar event does not occur again and that system problems are addressed. Coaching of physicians in appropriate communication strategies should be available. Organizations that have formal CRP programs conduct training of physicians in the best approaches to communication. Organizations with CRP programs often have established peer support programs. The work of Shapiro at Brigham and Women's Hospital has shown that the support of a trusted and trained colleague is beneficial to the surgeon when a severe adverse event has occurred [21]. Given increasing regulatory requirements for disclosure, these events should be tracked using performance improvement tools (see Table 18.2).

Surgeons have been leaders in the patient safety movement because of a long-standing commitment to analyzing and remediating error. Grounded in the tradition of an honest and forthright morbidity and mortality conference, it is not surprising that surgeons are at the forefront of the movement to disclose error.

TABLE 18.2 Key elements of the safe practice of disclosing unanticipated outcomes to patients

Content to be disclosed to the patient and family
Provide facts about the event
Results of event analysis to support informed decision-making by the patient
Presence of error or system failures if known
Express regret for unanticipated outcome
Give formal apology if unanticipated outcome caused by error or system failure
Institutional requirements
Integrate disclosure, patient safety, and risk management activities
Establish disclosure support system
Provide background disclosure education
Ensure that disclosure coaching is available at all times
Provide emotional support for healthcare workers, administrators, patients, and families
Use performance improvement tools to track and enhance disclosure

Selected Reading

1. Cook RI, Woods DD. Operating at the sharp end: the complexity of human error. In: Bogner MS, editor. Human errors in medicine. Hillsdale: NJL Erlbaum; 1994. p. 255–310.
2. Pronovost PJ, Armstrong C, et al. Creating a high-reliability health care system: improving performance on core processes of care at Johns Hopkins Medicine. Acad Med. 2015;90(2):165–72.
3. Kohn LT, Corrigan JM, Donaldson MS, editors. To err is human. Washington, DC: National Academy; 1999.
4. Reason JT. Human error. New York: Cambridge University; 1990.

5. Thomas EJ, Brennan TA. Errors and adverse events in medicine: an overview. In: Vincent C, editor. Clinical risk management. London: BMJ Books; 2001. p. 32.
6. Bosk CL. Forgive and remember: managing medical failure. Chicago: University of Chicago; 1979. p. 36–70.
7. The Joint Commission. Hospital accreditation standards. Oakbrook Terrace: Joint Commission Resources; 2007.
8. Safe practices for better healthcare. Washington, DC: National Quality Forum; 2007. http://www.qualityforum.org/projects/completed/safe_practices/.
9. Online: Disclosure of Errors. AHRQ' online. https://psnet.ahrq.gov/primer/disclosure-errors. 27 Aug 2020.
10. Frangou C. The art of error disclosure. Gen Surg News. 2007;34:1–22. Hobogood C, Peck CR, Gilbert B, Chappell K, Zou B. Medical errors-what and when: what do patients want to know? Acad Emerg Med. 2002;9:1156–61.
11. Online: Code of Medical Ethics Opinion 8.6. 14 Nov 2016. https://www.ama-assn.org/delivering-care/ethics/promoting-patientsafety#:~:text=(a)%20Disclose%20the%20occur-rence%20of,decisions%20about%20future%20medical%20care. 29 Aug 2020.
12. Gallagher TH, Studdert D, Levinson W. Disclosing harmful medical errors to patients. NEJM. 2007;356:2713–9.
13. Mazor KM, Simon SR, Yood RA, Martinson BC, Gunter MJ, Reed GW, et al. Health plan members views about disclosure of medical errors. Ann Inter Med. 2004;140:409–18.
14. Wu AW, Folkman S, McPhee SJ, Lo B. Do house officers learn from their mistakes? JAMA. 1991;265:2089–94.
15. Gallagher TH, Waterman AD, Garbutt JM, Kapp JM, Chan DK, Dunnagan WC, et al. US and Canadian physicians attitudes and experiences regarding disclosing errors to patients. Arch Intern Med. 2006;166:1605–11.
16. Loren DJ, Garbutt J, Dunagan WC, et al. Risk managers, physicians and disclosure of harmful medical errors. Jt Comm J Qual Patient Saf. 2010;36:99–100.
17. Boothman RC, Blackwell AC, Campbell DC, Commiskey E, Anderson S. A better approach to medical malpractice claims: the University of Michigan experience. J Health Life Sci Law. 2009;2:125–60.
18. Kraman SS, Hamm G. Risk management extreme honesty may be the best policy. Ann Intern Med. 1999;131:963–7.

19. Chan DK, Gallagher TH, Reznick R, Levinson W. How surgeons disclose medical errors to patients: a study using standardized patients. Surgery. 2005;138:851–8.
20. Michelle M, Mello J, et al. The medical liability climate and prospects for reform. JAMA. 2014;312(20):2146–55. https://doi.org/10.1001/jama.2014.10705.
21. Shapiro J, Galowitz P. Peer support for clinicians: a programmatic approach. Acad Med. 2016;10:1200–4.
22. The Michigan Model: Medical Malpractice and Patient Safety at UMHS. Retrieved from: http://www.uofmhealth.org/michigan-model-medical-malpractice-and-patient-safety-umhs.
23. Kachalia A, et al. Liability claims and costs before and after implementation of a medical error disclosure program. Ann Intern Med. 2010;153(4):213–21.
24. Mello MM, et al. Communication and resolution programs: the challenges and lessons learned from six early adopters. Health Aff. 2014;33(1):20–9.
25. Gallagher T, et al. Making communication and resolution programmes mission critical in healthcare organizations. BMJ Qual Saf. 2020;29(11):01–4.
26. Peto R, et al. One system's journey in creating a disclosure and apology program. Jt Comm J Qual Saf. 2009;35(10):487–96.
27. Mello MM, et al. Outcomes in two Massachusetts hospital systems give reason for an optimism about communication-and-resolution programs. Health Aff. 2017;36(10):179501803.
28. Mello MM, et al. Challenges of implementing a communication-and-resolution program where multiple organizations must cooperate. Health Serv Res. 2016;51:2550–68.
29. Massachusetts Alliance for Communication and Resolution following Medical Injury. 2020. https://www.macrmi.info/. Accessed 14 Sept 2020.
30. Gallaher TH, Mello MM, Sage W, et al. Can communication-and-resolution programs achieve potential? Five key questions. Health Aff. 2018;37:1845–52.
31. McDonald TB, Van Niel M, Gocke H, et al. Implementing communication and resolution programs: lessons learned from the first 200 hospitals. J Pat Saf Risk Manag. 2018;23:73–8.
32. Kachalia A, Kaufman SR, Boothman R, et al. Liability costs before and after implementation of a medical error disclosure program. Ann Intern Med. 2010;153(4):213–21.

33. Moore J, Bismark M, Mello MM. Patients' experience with communication-and- resolution programs after medical injury. JAMA. 2017;177(11):1595–603.
34. Agency of Healthcare Research and Quality. Communication and Optimal Resolution (CANDOR) toolkit. https://www.ahrq.gov/patient-safety/capacity/candor/modules.html. Accessed 16 Sept 2020.
35. Mello MM, et al. Ensuring successful implementation of communication-and-resolution programmes. BMJ Qual Saf. 2020;29:1.

Chapter 19
Avoidance of Complications

Prashant Sinha

The desire to avoid complications is embedded in the Hippocratic Oath and well precedes the often cited Institute of Medicine report from 1999 [1]. Our training, both cognitive and technical, has been passed down with rigorous discipline; our knowledge disseminated in journals and conferences and our colleagues critiqued weekly in morbidity and mortality serve as continual reminders of this profound desire. The Institute of Medicine report and many others preceding it and following it have changed the way we think about medical errors and will continue to shape the way we think about preventing them. This chapter will identify the methods and, when available, the evidence behind modern strategies taken to prevent complications. While these approaches must necessarily be applied to their specific clinical frameworks to affect a specific outcome, I hope to stimulate new thinking about the problem of surgical complications with a novel set of tools.

P. Sinha (✉)
Department of Surgery, NYU Langone Medical Center,
Brooklyn, NY, USA
e-mail: prashant.sinha@nyumc.org; http://nyulangone.org/

© The Author(s), under exclusive license to Springer Nature   373
Switzerland AG 2022
J. R. Romanelli et al. (eds.), *The SAGES Manual of Quality,*
Outcomes and Patient Safety,
https://doi.org/10.1007/978-3-030-94610-4_19

Morbidity and Mortality

This conference has been applied across every medical specialty from psychiatry and family medicine to all surgical specialties. Over the past two decades, however, calls to restructure this conference have centered around multiple themes. A PubMed search for "morbidity and mortality conference" was conducted, and 500 results were reviewed for relevance yielding 84 articles. Thirty-one articles were dated before 2010. Thematically, morbidity and mortality (M&M) conferences were critiqued for not using evidence, not linking the conference to performance improvement, and being accusatory rather than systematic. The redesign of M&M envisions a learning environment linked with system-level quality improvement at the hospital and even national level. Redesign also places the objectives of the ACGME at the front and sustainability for lessons learned. The objectives of improving M&M were best achieved with structured datasets relevant to national population trends or local hospital system quality objectives that are tracked and analyzed, presented in a standardized manner, and moderated with experts, with interactive assessment captured for evidence of learning.

The reimagined M&M is evidence-based, includes local data to review overall performance in areas of interest, and uses a system-based approach to deconstruct a complication into the errors or variations in care that led to the complication. In order to create a learning system, the rich discussion that often accompanies case level discussions and its context in the local healthcare system should be captured. Impactful complications and complications that occur at a higher than desired frequency deserve further attention beyond M&M. The hand-off from M&M to a process improvement team is critical to ensure that the mistakes are not repeated and that the learning is sustained. Risk adjustment and unexpected outcomes, both good and bad, can be found in large datasets, and both types of variations can serve as a more impactful case selection tool for M&M and subsequent performance improvement as described by Bohnen et al. [2].

Reporting Bias

The natural human tendency to hide from error is so pervasive that it creates a strong implicit bias even in our published literature [3]. The positive outcome bias reflects a tendency of editors to strongly prefer novel and positive findings over mundane or negative findings. This bias unfortunately reduces the reliability and impact of our data and gives lesser credence to low value interventions. It increases the chances that low value interventions or, worse, potentially damaging interventions are repeatedly used. In order to counteract this bias, the opposite should occur. There is value in repeating experiments and collating larger datasets. Research is sometimes reactive, revealing comparative effectiveness only after provocative studies stimulate additional research. In effect, researchers should encourage debate and scrutiny to arrive at the best conclusions. A relatively recent example is the practice of combining mechanical bowel preparation with oral antibiotics before elective colon surgery. This practice, called into question, led to its study at the same time CMS increased its scrutiny on infections after colon surgery. After some debate, the scrutiny and increasing literature has led us back to the older practice, with large datasets culminated from both positive and negative studies. SAGES has historically used the voice of its Presidency and its Board to drive large-scale change in a positive way, for example, in identifying the dangers of using synthetic mesh in hiatal hernia repair and in creating a consensus conference to address the continued problem of bile duct injury. Reactive research, regulatory bodies, and national societies are important tools to affect change, but these tools take time and require a great deal of deliberation for their output.

Clinical data registries (CDR), including regional collaboratives, are an alternative. They are an increasingly used instrument of process improvement that are faster and more specific to their various specialties. There is no assumption a priori of either positive or negative outcomes in such a registry. The outcomes over time generate both positive and negative signals that are detected statistically and whose relevance is then assessed. The Society for Thoracic Surgery (STS) cardiothoracic database set a high bar with their data registry, and the detailed and comprehensive collection has been invaluable in improving performance across the nation. Numerous advances have been achieved from analysis of this national registry including reduced transfusions, earlier mobility, reductions in cardiopulmonary bypass time, and reduced length of stay following coronary bypass surgery. The ASMBS database for bariatric surgery, the ACS' National Surgical Quality Improvement Program, Vascular Quality Initiative, Americas' Hernia Society Quality Collaborative, and the like have been empowering research that is driven from large datasets with wide ownership. CDRs can help drive improvements in clinical outcomes, by identifying specific targets for reducing variability. Variables in large datasets that demonstrate high variability can indicate the best targets for process improvement and can subsequently lead to better outcomes and better cost containment. Calls for national registries in inflammatory bowel disease, emergency general surgery, and other specialties are gaining traction and will continue to aid this effort. The progress toward more collected data is slow, as the initial effort to build a registry and its infrastructure is both large and expensive, and ongoing data collection requires training and dedicated personnel. Widespread participation in national registries has been hampered by their maintenance cost, and hospital systems have to weigh those costs against the future gains in performance promised by participation. Mandatory reporting, as required by local or national health authorities, may increase adoption of registries that have delivered the most value, while grants and local funding sources may help others gain traction, but the registries will increasingly play a pivotal role in aiding the goal of performance improvement [4].

Checklists to Bundles

Atul Gawande reached across disciplines to use process engineering tools. He asked whether checklists could be used in medicine to reduce errors. Most of us have benefitted from the use of these checklists when we perform central line insertions or to verify allergies, antibiotics, and laterality before an operative procedure. Checklists have been shown to reduce mortality and complications; however, they are best used when the complexity of a process can be readily broken down into quantifiable steps. Variability in medicine and in surgery can occur from many different areas. In order to reduce variability, one has to know where to look. An entire process does not need to be deconstructed, but one only need to know where variability can affect outcomes. A visible marker of variability is surgical site infections following colon procedures. The literature has an enormous volume treating this one area, and more recently, the approach to reducing these postop infections has taken the broad learnings and has combined them into a readily deployable process: the bundle. This is a departure from the checklist philosophy that seeks to control all the steps and factors in a given process. The colorectal literature has indicated that for any given patient, it is not always known which combination of factors will contribute to an infection. In this case, a care bundle is an approach that uses many elements all at once to modify multiple host and environment factors in parallel to achieve a better and more consistent result for most patients. Having embarked on a PI project to reduce colon SSI at three different hospitals, I can attest to the complexity of the challenge. At one hospital, prolonged operative times and hypothermia appeared to be risk factors. At another hospital, increasing adherence to an ERAS bundle was important, and at a third, changing antibiotic prophylaxis and enforcing the use of clean wound closure trays made a difference. Ultimately, a bundled approach that uses techniques from early recovery pathways, wound care techniques, microbial surveillance, and preoperative preparation can consistently address the variety of factors that can lead to postoperative infections. The strength of evidence supporting a bundle approach is significant – the more elements of a care bundle that are adhered to, the better the patient outcome [5]. The bundle approach to infection prevention has now expanded across many high-risk procedures.

Professionalism and Competency

No student embarks on a career in medicine or surgery believing that they will provide anything but the best care. The long duration of training attests to the surgeon's dedication as a clinician, scientists, and humanitarian, but, in spite of that time, variability in the individual still occurs. A widely cited finding in the *New England Journal of Medicine* identified that malpractice claims were concentrated into a few physicians. Only 6% of the over 900,000 physicians had a claim and 1% of physicians, having at least two paid claims, accounted for 32% of all claims. Apart from an increased risk for males and later stages of practice, repeat claims strongly predicted additional claims, raising the concern for individual behaviors. While the claims inherently are not a great correlate of substandard care, these findings suggest a behavioral component [6].

In another study, a comparison of malpractice claims against 360-degree peer evaluations demonstrated a strong correlation for certain types of negative and positive behaviors. Five behaviors were listed as having the highest odds ratios for malpractice claims: "snaps at others when frustrated," "talks down," "considers suggestions," "pays attention," and "informs others." Personal behaviors can be associated with malpractice claims, and this among other research illustrates that a few individuals can have measurable and negative effect on patients, peers, and their healthcare systems [7]. Medical education curricula have therefore included aspects of professionalism for young physician degree candidates and postgraduate trainees.

Missing, unfortunately, is a body of evidence that can prospectively identify or modify those behaviors. However, there are important areas such as prompt and transparent disclosure of errors that are beneficial to both patient and practitioner, even if they do not prevent error. Consequently, there has been a focus on this in board certification and maintenance of certification and whether either has value. A study evaluating almost two million procedures by 14,598 surgeons revealed that achieving board certification was associated with 21% less chance of having outlier complication rates. However, board certification and maintenance of certification did not correlate with exemplary complication rates; exemplary surgeons had higher volumes and affiliations with larger hospitals [8].

Without wading into the considerable debate around board certification, it suffices to say that it is important to expect and independently assess a basic level of cognitive and ideally technical proficiency. It is also important to expect a level of professionalism and to educate our trainees about the dangers of disruptive behaviors. The ACGME is moving toward addressing these gaps in assessment through the use of entrustable professional activities (EPA). Rather than redefining competencies, EPAs serve as a framework to set trainee expectations and guide a supervisor's assessment in order to allow an entrustment decision [9]. An entrustment decision may be unsupervised completion of an appendectomy, for example. This level of entrustment would require a trainee to demonstrate certain knowledge, skills, and attitudes. An instructor would be required to assess consistent achievement of the same in order to allow an entrustment decision, whether it be direct supervision or unsupervised. This framework could be applied to junior faculty but logistically has significant challenges [10].

We do not yet know the impact of EPAs and other tools for competency assessment on patient outcomes. Specifically, can we help our colleagues avoid complications through structured evaluation during training and early practice? The prevalence of surgeon variability coupled with decreased time in training in this era of reduced work hours will ensure that competency assessment tools will continue to evolve. The ultimate goal will be to reduce the variability of our trainees entering the workforce. Until then, post hoc assessments based on outcomes will continue to drive how we identify outliers.

Simulation and Skill Assessment

Inescapable is the desire to understand the technical skill level of a given surgeon. This might be one of the most mysterious statistics in medicine. On the face of it, one could scoff at the notion of trading "baseball cards" of surgeons, but perhaps many people actually desire this for different reasons. The public has little objective data by which to choose a surgeon, hospitals may believe this to be an important measure of efficiency, and certainly the risk managers and attorneys would find these measures too helpful. Most things in medicine cannot however be distilled to the skills used in an operating room, but those skills certainly matter. Simulated and real-world skill assessments, just like checklists, have to be complete in capturing the process that they try to distill. The transferability of simulation, the validity of simulation, and the ease and reproducibility of scoring can be variable and highly dependent on the skill being studied. However, when correlates of high volume on good outcomes abound in the literature, particularly in highly complex procedures, a tendency to focus on the practitioner rather than the entire environment is hard to avoid. A number of validated skills ratings systems do exist such as Fundamentals of Laparoscopic Surgery (FLS), Fundamentals of the Use of Safe Energy (FUSE), Objective Structured Assessment of Technical Skills(O-SATS), Global Operative Assessment of Laparoscopic Skills (GOALS), Global Evaluative Assessment of Robotic Skills(GEARS), and Crowd-Sourced Assessment of Technical Skills (C-SATS). The process of rating is resource intensive, and, even with the use of a tool such as C-SATS that uses crowd-sourcing review of video, the results can reliably distinguish less skilled surgeons but currently have not been well studied against hard outcomes data [11]. Furthermore, most of the excellent work done on assessment remains in specific fields such as urology or with specific tools such as laparoscopy or robotic surgery. Nevertheless, some assessments now serve as validated competency assessments including FLS and FUSE. The future of these objective scores remains open and will serve as an added data point for performance improvement. Ultimately, research remains to understand the degree of effect technical skills have on outcomes and on defining the correct skills to focus on that can be readily and easily measured, for each procedure. It seems like a daunting task, but progress toward reproducible measurements is exciting and may continue to provide achievable milestones that will benefit patient care.

High Reliability

All the aforementioned tools, training, and assessments need to be placed into a framework that can be readily used in any healthcare system. The ultimate goal of high performance, which can be measured, is the reduction of variability. The aphorism attributed to various physicians and famous individuals that good judgment comes from experience and experience from bad judgment need not be so. Surgeons are trained with time and volume requirements that enable them to obtain the proper experience and judgment. At least, we believe this to be the case within our system that has been developed and refined over time. Those achieving board certification have gained the cognitive skills to perform reasonably well. Those that maintain a high volume of practice are expected to perform at higher levels, unless they have exhibited disruptive behaviors that increase their chances of repeated malpractice claims. The future, however, is driven by an aversion to risk. We seek a better educational system that sequentially graduates surgeons through competency and skills-based assessments. Until we can consistently perform and intervene on these types of assessments, we must use system-level tools that are providing solutions that appear to work to reduce variability and error. "System failures are errors in the design, organization, training, or maintenance that lead to operator errors. Those failures involving direct contact with the patient – human failures – are often part of the proximate cause of an event" [12]. The best way to avoid errors is to prevent humans from making them, through structural barriers like checklists, bundles, and pathways. Identifying where to look next for interventions must come from large and shared datasets. The signals that we seek are not from mortality but from subtler and earlier signs and symptoms; this requires specialty-specific intelligence. Finally, there has to be an appetite to invest in the data systems that can help identify and then correct areas of variability. Alignment of goals within a hospital, hospital network, and region or across the nation can facilitate this. CMS has already learned that financial rewards and punishments are helpful, but only go so far. James Reason, famously known for the Swiss cheese model of error, acknowledged long ago, "Measures that involve sanctions and exhortations (that is, moralistic measures directed to those at the sharp end) have only very limited effectiveness, especially so in the case of highly trained professionals" [13].

Hospital systems that have chosen to take these lessons seriously understand that implementation is the next important challenge. Their next evolution is into a high reliability organization (HRO). An entire book can be devoted to this, but the basic principles can be outlined as follows: All members of an organization are called upon to act together on shared goals. For example, a medical-surgical floor team may discuss interventions that can help prevent patient falls; any staff walking past a room should stop and respond to a patient that is calling out or has rung a bell for assistance. This example illustrates important concepts in an HRO. Hierarchy is removed, accountability is given to everyone, a specific action is defined, and a specific result is measured and tracked. An HRO takes hundreds of these measurable tasks, studies them, and refines their interventions until a sustainable reliable outcome is achieved. A cultural transformation is required to move toward an HRO. The five principles that define a high reliability organization are as follows: (1) preoccupation with failure, (2) reluctance to simplify interpretations, (3) sensitivity to operations, (4) commitment to resilience, and (5) deference to expertise. Effectively an HRO constantly monitors for safety issues and errors, adjusts accordingly, and maintains the operations that keep the organization safe while recognizing that anyone with expertise is valued. A complex operation will inevitably have errors, but the goal is recovery, learning, and anticipation of these errors. A healthcare system that aims to become a high reliability organization can begin immediately but to perform well must continue to practice and mature [14]. The maturity is best seen as a system first learns to react to errors and eventually begins to look for weaknesses and proactively fix them.

Conclusion

Can we avoid complications? Yes. Can we help all trainees consistently avoid complications? Maybe. Reviewing lessons learned from individual cases should never stop, as a great deal of detail and insight can be gained through critical analysis of a single event. In most root cause analyses, the individual practitioner usually holds a small portion of accountability relative to the flaws in the systematic framework in which they work. In order to move our safety systems forward, the framework of accountability that follows the principles of a high reliability organization may prove to be the most effective. Within it, the individual strategies employed to improve safety and avoid complications are varied but may include aspects of training, assessments of skill and competency, attitudes, and behavior, coupled with targeted statistical analysis using large datasets and structured interventions. Surgeons are well suited to improving quality and preventing complications by adopting these among other quality tools. Armed with data and a desire for continuous improvement, surgeons can improve their outcomes with more than a scalpel.

References

1. Institute of Medicine (US) Committee on Quality of Health Care in America. In: Kohn LT, Corrigan JM, Donaldson MS, editors. To err is human: building a safer health system. Washington, DC: The National Academies Press; 2000. p. 312.
2. Bohnen JD, Chang DC, Lillemoe KD. Reconceiving the morbidity and mortality conference in an era of big data: an "unexpected" outcomes approach. Ann Surg. 2016;263(5):857–9.
3. Callaham ML, et al. Positive-outcome bias and other limitations in the outcome of research abstracts submitted to a scientific meeting. JAMA. 1998;280(3):254–7.
4. Romanelli JR, et al. Public reporting and transparency: a primer on public outcomes reporting. Surg Endosc. 2019;33(7):2043–9.
5. Jaffe TA, et al. Optimizing value of colon surgery in Michigan. Ann Surg. 2017;265(6):1178–82.
6. Studdert DM, et al. Prevalence and characteristics of physicians prone to malpractice claims. N Engl J Med. 2016;374(4):354–62.
7. Lagoo J, et al. Multisource evaluation of surgeon behavior is associated with malpractice claims. Ann Surg. 2019;270(1):84–90.
8. Xu T, et al. Association between board certification, maintenance of certification, and surgical complications in the United States. Am J Med Qual. 2019;34(6):545–52.
9. Ten Cate O. Nuts and bolts of entrustable professional activities. J Grad Med Educ. 2013;5(1):157–8.
10. Hoops HE, Deveney KE, Brasel KJ. Development of an assessment tool for surgeons in their first year of independent practice: the junior surgeon performance assessment tool. J Surg Educ. 2019;76(6):e199–208.
11. Ghani KR, et al. Measuring to improve: peer and crowd-sourced assessments of technical skill with robot-assisted radical prostatectomy. Eur Urol. 2016;69(4):547–50.
12. Chang A, et al. The JCAHO patient safety event taxonomy: a standardized terminology and classification schema for near misses and adverse events. Int J Qual Health Care. 2005;17(2):95–105.
13. Reason J. Understanding adverse events: human factors. Qual Health Care. 1995;4(2):80–9.
14. Chassin MR, Loeb JM. High-reliability health care: getting there from here. Milbank Q. 2013;91(3):459–90.

Chapter 20
Safe Introduction of Technology

Kathleen Lak

Introduction

Technology in medicine is expanding at a rapid pace. The ability to safely adopt and implement new surgical technologies can be challenging at both provider and hospital system levels. Patient safety and quality are often the basis of technological advancements, but a systematic method for verifying the intended and unintended consequences of new technologies has been overshadowed in the past by the swift implementation and mass use. In this chapter, we will discuss how surgical technology has been introduced to widespread use in the past, what kind of challenges or missteps were made along the way, and where we are headed as far as assessments for safe introduction of technology in the future.

K. Lak (✉)
Bariatric and Minimally Invasive Gastrointestinal Surgery, Medical College of Wisconsin, Milwaukee, WI, USA
e-mail: klak@mcw.edu

© The Author(s), under exclusive license to Springer Nature Switzerland AG 2022
J. R. Romanelli et al. (eds.), *The SAGES Manual of Quality, Outcomes and Patient Safety*,
https://doi.org/10.1007/978-3-030-94610-4_20

385

Introduction of Surgical Technology in the Past: Laparoscopic Cholecystectomy

Since the time of barber shop bloodletting in the fourteenth and fifteenth centuries, the field of surgery has been evolving. In a major leap of innovation, laparoscopic surgery entered the arena in the late twentieth century and changed the approach to surgery as we know it. The introduction of the laparoscopic cholecystectomy highlights what is thrilling about innovation in the surgical field and what is dangerous in unchecked dissemination of that innovation. Prior to its use in general surgery, laparoscopic approaches were mainly used in gynecology. In 1985, the first laparoscopic cholecystectomy was performed by Erich Mühe of Germany [1]. Mühe developed the technique after many years of interest in laparoscopy and abdominal endoscopy. After laparoscopic appendectomy was performed in 1980, his interest was further ignited in the application of the technology for cholecystectomy. He went on to learn the basics of laparoscopy from a gynecologic surgeon, and 5 years later Mühe performed his first laparoscopic cholecystectomy. He presented his work in 1986 at the German Surgical Society Congress and again at the Lower Rhine-Westphalian Society. At that time, his achievement was not met with enthusiasm. Philippe Mouret of France performed the procedure in 1987 followed by Dubois in 1988. Despite a slow start, the technique spread across the Atlantic, and the first laparoscopic cholecystectomy was performed in the USA in 1988 by McKernan and Saye. Over the course of these first years, the procedure was being modified, tweaked, and improved upon. Mühe began with a side-viewing scope at the umbilicus with pneumoperitoneum fashioned out of bicycle tubing and later transitioned to a subcostal incision with no pneumoperitoneum.

The history behind the laparoscopic cholecystectomy is inspiring with the leap in innovation and the passion behind bringing the technology to the mainstream. From its inception, the technology quickly progressed to the standard of care. In what might be an inspiring tale of innovative success, the actual and potential dangers of this unfettered progress cast a dark shadow. Over the following several years after Mühe introduced the technique, the laparoscopic approach quickly became adopted as the most standard method for cholecystectomy, replacing the open technique. By 1992, the National Institute of Health (NIH) issued a consensus statement citing that approximately 80% of cholecystectomies were being treated laparoscopically [2]. This consensus statement declares that the laparoscopic cholecystectomy is safe and effective although reports of common bile duct injuries at that time were reportedly higher. The procedure was advertised as a marrying of two safe, proven treatments – that of the open cholecystectomy and laparoscopic surgery, safely used by gynecologists for decades prior [3, 4]. The more than twofold increase in the incidence of biliary injuries was not initially known for a number of reasons [2].

The widespread use of laparoscopic cholecystectomy is said to have been propelled by several factors, one strong factor being market demand. Patients at that time were interested in the procedure as it gave an alternative to the open cholecystectomy known for longer hospital stays and recovery time. Surgeons at the time were reportedly pressured to adopt the procedure swiftly or risk losing patients to competitors [2, 5]. In a patient-driven market, surgeons were quick to adopt the relatively untested procedure with little objective data on outcomes. The market pressure and competition complicated accurate reporting of morbidity or mortality in the first years after its introduction. Case series from providers' early experience and rare randomized trials comparing open to laparoscopic cholecystectomy were trickling in at the time, but most were insufficiently powered to detect the difference in biliary complications. While medical centers reported low rates of bile duct injury, registry data drew a different picture with increased referrals for complex biliary reconstructions [2]. Biliary strictures, which may present months or years after surgery, were also presumed to be increased with the new innovation, but little data was available due to a lack of long-term studies following the innovation over time.

The actual training of surgeons on the technique cannot be understated either. Surgeons were met with a different visualization of the surgical field and different instruments and required a different skill set compared to open cholecystectomy, which had been the favored technique for a century before. The first surgeons to perform and market the technique in the USA organized courses outside of a university setting and brought the application of laparoscopy across the country [6]. The NIH acknowledged in their 1992 consensus statement that adequate physician training is paramount to achieving good outcomes – although what constitutes that training had yet to be determined, regulated, or tracked [2]. For many years, laparoscopic cholecystectomy was performed around the country without a requirement of institutional review board involvement or other oversight. Surgeons had variable instruction, training, and technical skills with the procedure, which leads to difficulty in interpreting data. When the morbidity associated with the procedure was ultimately recognized, it was initially attributed to the surgeon "learning curve," inadequate training, or insufficient credentialing [3, 4, 7].

The introduction of laparoscopic cholecystectomy and its brisk adoption brings up themes illustrating the benefits as well as risks associated with new innovations and their implementation. Even in the 1990s, the lack of objective assessment of the innovative procedure was acknowledged, but it was stated that controlled studies will likely be unable to be performed due to patient's refusing to forego the most modern treatment available [2]. Further, because bile duct injuries are fortunately infrequent, the number of patients needed to adequately power such a study renders the creation of such studies moot. These deterrents to real-time study of new innovation still complicate the introduction of new therapies, equipment, and techniques today.

Introduction of Surgical Technology in the Present: Introduction of the Robotic Platform

The evolution of the safe introduction of technology from the introduction of laparoscopy for cholecystectomy to the present can be described in part by the example of the use of the robotic platform in surgery. Like the laparoscopic cholecystectomy, the introduction and expansion of robotic technology in the field of surgery has been swift and widespread.

Robotic technology has become a usable adjunct to surgical practice to any surgeon with the interest and wherewithal to complete the steps necessary for implementation. These steps vary and differ from hospital to hospital. The necessary steps to credentialing and obtaining privileges are based on hospital's specific processes for assessing the provider's qualifications for a given service. This can be a challenging requirement set forth by the Joint Commission as leaders in healthcare administration are given little guidance on what constitutes proficiency in new technology [8]. The Society of American Gastrointestinal and Endoscopic Surgeons (SAGES) and the Minimally Invasive Robotic Association (MIRA) produced a document outlining consensus on several key topics regarding use of the robotic platform in surgery – in part outlining suggested training and credentialing requirements [6]. Published in 2007, the document outlines minimum requirements for granting privileges to providers in several scenarios of training. While the document does provide a general outline, individual institutions are required to define what constitutes a "structured training curriculum," what role the proctor will have in precepted cases, and how many cases are required for competency. Credentialing committees for new technology develop these criteria.

In the past, research and development of new medical technology was a distinctly different arena from that of determination of physician credentialing and granting of privileges; however, with the introduction of the robotic platform, companies such as Intuitive Surgical began to permeate surgical skills training. What followed was that a private company, which invested in the expansion of the use of their product, was now involved with determination of whether providers were felt to be safe and competent to proceed with use of their product. This changed in 2017 with a Supreme Court's reversal of a lower court's decision in Taylor vs. Intuitive. In this case, Intuitive Surgical was found liable for a poor patient outcome based on failure to warn or inform the *hospital,* in addition to the surgeon, of the risks associated with use of the technology. In this ruling, the liability of implementing new technology is now shared with the private company promoting the technology as well as the hospital aiming to use it. Prior to this ruling, Intuitive Surgical made recommendations on proctoring of cases and surgical competency – this was subsequently eliminated to leave these decisions in the hands of local credentialing committees [9, 10]. The ruling in 2017 intervened on this potential avenue for conflict of interest. Now that the liability is shared by all those involved, a collaborative but distinct consensus is suggested to remove any conflict of interest from the discussion on surgical credentialing for individual providers in the case of robotic surgery.

The determination of what constitutes adequate training for credentialing of a new provider in robotic surgery or a physician in practice gaining additional skills in the field is highly variable and fraught with individual characteristics that produce challenges. Several private companies offer web-based training programs, while others have on-site hands-on instruction [11]. The advancement of virtual reality simulation in the robotic surgery training paradigm has allowed instruction to take place prior to touching patients [12, 13]. This feature allows for improvement in surgeon comfort with the technology as well as proficiency in skills and overall efficiency. Some hands-on training programs incorporate mentorship by expert robotic-surgeon trainers to allow for constructive feedback in real time. Credentialing or new technology committees at individual institutions determine the requirements needed to grant physician privileges. Validation of these methods is forthcoming.

The introduction of the robotic platform improved upon many of the missteps from the introduction of laparoscopic cholecystectomy. Training programs are bolstering the preparation of surgeons in didactic curricula, hands-on instruction, and virtual reality. Credentialing and new technology committees are the gatekeeper to physician privileging for use of robotic surgery. The gaps in training and our ability to define what constitutes an able and knowledgeable surgeon for the technology as well as evidence-based guidelines to oversee use of the technology are yet to be determined. In the setting of frequent new devices hitting the market, strategies such as these to guide the safe implementation of innovation outside the scope of robotic surgery are needed now more than ever.

Introduction of Surgical Technology: Proposals for the Future

Defining Innovation

Progress in the field of surgery over the past 100 years has been extensive. The giant leaps in the development of the surgical standard of care for common surgical ailments were for the most part not bolstered by randomized controlled trials and long-term outcomes. Evaluation of evolving procedures or technology in the operating room was not commonplace in decades past in lieu of essentially trial and error with patients on the receiving end [14]. This is not to say that there were not altruistic intentions of improving patient care, but evidence-based medicine as we know it did not yet exist. With each trip to the operating room, surgeons are met with unique situations at hand which demand action. What begins as a variation in the way a surgical problem is addressed may develop into a new technique altogether. There is little clarity of what constitutes surgeon discretion, from innovative trial and error to experimental technique.

The surgical minutia is not played out in an informed consent process as much of this detail is not considered experimental but nonetheless is a form of untested innovation. The example described in our first section on the introduction of laparoscopic cholecystectomy is one example of untested innovation becoming widely disseminated. What began as a disruptive use of technology in a different way became mainstream prior to objective short- or long-term testing. This inevitably leaves potential for unintended consequences without oversight.

Fast forward to the twenty-first century; we now have sharing of surgical techniques daily on social media platforms and private surgical groups such as Twitter or Facebook. There is instantaneous sharing of cases, techniques, intraoperative decisions, and resulting discourse between surgeons worldwide. This arena is bolstered by real-time experience with those sharing often seeking feedback or critiques. This form of information dispersion is far from the randomized controlled trials that garner objective evidence, but it does hold the potential to influence the way surgery is practiced.

In the information age, we now look toward reproducible scientific methods to thoroughly evaluate the quality, safety, and short- and long-term efficacy of modifications to the surgical standard of care. When these modifications are in the form of pharmaceuticals, a regimented system for evaluation is required. However, when that modification is a surgical innovation, technique, or product, the playing field is largely unregulated.

Evaluation of Innovation in Pharmaceuticals and Surgery

To adequately envision a framework for the safe introduction of surgical innovation, the pharmaceutical industry's method is often described. Assessment of the safety and efficacy of pharmaceuticals involves a regulated process overseen by the US Food and Drug Administration (FDA). Initial steps include animal studies for safety with dosing in phase 0. Prior to moving on to human studies, FDA approval of an Investigational New Drug (IND) application must be met. What follows are three additional phases of trials for clinical safety and efficacy in humans. Randomized placebo-controlled trials are required, which adds a measure of complexity and expense to the process. The phases of pharmaceutical development are generally in succession requiring a predictable prolonged duration of analysis prior to achieving completion of the monitoring phase 4.

Each phase in this process has been defined and developed with the aim of patient safety and quality in mind. Phase 1 human studies are conducted on a small cohort of healthy volunteers. A tolerable dose range is determined as well as the safety with a limited number of doses. Phase 2 studies are generally randomized controlled trials (RCTs), and this is the first time the IND is used on the targeted patient population. Markers assessing for efficacy are often assessed at this stage. Phase 3 studies expand this research to include thousands of patients and are designed to assess the safety and efficacy of the drug using predefined endpoints [15]. The outcomes of these studies are used to apply for market approval through the FDA. Phase 4 studies are generally post-market studies which continually assess for long-term adverse outcomes or use in alternative populations.

What should be taken from this concise description of the rigorous process for safe implementation of pharmaceuticals is its direct comparison to the process for safe implementation of new surgical technologies and innovation: that no such process exists. At this point in our history, surgical technology is arguably advancing at a higher speed than ever. The introduction of these technological advances is unstandardized, not systematically regulated, and largely unstructured. Where the FDA holds an oversight of new pharmaceutical products, no overseeing body has defined what constitutes safe introduction of surgical technology. This is not to say that individuals, surgical groups, technology companies, and leaders within the field have not provided suggestions in this arena.

The pharmaceutical industry's systematic approach to new drug development and its path to the clinical market was not always as regimented as it is today. The history of new drug development began with failures as well – namely, drugs brought into clinical use and later withdrawn or restricted due to unforeseen side effects [14]. The regulation that followed led to the current system overseen in the USA. The oversight of surgical innovation in the form of surgical technology is less stringent, and oversight of innovation in the form of therapies or techniques does not exist. The role that the FDA plays with regard to surgical innovation is small. The process begins with a determination of how novel the new product is compared to that already on the market. New innovations, as opposed to pharmaceuticals, can achieve pre-market approval without the strict degree of evidence required by new drugs coming to the market. A fast-track assessment process is used if the device or innovation is "substantially equivalent" to a predicate device. Innovative procedures or techniques have no place within the FDA's regulatory process unless submitted as a research study. Often surgical techniques or procedures are developed in the clinical setting with reporting of the successes or failures in the form of non-comparative trials, retrospective cases series, or case reports.

An example of this process is use of radiofrequency (RF) ablation for metastatic colorectal malignancy in the liver. The device itself offers treatment of non-resectable liver tumors and has broadened the treatment algorithm for metastatic colorectal cancer. The technology involves use of a novel device, so FDA approval was required prior to its introduction into the surgical marketplace. The requirement for FDA approval for clinical use was to show that the device could safely ablate hepatic tissue – which it did. The questions that remained unanswered at the time of its introduction included whether the technique was equally effective in the treatment of resectable lesions. Was this treatment recommended for patients with only otherwise unresectable disease, or was this an option for patients with resectable disease as well? In this example, we see consideration for research into the indications for the use of the device. Expanding its use would intuitively require oversight, informed consent, and tracking. Offering the technique to patients with resectable lesions, those interested in a less invasive procedure, for example, would be putting the patient in harm's way as a proven effective open procedure is known. The potential for patient harm is clear, but the device as approved by the FDA is now in use with little oversight into patient selection and reporting of results. The limitations of our assessment of the technology are evident. Likewise, in the introduction of the adult-to-adult live donor liver transplantation, there was not insignificant risk of major morbidity in the donor, but the procedure moved forward at many institutions around the country with variable involvement of institutional review boards (IRB) or oversight committees [3, 14]. In each example, the innovation has massive potential for patient benefit and leaps forward in our treatment of complex clinical scenarios, but would a regulated approach with a pause for evidence-based analyses protect our patients in the process? In these examples, the ability to protect patients and weigh the benefits and harms of a new innovation lies with the provider.

As described by Strasberg et al., patients who undergo innovative procedures have no protection from the uncertainties of that procedure; those who undergo procedures with innovative devices approved by the FDA, based on predicate devices, have no guarantee that the device can meet the intended goals [3]. We have caught up to the limitations of our regulatory bodies. An ideal solution would be one that offers protection to patients without dampening innovation. Regulation and bureaucracy may have the consequence of adding significant time and money to the innovative process. Delaying significant advances in medicine and surgery could impact innumerable patient lives when potential therapies are stuck in red tape.

As mentioned previously, when the technology or advancement is in the form of a surgical procedure, the process for safe implementation is even less clear. The definition of an innovative surgical procedure is "a new or modified procedure that differs from currently accepted local practice, the outcomes of which has not yet been described, and which may entail risk to the patient" [16]. Innovations are further defined by taxonomy such as simple tool modification, revolutionary changes in tools such as laparoscopy, or revolutionary changes in science such as aseptic technique. How we communicate about these levels of innovation is important when determining the best methods for evaluation. The Belmont report, published in 1979, aimed in part to protect patients from a trial-and-error type of research at the clinical level [17]. What constitutes research remains a gray area in procedural specialties. A surgeon's modification of technique over time – even the slightest adaptation of method – would certainly not constitute a research study; however, when a provider strays in "a significant way" from the standard practice, then a research study should be encouraged. This lack of ability to define innovation by regulatory bodies inevitably leaves the decision-making in the hands of surgeon discretion.

A Proposal for the Future: The IDEAL Framework

The IDEAL framework was first introduced in 2009 in a pivotal *Lancet* series on surgical innovation and evaluation [14, 18]. The concept of innovation, development, exploration, assessment, and long-term study was born out of a need for a standardized framework for assessment of new technology in surgery.

An outlined pathway for the safe introduction of surgical innovation was described by Barkun et al. in a 2009 pivotal *Lancet* series on surgical innovation and evaluation [14]. Aptly named the "IDEAL" paradigm – innovation, development, exploration, assessment, and long-term study – the model follows a framework similarly outlined in the pharmaceutical industry for drug development and assessment. As this process has not clearly been defined in the past, the

IDEAL framework acts to define its commonly encountered stages with efforts to systematically assess innovation with the goal of patient protection and improvement in care. A heavy burden of logistical hoops has the potential to stifle innovation. Development and fostering of innovation as described by the authors attempts to do just the opposite. The development of a process to assess surgical innovation is tailored to the creative, entrepreneurial, holistic, and passionate providers who are driving it.

In the first stages of innovation, the method, technique, or technology would be used in prehuman research and development. This may include simulation or animal studies. Stage 1 of the IDEAL framework includes the first time the innovation is used in humans. The authors point out that due to the often intangible nature of innovation in surgery, some innovation may skip steps in the IDEAL paradigm, whereas others will follow sequentially through the steps. Innovation in surgery often is born from a difficult patient problem. If not in an emergency setting, when the surgeon has the benefit of time, then it is suggested that the surgeon inform the hospital of the intent to perform a new procedure and informed consent should reflect it. A formal centralized system should be developed to track these innovative techniques or procedures, and adverse events, failures, and successes should be tracked. The ability for the system such as this to thrive would include a culture shift. The reporting of adverse events centrally may require an anonymous reporting system to encourage participation; without such a system in place, it is easy to imagine the same failed innovations occurring in isolation, repeatedly, to patients around the world. A centralized system would aim to collect this information and distribute the successes and failures for collective and prospective review. Historically, innovation may first come to peer review as described in the form of retrospective case series – this method has obvious detriments when it comes to evidence-based medicine. Case series, which make up the majority of original research, are prone to uncontrolled bias and confounding factors which make the data arguably of little value

[19]. A prospective system with organized and predefined selection criteria and defined outcome values should be agreed upon centrally, outside of the parent institution, and undergo ethical review – all prior to patient recruitment.

Stage 2 involves more providers and few select patients. This is the stage when early adopters of innovation get involved. This stage would ultimately include a learning curve for providers and will require ethical consent from patients. How exactly providers are ushered through their learning curve is a matter of discussion. Mentorship and simulation have been proposed, but ultimately, all patients involved in this stage would be followed for complications with meticulous documentation. In addition to standard Institutional Review Board approval, there should be defined criteria on who will monitor and oversee patient safety. The indications, potential benefits, and harms are delineated, and the definitions for trackable outcome measures for long-term efficacy are refined, edited, and agreed upon. This system may mimic prior reporting as described in the CONSORT statement for effective, understandable, and reproducible standards of documentation [20]. The STROBE recommendations likewise laid out standards for clear data communication [21]. The recommendations in either of these statements may be used as a guide to develop a centralized way of prospectively following innovation throughout its development and introduction into widespread use.

In stage 2b the innovation is furthered by inclusion of a wider breadth of patients. More providers and institutions may have interest in the innovation and planning for a randomized, controlled trial (RCT) can be undertaken. Concurrent prospective uncontrolled trials may be initiated as well. The timing of when an RCT would be appropriate is another topic of debate, as provider involvement during their learning curve may be challenging. Data on providers, patients, and their disease process should be tracked. Likewise, it would be advantageous to allow for databases to be disease-centric rather than procedure- or treatment-based. This change in focus would allow for tracking of patients who follow traditional pathways and those who are elective for innovative treatment.

Stage 3, the assessment stage, may foster rapid adoption of the innovation, often driven by market demand. Individual providers may be learning the nuances of the technique, but the innovation has the perception of no longer being experimental. RCTs during this stage are ideal but often may be impractical. If the innovation has clear advantages without foreseeable bias, then RCT may be unnecessary or unethical, and attempts at performing such a trial would run into complicating factors of recruitment. When RCTs are not feasible, then alternative study designs may be implored which carry more weight than case series – such as parallel group non-randomized studies.

In stage 4, the long-term outcomes are assessed including any late complications or indications not originally included or those needing modification. Long-term patient benefit with the innovation should be assessed head-to-head with the prior standard of care. This proposed outline of safe introduction of technology shows inspiration from the systematic approach to the introduction of pharmaceuticals. Since the introduction of the IDEAL framework, modifications and applications have been made to it which encourage its applicability to different subsets of technology and different patient populations [22, 23]. Marcus et al. describe a new algorithm for assessment of surgical technology that expedites the process locally while maintaining an environment that is patient centered [24]. Quality outcomes and informed consent are a priority, and a streamlined process makes it a reality conducive to encouraging surgical innovation. Moving beyond device or technology safety and efficacy, procedural specialties have unique challenges inherent to the providers themselves – challenges not encountered in new drug development: the learning curve.

Unique Challenges: Surgeon Learning Curve

Inherent to the safe introduction of new innovation in surgery is the training and proficiency of those using the technology. Accounting for a learning curve is difficult, as criteria for proficiency are lacking. Ideally, providers would be outside of their learning curve during a comparative trial; however, this could ultimately delay ability to perform trials for innovation on a timely basis. Barrie et al. assessed the methods for determining surgeon learning curves for comparative analysis of laparoscopic- and robotic-assisted colectomies for colorectal cancer in efforts to define competency [25]. In this analysis, nearly one-third of laparoscopic studies used a single qualifier to determine competency – often an arbitrary number of cases performed by the surgeon, a defined operative case time or plateau in case time, or a case-conversion rate. Another one-third of studies used multiple parameters to define the learning curve, and others used cumulative sum (CUSUM) analysis. It is interesting to note that CUSUM analysis demonstrated that case number to competency was largely variable with some providers demonstrated to be competent in as few as 5 cases and others at as high as 310 cases. This variability highlights the unreliable nature of a single value such as case number in the assessment of surgeon competency. Operative time alone is a difficult marker of proficiency as faster operations do not necessarily correlate with better patient outcomes [25]. As surgeons progress in their skills, they also may be more likely to take on more challenging cases, and operative time may reflect patient properties rather than surgeon technique. This is also the problem when conversion to open is used as a marker of surgeon proficiency. Additional challenges in proficiency are seen when surgical trainees are engaged.

When looking at laparoscopic rectal cancer or robotic-assisted procedures, the cases required to achieve proficiency vary and likely depend on factors that are not tracked well in databases – such as training methods and mentorship. A study published in *Harvard Business Review* in 2001 followed cardiac surgeons as they adopted a new minimally invasive technique [26]. After completion of the same 3-day training sessions, the teams were followed on their surgical times over the course of the first 50 cases. Analyzing the data from 16 teams at respected institutions around the country, what was evident was that the learning curve was vastly different between teams. Experience did not equal speed of adoption – as a surgeon early in their practice was among the highest-achieving, fast learning curve. This study highlighted factors associated with fast adoption and found that a team-based approach was paramount and likely synergistic to surgeons' technical proficiency with the technology.

Accurate and thorough reporting of outcomes despite inevitable learning curves is necessary for transparency and for accurate assessment of the data. What makes this confounding factor challenging is the variable duration of learning curve between providers based on the innovation at hand. Monitoring results over time, especially in the event of new technology, can be done with the CUSUM. Definitions of failures and successes, their acceptable rates, and the false-positive and false-negative probabilities are made and agreed upon prior to initiation. These variables are then tracked over time from the moment the innovation is introduced allowing for oversight [27].

In the presidential address by Dr. Ralph Damiano for the International Society for Minimally Invasive Cardiothoracic Surgeons he describes physician groups taking responsibility for patient quality and safety by stating that if this is left to industry, the FDA, or individual surgeon discretion, then multifaceted conflicts of interest or burdensome bureaucracy can put our patients at risk.

Conclusion

In this age of innovation, we have discussed examples of fast adoption of surgical technology. Laparoscopic cholecystectomy is only one example of widespread change in mainstream surgical practice that occurred without rigorous scientific study. While its use is now substantiated, the potential patient harm in its early phases warrants careful examination of our practices and modifications and safeguards to prevent this from recurring. With the widespread minute to minute dissemination of ideas, knowledge, and experience, a new challenge has arisen as new innovation in the operating room may all too often bypass a peer-reviewed process. Surgeons with good intentions may look to adopt new methods, without the rigor of science proving their utility, safety, and efficacy over time. Damiano et al. warn against the cycle of innovation, fast adoption, and subsequent discrediting after systematic data collection [27]. As the ultimate burden for patient outcomes falls on the surgeon, it is our responsibility to wield prudence and tempered decision-making when it comes to surgical innovation that makes it to the operating room. Use of virtual reality, simulation, didactic courses, mentorship, and preceptorship may be some of the methods used and will depend on the type of innovation. We owe our patients a systematic, but expeditious, assessment process to ensure the safety of our patients as novel and promising therapies are introduced.

References

1. Laparoscopic cholecystectomy - a SAGES Wiki Article. Accessed 30 Nov 2020. https://www.sages.org/wiki/laparoscopic-cholecystectomy/.
2. Gollan JL, Bulkley GB, Diehl AM. Gallstones and laparoscopic cholecystectomy. JAMA J Am Med Assoc. 1993;269(8):1018–24. https://doi.org/10.1001/jama.1993.03500080066034.
3. Strasberg SM, Ludbrook PA. Who oversees innovative practice? Is there a structure that meets the monitoring needs of new techniques? J Am Coll Surg. 2003;196(6):938–48. https://doi.org/10.1016/S1072-7515(03)00112-1.
4. Shamiyeh A, Wayand W. Laparoscopic cholecystectomy: early and late complications and their treatment. Langenbecks Arch Surg. 2004;389(3):164–71. https://doi.org/10.1007/s00423-004-0470-2.

5. Tang CL, Schlich T. Surgical innovation and the multiple meanings of randomized controlled trials: the first RCT on minimally invasive cholecystectomy (1980–2000). J Hist Med Allied Sci. 2017;72(2):117–41. https://doi.org/10.1093/jhmas/jrw027.

6. SAGES/MIRA consensus document on robotic surgery - a SAGES Publication. Accessed 14 Oct 2020. https://www.sages.org/publications/guidelines/consensus-document-robotic-surgery/.

7. Rutledge R, Fakhry SM, Baker CC, Meyer AA. The impact of laparoscopic cholecystectomy on the management and outcome of biliary tract disease in North Carolina: a statewide, population-based, time-series analysis. J Am Coll Surg. 1996;183(1):31–45.

8. Quick Safety 3: potential risks of robotic surgery | The Joint Commission. Accessed 30 Nov 2020. https://www.jointcommission.org/resources/news-and-multimedia/newsletters/newsletters/quick-safety/quick-safety-issue-3-potential-risks-of-robotic-surgery/potential-risks-of-robotic-surgery/.

9. Pradarelli JC, Campbell DA, Dimick JB. Hospital credentialing and privileging of surgeons: a potential safety blind spot. JAMA J Am Med Assoc. 2015;313(13):1313–4. https://doi.org/10.1001/jama.2015.1943.

10. Pradarelli JC, Thornton JP, Dimick JB. Who is responsible for the safe introduction of new surgical technology?: An important legal precedent from the da vinci surgical system trials. Surgery. 2017;152(8):717–8. https://doi.org/10.1001/jamasurg.2017.0841.

11. Chen R, Rodrigues Armijo P, Krause C, Siu KC, Oleynikov D. A comprehensive review of robotic surgery curriculum and training for residents, fellows, and postgraduate surgical education. Surg Endosc. 2020;34(1):361–7. https://doi.org/10.1007/s00464-019-06775-1.

12. Intuitive | Products Services | Education Training. Accessed 30 Nov 2020. https://www.intuitive.com/en-us/products-and-services/da-vinci/education#.

13. RobotiX Mentor | Simbionix. Accessed 30 Nov 2020. https://simbionix.com/simulators/robotix-mentor/.

14. Barkun JS, Aronson JK, Feldman LS, Maddern GJ, Strasberg SM. Evaluation and stages of surgical innovations. Lancet. 2009;374(9695):1089–96. https://doi.org/10.1016/S0140-6736(09)61083-7.

15. Sweet BV, Schwemm AK, Parsons DM. Review of the processes for FDA oversight of drugs, medical devices, and combination products. J Manag Care Pharm. 2011;17(1):40–50. https://doi.org/10.18553/jmcp.2011.17.1.40.

16. Biffl WL, Spain DA, Reitsma AM, et al. Responsible development and application of surgical innovations: a position statement of the Society of University Surgeons. J Am Coll Surg. 2008;206(6):1204–9. https://doi.org/10.1016/j.jamcollsurg.2008.02.011.

17. Belmont. The Belmont Report. In: Office of the Secretary; 1979.

18. McCulloch P, Altman DG, Campbell WB, et al. No surgical innovation without evaluation: the IDEAL recommendations. Lancet. 2009;374(9695):1105–12. https://doi.org/10.1016/S0140-6736(09)61116-8.

19. Horton R. Surgical research or comic opera: questions, but few answers. Lancet. 1996;347(9007):984–5. https://doi.org/10.1016/S0140-6736(96)90137-3.

20. Altman DG. Better reporting of randomised controlled trials: the CONSORT statement. Br Med J. 1996;313(7057):570–1. https://doi.org/10.1136/bmj.313.7057.570.

21. Vandenbroucke JP, von Elm E, Altman DG, et al. Strengthening the reporting of observational studies in epidemiology (STROBE): explanation and elaboration. PLoS Med. 2007;4(10):e297. https://doi.org/10.1371/journal.pmed.0040297.

22. Schwartz JAT. Innovation in pediatric surgery: the surgical innovation continuum and the ETHICAL model. J Pediatr Surg. 2014;49(4):639–45. https://doi.org/10.1016/j.jpedsurg.2013.12.016.

23. Sedrakyan A, Campbell B, Merino JG, Kuntz R, Hirst A, McCulloch P. IDEAL-D: a rational framework for evaluating and regulating the use of medical devices. https://doi.org/10.1136/bmj.i2372.

24. Marcus RK, Lillemoe HA, Caudle AS, et al. Facilitation of surgical innovation: is it possible to speed the introduction of new technology while simultaneously improving patient safety? Ann Surg. 2019;270(6):937–41. https://doi.org/10.1097/SLA.0000000000003290.

25. Barrie J, Jayne DG, Wright J, Murray CJC, Collinson FJ, Pavitt SH. Attaining surgical competency and its implications in surgical clinical trial design: a systematic review of the learning curve in laparoscopic and robot-assisted laparoscopic colorectal cancer surgery. Ann Surg Oncol. 2014;21(3):829–40. https://doi.org/10.1245/s10434-013-3348-0.

26. Speeding Up Team Learning. Accessed 18 Oct 2020. https://hbr.org/2001/10/speeding-up-team-learning.

27. Damiano RJ. Surgical innovation in the information age the heavy burden of great potential; 2011.

Part III
Surgical Safety

Chapter 21
Quality, Safety, and the Electronic Health Record (EHR)

Eunice Y. Huang and Gretchen Purcell Jackson

Electronic health records (EHRs) have experienced increased adoption over the last several decades, prompted by advances in health information technologies; growth in requirements for documentation and quality reporting, which can be supported by EHRs; and regulatory pressures, such as the Health Information Technology for Economic Clinical Health (HITECH) Act, which provided first incentives for

E. Y. Huang
Departments of General and Thoracic Surgery, Monroe Carell Jr. Children's Hospital at Vanderbilt, Nashville, TN, USA
e-mail: eunice.huang@vumc.org

G. P. Jackson (✉)
Departments of General and Thoracic Surgery, Monroe Carell Jr. Children's Hospital at Vanderbilt, Nashville, TN, USA

Intuitive Surgical, Sunnyvale, CA, USA
e-mail: gretchenpurcell@stanfordalumni.org

J. R. Romanelli et al. (eds.), *The SAGES Manual of Quality, Outcomes and Patient Safety*,
https://doi.org/10.1007/978-3-030-94610-4_21

implementation and then penalties for failure to achieve Meaningful Use of EHRs. While EHRs have shown promise in the ability to support quality and safety in surgical specialties, significant challenges remain. This chapter provides an overview of how EHRs can be leveraged to determine and improve the quality and safety of surgical care.

Best Practices for EHR Implementation

Implementation and maintenance of EHRs are complex endeavors that require full engagement of organizational leadership and the healthcare personnel who work within the environment. Substantial investments in hardware, software, and technical support are necessary. Furthermore, workflow redesign, employee education, and ongoing process evaluations and adjustments should be expected. Implementation of an EHR presents opportunities to improve effective and efficient delivery of patient care, which can enhance quality and safety. However, if poorly planned and executed, the implementation process can also negatively impact quality and safety in both inpatient and outpatient settings. This section will discuss principles for surgeons to follow during EHR implementation.

An EHR implementation process can be divided into three phases: pre-implementation, implementation, and post-implementation [1]. Surgeons should actively seek to be integral members of the leadership team and participate in all three phases. To support such engagement, organizational leadership should create time for and appropriately compensate individuals who contribute to this critical undertaking. Without appropriate representation, the unique needs and workflows of surgical practice can be overlooked or misunderstood, with disruptive consequences when the EHR is launched.

The pre-implementation focus is developing an institutional framework for the project, including articulating institutional strengths, weaknesses, needs, and priorities. In addition, creating operating procedures for communication, identifying outcome measurements, and articulating deliverables and timelines are necessary. During implementation, surgeons should engage in workflow redesign. This process involves specifying existing workflows, adapting them to appropriate EHR workflows, and elucidating the technical and structural requirements for implementation and transition. This process may involve numerous iterations, as surgeons work across highly varied settings, from operating rooms, ambulatory surgery centers, and endoscopy suites to clinics, emergency departments, and intensive care units. After initial design, surgical leaders should participate actively in testing the EHR environment, address critical errors and oversights, and engage in the training of their peers [2]. During post-implementation, surgical leaders should track adoption, assess outcomes, assist in optimization, and support adaptations to the ever-changing healthcare environment.

Effective health information technology leaders must have expertise in EHR implementation and management, knowledge of evolving technologies and associated regulations, and awareness of privacy and security threats. Maintaining competence across these dimensions can be challenging. Developing a workforce of surgeon clinical informaticists who have practical clinical experience and formal informatics training is of great value to the surgical community and can enable optimal utilization of all technologies, including EHRs [3].

Leveraging the EHR to Measure and Optimize Quality and Safety

EHRs provide many opportunities to deliver knowledge, standardize care, reduce errors, measure compliance, and track quality in surgical practice. Examples include using visual cues on patient dashboards to inform medication dosing [4], creating electronic pathways to direct complex care across multiple encounters [5], and supporting rapid capture and delivery of quality improvement data to improve compliance [6].

Implementation, management, and use of EHRs are accompanied by significant institutional administrative and financial burdens. Therefore, it is important to continually assess whether EHRs are delivering on the promise of providing higher quality and safer care to patients. Several studies have evaluated the global impact of EHR adoption and its effects on quality and patient safety in surgery. Furukawa examined the association of hospital EHR implementation and adverse event occurrence rates using the Medicare Patient Safety Monitoring System. In patients admitted for acute cardiovascular disease, pneumonia, or conditions requiring surgery, those exposed to a fully electronic EHR were less likely to experience inhospital adverse events [7]. A systematic review was conducted by Robinson to assess the impact of EHRs, computerized physician order entry (CPOE), and patient portal adoption on surgical practice, and it identified three trends with use of these EHR-supported technologies: improvements in the quality of surgical documentation, increased adherence to guidelines for medication administration, and enthusiastic adoption of communication technologies such as patient portals [8]. Another systematic review by Borab found that computerized clinical decision-support systems increased the likelihood of ordering appropriate venous thromboembolism prophylaxis and reduced the occurrence of thromboembolic events [9]. A systematic review and meta-analysis performed by Campanella showed that, when properly implemented, EHRs can improve healthcare quality, increase efficiency and guideline adherence, and reduce medication errors and adverse drug events [10]. These studies provide compelling evidence of the quality and safety benefits that EHR adoption can offer in surgical specialties.

One emerging area of research is the use of artificial intelligence techniques, such as natural language processing and machine learning, to support identification or automatically determine measures of quality and safety within EHRs. Data registries and surveillance systems, such as the American College of Surgeons National Surgical Quality Improvement

Program (NSQIP), have been the foundation of quality and safety initiatives in surgery. These approaches are limited in scalability as they require time-consuming and costly manual abstraction and data entry, which can be prone to inconsistencies and errors. Quality criteria, such as the Agency for Healthcare Research and Quality (AHRQ) Patient Safety Indicators (PSIs), utilize diagnostic codes, which are easily collected from EHRs and administrative databases to identify adverse events. However, the quality of medical coding is highly variable, and it is not always possible to determine from a diagnostic code whether the condition was present on admission or acquired during hospitalization [11].

Surgeons have taken several approaches leveraging advance analytics and artificial intelligence to identify quality and safety metrics. Hu and colleagues developed machine learning models that predicted surgical complications including site infections, urinary tract infections, pneumonia, sepsis, and shock, with high specificity, based on structured EHR data [12, 13]. Murff and colleagues used natural language processing to identify surgical complications including acute renal failure requiring dialysis, pulmonary embolism, deep vein thrombosis, sepsis, pneumonia, and myocardial infarction from textual notes and reports in a comprehensive EHR across six Veterans Health Administration medical centers [14]. This system identified most of these complications with significantly higher sensitivity but lower specificity than AHRQ PSIs, which are based on discharge diagnostic codes. Bucher and colleagues developed a surveillance system that analyzed computerized orders entered from days 2 to 30 after a procedure to detect postoperative complications including superficial, deep, and organ-space surgical site infections, urinary tract infections, pneumonia, sepsis, septic shock, deep venous thrombosis requiring treatment, and pulmonary embolus [15]. This approach was able to identify individual complications with a negative predictive value of 98.7–100%, and it performed well for both inpatient and outpatient procedures. This methodology was proposed as an initial screening process to reduce the burden of manual review.

Although these approaches hold some promise in the use of analytics and artificial intelligence to support measurement of quality and safety, there remain barriers to widespread adoption. First, these approaches require comprehensive EHRs with high-quality data. Second, such algorithms may depend on organizational data structures and local documentation conventions, and thus, their performance may not necessarily be able to be replicated at other institutions. Third, the lack of inter-operability of EHRs significantly holds back the transfer of information between health systems, and if that problem were solved, the artificial intelligence burden would be significantly lessened. Fourth, many care providers document using "free text" fields, rather than mapping to coding systems such as ICD-10, CPT, or SNOMED, leading to a lower discovery rate of the information. Finally, algorithm performance varies and may not yet be sufficient to replace manual processes. Nonetheless, these approaches have the potential to augment human abstractors and decrease the burden of manual review.

Improving Surgeon-Patient Communication Using the EHR

Effective communication is critical to the successful delivery of safe, high-quality medical care. Many organizations have used functionalities within or in combination with their EHR to support communication between surgeons and their patients, including solutions for telemedicine and patient portals. Telemedicine or telehealth, defined as the use of information technology to deliver clinical healthcare from a distance [16], been modestly embraced by surgeons and patients. Telemedicine has been shown to be an effective tool for delivering postoperative care, to have high patient and physician satisfaction, and to reduce cost for patients [17]. Recently, telemedicine has experienced a dramatic growth in use as a result of the COVID-19 pandemic. Telemedicine visits have allowed patients to interact with their surgeons while minimizing risks for infection [18]. A recent survey study showed that the public viewed telemedicine as an acceptable substitute for in-person visits and would choose that option over an in-person visit during the pandemic [19]. Nevertheless, a greater number of respondents still preferred in-person interactions for surgical consultation outside the context of the pandemic. The reasons cited were the desire to meet their surgeon in person and to have the surgeon examine them prior to surgery. Although telemedicine may be a robust tool for some aspects of surgical care, it is unlikely to fulfill all the needs of the surgeon-patient relationship.

Patient portals are health-related online applications that allow patients to access their health information and to interact with healthcare organizations. Patient portal adoption increased markedly as a result of the American Recovery and Reinvestment Act of 2009 and the implementation of Meaningful Use. Most EHR solutions offer patient portals, which typically include a secure messaging functionality that enables patients to exchange messages with healthcare providers. Although patient portals were initially developed for primary care and medical specialties, several studies have shown avid adoption by surgical patients and providers [20, 21]. Analyses of portal messaging between surgeons, patients, and their caregivers have shown rich interactions, with most exchanges involving the delivery of medical care, including addressing new or worsening problems, adjusting treatment plans, requesting new consultations, and scheduling testing or therapeutic procedures [22, 23].

There is a growing evidence that use of patient portals through EHRs can enhance the quality and safety of surgical care. In a cohort of patients undergoing elective general surgery procedures, a combination of online surveys and patient portal communications was employed for postoperative follow-up [24]. Most patients were satisfied with this method of online follow-up; such visits took less time, and no complications were missed. In a study of patients undergoing orthopedic surgery procedures, patient portal use was associated with lower no-show rates and increased satisfaction [25]. In urology patients, patient portal users compared with nonusers had decreased rates of postoperative emergency department visits, unscheduled clinic encounters, and surgical complications [26].

Several studies have shown significant racial and socioeconomic disparities in adoption of patient portals in surgical patients [21, 27], highlighting the need to ensuring that such technologies do not exacerbate health inequities in access to and quality of care. A systematic review assessing barriers to portal adoption identified negative attitudes (in both patients and providers), interface challenges, lack of appropriate training, and privacy concerns [28]. The most common solutions included promotion of increased computer and Internet access, targeted marketing toward disadvantaged populations to articulate benefit, and redesign and standardization of portal interfaces.

Summary

EHRs are now widely adopted in surgical practice and offer numerous opportunities for enhancing the quality and safety of surgical practice. To maximally leverage these technologies for quality and safety, comprehensive and widely adopted EHRs with high-quality data are needed. Surgeons should be actively engaged in EHR design, implementation, and maintenance to ensure surgical needs and perspectives are represented. A growing body of evidence suggests that once adopted, use of EHRs and their associated technologies can reduce adverse events, increase guideline adherence, and improve the quality of surgical documentation. Advanced analytics and artificial intelligence techniques are showing promise in the ability to automate or augment manual processes for identifying measures of quality and patient safety in surgery. Communication technologies often delivered through or integrated with EHRs, such as telehealth applications and patient portals, offer attractive alternatives to in-person care. Some evidence suggests that patient portal interactions can enhance satisfaction, decrease urgent or emergent postoperative visits, and improve patient outcomes. Well-trained surgeon informaticians are critical to optimizing the implementation and utilization of EHRs to support quality care and patient safety.

Selected Reading

1. Irizarry T, Barton AJ. A sociotechnical approach to successful electronic health record implementation: five best practices for clinical nurse specialists. Clin Nurse Spec. 2013;27(6):283–5.
2. Aguirre RR, et al. Electronic health record implementation: a review of resources and tools. Cureus. 2019;11(9):e5649.
3. Zhao J, et al. The value of the surgeon informatician. J Surg Res. 2020;252:264–71.
4. Hincker A, et al. Electronic medical record interventions and recurrent perioperative antibiotic administration: a before-and-after study. Can J Anaesth. 2017;64(7):716–23.
5. Austrian JS, et al. The financial and clinical impact of an electronic health record integrated pathway in elective colon surgery. Appl Clin Inform. 2020;11(1):95–103.
6. Fisher JC, et al. A novel approach to leveraging electronic health record data to enhance pediatric surgical quality improvement bundle process compliance. J Pediatr Surg. 2016;51(6):1030–3.
7. Furukawa MF, et al. Electronic health record adoption and rates of in-hospital adverse events. J Patient Saf. 2020;16(2):137–42.
8. Robinson JR, Huth H, Jackson GP. Review of information technology for surgical patient care. J Surg Res. 2016;203(1):121–39.
9. Borab ZM, et al. Use of computerized clinical decision support systems to prevent venous thromboembolism in surgical patients: a systematic review and meta-analysis. JAMA Surg. 2017;152(7):638–45.
10. Campanella P, et al. The impact of electronic health records on healthcare quality: a systematic review and meta-analysis. Eur J Pub Health. 2016;26(1):60–4.
11. Romano PS, et al. Validity of selected AHRQ patient safety indicators based on VA National Surgical Quality Improvement Program data. Health Serv Res. 2009;44(1):182–204.

12. Hu Z, et al. Accelerating chart review using automated methods on electronic health record data for postoperative complications. AMIA Annu Symp Proc. 2016;2016:1822–31.

13. Hu Z, et al. Automated detection of postoperative surgical site infections using supervised methods with electronic health record data. Stud Health Technol Inform. 2015;216:706–10.

14. Murff HJ, et al. Automated identification of postoperative complications within an electronic medical record using natural language processing. JAMA. 2011;306(8):848–55.

15. Bucher BT, et al. Use of computerized provider order entry events for postoperative complication surveillance. JAMA Surg. 2019;154(4):311–8.

16. *Telehealth.* [cited 2021 March 14, 2021]; Available from: https://www.ama-assn.org/topics/telehealth.

17. Huang EY, et al. Telemedicine and telementoring in the surgical specialties: a narrative review. Am J Surg. 2019;218(4):760–6.

18. Contreras CM, et al. Telemedicine: patient-provider clinical engagement during the COVID-19 pandemic and beyond. J Gastrointest Surg. 2020;24(7):1692–7.

19. Sorensen MJ, et al. Telemedicine for surgical consultations - pandemic response or here to stay?: a report of public perceptions. Ann Surg. 2020;272(3):e174–80.

20. Cronin RM, et al. Growth of secure messaging through a patient portal as a form of outpatient interaction across clinical specialties. Appl Clin Inform. 2015;6(2):288–304.

21. Shenson JA, et al. Rapid growth in surgeons' use of secure messaging in a patient portal. Surg Endosc. 2016;30(4):1432–40.

22. Riera KM, et al. Care delivered by pediatric surgical specialties through patient portal messaging. J Surg Res. 2019;234:231–9.

23. Robinson JR, et al. Complexity of medical decision-making in care provided by surgeons through patient portals. J Surg Res. 2017;214:93–101.

24. Kummerow Broman K, et al. Postoperative care using a secure online patient portal: changing the (inter)face of general surgery. J Am Coll Surg. 2015;221(6):1057–66.

25. Varady NH, d'Amonville S, Chen AF. Electronic patient portal use in orthopaedic surgery is associated with disparities, improved satisfaction, and lower no-show rates. J Bone Joint Surg Am. 2020;102(15):1336–43.

26. Kachroo N, et al. Does "MyChart" benefit "my" surgery? A look at the impact of electronic patient portals on patient experience. J Urol. 2020;204(4):760–8.

27. Wedd J, et al. Racial, ethnic, and socioeconomic disparities in web-based patient portal usage among kidney and liver transplant recipients: cross-sectional study. J Med Internet Res. 2019;21(4):e11864.
28. Zhao JY, et al. Barriers, facilitators, and solutions to optimal patient portal and personal health record use: a systematic review of the literature. AMIA Annu Symp Proc. 2017;2017:1913–22.

Chapter 22
Checklists, Surgical Timeout, Briefing, and Debriefing: Safety in the Operating Room

Amelia T. Collings and Dimitrios Stefanidis

It is no surprise that that the magnitude of healthcare permeates the lives of hundreds of millions of Americans every year and the benefits provided are unmeasurable. There were 883.7 million doctors' office visits in 2016 and, in 2019, more than 4.38 billion retail prescriptions were filled [1, 2]. According to the National Quality Forum (NQF), there was a 300% increase in the number of procedures performed in the United States from 1996 to 2006 [3]. In 2010, 51.4 million surgical and nonsurgical procedures were performed [3]. Despite the innumerable benefits our healthcare system provides, it does not do so without considerable risk and even some harm to patients. In 1999, the Institute of Medicine released a landmark paper, reporting nearly 100,000 deaths per year as a result of medical errors [4]. Never before had medical errors been so publicly and comprehensively

---
A. T. Collings (✉) · D. Stefanidis
Department of Surgery, Indiana University School of Medicine, Indianapolis, IN, USA
e-mail: amroge@iu.edu; dimstefa@iu.edu

© The Author(s), under exclusive license to Springer Nature   419
Switzerland AG 2022
J. R. Romanelli et al. (eds.), *The SAGES Manual of Quality, Outcomes and Patient Safety*,
https://doi.org/10.1007/978-3-030-94610-4_22

reported. It stimulated a change in mindset to make medical errors a public health issue and called to fix system-wide errors. Surgery is not exempt from this problem. It is estimated that about 25–50% of all adverse events after surgery are due to medical errors [5, 6].

A number of organizations are focused on improving patient safety in healthcare. The NQF is an organization dedicated to providing Americans with high-quality and safe healthcare. It has developed a list of 28 "Serious Reportable Events (SERs)" that colloquially are known as "Never Events" and aim to prevent devastating iatrogenic injuries (Table 22.1) [7]. These have been deemed reportable, grave in nature, and largely preventable. The NQF's goals are supported by the Centers for Medicare & Medicaid Services (CMS) which has significantly reduced reimbursements for these events in an effort to attract attention to them and promote solutions [8]. Within the NQF's surgical domain, there are three main types of severe, yet preventable, events: wrong site surgery, retained foreign bodies, and the death of an ASA class I patient. The most commonly occurring errors are *wrong site surgery* and *retained foreign bodies*. Wrong site surgery also includes wrong patient and wrong side, in addition to wrong site.

The Joint Commission was created to help organizations increase their safety and reliability, and participating healthcare organizations are required to report certain sentinel events. A sentinel event is defined as an incident that causes death, permanent harm, or severe temporary harm and intervention required to sustain life [9]. These sentinel events then undergo root cause analyses to determine how and why the errors occurred. From the results of root cause analyses, surgical timeouts were created to decrease error occurrence [9]. The Joint Commission defines a surgical timeout as "an immediate pause by the entire surgical team to confirm the correct patient, procedure, and site." [10].

Both retained foreign bodies and wrong site surgeries are considered sentinel events by the Joint Commission. In 2018, the Joint Commission had a total of 112 sentinel events

TABLE 22.1 NQF's serious reportable events

Surgical events

Surgery performed on the wrong body part

Surgery performed on the wrong patient

Wrong surgical procedure performed on a patient

Unintended retention of a foreign object in a patient after surgery or other procedure

Intraoperative or immediately postoperative death in a ASA class I patient

Product or device events

Patient death or serious disability associated with the use of contaminated drugs, devices, or biologics provided by the healthcare facility

Patient death or serious disability associated with the use or function of a device in patient care in which the device is used or functions other than as intended

Patient death or serious disability associated with intravascular air embolism that occurs while being cared for in a healthcare facility

Care management events

Patient death or serious disability associated with a medication error (e.g., errors involving the wrong drug, wrong dose, wrong patient, wrong time, wrong rate, wrong preparation, or wrong route of administration)

Patient death or serious disability associated with a hemolytic reaction due to the administration of ABO/HLA – Incompatible blood or blood products

Maternal death or serious disability associated with labor or delivery in a low-risk pregnancy while being cared for in a healthcare facility

Patient death or serious disability associated with hypoglycemia, the onset of which occurs while the patient is being cared for in a healthcare facility

(continued)

TABLE 22.1 (continued)

Death or serious disability (kernicterus) associated with failure to identify and treat hyperbilirubinemia in neonates

Stage 3 or 4 pressure ulcers acquired after admission to a healthcare facility

Patient death or serious disability due to spinal manipulative therapy

Artificial insemination with the wrong donor sperm or wrong egg

Environmental events

Patient death or serious disability associated with an electric shock while being cared for in a healthcare facility

Any incident in which a line designated for oxygen or other gas to be delivered to a patient contains the wrong gas or is contaminated by toxic substances

Patient death or serious disability associated with a burn incurred from any source while being cared for in a healthcare facility

Patient death or serious disability associated with a fall while being cared for in a healthcare facility

Patient death or serious disability associated with the use of restraints or bedrails while being cared for in a healthcare facility

Criminal events

Any instance of care ordered by or provided by someone impersonating a physician, nurse, pharmacist, or other licensed healthcare provider

Abduction of a patient of any age

Sexual assault on a patient within or on the grounds of a healthcare facility

Death or significant injury of a patient or staff member resulting from a physical assault (i.e., battery) that occurs within or on the grounds of a healthcare facility reported for wrong site surgeries; however, due to underreporting, they estimated that these most likely occur as often as 40–60 times per week across the nation [11,12]. Furthermore, in 2018, there were 131 retained foreign body events reported [11]. These figures, although high, are likely underestimated as oftentimes there is inconsistent reporting due to fear of litigation. In addition, these incidents are not benign in nature. In a 2018 study by Steelman et al., 308 patients with unintentional retained foreign bodies were analyzed, and they found almost 2% of patients had died as a direct result of the foreign body [12]. In addition, almost half of foreign bodies are discovered after the patient is discharged, leading to increased inpatient days, additional procedures, and opportunities for more errors to occur [13].

There are a multitude of factors that increase the risk of these errors occurring. In 2009, after root cause analysis, the Joint Commission identified 29 factors that contributed to wrong site surgeries (Table 22.2) [14]. The top three factors of both wrong site surgery and retained foreign bodies were related to leadership, human factors, and communication [12, 15]. The variables that contribute to these sentinel events are far reaching and diverse; they involve every aspect of the continuum of patient care. Therefore, the solutions need to include every participant involved in patient care and have the perspective of a system-wide approach. Surgical teams work in highly stressful environments. They experience many interruptions, most often from equipment failures, and must multitask while performing complex technical skills [16]. These interruptions increase both the workload and stress of the entire surgical team [17]. This in turn negatively impacts the technical skills of the surgeon [18].

System-wide flaws leading to errors are not a unique problem to the medical field. Other complex, high-risk fields, such as nuclear power and aviation, face similar issues and have implemented checklists to decrease errors from human factors and poor communication [19]. Checklists help remind a team of people of the minimum, routine steps required and can help close the loop in communication and verify that

TABLE 22.2 The Joint Commission's 29 main causes of wrong site surgery

Scheduling

1. Booking documents not verified by office schedulers

2. Schedulers accept verbal requests for surgical bookings instead of written documents

3. Unapproved abbreviations, cross-outs, and illegible handwriting used on booking form

4. Missing consent, history and physical, or surgeon's orders at time of booking

Pre-op holding/holding

5. Primary documents (consent, history and physical, surgeon's booking orders, operating room schedule) missing, inconsistent, or incorrect

6. Paperwork problems identified in pre-op but resolved in a different location

7. Inconsistent use of site marking protocol

8. Someone other than surgeon marks site

9. Surgeon does not mark site in pre-op/holding

10. Site mark made with non-approved surgical site marker

11. Stickers used in lieu of marking the skin

12. Inconsistent site marks used by physicians

13. Inconsistent or absent timeout process for regional blocks

14. Rushing during patient verification

15. Alternate site marking process does not exist or is not used

16. Inadequate patient verification by team

Operating room

17. Lack of intraoperative site verification when multiple procedures performed by the same provider

18. Ineffective hand-off communication or briefing process

TABLE 22.2 (continued)

19. Primary documentation not used to verify patient, procedure, site, and side

20. Site mark(s) removed during prep or covered by surgical draping

21. Distractions and rushing during timeout

22. Timeout process occurs before all staff are ready or before prep and drape occur

23. Timeout performed without full participation

24. Timeouts do not occur when there are multiple procedures performed by multiple providers in a single operative case

Organization culture

25. Senior leadership is not actively engaged

26. Inconsistent organizational focus on patient safety

27. Staff is passive or not empowered to speak up

28. Policy changes made with inadequate or inconsistent staff education

29. Marketplace competition and pressure to increase surgical volume lead to shortcuts and variation in practice

pivotal jobs have been completed. For example, pilots and flight attendants use checklists to verify engine readiness before takeoff. Borrowing from that experience, many different facets of healthcare have begun to adopt checklist tools to prevent devastating errors.

In 2002, the Veterans Affairs National Center for Patient Safety developed a protocol called Ensuring Correct Surgery [20]. This protocol employed a five-step process aimed at reducing operations performed at the incorrect site and on the incorrect patient or performing the incorrect procedure. It starts with confirmation of the correct patient and correct procedure during the consent process. Next, the operative site is marked. Then, the patients themselves state multiple items of identification (i.e., name, date of birth, social security number, etc.). Next, two members of the team confirm the correct imaging is readily available. Lastly, a timeout is performed attesting that the previous steps have been completed and are correct [20].

In 2004, the Joint Commission developed the Universal Protocol in an effort to decrease, if not eliminate completely, wrong site surgeries (Fig. 22.1) [21]. The three main steps of the Universal Protocol are preoperative verification process, marking the operative site, and a timeout immediately before the procedure. Their goal was to encourage communication and thus improve teamwork leading to better outcomes. In 2010, with the results from a root cause analysis on wrong site surgeries (Table 22.2), the Joint Commission expanded upon their Universal Protocol and developed a program called Safe Surgery. In this program, they offer solutions to the most common causes of wrong site surgery in each of the four phases of surgical care (scheduling, pre-op/holding, operating room, organizational culture) [9].

Each year surgical interventions contribute about 13% of the world's total disability-adjusted life years, and, in some developing nations, the mortality rate from general anesthesia can be as high as 1 in 150 [22]. Thus, the World Health Organization (WHO) developed the first globally accepted

Conduct a pre-procedure verificaiton process

Address missing information or discrepancies before starting the procedure.

- Verify the correct procedure, for the correct patient, at the correct site.
- When possible, involve the patient in the verification process.
- Identify the items that must be available for the procedure.
- Use a standardized list to verify the availability of items for the procedure. (It is not necessary to document that the list was used for each patient.) At a minimum, these items include:
  - ☐ relevant documentation
    Examples: history and physical signed consent form, preanesthesia assessment
  - ☐ labeled diagnostic and radiology test results that are properly displayed
    Examples: radiology images and scans, pathology reports, biopsy reports
  - ☐ any required blood products, implants, devices, special equipment
- Match the items that are to be available in the procedure area to the patient.

FIGURE 22.1 The Joint Commission's Universal protocol

Mark the procedure site

At a minimum, mark the site when there is more than one possible location for the procedure and when performing the procedure in a different location could harm the patient.

- For spinal procedures: Mark the general spinal region on the skin. Special intraoperative imaging techniques may be used to locate and mark the exact vertebral level.
- Mark the site before the procedure is performed.
- If possible, involve the patient in the site marking process,
- The site is marked by a licensed independent practitioner who is ultimately accountable forthe procedure and will be present when the procedure is performed.
- In limited circumstances, site marking may be delegated to some medical residents, physician assistants (P.A.), or advanced practice registered nurses (A.P.R.N.).
- Ultimately, the licensed independent practitioner is accountable for the procedure — even when delegating site marking.
- The mark is unambiguous and is used consistently throughout the organization.
- The mark is made at or near the procedure site.
- The mark is sufficiently permanent to be visible after skin preparation and draping.
- Adhesive markers are not the sole means of marking the site.
- For patients who refuse site marking or when it is technically or anatomically impossible or impractical to mark the site (see examples below): Use your organization's written, alternative process to ensure that the correct site is operated on. Examples of situations that involve alternative processes:
  - ☐ mucosal surfaces or perineum
  - ☐ minimal access procedures treating a lateralized internal organ, whether percutaneous or through a natural orifice
  - ☐ teeth
  - ☐ premature infants, for whom the mark may cause a permanent tattoo

FIGURE 22.1 (continued)

Perform a time-out

The procedure is not started until all questions or concerns are resolved.

- Conduct a time-out immediately before starting the invasive procedure or making the incision.
- A designated member of the team starts the time-out.
- The time-out is standardized.
- The time-out involves the immediate members of the procedure team: the individual performing the procedure, anesthesia providers, circulating nurse, operating room technician, and other active participants who will be participating in the procedure from the beginning.
- All relevant members of the procedure team actively communicate during the time-out.
- During the time-out, the team members agree, at a minimum, on the following:
  - ☐ correct patient identity
  - ☐ correct site
  - ☐ procedure to be done
- When the same patient has two or more procedures: Ifthe person performing the procedure changes, another time-out needs to be performed before starting each procedure.
- Document the completion of the time-out. The organization determines the amount and type of documentation.

FIGURE 22.1 (continued)

surgical safety checklist, in an effort to decrease unnecessary surgical deaths and complications across the world in their Safer Surgery Initiative [22]. Their tool is a 19-item checklist involving three phases of care for a surgical patient: before anesthesia, before skin incision, and before the patient leaves the operating room (see Fig. 22.2 for complete details) [23]. Before implementation, the WHO's Surgical Safety Checklist was prospectively studied in a multi-institutional, multinational study that included both developed and developing nations. They showed a significant decrease in complications, but, more importantly, decreased patient mortality rate by almost 50% [24].

Following the advent of these two landmark surgical safety checklists, numerous iterations have been developed and published. For example, in England and Wales, they use a process called "Five Steps to Safer Surgery" (Table 22.3) [25].

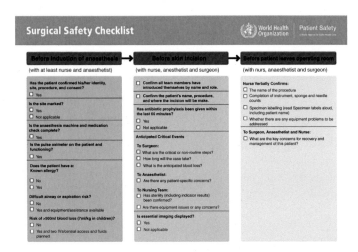

FIGURE 22.2 WHO surgical safety checklist

This checklist includes the concept of briefing and debriefing, in addition to the surgical timeout. A briefing prepares the team for the upcoming operation by verifying that all the necessary equipment and personnel are available and attempt at anticipating potential problems before they arise. A debrief reviews aspects that did not go as anticipated, as discussed in the briefing, and brainstorm solutions for future cases. The concept of debriefing originated in the military. During World War II, S.L.A. Marshall noticed that while recording the experiences of soldiers that they were able to receive social support and ultimately emotional healing through this process [26]. Marshall observed a restored sense of cohesion in the unit and readiness to return to combat [26]. This has since been incorporated throughout all branches of the military in an effort to decrease post-traumatic stress disorder. Briefing also has military roots. They have a specific, predefined formula to communicate critical information in a clear, concise manner [27]. The purpose of both a brief and debrief is to flatten the slope of hierarchy, consequently creating an environment of open communication, free from fear of reprisal.

TABLE 22.3 Five steps to safer surgery

Step	Timing of intervention	What to discuss (summary)	Comments/challenges
1. Briefing	Before list or each patient (if different staff for each patient, e.g., emergency list)	Introduction of team/ individual roles	Local arrangements will determine when the first patient on list is sent for May also include aspects from steps 2 and 3
		List order	
		Concerns relating to staff/equipment/surgery/ anesthesia	Could be an opportunity to discuss anticipated breaks during the list (e.g., lunch)
			May be difficult to get the team together
2. Sign-in	Before induction of anesthesia	Confirm patient/procedure/ consent form	Aspects of step 3 may be done here
		Allergies	Surgical site marking should be checked by the surgeon at this point
		Airway issues	

		Anticipated blood loss
		Machine/medication check
3. Timeout (stop moment)	Before the start of surgery	In practice most of this information is discussed before, so this is used as a final check
	Team member introduction	Surgeons may use this opportunity to check that antibiotic prophylaxis has been administered
	Verbal confirmation of patient information	
	Surgical/anesthetic/nursing issues	
	Surgical site infection bundle	
	Thromboprophylaxis	

(continued)

Table 22.3 (continued)

Step	Timing of intervention	What to discuss (summary)	Comments/challenges
	Imaging available		
4. Sign out	Before staff leave theatre	Confirmation of recording of procedure: Instruments, swabs, and sharp correct	Should include all team members (including surgeons and anesthetists)
		Specimens correctly labelled	
		Equipment issues addressed	
		Postoperative management discussed and handed over	
5. Debriefing	At the end of the list	Evaluate list	Can be difficult to gather people together to do this
		Learn from incidents	Evaluation of the list includes a discussion of what went well
		Remedy problems, e.g., equipment failure	
		Can be used to discuss five-step process	

During the briefing step, every member of the team introduces themselves and their role. Concerns for the day or the individual procedure are discussed, including equipment needs, patient factors, or staffing issues. By taking the time to brief as a team, a feeling of cohesion and equality is nurtured so that every member feels comfortable to speak up if they have concerns. During the debrief stage, the team again convenes to talk about the strengths and weaknesses of the day or of an individual case. They discuss what went wrong and why, in order to prevent that same issue from recurring.

Numerous studies have shown that using a team-based, preoperative checklist can not only decrease communication failures but also decrease complications and even mortality [24, 28, 29]. Lingard et al. prospectively studied a busy Canadian hospital before and after initiating a preoperative briefing session guided by a checklist. Overall the total number of communication failures observed decreased after implementing the briefing session [28]. Furthermore, there was a 64% reduction in communication failures with at least one visible negative consequence [28]. Examples of negative consequences included inefficiency, team tension, resource waste, workaround, delay, patient inconvenience, and procedural error. Likewise, Haynes et al. showed that use of the WHO checklist significantly decreased both complications and mortality in eight different institutions in eight different countries (Canada, India, Jordan, New Zealand, Philippines, United States, Tanzania, and United Kingdom) [24]. This shows that even in a diverse set of cultural and socioeconomic settings, the WHO Surgical Safety Checklist is able to affect real change.

Application of the Universal Protocol is mandatory to receive accreditation by the Joint Commission, which in turn results in reimbursements from CMS [30]. The Accreditation Association for Ambulatory Health Care (AAAHC) certifies ambulatory surgery centers and also mandates the use of surgical timeout safety checklists. This accreditation is linked with CMS reimbursements as well [31]. The American College of Surgeons (ACS) recommends following the

Universal Protocol and the WHO's Safe Surgery Checklist in order to deliver high-quality surgical care [32].

Given that there has been extensive evidence supporting the efficacy of checklists, timeouts, and briefs/debriefs, these practices should be incorporated into every operating room. It is important for surgeons to recognize that the goal of all these approaches is to enhance patient safety by helping the team prepare for and focus on the task at hand, minimize ambiguity, and empower all team members to voice any concerns that arise. Checklists ensure that all important elements of the task have been addressed and none has been omitted and timeouts ensure that the team is focused when checklist and other items are being addressed. Briefings help prepare teams for what to anticipate during task performance and share a common mental model, while debriefs close the loop by reviewing what happened and learning from any deviations from the anticipated and errors that may have occurred to minimize them in subsequent iterations of the same task.

Utilization of checklists permeates multiple other areas of medicine besides the operating room. In critical care, checklists were found to increase confidence in unfamiliar tasks, but required a positive attitude by senior physicians for successful implementation [33]. In emergency medicine, checklists have been shown to increase guideline compliance and improve outcomes in airway management [34]. In addition, checklists have been shown to increase the accuracy in handoff communication [35]. Lastly, checklists are used for more than preventing sentinel events, but in fact improve surgical care in other ways as well. They help increase compliance with antibiotic timing, keep patients normothermic, and decrease blood transfusions [36, 37].

There are challenges to studying the efficacy of surgical checklists and timeouts. Firstly, not only do results depend on initiation and adherence, but murkier elements such as participant attitude and initial culture of the institution influence the results. In addition, wrong site surgeries and retained foreign bodies are not common events and so require the observation of a large number of procedures over time.

Rarely are these studies powered adequately to detect the change they are looking for. On the other hand, those that are powered appropriately must be conducted over such a long time period that their results are confounded by the changes in practice patterns. Several systematic reviews have been done analyzing the effectiveness of surgical checklists and timeouts and the results are mixed. Although some studies observed a decrease in complications and mortality, many saw no change, and even some studies actually reported an increase in complications [38, 39]. It appears that developing nations and high-risk procedures are settings where checklists and timeouts have shown the greatest benefit [38, 39].

Outside of research, even with the best of intentions, there are challenges to implementing surgical safety checklists. Several studies show that implementation and continued use over time requires stakeholder involvement from the beginning [40, 41]. In addition, adherence is dependent on the presence of all critical team members and their attention during the timeout process [41]. With decreasing reimbursements and increasing amounts of paperwork, surgeons are expected to perform more procedures while having less time to do so. Although this time pressure leads to increased errors, like wrong site surgeries and retained foreign bodies, it also makes the surgeon less likely to want to stop for a brief, timeout, and debrief. Emergency operations create another complicating factor in adherence to surgical timeouts. Further, the repetitive, routine nature of the timeout can lead to complacency, leaving the process open to preventable errors. Lastly, execution of a new process requires a new mentality and, subsequently, a change in culture. In order for the brief/debrief to be effective, complete buy-in from all parties involved is needed. It is not enough to tell people they are free to speak up, unless they truly feel safe to do so. This change in culture oftentimes comes from the leadership of the team, which consequently is also one of the top reasons for wrong site surgeries, according to the Joint Commission. If the leadership of the operating room, most commonly the attending surgeon, does not believe in the necessity or the importance of the surgical timeout, then the rest of the team will follow suit.

Each organization must address their specific barriers to implementation and participation before they can expect to change their culture of safety. Making sure that everyone from the team is present and attentive before starting a time-out or briefing is critical. This may mean waiting to drape the patient or keeping the instruments away from the table until the timeout has been completed. In addition, everyone needs to feel that they can speak up, and this means listening and acknowledging, without belittlement, every team member when they speak. As we have discussed, issues with leadership are a major cause of wrong site surgeries and retained foreign bodies, thus with a commitment toward safety from the leadership this is able to change. The rest of the team will follow the example that is set by the primary surgeon.

From an organizational perspective, patient safety has to be critical to the mission, more so than productivity. They should support their staff's efforts to take the dedicated time, unhurried and without distraction, in order to thoroughly complete all the steps of the brief, pre-procedure verification, timeout, and debrief. On average, a surgical timeout takes about 60 sec to complete [42]. Policy should reflect this commitment and they should invest in ample education for staff on the importance and practicality of application. The Association of periOperative Registered Nurses (AORN) has developed, in conjunction with the Joint Commission, a tool kit to help organizations implement the Universal Protocol. It includes an educational component for staff, resources for facilities to create their own policies, reference tools, and patient education materials [43]. AORN has also recommend involving patients and their families when marking the correct site and using a specified, indelible, unequivocal marking of the correct site. AORN's verification checklist before surgery should include the following: verbal communication with the patient, complete medical record review, review of informed consent and all available imaging, direct observation of marked surgical site, and verbal verification with surgical team. Lastly, it is critical that quality control initiatives be in place to monitor protocol compliance [44].

Operating room teams work in high stress, high stakes environments daily, and there are countless distractions on their attention and time. So, even with the utmost attention to detail, human errors including errors in communication occur, and the results can be disabling or even life threatening. Therefore, it is in the best interest of the patients and the members of the team to have systems in place that are reliable, effective, and safe. With a small investment in time and energy, the implementation of surgical timeouts and briefs/debriefs will not only improve the communication within the operating room, but prevent devastating errors causing patients real harm.

References

1. Centers for Disease Control and Prevention. FastStats - Physician Office Visits. Centers for Disease Control and Prevention, 10 Oct 2019. www.cdc.gov/nchs/fastats/physician-visits.htm.
2. Shahbandeh M. Total number of retail prescriptions filled annually in the U.S. 2013–2025. Statista, 28 Aug 2020. www.statista.com/statistics/261303/total-number-of-retail-prescriptions-filled-annually-in-the-us/.
3. Surgery 2015–2017 Final Report. *NQF: Surgery 2015–2017 Final Report*, National Quality Forum, 20 Apr 2017. www.qualityforum.org/Publications/2017/04/Surgery_2015-2017_Final_Report.aspx.
4. Kohn LT, et al. To err is human building a safer health system. Washington D.C., USA: National Academy Press; 2000.
5. Krizek TJ. Surgical error: ethical issues of adverse events. Arch Surg. 2000;135(11):1359. https://doi.org/10.1001/archsurg.135.11.1359.
6. Suliburk JW, et al. Analysis of human performance deficiencies associated with surgical adverse events. JAMA Netw Open. 2019;2(7). https://doi.org/10.1001/jamanetworkopen.2019.8067.
7. Serious Reportable Events in Healthcare–2006 Update. NQF: Serious Reportable Events in Healthcare–2006 Update. National Quality Forum, 2007. www.qualityforum.

org/Publications/2007/03/Serious_Reportable_Events_in_ Healthcare%E2%80%932006_Update.aspx.

8. Fact Sheet ELIMINATING SERIOUS, PREVENTABLE, AND COSTLY MEDICAL ERRORS - NEVER EVENTS. *CMS.gov*, Centers for Medicare and Medicaid, 18 May 2006. www.cms. gov/newsroom/fact-sheets/eliminating-serious-preventable-and- costlymedical-errors-never-events.

9. Safe Surgery. Center for Transforming Healthcare. The Joint Commission. www.centerfortransforming- healthcare.org/improvement-topics/safe-surgery/?_ ga=2.92660317.1584263004.1596126705-525192084.1596126705.

10. Pellegrini C. Time-outs and their role in improving safety and quality in surgery. Bull Am Coll Surg. 2017. https://bulletin.facs. org/2017/06/time-outs-and-their-role-in-improving-safety-and- quality-in-surgery/.

11. Summary Data of Sentinel Events Reviewed by the Joint Commission. The Joint Commission, The Joint Commission, 1 July 2019. www.jointcommission.org/-/media/tjc/documents/ resources/patient-safety-topics/sentinel-event/summary- 2q-2019.pdf.

12. Steelman VM, et al. Unintentionally retained foreign objects: a descriptive study of 308 sentinel events and contributing fac- tors. Jt Comm J Qual Patient Saf. 2019;45(4):249–58. https://doi. org/10.1016/j.jcjq.2018.09.001.

13. Steelman VM, et al. Retained surgical sponges: a descriptive study of 319 occurrences and contributing factors from 2012 to 2017. Patient Saf Surg. 2018;12(1) https://doi.org/10.1186/ s13037-018-0166-0.

14. Joint Commission identifies 29 main causes of wrong-site surgery, offers solutions. Becker's ASC Review, 30 June 2011. www.beckersasc.com/asc-accreditation-and-patient-safety/joint- commission-identifies-29-main-causes-of-wrong-site-surgery- offers-solutions.html.

15. 10 most common causes of wrong-site surgeries, according to the Joint Commission: Incidents involving wrong-patient, wrong-site or wrong-procedure errors were the sixth most common sentinel events reported to the Joint Commission last year. Becker's Hospital Review. www.beckershospitalreview.com/quality/10- most-common-causes-of-wrong-site-surgeries-according-to-the- joint-commission.html.

16. Göras C, et al. Tasks, multitasking and interruptions among the surgical team in an operating room: a prospective obser-

vational study. BMJ Open. 2019;9(5). https://doi.org/10.1136/bmjopen-2018-026410.

17. Bretonnier M, et al. Interruptions in surgery: a comprehensive review. J Surg Res. 2020;247:190–6. https://doi.org/10.1016/j.jss.2019.10.024.

18. Arora S, et al. The impact of stress on surgical performance: a systematic review of the literature. Surgery, 2010;147(3). https://doi.org/10.1016/j.surg.2009.10.007.

19. Systems approach. PSNet, AHRQ, 7 Sept 2017. psnet.ahrq.gov/primer/systems-approach.

20. VA.gov: Veterans Affairs. Ensuring Correct Surgery, 5 Dec 2013. www.patientsafety.va.gov/media/correctsurg.asp.

21. The universal protocol for preventing wrong site, wrong procedure, and wrong person surgery. The Joint Commission, www.jointcommission.org/-/media/tjc/documents/standards/universal-protocol/up_poster1pdf.pdf.

22. Safe Surgery. *World Health Organization*, World Health Organization, 13 June 2017, www.who.int/patientsafety/topics/safe-surgery/en/.

23. "Implementation manual surgical safety checklist." World Alliance for Patient Safety, The World Health Organization, 2008., www.who.int/patientsafety/safesurgery/tools_resources/SSSL_Manual_finalJun08.pdf?ua=1.

24. Haynes AB, et al. A surgical safety checklist to reduce morbidity and mortality in a global population. N Engl J Med. 2009;360(5):491–9. https://doi.org/10.1056/nejmsa0810119.

25. Vickers R. Five steps to safer surgery. Ann R Coll Surg Engl. 2011;93(7):501–3. https://doi.org/10.1308/147870811x599334.

26. Koshes R, et al. Debriefing following combat. In: Jones FD, editor. War psychiatry. Office of the Surgeon General, United States Army; 1995. p. 271–90.

27. United States, Congress, Marine Corps Training Command. Military briefing W3S0005 student handout, United States Marine Corps, pp. 1–14.

28. Lingard L. Evaluation of a preoperative checklist and team briefing among surgeons, nurses, and anesthesiologists to reduce failures in communication. Arch Surg. 2008;143(1):12. https://doi.org/10.1001/archsurg.2007.21.

29. Mazzocco K, et al. Surgical team behaviors and patient outcomes. Am J Surg. 2009;197(5):678–85. https://doi.org/10.1016/j.amjsurg.2008.03.002.

30. State Recognition. The Joint Commission, 2020. www.jointcommission.org/accreditation-and-certification/state-recognition/.
31. Ambulatory Surgery Centers (ASCs). AAAHC, 2020. www.aaahc.org/accreditation/ambulatory-surgery-centers-ascs/.
32. American College of Surgeons (ACS) Committee on Perioperative Care. Revised statement on safe surgery checklists, and ensuring correct patient, correct site, and correct procedure surgery. American College of Surgeons. 2016. www.facs.org/about-acs/statements/93-surgery-checklists.
33. Thomassen Ø, et al. Checklists in the operating room: help or hurdle? A qualitative study on health workers' experiences. BMC Health Serv Res. 2010;10(1). https://doi.org/10.1186/1472-6963-10-342.
34. Chen C, et al. Use and implementation of standard operating procedures and checklists in prehospital emergency medicine: a literature review. Am J Emerg Med. 2016;34(12):2432–9. https://doi.org/10.1016/j.ajem.2016.09.057.
35. Jullia M, et al. Training in intraoperative handover and display of a checklist improve communication during transfer of care. Eur J Anaesthesiol. 2017;34(7):471–6. https://doi.org/10.1097/eja.0000000000000636.
36. Haugen AS, et al. Causal analysis of World Health Organization's surgical safety checklist implementation quality and impact on care processes and patient outcomes. Ann Surg. 2019;269(2):283–90. https://doi.org/10.1097/sla.0000000000002584.
37. White MC, et al. Sustainability of using the WHO surgical safety checklist: a mixed-methods longitudinal evaluation following a nationwide blended educational implementation strategy in Madagascar. BMJ Glob Health. 2018;3(6). https://doi.org/10.1136/bmjgh-2018-001104.
38. De Jager E, et al. Postoperative adverse events inconsistently improved by the World Health Organization surgical safety checklist: a systematic literature review of 25 studies. World J Surg. 2016;40(8):1842–58. https://doi.org/10.1007/s00268-016-3519-9.
39. Lagoo J, et al. Effectiveness and meaningful use of paediatric surgical safety checklists and their implementation strategies: a systematic review with narrative synthesis. BMJ Open. 2017;7(10). https://doi.org/10.1136/bmjopen-2017-016298.
40. Van Schoten SM, et al. Compliance with a time-out procedure intended to prevent wrong surgery in hospitals: results of a National Patient Safety Programme in the Netherlands. BMJ Open. 2014;4(7). https://doi.org/10.1136/bmjopen-2014-005075.

41. Schwendimann R, et al. Adherence to the WHO surgical safety checklist: an observational study in a Swiss Academic Center. Patient Saf Surg. 2019;13(1). https://doi.org/10.1186/s13037-019-0194-4.
42. Russ S, et al. Measuring variation in use of the WHO surgical safety checklist in the operating room: a multicenter prospective cross-sectional study. J Am Coll Surg. 2015;220(1). https://doi.org/10.1016/j.jamcollsurg.2014.09.021.
43. Mulloy D. Wrong-site surgery: a preventable medical error. In: Hughes R, editor. Patient safety and quality: an evidence-based handbook for nurses. Agency for Healthcare Research and Quality, U.S. Dept. of Health and Human Services; 2008.
44. AORN Develops Correct Site Surgery Kit. Imaging Technology News, 4 June 2007. www.itnonline.com/content/aorn-develops-correct-site-surgery-kit.

Chapter 23
Creating Effective Communication and Teamwork for Patient Safety

Pascal Fuchshuber and William Greif

Effective Communication Within a Culture for Patient Safety

> Healthcare culture does not support high performing teamwork (…and culture eats strategy for lunch) (IHI)

Patient safety culture exists within a conducive set of behavioral norms. Teamwork and effective communication are part of a multidimensional framework that determines safety culture and ultimately the quality of care (Figs. 23.1 and 23.2). Good teamwork and effective communication rely on mutual respect, problem solving, and sharing of ideas. Without these

P. Fuchshuber (✉)
Sutter East Bay Medical Group, UCSF-East Bay,
Oakland, CA, USA

W. Greif
The Permanente Medical Group, Kaiser Walnut Creek Medical Center, Walnut Creek, CA, USA
e-mail: William.Greif@kp.org

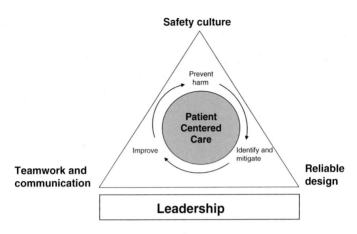

FIGURE 23.1   Delivering safe care – Institute for Healthcare Improvement model (IHI Boston Patient Safety Officers Curriculum, 2010)

The top 5 most commonly identified contributing factors of preventable adverse outcomes

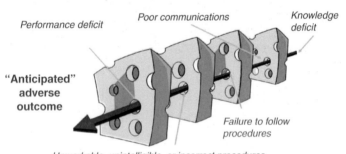

FIGURE 23.2   Effective communication is one of the five basic tools to prevent patient harm. (Source – 2009 SERCIT report on Care and Treatment (Emily Sandelin, CO; Mark Littlewood, Permanente Federation; Doug Bonacum, Dept Care and Service Quality))

essential elements, care cannot be delivered in a safe and reliable way. Unfortunately, this dynamic is far from being the norm in today's healthcare environment. Many healthcare providers – especially physicians – lack deep understanding of good communication skills and ignore opportunity to improve when they fall short. Today, many members of healthcare teams will admit that their ability to communicate is hindered and that they would be hesitant to point out mistakes made by their leaders (again in particular physicians) even though they judge good teamwork by their ability to speak up. Conversely, physicians see good teamwork and communication as the ability and effectiveness to tell others what to do and get it done.

This chapter describes how to overcome these barriers and use the tools of effective communication as the basis for delivery of safe patient care. Failed communication is the most common reason for harm to the recipient of healthcare. In the context of a clinical setting, effective communication is the accurate transfer of information between two or more providers. Communication fails when it is incomplete, ineffective, or inappropriate. The result is patient harm, i.e., substandard care because of missing and inadequate information. The importance of understanding why this happens and what is the context of communication within healthcare organizations cannot be overemphasized.

The primary root causes of failed communications are (1) poor handoffs, i.e., the failure to read back and confirm the information given, (2) the inability to share information due to fear of authority and retaliation, and (3) the assumption that outcome and safety of care is as expected and does not need to be checked.

The most important foundation of effective communication is one that (1) fosters an environment that promotes consistent high-quality care, (2) is free of retaliation and blame, (3) encourages learning from mistakes, and (4) supports interactions between patients, families, and providers within a safe, satisfying, and rewarding workplace.

There are many reasons why these are difficult to achieve within a healthcare organization. Briefly, some of the fundamental and pervasive issues are as follows:

(a) *Teamwork* – Clinical medicine is a very complex environment with quickly changing parameters, unpredictability, incomplete data, and frequent task interruptions. Building on teamwork does largely mitigate the negative impact of these circumstances, thus the strong impetus to build a team approach to patient safety and care delivery.

(b) *Leadership* – Failure of leadership to recognize the importance and prioritize the implementation of effective communication and teamwork.

(c) *Training* – Failure to create and train providers to form teams that can effectively interact and are accountable for maintaining effective communication skills.

(d) *Culture* – Creating "buy-in" and the organizational value for team approaches over individual expert-thinking, particularly among healthcare providers steeped in autonomy and lacking effective leadership training.

(e) *Hierarchy/psychological safety* – Psychological safety is a belief that one will not be punished or humiliated for speaking up with ideas, questions, concerns, or mistakes. Hierarchical barriers are inherent to healthcare systems based on vertical authority and prevent people from "speaking-up" when a decision is questionable, or a problem arises. Effective leadership by a surgeon should emphasize "flat hierarchy" by (1) using a person's name, (2) sharing the plan of action, (3) inviting other team members to participate in the communication, and (4) asking people directly to share questions or concerns.

Psychological safety matters most in systems with a rapidly changing knowledge base, a high need for collaboration, and a short decision time – classic attributes of a modern healthcare organization.

(f) *Lack of structure* – Absence of processes that include a structured "handoff" template to ensure completeness of information, maintain respect for all participants, and ensure engagement in effective communication.

(g) *Abusive and disrespectful behavior* – Failure to create a culture of universal mutual respect leads to increased risk as recognized in the Joint Commission "Sentinel Event Alert" [1]: "Intimidating and disruptive behavior can foster medical errors, contribute to poor patient satisfaction and to preventable adverse outcomes, increase the cost of care, and cause qualified clinicians, administrators, and managers to seek new positions in more professional environments." For example, if a surgeon loses his or her temper in the OR and treats the team with disrespect, leadership must intervene and ensure psychological safety for the members of the team. This is best done by timely intervention and demonstrating that disrespectful behavior is not tolerated within the organization. The CEO, Chief Medical Officer, or Patient Safety Officer is responsible for reinforcing desired behavior with disregard to the vertical hierarchy of the team. For example, a surgeon behaving rudely and disrespectful in the OR is required to apologize to the team and nursing staff as soon as possible. This "culture" requires the leadership to adhere to fundamental common and nonnegotiable principles of interpersonal communication and behavior made transparent and clear to all members of the healthcare team.

(h) *Setting the tone* – Negative Example: *A surgeon runs into the OR loudly announcing that he has a meeting he cannot miss in 3 hours and a whole lot of cases to do. "Get going!"* Setting the stage and tone occurs within a few seconds from the beginning of a verbal communication and has a profound effect on the effectiveness of communication. It is an important, trainable leadership skill for the surgeon [2]. Ideally, the surgeon as a leader tries to create a positive tone immediately by greeting each person by name and setting the stage by communicating that the common value is the care of the patient, the team effort, and respectful, open collaboration. Nonnegotiable mutual respect in every interaction every day and accessibility, humility, and determination to get things done right are key elements of a successful surgeon team leader.

Structured Communication, Handoffs, and SBAR – The Tools of the Trade

In order to assure effective communication in situations where specific and complex information must be exchanged and acted upon in a timely manner, structured communication techniques become essential tools. Below is a brief list of such structured communication tools with a description of their definition and use. Some of these tools are described in more detail in other chapters of this manual:

(a) *Briefings* – concise exchange of information essential to operational effectiveness involving others by (1) asking for their input, (2) using first names to encourage familiarity and lower barriers to speak up, and (3) making eye contact and facing the other person to reinforce their contribution and value. Briefings are most effective in procedural areas (OR, ICU, ambulatory care, etc.). It may be difficult to gain "buy-in" for briefings in the OR, particularly from surgeons inherently adverse to interference with what they perceive as their "realm." Getting physician support for briefings may be facilitated by team-training exercises in the OR, by showing the particular provider how briefings will increase the likelihood for an effective day in the OR (correct equipment, more engagement by other team members, faster turnaround) and greater patient safety by ensuring correct side surgery and consequently lower malpractice risk.

(b) *Debriefings* –should occur at the end of procedures to allow learnings from what happened during the process and set the stage for the next procedure. Briefings and debriefings depend on each other and both should be as specific and detailed as possible. Typical debriefing questions:
   - What was the procedure? Wound classification?
   - Are specimens correct?
   - What went well?
   - What could have gone better?

- What are the next steps for this patient?
- What did we learn?
- How did we document (specimen, wound class, etc.)?
- What do we need for the next case?

(c) *Assertive Language* – this refers to a communication for members of the team to "speak up" and to state the information with appropriate persistence until there is resolution. The lack of assertive language skills may lead to patient harm, particularly when it is paired with the pervasive vertical authority encountered in healthcare organizations. It is known that up to 40% of nurses report hesitance to speak up about mistakes in Safety Attitude Questionnaires. Because of these barriers, information is typically communicated in an unclear, oblique, and indirect manner with a "hint of hope that what I said must have been heard" and "something didn't seem right, but a proposed action did not occur." Effective assertion does not mean aggressive and confrontational communication but rather a polite form of making sure one is heard in a timely and clear manner. Training and practice among team members in assertive language can be very helpful. A typical checklist to help understand the meaning and technique of assertive language is shown here:

- Get the attention of the other(s).
- Use names.
- Use eye contact.
- Face the other person.
- State the problem concisely.
- State your concern.
- Propose an action.
- Recheck if concern and action were understood.
- Reassert if necessary.
- Expect a decision that is understood by all members of the team.
- Escalate if no result.

Assertive communication skills can be trained and are very helpful in creating a culture of safety and effective communication.

(d) *Critical Language* – briefly, this is the ability to use language during a stressful and dangerous situation to avert patient harm. Again, this will work best if a flattened hierarchy has already been established. Typical sentences to illustrate this type of language are "I am concerned/scared," "may I have a little clarity," or "let's hold for a minute and make sure we are all on the same page." Ultimately, this may translate into "excuse me, doctor, but I need some clarity about which breast you are going to do the mastectomy..." after the fourth or fifth breast case of the day One can easily imagine the potential benefit of critical language used by a nurse when a tired surgeon is about to operate on the wrong side, when a flattened hierarchy has been established.

(e) *Common Language* – this communication tool describes a specific language around a specific event of clinical setting that is adopted and understood by all team members. It creates a "benchmark" of how to communicate around certain events. A good example is the standardized terminology and language describing fetal heart rates by the National Institute of Child Health and Human Development (NICHD). This assures good understanding by all providers in the clinical setting of the fetal heart tracing [3]. An agreed upon language around checklists and timeout procedures is another example of the use of common language to assure reliable and effective communication.

(f) *Closed Communication Loops* – it consists of the use of read-back, whereby the recipient repeats back the concisely stated information by the sender and the sender in turn acknowledges the read-back. Corrections are made as necessary to the communicated content. This type of communication is mandatory when critical content cannot be lost, for example, when communicating in a dangerous and complex environment such as a nuclear submarine. Think of clinical settings as equivalent to that of a submarine; for example, use read-back when confirming the sponge count, giving telephone orders for medications, or confirming consent and operative site. This is recognized by the Joint Commission which requires a read-back process for verbal or telephone orders as defined in the National Patient Safety Goals [2].

(g) *Callouts* – surgeons commonly use this communication technique in the OR to clearly indicate the timeline of the procedure in progress. Callouts should be communicated in clearly and loudly spoken simple phrases so that all team members can understand and hear. Good examples are "we are closing," "we are having difficulty and will convert to open procedure in 5 minutes," "we will be closing in 15 minutes," "start the sponge count," and "I will need the ultrasound machine in 30 minutes."

(h) *Handoffs* – "Gentlemen, it is better to have died as a small boy than to fumble this football" – John Heisman (1869–1936). Handoffs or the transfer of information from one team to another is an essential part of effective communication. This occurs innumerable times each day in hospitals, offices, and laboratories. These critical moments of transition of care are prone to error and can be dangerous as each handoff carries the potential for information loss or misinterpretation. Errors at the time of transition of care are among the most common and consequential errors in healthcare. Handoffs occur between different providers (change of shift in the ER, change of call provider on the floor) or can involve the physical location change of a patient (transfer from floor to ICU, from hospital to skilled nursing facility, discharge home). The key for a successful handoff is accuracy and completeness, preferably through standard protocols. Common aspects of a good handoff are interaction, timeliness, appropriate information content, review of relevant data, and lack of interruptions. To achieve that goal, it is helpful to designate specific times and locations for handoffs to minimize distraction, cover all possible scenarios, and use structured language and checklists. Within the National Patient Safety Goals, the Joint Commission requires a structured process for patient handoffs. Table 23.1 depicts a simple mnemonic for a safe and effective handoff [4].

TABLE 23.1 Mnemonic for safe and effective handoffs: "ANTICipate"

*A*dministrative:	Name and location of patient
*N*ew information:	Update of clinical situation, brief H+P, problem list, meds, current status, significant events
*T*asks:	To-do list (use "if/then" statements)
*I*llness:	Assessment of the severity of current illness
Contingency plan(s):	Prepare cross coverage for best way to manage based on what did and did not work in the past

Modified from [4]

(i) *SBAR (Situation, Background, Assessment, Recommendation)* – SBAR is a communication technique using a standardized template similar to the SOAP model (subjective/objective/assessment/plan) as shown in Table 23.2. It can be used in verbal and written communications to set the expectations within a dialogue. Its structure assures that relevant and critical informational content is communicated every time a patient or an issue is discussed. It forces the communicators to acknowledge the goals of all involved parties – as they may diverge. For example, physicians tend to focus on problem solving ("what do I need to do" – "in a nutshell, this is the problem"), while nurses are trained to be narrative and descriptive. They may need to understand the background and more specific aspects of the problem. Similarly, when used in a performance improvement project, written communication by SBAR will concisely communicate the fundamental framework and context of a project and describe its goal and how to achieve it (Table 23.2). To be effective and enhance predictability of the communication, SBARs need to be crisp and to the point and promote critical thinking.

TABLE 23.2 SBAR – Situation, Background, Assessment, Recommendation. A situational briefing tool. Three examples in clinical practice

S – SITUATION: WHAT IS THIS ABOUT? ESTABLISH THE TOPIC OF THE COMMUNICATION (PUNCH LINE)

B – BACKGROUND: WHAT INFORMATION IS NEEDED; WHY ARE WE TALKING ABOUT THIS? (CONTEXT)

A – ASSESSMENT: DESCRIBE AND STATE THE PROBLEM/SITUATION (PATIENT STATUS, PROBLEM)

R – RECOMMENDATION: WHAT SHOULD WE DO? WHEN ARE WE DOING IT (CLARIFY ACTION)?

KAISER PERMANENTE, SBAR (SITUATION, BACKGROUND, ASSESSMENT, RECOMMENDATION) TOOL, 2002

SBAR – a technique for communicating critical information that requires immediate attention and action concerning a patient's condition

Situation – What is going on with the patient? "I am calling about Mrs. Joseph in room 251. Chief complaint is shortness of breath of new onset."

Background – What is the clinical background or context? "Patient is a 62-year-old female post-op day 1 from abdominal surgery. No prior history of cardiac or lung disease."

Assessment – What do I think the problem is? "Breath sounds are decreased on the right side with acknowledgment of pain. Would like to rule out pneumothorax."

Recommendation – What would I do to correct it? "I feel strongly the patient should be assessed now. Are you available to come in?"

Source: Institute for Healthcare Improvement. Guidelines for communicating with physicians using the SBAR process. http://www.ihi.org/IHI/Topics/PatientSafety/SafetyGeneral/Tools/SBARTechniqueforCommunicationASituationalBriefingModel.htm. Accessed Sept 14, 2020

Clinical examples for SBAR:

S – State patient name and call out problem: "Doctor, I am worried about Ms. Flagherty's wound. I think it is infected."

B – State the pertinent medical history and treatment to date: "She is diabetic and had a colon resection 2 days ago."

A – What is your assessment and what is the clinical picture: "I am concerned because her wound is red and she had a high temperature and chills last night."

(continued)

TABLE 23.2 (continued)

R – State what you would like to see done: "I think she needs her wound to be opened. I need you to come and see her."

S – "Jim, I know you are getting ready to wake up the patient, but the instrument count is wrong."

B – "We looked and counted two times, but it is still incorrect. We need to find the missing instrument."

A – "The count is incorrect; thus, we need an X-ray."

R – "Don't wake the patient up until we have done the X-ray and the radiologist has seen it. Let's get the film now."

Performance improvement example for SBAR:

S – Finding the standard for surgical prep solution to reduce surgical site infections.

B – We do not have a standard for adult surgical skin prep solutions. Evidence suggest solutions A and B are superior than Y and Z.

A – The most common prep solution we use is Y and Z. Infection rate is measurably less when using prep solutions A and B.

R – Use of prep solutions A and B for all adult skin prep. Eliminate solutions Y and Z from OR and procedure rooms. Exceptions listed.

In addition to the above list of communication tools, organizations may want to use communication structures such as *multidisciplinary rounds* and *red rules*.

Multidisciplinary rounds assemble all members of the care team for walk rounds on each patient. Teams are encouraged to use structured communication tools such as SBAR and briefings to enhance their ability to effectively speak to each other about the current care issues. The success of such multidisciplinary rounds depends largely on the ability of the leadership to create a culture of safety and flattened hierarchy that gives every team member the confidence to speak up. Further, such tools can effectively allow the healthcare team to present a unified plan of care to the patients, who are often confused and frustrated by multidisciplinary failures in communication.

Red rules are adopted from the nuclear power industry to provide nonnegotiable rules when necessary. In a healthcare environment, these might be "always do a time-out," "always check sponge count before closing," "always wash hands before and after entering a patient's room". These hard rules need to have the "buy-in" of everybody, should be nonambiguous, and carry immediate consequences for violating them. Because of this stringent normative setting, the number of red rules within an organization should be limited.

Structured communications, handoffs, and SBARs are part of effective teamwork and communication skills that are not inherent to the nature of healthcare providers. They require specific training and practice that should be provided by any healthcare organizations striving for best outcomes in patient care and safety. Specific teamwork training sessions should include all members of a care team and be led by a trained professional (e.g., Institute of Health Improvement-trained Patient Safety Officer). Key elements of these training sessions are realistic scenarios to provide education on team behavior, communication strategies, and safe culture. Essential attributes of a team include nonnegotiable mutual respect, inclusiveness of all concerns and acknowledgment of failure, thrive for excellence, conflict resolution, and use of structured communication tools. Assessment of effective communication provides critical feedback, and observation of team climate, behavior, and work is essential to continued improvement (see Chap. 26 on Culture of Safety and 28 on Team Training).

Rapid Response Team

The purpose of a rapid response team (RRT) is to assemble a team of experts around the bedside of a patient within minutes anytime there is a concern because:

- A staff member is worried
- There is an acute change in vital signs such as change in systolic blood pressure (<90), heart rate (<40 >130), and respiratory rate (<8 >30)

- There is an acute change in oxygen saturation <90%
- There is a change in mental status
- There is drop in Urine Output to <50 mL in 4 hours

The team consists typically of a hospitalist or intensivist, an ICU nurse, and a respiratory therapist. The team can be called upon by anyone involved in the patient's care including clinicians, nurses, patients, and family members, whenever the patient meets certain criteria posted throughout the hospital.

The role of the RRT is to:

- Assess the health status of the patient
- Stabilize the patient
- Communicate with all involved healthcare providers and nurses
- To make sure the primary attending is notified
- Provide support and expertise for the staff caring for the patient
- Assist with transfer to a higher level of care when necessary

Good RRTs are allotted time by their organization to make rounds on all patients assigned to them so potential problems and harm can be anticipated and acted upon. It helps foster a good relationship between floor staff and the RRT. Use of the RRT should be encouraged. Essentially, there is no "bad" reason to call on the RRT, and the willingness of the team to help in any situation should never be called into question. The characteristic of a good RRT is a positive attitude: always ask, "how can I help?" with a smile! This is increasingly important as nursing shortages, inexperienced staff, and the higher acuity of inpatients in hospitals today have created the need for rapid availability of care expertise at the bedside of a deteriorating patient. By creating an RRT, organizations can provide patients the care they need when they need it [5].

Good Teamwork Through Collaboration

A key strategy to achieve patient safety is to take advantage of the complimentary roles of the providers within the healthcare team. Forming a collaborative approach and formulating goals that include the diverse responsibilities and problem-solving abilities of each healthcare team member accomplishes several important objectives [6]:

1. Increase awareness of each other, thereby strengthening the team's efficiency and impact.
2. Make siloed knowledge and skills available to everybody on the team.
3. Improve the final decision-making through integration of the inherent team diversity.

Ultimately, collaboration adds another pillar besides trust and respect to the effectiveness of teamwork. In healthcare, this is equivalent to an interdisciplinary approach to the problem of patient safety. Interdisciplinary should not be confused with multidisciplinary. Again, the former is used to integrate diverse approaches and cultures within the team for the betterment, whereas the latter subdivides the team in separate areas of responsibility and task assignment.

From a patient perspective, the communication with a team that has integrated through collaboration is much easier and effective. Likewise, a collaborative team will excel at formulating an individual care approach for each patient that considers all facets of safety and optimization.

In order to achieve good collaboration, all team members should be made aware of the many barriers to interdisciplinary communication. The most important are (1) understanding personal expectations and principles and (2) acknowledging hierarchical structures; (3) ethnic and generational differences; (4) gender, language, and professional and status differences; (5) fears regarding loss of autonomy, identity, and situational safety; and (6) hidden biases due to differences in payment and rewards.

Good teamwork communication through collaboration is characterized by open communication in a tolerant, nonpunitive environment. Each team member needs to be assigned direction and roles that are clear, well defined, and known to all others. When a fair balance of assignments and shared responsibility is established, respect and mutual support come easy. Hierarchy within the team must be outlined clearly and understood by everyone. Regular feedback and audits should be implemented and discussed regularly. Appropriate access to resources should be verified and assured [7–9].

One of the earliest and most influential realizations that effective team management is the basis for safety and communication is the development of the Crew Resource Management (CRM) safety training in aviation in 1979 [10]. In a landmark study by Sexton et al., the leanings of this program were studied on and applied to operating room teams [11]. Out of this came the VA Palo Alto Health Care System and Stanford-led Anesthesia Crisis Resource Management (ACRM) model and adoption of CRM by the Kaiser Permanente Medical Group [12, 13]. Many other hospital systems have since adopted and modified CRM to their specific system and studied outcomes. In summary, the adoption of the CRM model to healthcare has led to the development and design of blame-free, nonpunitive approaches to safety processes and procedures. Debriefing of all safety events and extracting improvement strategies from near misses and never-events has become standard to good healthcare safety practice. Ongoing risk identification, compliance training, redundant and standardized checklists, and implementation of prevention programs are now common goals of any healthcare system trying to achieve effective communication for patient safety.

References

1. Joint Commission Sentinel Event Alert 40, 9 July 2008. http://www.jointcommission.org/sentinelevents/sentineleventsalert/sea_40.htm.
2. Mazzocco K, Petitti DB, Fong KT, et al. Surgical team behaviors and patient outcomes. Am J Surg. 2009;197(5):678–85.
3. Fox M, Kilpatrick S, King T, et al. Fetal heart rate monitoring: interpretation and collaborative management. J Midwifery Womens Health. 2000;45(6):498–507.
4. Vidyarthi AR. Triple handoff. AHRQ WebM&M (ersial online), September 2006. Available at: http://www.webmm.ahrq.gov/case/aspx?caseID=134.
5. Joint Commission Resources. Best practices in medical emergency teams. Oakbrook Terrace: The Joint Commission; 2006.
6. O'Daniel M, Rosenstein AH. Chapter 3: Professional communication and team collaboration. In: Hughes RG, editor. Patient safety and quality: an evidence-based handbook for nurses. Rockville: Agency for Healthcare Research and Quality (US); 2008.
7. Baldwin DC. The role of interdisciplinary education and teamwork in primary care and health care reform. Rockville: Bureau of Health Professions, Health Resources and Services Administration; 1994. Order No 92–1009.
8. Hackman JR, editor. Groups that work (and those that don't): creating conditions for effective teamwork. San Francisco: Jossey-Bass; 1990.
9. Bernard M, Connelly R, Kuder LC, et al. Interdisciplinary education. In: Klein S, editor. A national agenda for geriatric education: white papers. Rockville: Bureau of Health Professions Health Resources and Services Administration; 1995. p. 57–80.
10. Cooper GE, White MD, Lauber JK. Resource management on the flight deck: proceedings of a NASA/industry workshop, NASA Conference Publication No. CP-2120. Moffett Field: NASA-Ames Research Center; 1980.
11. Sexton JB, Thomas EJ, Helmreich RL. Error, stress, and teamwork in medicine and aviation: cross sectional surveys. BMJ. 2000;320:745–9.

12. Howard SK, Gab DM, Fish KJ, et al. Anesthesia crisis resource management training: teaching anesthesiologists to handle critical incidents. Aviat Space Environ Med. 1992;63:763–70.
13. Leonard M, Graham S, Bonucom D. The human factor: the critical importance of effective teamwork and communication in providing safe care. Qual Saf Health Care. 2004;13(Suppl 1):185–90.

Selected Reading

Edmondson AC. Learning from failure in health care: frequent opportunities, pervasive barriers. Qual Saf Health Care. 2004;13(Suppl II):ii3–9. https://doi.org/10.1136/qshc.2003.009597.

Frankel A, Leonard M, Simmonds T, Haraden C, Vega B. The essential guide for patient safety officers. Institute for Healthcare Improvement, Joint Commission Resources; 2009.

Haig KM, Sutton S, Whittington J. SBAR: a shared mental model for improving communication between clinicians. Jt Comm J Qual Patient Saf. 2006 Mar;32(3):167–75.

Leape L, Berwick D, Clancy C, et al. Transforming healthcare: a safety imperative. Qual Saf Health Care. 2009;18(6):424–8.

Makary MA, Sexton JB, Freischlag JA, et al. Operating room teamwork among physicians and nurses: teamwork in the eye of the beholder. J Am Coll Surg. 2006;202:746–52.

Nundy S, Mukherjee A, Sexton JB, et al. Impact of preoperative briefings on operating room delays: a preliminary report. Arch Surg. 2008;143(11):1068–72.

Yates GR, Hochman RF, Sayles SM, et al. Sentara Norfolk General Hospital: accelerating improvement by focusing on building a culture of safety. Jt Comm J Qual Saf. 2004;30(10):534–42.

Chapter 24
Energy Safety in the Operating Room

Timothy Fokken and Sharon Bachman

Introduction

The use of energy in surgery has become an indispensable tool over the past century. As new technologies become available to the surgeon, so should the understanding of the risks those technologies impose. From inducing unintended defibrillation to morbid burns and perforation of a hollow viscus, the use of energy in surgery carries the burden of life-threatening injury despite the obvious benefits. The ethical onus is on the developer and operator of these devices to mitigate risk to the patient. Unfortunately, the preponderance of both anecdotal and objective evidence indicates that there is a perpetual gap between technological advancement and user understanding of surgical technology. Within this gap lies unintended injury to the patient. A striking demonstration of this educational lacuna was documented in a study conducted by the Society of American Gastrointestinal and Endoscopic Surgeon (SAGES). Recognizing a lack of standardized education regarding surgical energy, a curriculum on

T. Fokken · S. Bachman (✉)
Department of Surgery, Inova Fairfax Medical Campus,
Falls Church, VA, USA
e-mail: Sharon.Bachman@inova.org

© The Author(s), under exclusive license to Springer Nature   461
Switzerland AG 2022
J. R. Romanelli et al. (eds.), *The SAGES Manual of Quality,
Outcomes and Patient Safety*,
https://doi.org/10.1007/978-3-030-94610-4_24

the Fundamental Use of Surgical Energy (FUSE) was developed by subject-matter experts and initially presented as a postgraduate course. In 2011, the course's 11-question pretest was administered to 48 surgeons from SAGES leadership to assess their baseline knowledge of surgical energy and safety group; the median score among this experienced cohort was 59% [1]. This data was presented at the national SAGES conference in 2012 and served as a call to arms against the technology and safety knowledge gap, and is the rationale for the FUSE curriculum.

Energy is used by all surgeons, across all disciplines. This chapter aims to provide the proceduralist with essential principles to safe energy use in terms of modalities, unseen energy dispersal, fire safety, and prevention. Finally, we will outline the FUSE curriculum that serves as a standard primer for electrosurgical principles and safety.

Surgical Energy

Cautery

In the early days of surgery (possibly as far back as 3000 B.C [2].), thermal cautery was the primary form of surgical energy. Cautery is defined as the passive transfer of heat from the instrument to the tissue. Before electricity, cauterization was performed with the use of fire-heated metal placed in direct contact with a wound or lesion. In the modern surgical lexicon, the term "electrocautery" is used often and incorrectly. Electrocautery uses direct current and generates resistance that heats the instrument and then the tissue via direct application of the device tip. Today, this is mainly limited to battery-powered disposable devices that no longer have a role in the operating room (but can be found in most emergency departments). The term "electrosurgery" is more accurate to describe the use of hemostatic instruments in today's operating rooms, which are powered by rapid alternating current and will be discussed below.

Monopolar

The most common form of electrosurgery used in the modern operating room (although by definition, all electrosurgery requires two electrodes) is what surgeons refer to as monopolar radiofrequency energy. The ancestor of modern devices was developed by scientist Dr. William Bovie, and first used clinically by Dr. Harvey Cushing in 1926 [3], and its progeny devices are known by the Bovie eponym in operating rooms around the world. The true name of the device in total is the "electrosurgical unit," or ESU, and entails a generator that augments a standard 60 Hz electrical alternating current to 500,000 Hz radiofrequency current and directs it to the hand-held surgical instrument ("Bovie," the active electrode) via an insulated cord and allows for energy parameters that can be altered by the surgeon to achieve the desired effect at the tissue. This rapid alternating flow of electrons forces the ionically charged intracellular proteins to equally rapidly realign their direction as the polarity of the alternating current continually reverses. The friction created by the movement of these large molecules then heats the cell (any heat at the tip of the instrument is secondary heating back from the tissue). This current then travels through the body through the path of least resistance to the dispersive electrode ("Bovie pad") attached to the patient and returns to the generator. This creates a closed circuit through the patient, and if the generator does not detect the same amount of energy returning that it disperses, the machine will stop generating energy as a safety precaution.[1] In summary, electromagnetic energy applied to the cells is converted to kinetic energy, which then becomes thermal energy [4].

---

[1] The colloquial term "grounding pad" harkens back to the early days of electrosurgery where a true electrical ground was used to disperse current, i.e., there was no closed loop circuit. With this arrangement, any other metal touching the patient can divert the current away from the grounding pad and travel through to the metal. This causes a "short" in the circuit and can lead to local tissue burns or electrocution. Therefore, true "grounding pads" are no longer used in modern surgery.

The surgeon is able to adjust many aspects of the energy that enters tissue. These include the waveform, amplitude, duty cycle, and current density. The waveform, amplitude, and duty cycle are all controlled by the electrosurgical unit and the handheld device. The pure "Cut" setting creates a constant (continuous current and duty cycle) sinusoidal wave pattern that is low amplitude (low voltage). This efficient energy flow leads to rapid intracellular heating, and the cytoplasmic water molecules convert to steam to their boiling point (100 C), vaporizing cells nearly instantaneously. This rapid phase change minimizes thermal spread to surrounding tissues. Comparatively, the same energy setting used on the "Coag" setting creates electron flow that is released in bursts (short duty cycle), leading to an infrequent, but high-voltage, active current. The high-voltage pulses of current application in this mode result in slower increases of intracellular temperatures rising to up to 200 C, which allows for coagulation, desiccation, and even carbonization of the superficial tissue surface over a relatively diffuse area [4].

It is important to mention current density and impedance when using either of these modes. In essence, the smaller the surface area in contact between the instrument and the tissue, the more focused the current transfer and the more localized the effect. The opposite end of the current density spectrum is fulguration, whereby holding the instrument just above the desired tissue necessitates a high-voltage waveform to overcome the impedance by the surrounding air; the arcing electrical current rapidly heats and cools the superficial surface of the tissue leading to coagulation.

All of these variables give the surgeon great control of the energy applied to the patient. The multitude of combinations of voltage, current, density, and technique necessitates a solid understanding of the above basic principles in order to achieve the desired effect with the least amount of energy applied to the patient.

The safety considerations regarding the use of monopolar instrumentation are discussed in the following sections.

Bipolar

While monopolar energy houses one electrode in the hand-held instrument and the other in the dispersive electrode pad, bipolar radiofrequency houses both electrodes within the handheld instrument itself. When tissue is grasped between the two electrode tips (coaptive coagulation), the current flows through only that tissue directly and not throughout the entire body to a distant dispersal pad. This reduces the voltage required to have a desired tissue effect and reduces the risk of current diversion. Early designs of bipolar instruments were limited by the development of impedance in the tissues as the coagulum developed. This can lead to incomplete sealing of a vessel and/or increased lateral thermal spread as energy is diverted away through pathways with less tissue resistance. Modern bipolar radiofrequency devices utilize computerized feedback systems that constantly measure tissue impedance and continually adjust the energy delivery for more efficient localized coagulation. Many of these bipolar vessel sealers are effective at controlling vessels up to 7 mm in diameter, and have the addition of a cutting blade that allows for ligation of the vessel once coagulation is completed.

While appropriate use of bipolar instruments can limit thermal spread and energy diversion, care should be taken to prevent buildup of coagulum between the two electrode jaws. As hemostasis relies on protein coagulation, bipolar devices should be used with caution in any patient with a condition that leads to protein changes or loss, including liver dysfunction, collagen vascular disorders, malnutrition, and atherosclerotic changes.

Ultrasonic Dissection

Ultrasonic devices convert electromechanical energy to mechanical energy by generating vibrations at a rapid frequency, which then are converted to thermal energy via friction at the instrument's effector end; thus, no current is transmitted through the patient. When activated, piezoelectrodes in the instrument's handle generate vibrations at an ultrasonic frequency ranging from 20 to 100 kHz which drives an attached solid shaft at the same rate. These vibrations are transmitted to the active jaw at the tip of the instrument, and when tissue is clamped between the active and passive jaw, the friction resulting from the oscillation between the jaws heats the instrument tip, thus heating the entrapped tissue. There are different settings for the distance of jaw excursion which can affect the rate of heating, leading to variable tissue effects, including vaporization or protein coagulation and tissue separation. Recent models of ultrasonic devices also utilize microprocessors with continuous feedback mechanisms to control protein denaturation, and some instruments allow vessels as large as 7 mm can be safely ligated with this method of electrosurgery.

Since the radiofrequency energy is limited to the handle of the device, ultrasonic dissectors do not require a dispersive electrode, and no stray energy is transmitted to the patient. They also function in wet environments that might limit the deployment of electrosurgery. Safety considerations include keeping the blade clean and keeping coagulum buildup from forming, and care must be taken to prevent thermal injury to surrounding structures when the instrument tip is hot. Although lateral thermal spread at the site of dissection is limited, inadvertently touching nearby bowel without quenching the hot tip can lead to delayed viscus perforation and subsequent patient sepsis.

Plasma Energy

Plasma coagulators' direct current to the desired tissue via a conductor is formed by a jet of inert gas, usually argon. Argon is ionized by the current, which creates a zone of low impedance between the electrode on the instrument and the tissue surface [4]. This allows for the device to avoid physical contact with the tissue but deliver a focused stream of energy to the tissue surface causing coagulation. Therefore, they are often used on diffusely bleeding (wet) surfaces that are unable to be coagulated with a monopolar or bipolar modality, commonly the liver or spleen.

Safety Consideration in Electrosurgery: Unseen Energy Dispersal

Open Surgery

Safe electrosurgery current dispersal is based on the positioning of the receiving dispersive electrode, and placement of the pad on the patient is not trivial. The large size of the pad increases the surface area of the electrode, thus decreasing the current density and preventing tissue injury. It is crucial to avoid pad placement on bony prominences that lead to pressure points, hair, and scars as these can serve as a path of reduced resistance and focus enough energy to cause thermal injury. Most importantly, unseen metal implants can also serve as conductors of current flow between the two electrodes. Placing a dispersive pad over a metal implant can focus the current to the point of causing an unseen thermal injury to the tissue surrounding the implant; no metal prostheses should be between the two electrodes. (The use of bipolar radiofrequency energy mitigates this risk.) Greater distance between the operative site and the pad allows for more opportunities for current diversion and injury to other parts of the body; thus, the pad placement should be as close as is feasible to the operative site [5].

Additionally, magnetic fields created by current passing through the insulated cords (antenna coupling), the device itself, and the dispersal pad can interfere with pacemaker or defibrillator function. When a monopolar device is activated, it can cause an implanted defibrillator to perceive an arrhythmia and deliver a shock. Mitigation strategies for this include use of bipolar energy, minimizing the power level of the ESU, using cut mode, using short bursts of energy on tissue, and placing the dispersal pad and associated cords away from the implanted cardiac device (running the cord from the feet) [6, 7]. In a laboratory model, antenna coupling has been demonstrated to increase the skin temperature at the site of nearby neuromonitoring and EKG leads when monopolar energy was used nearby; this was mitigated by decreasing the ESU wattage used and by separating all cords and cables 15 cm from each other [8].

Once starting dissection with an electrosurgery device, technique becomes paramount to fire safety and burn prevention. Storing the instruments in holsters prevents inadvertent activation, residual heating of drapes, or ignition of alcohol-based preps. Proper retraction places tissue on tension and decreases the amount of energy required to coagulate or cut. Proper exposure prevents inadvertent damage to surrounding structures, particularly in deep dissections.

In open surgery, direct contact and direct coupling are the most likely sources for inadvertent thermal injury to the patient. Direct contact injury is a result of activation of the instrument while it is in contact with tissue. Direct coupling is either the intentional activation of another metal instrument to transmit current to tissue such as with forceps grasping a bleeding vessel or the unintentional contact between the activated instrument and clamps or retractors that can then cause injury outside the desired field of dissection. These patterns of injury can be avoided by using the appropriate holsters and only activating the instrument when it is in full view from the users hand to the tip and noted to be in contact with only the intended tissue.

Residual heat is a third modality of electrosurgical injury that, while common in open surgery, applies to all forms of surgery using energy. Simply put, heat acquired by or generated from the device lingers beyond the point of deactivation, and when combined with direct contact, unanticipated thermal injury can occur if the device has not sufficiently cooled. Each type of electrosurgical device has a characteristic period of time at which it remains a thermal risk. A 2011 study on the residual heat of laparoscopic instruments demonstrated that ultrasonic instruments had both the highest peak temperature (173 °C) and longest delay in return to normal temperature (remained 24 °C above baseline temperature at 20 seconds). Monopolar, bipolar, and argon beam modalities had considerably lower residual heat parameters [9].

A final note should be made regarding the situational awareness required when metal becomes part of the surgical field. Surgical clips and staples are commonly used in all types of surgery for hemostasis and bowel anastomoses; however, acknowledgment of the inherent burn injury risk these tools carry is often underappreciated. For instance, direct contact between an active instrument and a staple line can heat the staple to nearly 1000 °C, beyond the melting point of the staple. Even less contact is required to cause clinically relevant morbidity as a partial thickness burn on small bowel can occur at temperatures as low as 75 °C and lead to perforation. Situational awareness is paramount once a staple or clip is placed.

Laparoscopic and Robotic Surgery

Laparoscopic and robotic surgeries require their own unique principles in understanding energy transfer in electrosurgery. Risk of inadvertent injury from direct contact, direct coupling, and residual heat is heightened in the laparoscopic realm primarily due to the fact that the entire instrument can easily fall out of the view of the camera. Additional considerations must be taken into account with minimally invasive surgery to mitigate electrosurgical risk. Unfortunately, data on laparoscopic sharp, blunt, or thermal injury remain ill-defined due to inconsistent reporting. In particular, cases of thermal injury as the mechanism of action for a missed enterotomy are difficult to quantify due to delay in diagnosis [10].

Antenna coupling is an insidious cause of electrosurgical injury that is now gaining more recognition and most commonly applies to minimally invasive approaches. Antenna coupling occurs when radiofrequency energy passes through insulated wire that is in close proximity to and in parallel configuration with other wires such as long tubular laparoscopic instruments, light cords, and camera power cords; these cords can augment that radiofrequency and generate heat that can burn the patient or ignite a fire. The higher wattage used and the closer the proximity of the source cord to these non-powered instruments, the more energy can transfer via antenna coupling. This phenomenon is a common cause for thermal injury in laparoscopy leading to unseen burns to the patient and even melted plastic across surgical drapes. With this in mind, it is recommended to keep the electrosurgical instrument and dispersal pad cords away from other light cords and wires that will be required for laparoscopic and robotic surgery.

Insulation failure is another source of inadvertent thermal injury. The insulation that surrounds laparoscopic instruments can break down over time with multiple rounds of sterilization. A study at four urban hospitals found one in five reusable laparoscopic instruments had an insulation failure, even at facilities that routinely tested for breaks. Overall they found that 19% of reusable instruments and 3% of disposable instruments had insulation breaks [11]. When breaks in the insulation do occur, current can escape and transfer charge to tissue that is touching or in close proximity to the break in insulation via arcing. Unfortunately, many defects cannot be appreciated by direct visualization, and the smaller the defect, the greater the risk for thermal injury as the energy dispersion is concentrated into a smaller surface area (increased current density). In addition to testing instruments for breaks between cases, active electrode monitoring systems are available which continuously monitor instruments for insulation failures during a procedure.

The final concerning phenomenon in minimally invasive electrosurgery is capacitive coupling. This occurs when there is an insulating or resistive material between two conductors and charge can be stored within the insulator, only to be discharged upon direct contact with another conductor.

Classically, this can be seen between two laparoscopic instruments using monopolar energy that touch along their insulation and then release charge from that insulation to viscera, usually outside the view of the surgeon. This can be avoided with proper trocar and instrument placement, along with careful attention to the length of the laparoscopic instrument and avoiding contact with viscera.

Robotic surgery offers new and unique opportunities for surgical technique. With this advancement, however, come new risks to the patient in terms of energy safety and fire risk. Metal trocar cannulas serve as points of direct contact to the abdominal wall or viscera beyond the point of view of the operating surgeon and can lead to thermal injury in cases where the ports are being used for bedside laparoscopy and monopolar energy is used, or by direct coupling or insulation failures. A study performed in 2011 demonstrated a prevalence of 32% of insulation failures in robotic instruments, with more occurring in bipolar instruments. The same study demonstrated the rate of insulation failures increased significantly after each of the ten uses, with a rate of up to 80% after the tenth use [12]. Just as in laparoscopy, cord management is essential in robotic surgery to avoid antenna coupling. Finally, the surgeon is far away from the operating field by design, thus reducing direct observation of the surgical field beyond the scope of the camera. Recognition of and extinguishing an operating room fire on or near the patient can be delayed with the operating surgeon located at the robotic console.

Endoscopy

Energy in endoscopy is not without its own risk and is worth mentioning. Snares require monopolar energy that is transferred down the endoscope in parallel with the camera circuitry. This allows for antenna coupling and heat transfer from the endoscope to the tissue. Capacitive coupling may occur when using monopolar energy, and this energy can be discharged to the opposing bowel wall outside the operator's view. Methods to reduce this risk include using short duration bursts of energy, using low-energy modes and reducing the power setting, and using an ESU that continuously monitors impedance and fully insufflating the bowel to provide the most distance between the endoscope and the bowel wall [13].

Operating Room Fires and Fire Prevention

Operating room fires are a rare event, reported up to 550–600 times per year in the United States alone and near-misses are likely underreported [14]. While rare, they carry a significant morbidity and mortality when they do occur and are likely to result in malpractice lawsuits [14]. This makes intraoperative fires an often-devastating outcome for both the patient and the surgeon, and leaves long-lasting physical and psychological sequelae. While the rarity of these events is reassuring, it can lead to complacency. Prevention begins with constant vigilance and situational awareness in spite of a perceived lack of danger.

Fires require three important factors in order to occur: (1) heat source or ignition, (2) fuel (3), and oxygen. In most instances, the ignition source is the handheld monopolar device. In fact, one case series implicated monopolar energy in 90% of operating room fires [15]. However, residual heat from a laparoscopic lens, drills, and ultrasound devices can also serve as a source. Fuel is ubiquitous in the operating field. Alcohol base preps, drapes, sponges, gowns, hair, and skin all serve as potential fuel sources once ignition begins. The normal oxygen saturation in the air is 21%; however, near the airway or in cases where nasal cannulas or face-masks are used, it can be substantially higher. An increase in ambient air oxygen saturation to >30% can cause nearly all objects to become fuel for fire [16], and time to ignition similarly decreases with increased oxygen concentration [17]. In a review of OR fire claims, 83% of electrosurgery-induced fires occurred during MAC or regional anesthesia; thus, these conditions require heightened attention to risks [15].

Due to the rarity of such catastrophic events, there is limited training at the surgeon level for what steps should be taken in the event of an operating room fire. The Emergency Care Research Institute (ECRI) provides the following recommendations for an operating room fire on the surgical patient [18]:

1. Stop the flow of all airway gases to the patient.
2. Immediately remove all burning materials and have another team member extinguish them.
   (a) If needed, use a CO_2 fire extinguisher to put out a fire on the patient.

3. Care for the patient:
   (i) Resume ventilation.
   (ii) Control bleeding.
   (iii) Evacuate the patient if there is still danger from smoke or fire.
   (iv) Examine the patient for injuries and treat accordingly.

4. If the fire is not quickly controlled:
   (i) Evacuate and isolate the room.
   (ii) Notify other operating room staff and the fire department.

The ECRI also has recommendations for extinguishing airway fires:

1. Remove the endotracheal tube.
2. Stop the flow of all gases to the airway.
3. Pour saline into the airway.
4. Care for the patient:
   (i) Re-establish the airway.
   (ii) Resume ventilation, and only switch to 100% FiO_2 when you are certain the fire has been extinguished.
   (iii) Examine airway and assess degree of injury and treat patient accordingly.

Fire mitigation risk begins before the patient is in the operating room. Fire extinguishers must be available in every room, and their location confirmed before every case. Sterile saline should be on the field at all times when an energy device is used. Special considerations should be made for surgery of the head and neck, trachea, bronchial tree, and upper chest. In these cases, closed oxygen delivery with an endotracheal tube or laryngeal mask airway is preferred. Additionally, deliver the minimum amount of required oxygen necessary, ideally less than 30% FiO_2 or 5–10 L/min in open systems. In these high-risk scenarios, it is recommended to soak gauze and coat facial hair with saline and surgical jelly, respectively, and to arrange drapes to avoid accumulation of oxygen near the surgical field.

FUSE Curriculum

The Fundamental Use of Surgical Energy (FUSE) curriculum was developed by SAGES to address the deficiencies in surgeon and trainee knowledge that pose risk to the patient. It is the first comprehensive educational tool designed to close the knowledge gap between surgical technology advancement and provider practice. The course covers 11 domains (Fig. 24.1) ranging from physical principles of the energy devices to their clinical applications and safe operation. The didactic content is free, and is available at www.

FIGURE 24.1 The FUSE Program curriculum

- Fundamentals of Electrosurgery
- Mechanisms and Prevention of Adverse Events
- Monopolar Devices
- Bipolar Devices
- Radiofrequency for Soft Tissue Ablation
- Endoscopic Devices
- Ultrasonic Energy Devices
- Microwave Energy Systems
- Energy Devices in Pediatric Surgery
- Integration of Energy Systems with Other Devices
- Prevention of OR Fires

fusedidactic.org. A high-stakes exam that certifies knowledge acquisition is available, as is CME credit. While there is no formal simulation-based assessment as with the laparoscopic and endoscopic fundamentals courses (FLS, FES), a hands-on, bench-top simulation developed by the FUSE authors demonstrated increased learning and retention of the FUSE curriculum up to 1 year after the teaching session [19, 20].

FUSE attempts to change the surgical energy teaching modality from an apprenticeship model that is not standardized to a formal curated curriculum that can be adapted as technology advances. From a purely ethical standpoint, it stands to reason that surgeons undergo formal education and assessment in the field of surgical energy and safety. The FUSE curriculum should become part and parcel of a complete surgical education to ensure the most up-to-date technology can be used with the least risk for the benefit of the patient.

References

1. Feldman LS, Fuchshuber P, Jones DB, Mischna J, Schwaitzberg SD, FUSE (Fundamental Use of Surgical Energy™) Task Force. Surgeons don't know what they don't know about the safe use of energy in surgery. Surg Endosc. 2012;26(10):2735–9.
2. Majno G. The healing hand; man and wound in the ancient world. Cambridge, MA: Harvard Press; 1991.
3. Cushing H, Bovie W. Electrosurgery as an aid to the removal of intracranial tumors. Surg Gynecol Obstet. 1928;47:751–84.
4. Munro MG. Fundamentals of electrosurgery part I: principles of radiofrequency energy for surgery. In: Feldman L, Fuchshuber P, Jones D, editors. The SAGES manual on the fundamental use of surgical energy (FUSE). New York: Springer; 2012.
5. Brunt LM. Fundamentals of electrosurgery part II: thermal injury mechanisms and prevention. In: Feldman L, Fuchshuber P, Jones D, editors. The SAGES manual on the fundamental use of surgical energy (FUSE). New York: Springer; 2012.
6. Govekar HR, Robinson TN, Varosy PD, Girard G, Montero PN, Dunn CL, Jones EL, Stiegmann GV. Effect of monopolar radiofrequency energy on pacemaker function. Surg Endosc. 2012;26(10):2784–8.

7. Robinson TN, Varosy PD, Guillaume G, Dunning JE, Townsend NT, Jones EL, Paniccia A, Stiegmann GV, Weyer C, Rozner MA. Effect of radiofrequency energy emitted from monopolar "Bovie" instruments on cardiac implantable electronic devices. J Am Coll Surg. 2014;219(3):399–406.

8. Townsend NT, Jones EL, Paniccia A, Vandervelde J, McHenry JR, Robinsons TN. Antenna coupling explains unintended thermal injury caused by common operating room monitoring devices. Surg Laparosc Endosc Percutan Tech. 2015;25:111–3.

9. Govekar HR, Robinson TN, Steigmann GV, McGreevy FT. Residual heat of laparoscopic energy devices: how long must the surgeon wait to touch additional tissue? Surg Endosc. 2011;25:3499–502.

10. Cassaro S. Delayed manifestations of laparoscopic bowel injury. Am Surg. 2015;81(5):478–82.

11. Montero PN, Robinson TN, Weaver JS, Stiegmann GV. Insulation failure in laparoscopic instruments. Surg Endosc. 2010;24(2):462–5.

12. Espada M, Munoz R, Noble BN, Magrina JF. Insulation failure in robotic and laparoscopic instrumentation: a prospective evaluation. Am J Obstet Gynecol. 2011;205(2):121.e1–5.

13. Jones EJ, Madani A, Overby DM, Kiourti A, Bojja-Venkatakrishnan S, Mikami DJ, Hazey JW, Arcomano TR, Robinson TN. Stray energy transfer during endoscopy. Surg Endosc. 2017;31(10):3946–51.

14. Choudhry AJ, Haddad NN, Khasawneh MA, Cullinane DC, Zielinski MD. Surgical fires and operative burns: lessons learned from a 33-year review of medical litigation. Am J Surg. 2017;213(3):558–64.

15. Mehta SP, Bhananker SM, Posner KL, Domino KB. Operating room fires: a closed claims analysis. Anesthesiology. 2013;118(5):1133–9.

16. Culp WC Jr, Kimbrough BA, Luna S. Flammability of surgical drapes and materials in varying concentrations of oxygen. Anesthesiology. 2013;119(4):770–6.

17. Goldberg J. Brief laboratory report: surgical drape flammability. AANA J. 2006;74(5):352–4.

18. https://d84vr99712pyz.cloudfront.net/p/pdf/solutions/afig/emergency-procedure-extinguishing-a-surgical-fire.pdf.

19. Madani A, Watanabe Y, Townsend N, Pucher PH, Robinson TN, Egerszegi PE, Olasky J, Bachman SL, Park CW, Amin N, Tang DT, Haase E, Bardana D, Jones DB, Vassiliou M, Fried GM, Feldman LS. Structured simulation improves learning of the Fundamental Use of Surgical Energy™ curriculum: a multicenter randomized controlled trial. Surg Endosc. 2016 Feb;30(2):684–91.
20. Madani A, Watanabe Y, Vassiliou MC, Fuchshuber P, Jones DB, Schwaitzberg SD, Fried GM, Feldman LS. Long-term knowledge retention following simulation-based training for electrosurgical safety: 1-year follow-up of a randomized controlled trial. Surg Endosc. 2016;30(3):1156–63.

Chapter 25
Patient Safety Indicators as Benchmarks

Stacy M. Ranson and Jonathan M. Dort

Quality Measures and Patient Safety

Patient safety and quality has increasingly garnered more attention over the last 20 years as healthcare delivery has focused on a more systematic way to ensure the implementation and execution of best practice guidelines. The Agency for Healthcare Research and Quality (AHRQ) is an integral part of measuring patient safety and outcomes. A greater emphasis on safety has been at the forefront of healthcare delivery since the Institute of Medicine released its landmark report "To Err Is Human: Building a Safer Health System" in 2000. In this important statement, the committee emphasizes the extent of medical errors, specifically preventable ones, with a goal to shift the focus "from blaming individuals for past errors to a focus on preventing future errors by designing safety into the system." [1] The shift in focus to improve sys-

S. M. Ranson
Inova Fairfax Medical Campus, Falls Church, VA, USA

J. M. Dort (✉)
Department of Surgery, Inova Fairfax Medical Campus, Falls Church, VA, USA
e-mail: Jonathan.dort@inova.org

© The Author(s), under exclusive license to Springer Nature Switzerland AG 2022
J. R. Romanelli et al. (eds.), *The SAGES Manual of Quality, Outcomes and Patient Safety*,
https://doi.org/10.1007/978-3-030-94610-4_25

tems models those already in place in other complicated markets such as the aviation industry. This treatise is centered on the belief that effective and quality healthcare delivery should be predicated on building safer systems built to avoid accidental injury from pitfalls in poor equipment design, communication issues, and other barriers to patient care.

Specifically, in the surgical community, adverse events can be devastating to a patient's postoperative recovery and, in some cases, life-threatening or lethal. In a comprehensive review by Ferraris et al., a review of over 1.9 million surgical patients found that 207,236 patients developed serious postoperative complications, and of these, death occurred in 21,731 (10.5%) and that these represented cases of failure to rescue. Further review showed that in these groups of patients, when stratified according to preoperative risk profiles, 90% of operative deaths occurred in the highest-risk quintile. Often, these patients suffered from several postoperative sequelae; only 31.8% had a single postoperative complication [2]. These findings underscore the massive impact postoperative adverse outcomes have on surgical patients. Additionally, in an observational study by Healy et al. from a single institution, a significant effect of adverse events was found to affect hospital costs and the financial burden on hospitals and payers. The overall complication rate for this cohort was 14.5% (744 of 5120) for all procedures, and for studied procedures, mean hospital costs were $19,626 (119%) higher for patients with complications compared with those without complications. Procedures included cholecystectomies, colectomies, proctectomies, small bowel procedures, and ventral hernia repairs. The data showed an overall profit margin that decreased from 5.8% for patients without complications to 0.1% for surgical patients with complications, further underscoring the monetary implications of adverse outcomes on the healthcare system at large [3].

In the last few decades, with an increased spotlight on patient safety, the culture of quality measurement has been further emphasized. Data have shown that this indeed has an impact on patient outcomes. A review from Mardon et al. showed a relationship between patient safety culture and outcomes. Findings from this study show that a more positive patient safety culture is associated with fewer adverse events. The data from 179 hospitals were reviewed including Hospital Survey on Patient Safety Culture (HSOPS) and Patient Safety Indicators (PSI). Hospitals with higher patient safety scores as indicated by the HSOPS tended to have fewer documented adverse events, such that for a hospital scoring 1 SD above the mean on the HSOPS, on average, would experience 0.64 fewer cases per 1000 patients for the PSI average than a hospital at the HSOPS mean [4]. Indeed, another study from the intensive care unit (ICU) setting regarding safety culture found that there was an important relationship between ICU personnel perception and patient outcomes. When looking at the ICU safety climate percent-positive score, for every 10% decrease in safety perception, there was a significantly increased length of stay (LOS) by 15%. Also, lower perceptions of management were significantly associated with higher hospital mortality [5]. A cross-sectional study of 91 hospitals collected data from a survey of hospital personnel and found hospitals with a better safety climate had lower incidence of PSIs, thereby further connecting climate to indicators of safety [6]. These data demonstrate that not only is quality measurement important, but that provider perception regarding safety has an objective impact on patient outcomes. Building a culture that encourages recognition of errors and learning from adverse events and outcomes at an organizational level to further improve safety in healthcare delivery is of paramount importance.

Patient Safety Indicators as a Measure of Quality

In the ever-present drive to enhance patient safety and improve systems, an objective measure of quality was formulated in order to track hospital outcomes in healthcare delivery. Patient Safety Indicators (PSIs) were formulated by the AHRQ in order to outline how well hospitals are performing when it comes to key measures and potentially preventable adverse events. There are four different forms of Quality

Indicator modules with which the AHRQ uses in order to measure efficacy of care delivery, including Patient Safety Indicators, Prevention Quality Indicators, Inpatient Quality Indicators, and Pediatric Quality Indicators. There are a total of 27 Patient Safety Indicators that evaluate complications and adverse events that are potentially preventable, often by evaluating potential barriers on a system level that impede exceptional care. Often, PSIs are used to track hospital and even provider outcomes, as well as drive payment and pay for performance models involving reimbursement.

Patient Safety Indicators are divided into two categories – provider-level and area-level PSIs. Provider-level PSIs include issues related to technical errors, difficulty with procedures, and obstetric or birth trauma. Other factors tracked include postoperative complications, including bleeding/hemorrhage, pulmonary embolism or deep vein thrombosis, sepsis, respiratory failure, hip fracture (from inhospital falls), accidental puncture or laceration, and issues relating to the birthing process. These are monitored by using secondary *International Classification of Diseases, Ninth and Tenth Revision* (ICD-9 and ICD-10) diagnosis codes. Some PSIs include complications that may occur after a patient's index admission during a different hospitalization. Such adverse outcomes include a foreign body left during a procedure, postoperative wound dehiscence in abdominopelvic surgical patients, accidental puncture or laceration, and postoperative hemorrhage or hematoma. These are deemed area-level PSIs and pertain to issues relating to safety within a hospital system. Importantly, area-level PSI tracking is needed to identify deficiencies within a system. This is necessary to ensure an environment of safety, and a review of processes, including best practices and standards of care, as well as departmental and multidisciplinary evaluations to ensure appropriate and streamlined delivery of that care.

Monitoring provider- and area-level PSIs may uncover deficiencies within the information technology realm and potential electronic medical record pitfalls leading to errors or adverse events. Many PSIs are related specifically to surgical outcomes because the associated ICD-9 and ICD-10 codes related to postoperative complications are readily captured and obtained. In contrast, quality measures related to chronic medical or psychiatric conditions are often comorbidities present on admission that are difficult to isolate and identify [7].

Area-level PSIs can be monitored by both ICD-9 and ICD-10 principal diagnosis codes and secondary diagnoses regarding the subsequent associated complication. Because PSIs are tracked primarily via clinician documentation and linked ICD-9 and ICD-10 codes, there is a dependency on the accuracy of that documentation and coding to capture correct PSIs. This is a major criticism of using PSIs as the way to measure quality and outcomes which has been studied at length. Many PSIs are often not captured due to incomplete documentation, and others may be incorrectly flagged as adverse events that were due to disease processes.

Efficacy of Using Patient Safety Indicators to Measure Quality and Surgical Outcomes

Patient Safety Indicators are an invaluable tool used to track quality outcomes and hospital and provider performance. Because they are captured via ICD-9 and ICD-10 codes that are entered by providers, PSIs are relatively easy to obtain; however, the accuracy of PSIs is then founded on accurate documentation which can be variable and unreliable. In a single institution study by Kubasiak et al., 136 surgical cases for 1 year were queried to evaluate target PSIs and whether a PSI event was inherent to the disease process and not a direct effect of the surgery, thereby not a marker of patient safety (false positive). The PSIs reviewed included iatrogenic pneumothorax (PSI-6), puncture or laceration (PSI-9), and postoperative hemorrhage (PSI-15). The cases were reviewed by senior patient safety officers, one with surgical training and one with medical training. The study found that in 11.8–33.3% of cases, the reviewers found the PSI was related to the disease process, not the procedure, and therefore a false positive. Further, the reviewers agreed that these events were not clinically significant in 11.8–30.4% of cases. There was moderate interrater reliability for the PSIs and clearly a high false-positive rate [8].

In addition to Patient Safety Indicators, other means of evaluating surgical outcomes have been utilized. The American College of Surgeons National Surgical Quality Improvement Program (ACS-NSQIP) is used to compare surgical data for general and vascular operations based on observed versus expected outcomes that was initially implemented in 1991 in the US Department of Veterans Affairs in order to improve quality surgical care and build consistent systems of care [9]. Unlike PSIs which use ICD-9 and ICD-10 codes inputted into the chart from providers, the data obtained for ACS-NSQIP outcomes is collected by trained abstractors using defined criteria for complications. A single institution study compared ACS-NSQIP and AHRQ-PSI methods for general and vascular surgical inpatients and found that ACS-NSQIP adverse events were identified in 564 (7.4%) patients and AHRQ-PSIs were identified in 268 (3.5%) patients. Of these cases, only 159 (2.1%) patients had inpatient postoperative events that were captured by both methods, and less than a third of the ACS-NSQIP clinically important events were identified by the AHRQ-PSI ICD-9 method, thus calling into question the sensitivity of PSIs as a reliable measure of capturing adverse events [10].

A large database review correlated PSIs to determine if there was a significant impact on length of stay, charges, and mortality according to 18 different PSIs. It was found that length of stay ranged from 0 to 10.89 days for injury to a neonate and postoperative sepsis, respectively. The cost associated with PSI ranged from $0 for obstetric trauma to $57,727 for postoperative sepsis. In terms of mortality, the range was from 0% for obstetric trauma to 21.96% for postoperative sepsis [11]. This analysis showed that Patient Safety Indicators are a valuable measure of patient outcomes; however, these outcomes vary widely in severity and clinical significance.

Limitations to Patient Safety Indicators

Many have argued that using PSIs to gauge quality and outcomes in the surgical realm may not be an accurate form of measurement. For instance, when evaluating PSI-9 (accidental puncture or laceration during a surgical procedure), a single-hospital institutional review for colorectal procedures found that 9.2% of cases included this indicator. However, there was a wide variability in the significance and outcome of that accidental laceration, such that this PSI includes serosal tear (47%), enterotomy (38%), and extraintestinal injury (15%). Notably, those with serosal tears (the majority of cases including this PSI) had no significant difference in their surgical outcome when compared to those without injury. Those cases that involved an enterotomy, however, did have longer operative times, some requiring resection or diversion, and increased lengths of stay. Similarly, those with extraintestinal injury had higher rates of reoperation and sepsis [12]. This study underscores the notion that not all Patient Safety Indicators are created equal and that there is a wide variability on the clinical impact of each PSI. Further, PSI definitions used are not necessarily specific enough in verbiage and thus can introduce human error into the equation as coders have to decide what qualifies for each PSI.

Another PSI (PSI 9), postoperative hemorrhage or hematoma (PHH), was evaluated to determine if this PSI qualifier is an accurate representation of outcomes by determining positive predictive value (PPV) and characterizing cases as true or false positives. True positives were identified in 84 cases, with a PPV of 75%, with a majority having a diagnosis of hematoma (63%) and hemorrhage (30%), and some with both diagnoses (7%). False positives included events that were present on admission, hemorrhage identified during the index operation and controlled, or postoperative hemorrhage/hematoma not requiring a further intervention/procedure [13]. Once more this demonstrates that there are indeed many limitations to using PSIs as an accurate measure of surgical outcomes.

A 2016 systematic review and meta-analysis of published studies from 1990 to 2015 sought to evaluate the validity of hospital-acquired condition (HAC) measures and PSIs. Only five measures, iatrogenic pneumothorax (PSI 6/HAC 17), central line-associated bloodstream infections (CLABSI) (PSI 7), postoperative hemorrhage/hematoma (PSI 9), postoperative deep vein thrombosis/pulmonary embolus (PSI 12), and accidental puncture/laceration (PSI 15), had sufficient data for pooled meta-analysis. Only accidental puncture/laceration (PSI 15) met the study criteria for validity, which was a positive predictive value (PPV) of >80%, but even this result was described as weakened by study heterogeneity. Utilizing the 80% threshold for PPV and sensitivity, the study found that there is limited validity for the HAC and PSI measures, and recommended that their use for public reporting and pay-for-performance should be re-evaluated [14].

The PSI data for many studies was previously based on the ICD-9 framework; however, with the introduction of the ICD-10 system, there is a new inclusion of chronicity and timing of diagnoses. When only relying on ICD-9 codes, there is an inability to differentiate a preexisting diagnosis from one arising during the course of the hospitalization. One review by McIsaac et al. found that the institution of timing with ICD-10 codes did not increase accuracy to correctly capture PSIs, but that future work is still needed to integrate and improve PSI indicator systems [15].

Conclusion

With an increasing emphasis on patient safety and quality, a meaningful and accurate way to measure healthcare delivery and outcomes has become a necessary component of improving systems at a national, hospital, and provider levels. Using the AHRQ's Patient Safety Indicators as a means of measuring efficacy of quality outcomes has many benefits. The PSI model relies on ICD-9 and ICD-10 codes in order to capture adverse events for hospitalized patients. Patient Safety

Indicators do, however, have limitations. Since PSI data is captured via clinical documentation, it relies heavily on the accuracy of inputting those diagnoses appropriately, and retrospective review has shown that many adverse events may go uncaptured. Additionally, many PSIs have a wide variability in their clinical impact for which some have a negligible role while others have a large part to play in a patient's overall recovery. For instance, as shown above, the PSI accidental laceration or puncture includes negligible surgical events such as repaired serosal tears, but also includes enterotomies which may have required a formal resection. In this case, these two events are classified the same, but have a vast difference in their clinical significance.

Overall, Patient Safety Indicators are a useful means to track hospital and provider performance when it comes to quality healthcare delivery. PSIs are useful for predicting relationships between mortality, length of stay, and cost. While PSIs are measured nationally and are an important component of hospital system reporting for payment and quality, they are also important within a hospital to identify and target potential areas for improvement. With an ongoing emphasis on quality and improved patient outcomes, particularly in the surgical realm, using PSIs will continue to be an integral part of striving toward streamlining systems and working to pinpoint preventable adverse events to further improve healthcare delivery.

References

1. To err is human: building a safer health system. National Academies Press; 2000:9728. https://doi.org/10.17226/9728.
2. Ferraris VA, Bolanos M, Martin JT, Mahan A, Saha SP. Identification of patients with postoperative complications who are at risk for failure to rescue. JAMA Surg. 2014;149(11):1103. https://doi.org/10.1001/jamasurg.2014.1338.
3. Healy MA, Mullard AJ, Campbell DA, Dimick JB. Hospital and payer costs associated with surgical complications. JAMA Surg. 2016;151(9):823. https://doi.org/10.1001/jamasurg.2016.0773.

4. Mardon RE, Khanna K, Sorra J, Dyer N, Famolaro T. Exploring relationships between hospital patient safety culture and adverse events. J Patient Saf. 2010;6(4):226–32. https://doi.org/10.1097/PTS.0b013e3181fd1a00.

5. Huang DT, Clermont G, Kong L, et al. Intensive care unit safety culture and outcomes: a US multicenter study. Int J Qual Health Care. 2010;22(3):151–61. https://doi.org/10.1093/intqhc/mzq017.

6. Singer S, Lin S, Falwell A, Gaba D, Baker L. Relationship of safety climate and safety performance in hospitals. Health Serv Res. 2009;44(2p1):399–421. https://doi.org/10.1111/j.1475-6773.2008.00918.x.

7. Barton A. Patient safety and quality: an evidence-based handbook for nurses. AORN J. 2009;90(4):601–2. https://doi.org/10.1016/j.aorn.2009.09.014.

8. Kubasiak JC, Francescatti AB, Behal R, Myers JA. Patient safety indicators for judging hospital performance: still not ready for prime time. Am J Med Qual. 2017;32(2):129–33. https://doi.org/10.1177/1062860615618782.

9. Henderson WG, Daley J. Design and statistical methodology of the National Surgical Quality Improvement Program: why is it what it is? Am J Surg. 2009;198(5):S19–27. https://doi.org/10.1016/j.amjsurg.2009.07.025.

10. Cima RR, Lackore KA, Nehring SA, et al. How best to measure surgical quality? Comparison of the Agency for Healthcare Research and Quality Patient Safety Indicators (AHRQ-PSI) and the American College of Surgeons National Surgical Quality Improvement Program (ACS-NSQIP) postoperative adverse events at a single institution. Surgery. 2011;150(5):943–9. https://doi.org/10.1016/j.surg.2011.06.020.

11. Zhan C. Excess length of stay, charges, and mortality attributable to medical injuries during hospitalization. JAMA. 2003;290(14):1868. https://doi.org/10.1001/jama.290.14.1868.

12. Kin C, Snyer K, Kiran R, Remzi F, Vogel J. Accidental puncture or laceration in colorectal surgery: a quality indicator or a complexity measure? Dis Colon Rectum. 2013;56(2):219–25.

13. Borzecki AM, Kaafarani H, Cevasco M, et al. How valid is the AHRQ patient safety indicator "postoperative hemorrhage or hematoma"? J Am Coll Surg. 2011;212(6):946–953.e2. https://doi.org/10.1016/j.jamcollsurg.2010.09.033.

14. Winters BD, Bharmal A, Wilson RF, et al. Validity of the agency for health care research and quality patient safety indicators and the centers for medicare and medicaid hospital-acquired conditions. Med Care. 2016;54(12):1105–11. https://doi.org/10.1097/MLR.0000000000000550.

15. McIsaac DI, Hamilton GM, Abdulla K, et al. Validation of new ICD-10-based patient safety indicators for identification of in-hospital complications in surgical patients: a study of diagnostic accuracy. BMJ Qual Saf. 2020;29(3):209–16. https://doi.org/10.1136/bmjqs-2018-008852.

Chapter 26
Culture of Safety and Era of Better Practices

Eileen R. Smith and Shaina R. Eckhouse

Introduction

While we traditionally consider surgeon skill and experience to be the major driving factor in surgical outcomes, a growing body of evidence demonstrates that the perioperative environment impacts patient safety and outcomes [1]. An organizational culture of safety is a key tool in the pursuit of excellence in patient safety and surgical outcomes [1, 2]. The Joint Commission defines safety culture as the sum of what an organization is and does in the pursuit of safety. A safety culture is the product of individual and group beliefs, values, attitudes, perceptions, competencies, and patterns of behavior that determine the organization's commitment to quality and patient safety [3]. In a culture of safety, the attitudes, values, and policies of an organization promote and elevate safety at all levels [1, 4]. Organizations must implement robust procedures and policies that support and sustain a just culture, which shifts error analysis and prevention toward a fair-

E. R. Smith (✉) · S. R. Eckhouse
Section of Minimally Invasive Surgery, Department of Surgery, Washington University School of Medicine, Saint Louis, MO, USA
e-mail: e.r.smith@wustl.edu

© The Author(s), under exclusive license to Springer Nature Switzerland AG 2022
J. R. Romanelli et al. (eds.), *The SAGES Manual of Quality, Outcomes and Patient Safety*,
https://doi.org/10.1007/978-3-030-94610-4_26

minded, systems-based approach that supports open reporting and accountability while avoiding individual blame [5].

Barriers to Achieving a Culture of Safety

It is clear that a culture of safety should be our goal as surgeons. However, the barriers to achieving this in reality are challenging in their scope and diversity. We identify four critical barriers to attaining a culture of safety: traditional hierarchical culture, communication disconnects, team dynamics, and increasing complexity of surgical services. Each of these concerns deserves special attention as we work to recognize and ultimately break down barriers to a culture of safety in surgical practice.

Hierarchy in Surgical Culture

The culture of general surgery has long been infused with a strong, hierarchical system representing a persistent obstacle to adopting a true culture of safety. Attending surgeons have traditionally been considered the leader in the operating room - the captain of the ship. In one study comparing medicine and the aviation industry, only 55% of surgeons were opposed to steep hierarchies, in which senior members are not open to input from junior members [6]. In fact, surgical training programs rely on this structure, and surgical residents perceive significant professional consequences to disrupting this hierarchy [7]. This culture, despite diminishing over time as workplace values have shifted, remains a key barrier to the open communication and accountability we seek in establishing a culture of safety. If trainees and our non-surgeon team members in the operating room feel intimidated by this hierarchical framework, they will be less likely to speak up about patient safety concerns [8–11].

Communication Disconnects

A storied history exists in the specialty of surgery in regard to poor communication and disruptive behavior. These communication and behavioral issues negatively impact patient outcomes [12–14]. Tense communications directly diminish teamwork quality [15]. Aside from specifically disruptive behavior, patient safety can be impacted by simple communication failures that result in the loss of information between team members [16]. One observational study of operating rooms documented a 30% rate of communication failure, with up to 36% of these failures having a measurable impact on patient safety [17]. Communications across disciplines – for instance, surgeon to nurse – remain particularly vulnerable to errors [18]. It should be noted that lead surgeons are frequently unaware of how effectively they communicate and the level of psychological safety their team members feel, with a significant difference in perception of safety culture when compared to other operating room staff such as nurses, scrub technicians, and anesthesiologists [19].

Team Dynamics

Today's operating room relies on a surgical team working effectively and efficiently in concert to deliver excellent patient care. Due to scheduling needs, operative teams may change in composition multiple times throughout the course of a single operation. This results in a lack of familiarity among team members and even a lack of familiarity with the operation to be performed. One example from cardiac surgery demonstrated that teams with less familiarity caused an increase in number of teamwork and communication related errors [20].

Team dynamics are additionally complicated by the effect of implicit biases and microaggressions in the workplace.

Despite the well-acknowledged advantages to a diverse workforce, diversity within medicine is still lacking in part due to implicit biases and microaggressions [21, 22]. Interestingly, women and minorities experience a significant amount of stress and anxiety as a result of microaggressions. These subtle discriminatory events contribute to an environment where these team members feel undervalued and delegitimized [23]. Recent evaluation of current surgical residents demonstrated a correlation between these experiences and risk of burnout [24]. These factors erode our ability to function as an effective team by pushing us away from a culture of safety and make it difficult to nimbly respond to patient safety concerns.

Increasing Complexity of Surgical Services

Delivery of surgical care, especially in the area of minimally invasive surgery, is now more complex than ever. Even routine operations can include a wide range of techniques and technologies, from surgical robots to advanced laparoscopic devices, instruments, and camera technologies. The introduction of these advanced technologies has increased the opportunity for error just due to the increasing number of complex devices involved [25, 26]. We must acknowledge that the complexity of surgery in the current era can lead to patient safety events.

The surgeon of today must also effectively manage their time to maintain the electronic medical record, respond to patient questions and concerns quickly, and negotiate with insurance groups. These varied demands contribute to an increased workload and pull the attention of the surgeon in many directions – potentially increasing the opportunity for errors and safety events if the appropriate infrastructure is not in place. We know that distraction can be a source of error, and in this period, the practicing surgeon has numerous demands on their time beyond traditional clinical care. Prior work has shown intraoperative phone calls can impact technical performance, and one observational study illustrated most distractions related to phone usage in the operating rooms are due to surgeons responding to calls [27, 28]. The introduction of the electronic medical record, while not without advantages, adds to the increased work burden for practicing surgeons. (This is discussed in more detail in Chap. 38.) More specifically, a recent investigation of surgeon workflow demonstrated that 30% of working time, representing a median of 23 hours per week, is spent managing the electronic medical record [29].

Strategies to Overcome Barriers and Establish a Culture of Safety

Despite these numerous challenges, it is possible to move the field of surgery toward a robust culture of safety. This chapter describes four key strategies to potentially address these barriers: event reporting, standardized communication, a focus on teamwork, and surgical leadership. Healthcare systems and surgical practices should adopt easy to access systems for reporting errors that take team member concerns seriously, regardless of their role. Surgeons and their teams should establish clear communication standards that work to flatten the hierarchy and make routine the solicitation of input from all team members. These standards should be utilized in concert with specific training with a focus on effective teamwork that includes mitigating bias and microaggressions in the workplace. Finally, surgeons must fully recognize their role as key leaders in the operating room with the important goal of promoting safety.

Event Reporting and Promotion of a Just Culture

In order to foster a culture of safety, there must be a clear and accessible mechanism for reporting safety concerns, and those elevated through the system should be considered with appropriate gravity, regardless of what role on the surgical team the reporting individual holds. It is important for event reporting systems to be agile and able to respond to concerns in a timely fashion, with investigations striving to promote a just culture and examine the role of both systems and individuals in safety errors. Finally, when individuals who occupy a more junior role express concerns about those in senior positions, there should be clarity and transparency regarding how those individuals will be held accountable. Organizations must support and protect those who identify safety concerns to ensure those who report will not experience any form of retaliation. Emphasizing an organizational culture of not just safety but accountability is key to optimizing safety event reporting system.

Standardized Communication

In addition to a positive and robust reporting system, adopting standardized communication methods positively impacts patient safety. Examples include standardized preoperative time-outs, postoperative debrief, or the use of checklists prior to performing complicated tasks. Work in the area of surgical checklists by the World Health Organization demonstrated the utilization of surgical checklists resulted in reduced mortality [30]. Utilization of communication tools such as a surgical time-out previously demonstrated improvement in team perception of safety culture [31]. Introducing standardizing communication tools aides in the mitigation of safety risks associated with the increasing complexity of surgical care and the challenging workload facing today's surgeon. Furthermore, adopting these techniques to establish a routine for communication helps to flatten the hierarchy in surgical care and creates a safe space for all team members to express concerns.

A Focus on Teamwork

A culture of safety cannot be achieved without a specific focus on team dynamics. The key report "To Err is Human" by the Institute of Medicine highlighted effective team functioning as one of its five values for creating safe hospitals [32]. All team members should participate in rigorous training efforts to increase skill in interprofessional communication and emphasize the value of team members across roles and levels of seniority. A team training approached previously studied by the Veterans Health Administration demonstrated a 17% reduction in surgical morbidity after implementation [33]. In addition to training on team dynamics, surgeons and those they work with closely in patient care environments should receive education on the impact of bias and discrimination in the workplace. Understanding the challenges women and underrepresented minorities experience in healthcare is critical to establishing a supportive workplace that promotes a culture of safety. Furthermore, recent formal recommendations by the American College of Surgeons Task Force on Racial Issues includes training on topics of diversity, equity, and inclusion for surgical departments [34].

Surgical Leadership

Though we have seen significant efforts to flatten hierarchy within surgery and discourage a perception that the surgeon is the sole leading voice in the operating room, it remains a reality that surgeons are in a critical leadership role on the operating room team. We have a tremendous ability to support a culture of safety in our operating rooms by setting clear expectations, communicating effectively, and modeling professional and respectful behavior. Effective surgical leadership can have a demonstrable impact on patient care; work by Dimick et al. found surgeons with constructive leadership styles had lower rates of adverse outcomes [35]. A key part of these efforts is soliciting feedback from team members and accepting responsibility for errors. Through these behaviors, surgeons can personally promote a culture of safety in their work environments.

Conclusion

There exist numerous and diverse barriers to achieving a true culture of safety and attaining best practices for patient safety within surgery. The culture of surgery itself with its emphasis on hierarchy and prior tolerance for difficult behavior makes it especially difficult for surgical specialties to create and sustain an environment where all team members feel their concerns will be heard. Surgery is only increasing in its complexity, and effective communication remains critical to avoiding poor outcomes. Despite these challenges, the surgical community can still rigorously pursue best practices. Adoption of strong organizational policies that work to flatten the hierarchy, support and promote reporting of safety events, and deliver training in areas of communication, leadership, and bias can help shift healthcare systems closer to that ideal culture of safety. These efforts can be furthered by utilizing standardized methods for communicating inside and outside the operating room that help to minimize loss of information during care and create ample opportunities for team members to voice concerns. By recognizing the key barriers to a culture of safety and working to overcome them, we can deliver care in an era of better practices while we pursue our ideal.

References

1. Fan CJ, Pawlik TM, Daniels T, et al. Association of safety culture with surgical site infection outcomes. J Am Coll Surg. 2016;222:122–8.
2. Odell DD, Quinn CM, Matulewicz RS, et al. Association between hospital safety culture and surgical outcomes in a statewide surgical quality improvement collaborative. J Am Coll Surg. 2019;229:175–83.
3. Commission J. 11 tenets of a safety culture.
4. Pronovost PJ, Berenholtz SM, Goeschel CA, et al. Creating high reliability in health care organizations. Health Serv Res. 2006;41:1599–617.
5. Boysen PG 2nd. Just culture: a foundation for balanced accountability and patient safety. Ochsner J. 2013;13:400–6.
6. Sexton JB, Thomas EJ, Helmreich RL. Error, stress, and teamwork in medicine and aviation: cross sectional surveys. BMJ. 2000;320:745–9.
7. Kellogg KC, Breen E, Ferzoco SJ, Zinner MJ, Ashley SW. Resistance to change in surgical residency: an ethnographic study of work hours reform. J Am Coll Surg. 2006;202:630–6.
8. Barzallo Salazar MJ, Minkoff H, Bayya J, et al. Influence of surgeon behavior on trainee willingness to speak up: a randomized controlled trial. J Am Coll Surg. 2014;219:1001–7.
9. Belyansky I, Martin TR, Prabhu AS, et al. Poor resident-attending intraoperative communication may compromise patient safety. J Surg Res. 2011;171:386–94.
10. Okuyama A, Wagner C, Bijnen B. Speaking up for patient safety by hospital-based health care professionals: a literature review. BMC Health Serv Res. 2014;14:61.
11. Bowman C, Neeman N, Sehgal NL. Enculturation of unsafe attitudes and behaviors: student perceptions of safety culture. Acad Med. 2013;88:802–10.
12. Rosenstein AH, O'Daniel M. Impact and implications of disruptive behavior in the perioperative arena. J Am Coll Surg. 2006;203:96–105.
13. Rosenstein AH, O'Daniel M. Disruptive behavior and clinical outcomes: perceptions of nurses and physicians. Am J Nurs. 2005;105:54–64; quiz 64–55.

14. Cooper WO, Guillamondegui O, Hines OJ, et al. Use of unsolicited patient observations to identify surgeons with increased risk for postoperative complications. JAMA Surg. 2017;152:522–9.

15. Keller S, Tschan F, Semmer NK, et al. "Disruptive behavior" in the operating room: a prospective observational study of triggers and effects of tense communication episodes in surgical teams. PLoS One. 2019;14:e0226437.

16. Christian CK, Gustafson ML, Roth EM, et al. A prospective study of patient safety in the operating room. Surgery. 2006;139:159–73.

17. Lingard L, Espin S, Whyte S, et al. Communication failures in the operating room: an observational classification of recurrent types and effects. Qual Saf Health Care. 2004;13:330–4.

18. Hu YY, Arriaga AF, Peyre SE, Corso KA, Roth EM, Greenberg CC. Deconstructing intraoperative communication failures. J Surg Res. 2012;177:37–42.

19. Magill ST, Wang DD, Rutledge WC, et al. Changing operating room culture: implementation of a postoperative debrief and improved safety culture. World Neurosurg. 2017;107:597–603.

20. ElBardissi AW, Wiegmann DA, Henrickson S, Wadhera R, Sundt TM 3rd. Identifying methods to improve heart surgery: an operative approach and strategy for implementation on an organizational level. Eur J Cardiothorac Surg. 2008;34:1027–33.

21. Cooper-Patrick L, Gallo JJ, Gonzales JJ, et al. Race, gender, and partnership in the patient-physician relationship. JAMA. 1999;282:583–9.

22. Traylor AH, Schmittdiel JA, Uratsu CS, Mangione CM, Subramanian U. The predictors of patient-physician race and ethnic concordance: a medical facility fixed-effects approach. Health Serv Res. 2010;45:792–805.

23. Torres MB, Salles A, Cochran A. Recognizing and reacting to microaggressions in medicine and surgery. JAMA Surg. 2019;154:868–72.

24. Hu YY, Ellis RJ, Hewitt DB, et al. Discrimination, abuse, harassment, and burnout in surgical residency training. N Engl J Med. 2019;381:1741–52.

25. Catchpole K, Perkins C, Bresee C, et al. Safety, efficiency and learning curves in robotic surgery: a human factors analysis. Surg Endosc. 2016;30:3749–61.

26. Mathew R, Markey K, Murphy J, Brien BO. Integrative literature review examining factors affecting patient safety with

robotic-assisted and laparoscopic surgeries. J Nurs Scholarsh. 2018;50:645–52.

27. Yang C, Heinze J, Helmert J, Weitz J, Reissfelder C, Mees ST. Impaired laparoscopic performance of novice surgeons due to phone call distraction: a single-centre, prospective study. Surg Endosc. 2017;31:5312–7.

28. Avidan A, Yacobi G, Weissman C, Levin PD. Cell phone calls in the operating theater and staff distractions: an observational study. J Patient Saf. 2019;15:e52–5.

29. Cox ML, Farjat AE, Risoli TJ, et al. Documenting or operating: where is time spent in general surgery residency? J Surg Educ. 2018;75:e97–e106.

30. Haynes AB, Weiser TG, Berry WR, et al. A surgical safety check-list to reduce morbidity and mortality in a global population. N Engl J Med. 2009;360:491–9.

31. McLaughlin N, Winograd D, Chung HR, Van de Wiele B, Martin NA. Impact of the time-out process on safety attitude in a tertiary neurosurgical department. World Neurosurg. 2014;82:567–74.

32. Institute of Medicine Committee on Quality of Health Care in A. In: Kohn LT, Corrigan JM, Donaldson MS, editors. To err is human: building a safer health system. Washington (DC): National Academies Press (US). Copyright 2000 by the National Academy of Sciences. All rights reserved; 2000.

33. Young-Xu Y, Neily J, Mills PD, et al. Association between imple-mentation of a medical team training program and surgical mor-bidity. Arch Surg. 2011;146:1368–73.

34. American College of Surgeons Task Force on Racial Issues: Report of Recommendations. 2020.

35. Shubeck SP, Kanters AE, Dimick JB. Surgeon leadership style and risk-adjusted patient outcomes. Surg Endosc. 2019;33(2):471–4.

Chapter 27
Learning New Operations and Introduction into Practice

Ugoeze J. Nwokedi, Lee Morris, and Nabil Tariq

Introduction

Surgery continues to be a rapidly innovative field. Over the last three decades, we have seen the widespread adoption of laparoscopy to span beyond general surgery, to include colorectal, urology, gynecology, and thoracic surgery, in addressing the burden of surgical disease. More recently, robotic technology has also been added to the surgical armamentarium of tools available for minimally invasive approach to patient care in the twenty-first century.

However, these rapid advancements in the field of gastro-intestinal and endoscopic surgery bring along new challenges that surgeons today must contend with. First, we need to define a common nomenclature around the adoption of what is considered a "new" procedure, surgical technique, or technology versus a modification or alternate use of existing device or technique. Hutchinson et al. in their work attempt

U. J. Nwokedi · L. Morris · N. Tariq (✉)
Department of Surgery, The Houston Methodist Hospital,
Houston, TX, USA
e-mail: LMMorris@Houstonmethodist.org;
ntariq@houstonmethodist.org

© The Author(s), under exclusive license to Springer Nature Switzerland AG 2022
J. R. Romanelli et al. (eds.), *The SAGES Manual of Quality, Outcomes and Patient Safety*,
https://doi.org/10.1007/978-3-030-94610-4_27

to lay out an original definition of the term "surgical innovation" (Table 27.1) that meets robust criteria that can be reliably and prospectively applied to both "new" techniques and devices [1]. They describe whether the innovative technique is entirely new to the field, new to an anatomic location, or new to a specific patient group. Similarly, they describe whether the innovative device is new to the field, new to an anatomical location, or new to a patient group. This is paired with a practical day-to-day survey termed the Macquarie Surgical Innovation Identification Tool (Fig. 27.1) that surgeons can utilize in identifying "new" innovation. This again differentiates if a procedure is new to the hospital, new to the surgeon, new to the field, or new to a particular patient group. This proposed theoretical framework could obviate the nuances surrounding the deployment of these specific terminologies in the field and help structure a standardized approach with regard to the introduction of surgical innovation from the industry.

Drawbacks of the aforementioned framework are reflected in its identification of "new" technique or technology. Most surgeons would agree that in daily practice, they repurpose existing technology or technique distinct from what is captured by the Macquarie Surgical Innovation Identification Tool. It is therefore important to describe the alternatives to "new" technique or technology as these may have practical implications, for example, with regard to credentialing and privileging at the institutional level and perhaps more importantly, patient safety.

In August 2014, the Society of American Gastrointestinal and Endoscopic Surgeons (SAGES) and its Board of Governors approved expert consensus statements outlining the adoption of new technology and techniques [2]. Outlined in these committee statements are further definitions of "new" and "modified" terminology to capture the breadth of possibilities that may arise in clinical practice. The SAGES Guideline Committee definitions are listed below and supplement the aforementioned framework:

TABLE 27.1 A definition of innovative surgery with illustrative examples

An innovative surgical procedure is any procedure that meets 1 or more of the following criteria:		
	Criteria	**Examples**
1	*Innovative technique*: The technique used is new or differs from the standard technique in one or more of the following ways:	Different incision position or size; combination of two procedures such as mastectomy and reconstruction; extension of microsurgical techniques; established procedure undertaken on a different category of patient
1a	Altogether new	Pioneering transplant surgery, e.g., first heart transplant, first face transplant, first uterus transplant; use of hypothermia for neurosurgery
1b	New to anatomical location[a]	Novel anatomical approach for existing procedure; use of established anastomotic techniques in new locations
1c	New to patient group	Expansion of indications to groups whose surgical outcomes may be different, such as children; people with comorbidities likely to influence surgical outcomes; patients of a different sex
or		
2	*Innovative device*: The tools or devices used are new, or the use differs from standard use in one of the following ways described:	Surgical robot; new hip prosthesis; implant made from new material; use of laparoscope to perform procedure usually done without one; use of adult device or tool on a child

(continued)

TABLE 27.1 (continued)

An innovative surgical procedure is any procedure that meets 1 or more of the following criteria:

	Criteria	Examples
2a	Altogether new	Invention of the da Vinci robot; first use of laparoscope; first use of the endotracheal tube for anesthesia
2b	New to anatomical location[a]	Application of laparoscopic instruments or robotic surgery to new organ or body cavity
2c	New to patient group	Use of device or tools in groups whose surgical outcomes may be different, such as children; people with comorbidities likely to influence surgical outcomes; patients of a different sex

From: Hutchinson et al. [1], with permission
[a]Here we exclude procedures, such as fixation of fractures, which are not standardized to a particular anatomical location

1. *Modified Device:* existing device the surgeon has experience with that has been altered to improve functionality or performance, e.g., a modified stapler, a new mesh, etc.
2. *New Device:* product of disruptive innovation or device that has not been previously used by surgeons. Includes modified devices that surgeons have no prior experience with, e.g., endoscopic hemoclips, when surgeons have not used similar clips before.
3. *Modified Procedure:* modification of known procedure or technique. Surgeons have experience with similar procedures/techniques, e.g., a surgeon experienced with laparoscopic Nissen wants to perform a laparoscopic Toupet fundoplication or a surgeon who performs a laparoscopic bypass wants to adopt laparoscopic sleeve gastrectomy.
4. *New Procedure:* novel technique that differs dramatically from what surgeons are used to or technique not previously

1. The **techniques, instruments and/or devices** to be used in the operation for which the patient has consented:

   1a. Have all been used before in this **hospital** ☐ Yes ☐ No
   1b. Have all been used before in this **surgeon** ☐ Yes ☐ No

   > *A `No' response for either of these item identifies first performance of the intervention by the surgeon, or introduction of the intervention to the institution. This may flag innovation if the intervention has never been performed elsewhere. Further details should be requested regarding requirements for training and supervision, change in resources, extent of patient communication, and prior experience of the intervention elsewhere.*

2. The conditions under which this operation will take place do not depart from those under which such a procedure would usually occur, for example the **techniques, instruments and/or devices** to be used in the operation for which the patient has consented are routinely used:

   2a. For this indication ☐ Yes ☐ No
   2b. In patients of this sex (where sex differences relevant) ☐ Yes ☐ No
   2c. In patients of this age (c.f. pediatric and elderly patients) ☐ Yes ☐ No
   2d. In patients with this comorbidity ☐ N/A ☐ Yes ☐ No

   > *A `No' response for any of these items suggests that innovation may be occurring. Further details should be requested regarding the surgeon's knowledge of likely outcomes of the procedure, whether the outcomes of the surgery are likely to be of interest to surgical peers (e.g. publishable) and whether special preparations are needed (such as training, or special instructions to the anesthetist or to the preoperative, perioperative or postoperative teams).*

FIGURE 27.1 Macquarie surgical innovation identification tool. This is a practical tool to identify potentially innovative procedures to prompt appropriate support. (*From*: Hutchinson et al. [1], with permission)

used by surgeons, e.g., POEM vs. laparoscopic myotomy or adaptation of a laparoscopic or robotic procedure by an open surgeon.

These definitions of specific terminology play a critical first step by providing language commonality for surgeons and administrators to utilize in developing policy and regulations around implementation of new procedures, techniques, or technology at the institutional level. The appropriate terminology could also redefine current procedural terminology (CPT) codes which invariably are tied to the healthcare reimbursements that hospitals and surgeons receive from insurance agencies. Therefore, appropriate designation of either "new" or "modified" terminology to surgical techniques and technology as it is incorporated into the clinical setting could have important financial implications as well.

Some of the criticisms of developing strict definitions around surgical innovation could be the ensuing regulatory oversight which ultimately gets translated into both privileging and credentialing processes for surgeons, as well as day-to-day practice [1, 3]. This inadvertently could potentially discourage the widespread adoption of these terms by surgeons. The reality today for surgeons undergoing the privileging and credentialing process is that in most institutions, it is more often than not cumbersome and time consuming. It is then not too surprising that in the era of increasing administrative responsibilities placed on surgeons, especially with tedious electronic medical record documentation and billing, this additional regulatory oversight is yet another aspect of patient care that the modern surgeon needs to balance with other clinical responsibilities. While it is safe to say no expeditious solutions to this dilemma exist, defining common terminology as we integrate surgical innovation into patient care is a necessary first step that carries both legal and patient safety ramifications for clinical practice. Thus, the ensuing discussion will employ these definitions to designate "new or innovative" or "modified" techniques and technology in our discussion.

Finally, as we continue to make progress in the ever-changing field of surgery, we ought to have in place specific pathways to guide practicing surgeons on how best to adapt to the modern practice of surgery. Not surprisingly, surgical societies often play a significant role as flagship organizations to further delineate these responsibilities. Invariably, surgeons adopting new technology and techniques have to abide by their institution-specific privileging and credentialing criteria. Paramount to the success of effective adoption of new technique and technology is addressing the knowledge gap in safely integrating these new technologies into day-to-day surgical practice while maintaining delivery of high-value and high-quality healthcare to our patients. In this chapter, we will highlight the hurdles met in instituting a uniform framework around incorporating surgical technology at the local level and provide some practical guidelines and checklists for practicing surgeons to utilize in establishing their implementation framework.

What Different Steps Need to Be Taken to Evaluate New Technology and Surgical Techniques?

Implementing new technology and surgical techniques (NT&T) into clinical medicine can be highly rewarding to both patients and care providers but may also cause harm if the technology or new surgical technique is not appropriately evaluated to determine its true safety and efficacy. Determining the safety and efficacy of a surgical technology or new procedure is a complex task as surgical research is difficult on many levels. To help assist the surgical innovator in evaluating NT&T, a general framework has been suggested to be of benefit.

The IDEAL (Idea, Development, Exploration, Assessment, Long-term monitoring) framework is one such paradigm to guide innovators in producing high-quality surgical studies for each stage of evolution of the particular NT&T. The IDEAL framework began in Oxford, England, from 2007 to 2009 to discuss the specific challenges of evaluating surgical innovation. These discussions resulted in a publication of a five-stage framework describing the natural stages of surgical innovation. The IDEAL framework was established to provide a pathway for evaluating surgical innovations at each stage of their development [4]. Each stage is defined by a key research question:

- Stage 1 (Idea): What is the new treatment concept and why is it needed?
- Stage 2a (Development): Has the new intervention reached a state of stability sufficient to allow replication by others?

- Stage 2b (Exploration): Have the questions that might compromise the chance of conducting a successful RCT been addressed?
- Stage 3 (Assessment): How does the new intervention compare with current practice?
- Stage 4 (Long-term study): Are there any long-term or rare adverse effects or changes in indications or delivery quality over time?

Various users and funders of research have acknowledged the utility of IDEAL; however, use has remained somewhat limited. For this reason, more recently, it has been updated to help clarify and offer more detailed guidance about how to implement the updated recommendations [5]. Updated descriptions of the IDEAL framework and stage appropriate study designs are briefly summarized as follows:

The Pre-IDEAL stage is research prior to first human trials of an innovation. Appropriate preclinical studies include material testing, simulator, cadaver, animal, modeling, and cost-effectiveness studies. Stage 1 (Idea) describes the first use of a new procedure or device in a patient. Appropriate studies involve a single case or a few cases. It is recommended that reports explain the need for the new treatment concept and why it might be better than currently available treatment. Video recording and sharing is highly recommended and can be part of online publication. Stage 2a (Development) involves modifying procedures toward a final stable version. Appropriate studies are small single center prospective trials. A typology which deconstructs interventions into their component parts may help with precise definition of procedures and clarify description of which parts of the procedure change as it is modified and updated. Stage 2b (Exploration) is a stage where the main purpose is to gain greater experience of the new intervention in a wider group of surgeons and patients. This will allow more information to be collected, which will determine whether and how to progress to a definitive comparison against current best treatment. Appropriate studies are typically collaborative multicenter prospective studies and determine the feasibility of a RCT. Stage 3 (Assessment) is a pivotal comparative evaluation stage that usually occurs against the current standard treatment. Appropriate studies are a multi-surgeon, multicenter RCT when feasible. Variants, including cluster-randomized or expertise-based RCTs or stepped wedge designs, may be appropriate. Stage 4 (Long-term study) proposes registries for data collection. Their strength lies in recognizing late or uncommon safety outcomes. Key design issues for registries center on the dataset and on fostering engagement. Datasets should be as small and cheap to collect as possible, while reliably capturing patient and device/procedure identity, diagnosis, and the key influences on outcome [5].

The IDEAL framework is just one example of a stepwise evaluation tool to help innovators evaluate more accurately the safety and efficacy of complex interventions or new technology. Tools such as this are widely accepted as necessary in evaluating NT&T and to prevent adverse events or wide adoption of NT&T that later proves to be harmful.

What Are the Surgeon's Responsibilities to Start NT&T?

Today, new technology and new and more advanced surgical procedures are being introduced with ever-increasing frequency. To prevent from being left behind, modern surgeons must stay aware of new therapies and technology and find ways to safely implement these changes into their practice. However, for busy practicing surgeons, learning new techniques and implementing them safely can be a challenging task. One of the initial steps after identification of the new technique for implementation is proper training in order to acquire competence and proficiency. Learning any new technique to the expert level requires time and dedication. The amount of time to adequately learn the NT&T and overcome the learning curve is often underestimated. Practicing surgeons must consider what tools are available to help them minimize the impact of a learning curve on their patient's outcomes.

Traditionally, short courses offered over weekends to accommodate practicing surgeons' busy schedules were the only training available. However, higher complication rates have been reported for such techniques as laparoscopic surgery when training was limited to short courses held over a weekend [6]. What additional options are then available to surgeons trying to modernize their practice or stay on the forefront of treatment options? SAGES has outlined additional modalities that may be helpful and beneficial to surgeons learning NT&T [2]. Some examples include informal familiarization of surgeon with device or procedure before introduction, review of existing data/literature, pursuit of expert input, video review of device use or procedure, practice on appropriate simulated models (e.g., realistic or virtual reality), practice on animate models, practice on cadavers or cadaveric tissues, participation at courses at society meetings (e.g., SAGES, ACS), participation in online courses, completion of formal training (e.g., fellowship), proctored initial cases, tele-proctoring of initial cases, and team training (if applicable). However, knowing where to start may be difficult and appropriate pathways are not well defined in many situations. Creating a learning contract has been suggested as a good place to start [7]. The learning contract starts with stating your goal. The learning contract includes your timeline, the steps you will take to learn the technique, and who you will engage to assist you with this task. The more modalities you implement as listed above, the greater the depth of your learning and the higher the likelihood that your implementation of NT&T will be successful.

Several barriers will inevitably need to be overcome to become competent in performing a new procedure. To illustrate this, we will outline a real-world example of the pathway one of the authors took to implement NT&T in their practice. As a relatively new faculty member, he set out to learn Per

Oral Endoscopic Myotomy (POEM) after completing a fellowship in minimally invasive surgery, which included only a limited number of therapeutic endoscopic cases but introduced our author to POEM (this procedure was still in the early phases of clinical experience). Our hospital had developed POEM privileging guidelines for the operating room, which also required surgeons to have upper endoscopy privileges in the general endoscopy center. The gastroenterologist-managed endoscopy center required a minimum of 200 upper endoscopies for privileging, which the author had not met despite the fellowship training and was unable to perform endoscopies at any other facilities as the author was an employed physician and this was not permitted under the hospital credentialing contract. So, in order to obtain privileges for POEM at our institution, additional POEM training was needed as well as credentialing for upper endoscopies in the GI endoscopy center. Through mentors within the department, a pathway was instituted that allowed for completion of the privileging requirements. The pathway was a program sponsored by SAGES and industry that offered advanced flexible endoscopy training to practicing surgeons. The program comprised two phases of training: first a 3-day hands-on training course in the USA with explant models, followed by a 2-week clinical hands-on advanced training at a high-volume international site, which included over 300 upper and lower endoscopies during the 2-week training period. Their POEM volume is also exceedingly high and on average a POEM per day was achieved with hands-on experience. Following completion of this program, credentialing requirements were met that then allowed for privileging for POEM after five proctored cases. This is just one of many possible pathways and no one pathway fits every surgeon or all NT&T. However, with adequate persistence and institutional support, a successful pathway can be managed and inevitable barriers overcome.

On the other hand, surgeons who want to incorporate a new technology into a procedure they already perform such as performing a procedure using a surgical robot in lieu of a laparoscopic approach may face fewer barriers to success. In order to ensure and maintain the highest level of care, SAGES has outlined guidelines for training and credentialing on this topic [8]. The basic premise for credentialing is that the surgeon must have the judgment and training to safely complete the procedure intended, as well as have the capability of immediately proceeding to an alternative therapy when circumstances indicate. There are two broad aspects to training with robotic systems. The first is technical training and capability. The second aspect of training involves the use of the robot for specific operations. Currently, the Food and Drug Administration (FDA) has in place a mandate that companies provide at least some of this training; at thus, at a minimum, surgeons must be trained to meet these FDA standards.

Training recommendations for surgeons without residency and/or fellowship training that included structured experience in therapeutic robotic procedures should mandate a structured curriculum. The curriculum should be defined by the institution and should include didactic education on the specific technology and an educational program for the specialty-specific approach to the organ systems. Hands-on training, which includes experience with the device in a dry lab environment as well as a specialty-specific model which may include animal, cadaveric, and/or virtual reality and simulation modeling, is necessary. Observation of live cases should be considered mandatory as well. Initial clinical experience on the specific procedure must be undertaken under the review of an expert and may include assisting and/or proctoring. An adequate number of cases to allow proficient completion of the procedure should be performed with this expert review. Criteria of competency as determined by the expert should be established in advance and should include evaluation of familiarity with instrumentation and equipment, competence in their use, appropriateness of patient selection, clarity of dissection, safety, and successful completion of the procedure [6].

What Are Institution-Level Responsibilities to Start NT&T?

As the pace of innovation is increasing, there are institutional-level responsibilities that have to be carried out as well. Institutional credentialing pathways have to keep up with the ability to introduce procedures that are either new to the institution or new to the field in general. These have to be anticipated in advance rather than coming up with last minute accommodations so appropriate balance can be struck between innovation and patient safety.

In the SAGES guidelines (which are based on available literature and expert opinion), the recommendation to the question of who should monitor the introduction of new procedures was given as follows:

> "To protect their patients, surgeons should demonstrate the highest level of professionalism and exercise self-assessment and self-regulation when introducing new technology and techniques in their practice. Besides the FDA, which regulates the production and sale of new devices, institutional credentialing and/or new technology committees and the IRB should monitor their introduction in clinical practice. The introduction of novel procedures should be overseen by the credentialing committee and/or the IRB, while the role of specialty societies and new technology committees needs further assessment." [2]

Who Approves and Monitors the Introduction of New Procedures?

Though self-assessment and self-regulation remains very important to ensure patient safety, it cannot be relied upon as one of the only safeguards. There are multiple factors that can influence the surgeon's decision to adopt a new procedure or using a new device/platform. These factors include pressures from industry or the healthcare systems, marketing pressures from patients and competing with colleagues, the novelty of a new procedure, or simply the desire to provide the most up-to-date care for their patients [2]. Due to these pressures, it's reasonable to conclude that someone other than the surgeons should also be involved in approval and subsequent monitoring of new procedures.

In the SAGES guidelines, for the device modification category, a majority agreed that surgeons themselves should be able to monitor the introduction of NT&T into their practice. For new devices, again it was surgeons themselves as well as the FDA that were considered the best options, with the credentialing committee and new technology committee monitoring new devices as well. For entirely new procedures, the credentialing committee of the institution would be the most important monitoring entity, followed by the surgeons and the IRB. Specialty societies could also play a role in this aspect, but it is unclear how they would do so at the local level. There are certain prerequisite elements that have been described as important for introduction of new procedures. This includes being credentialed by the local institution to perform procedures on the affected organ system.

What Should Be Assessed Before and After Introduction of a New Procedure?

It is important to establish safety, efficacy, and cost-effectiveness of any new procedure that is going to be adopted. Currently, one of the tools used for this assessment is health technology assessments (HTAs) [9]. These include effectiveness compared to alternative treatments or procedures, the safety profile, the cost compared to existing therapies, and patient outcomes. National societies such as SAGES have now created committees such as the Technology and Value Assessment Committee (TAVAC) that have been tasked to generate HTAs for minimally invasive surgery.

It is important to distinguish between the introduction of new technology and a new technique or procedure. The pathways for introduction and subsequent monitoring for a modified device versus a new device or technology and that of a new procedure will be different. It is also relevant whether that it is new procedure for the field or just new procedure locally for the surgeon as previously described.

In an academic setting, the Surgery Department Chair plays an important role in approving and/or recommending the initiation of a new procedure or technology at the hospital, as well as signing off on privileges for the practitioner. They may know and understand the current capabilities of the requesting surgeon and may have a better understanding of the training and courses taken thus far in preparation for the new procedure. They will also be able to follow the early experience closely and review the early patient outcomes closely as well. In smaller private and community hospitals, however, this can be less relevant. The Surgery Chair may be someone related to a completely different specialty (i.e., orthopedic surgery) and may not have the administrative setup or know-how to make a judgment on the practitioner's training and courses thus far and to follow the outcomes as closely.

Though national organizations and societies can provide guidelines regarding credentialing and privileging to perform a new procedure, this still largely remains the local institution's responsibility. They are responsible for verifying the requesting practitioner's training and determining its relevance and adequacy. Each institution may have its own system of privileging related to new procedures. The committee responsible needs to take into account guidance from existing literature as to what constitutes a completely new procedure or use of a completely new device versus what's a modified device in a modified or adaptation of a procedure and where there is overlap. Care must be taken to keep the credentialing and privileging process as objective as possible, as not to allow competing groups and local hospital politics to creep into the decision-making. Ultimately, each surgeon and institution bear the primary responsibility for establishing an appropriate and fair system that strikes the right balance between innovation and ensuring patient safety. Both the surgeon and institution have the most "skin in the game," aside from the patient, to ensure this is done appropriately as they may also have the highest liability risk.

What Is the Pathway to Surgeon Credentialing and Privileging for NT&T?

Utilizing correct terminology is very important. Credentialing refers to the verification of the surgeon's training, education, malpractice claims, professionalism, etc. Privileging was defined as the surgeon's scope of practice and the clinical services they can provide [9]. Since there isn't good data available to guide the privileging committees regarding the number of procedures needed for competency in most of the new procedures, and taking into account differing learning curves of surgeons, it is difficult to set a minimum number of procedures with confidence. As mentioned earlier, apart from having the privileges of working in that specific organ system, the level of training obtained and verified will depend on the complexity of the procedure and new technology. The Society of Thoracic Surgery (STS) task force suggested that due to the variability in complexity of new procedures and technology, it is difficult to set a defined pathway that can be applied to all new privileges being requested. A better approach would be to stress the importance of preparation to align the surgeon's existing skill set with the complexity of the new procedure or technology being implemented [9]. The hospital's normal credentialing and privileging process may not include the ability or expertise to pass judgment on a new technology or procedure being requested. Larger institutions may have an innovation/new technology committee or a specialty committee that can collaborate. Smaller institutions may need to seek guidance from a local or regional larger institution as a consulting service.

The American College of Surgeons (ACS) has defined a five-level verification model for documenting a surgeon's participation in educational programs and assessment of their knowledge and skills [6, 9]. These five levels include verification of attendance, verification of satisfactory completion of course objectives, verification of knowledge and skills, verification of preceptor experience, and demonstration of satisfactory patient outcomes. Building upon these levels,

Blackmon et al. proposed five levels of supervision when training for new procedures as shown in Table 27.2 [9]. These levels can be used to standardize educational course certifications to better understand the depth of training and verification the participant went through. The Joint Commission recommends that practitioners applying for new privileges undergo a focused professional practice evaluation (FPPE) [9]. This in turn can be used by hospital credentialing and privileging committees to assess readiness. Most of the time, if a FPPE is requested, data will have to be collected prospectively, and institutional review board (IRB) approval and safety monitoring will be needed. This is recommended by most when performing a new procedure that is new to the field not just new to the institution. This is needed when performing research comparing the new technique or technology

TABLE 27.2 Five levels of supervision when training for new technology and advanced procedures

Level 1	Certifies the learner attended a lecture or completed a lecture format course (no verification of skills)
Level 2	Certifies the learner completed a course and was assessed with a test or other evaluation of training and was provided feedback regarding their assessment score (a better model incorporates a minimum pass rate)
Level 3	Certifies the instructor observed the learner perform a skill and verified completion of task(s). Alternatively, the learner completed a course and participated in a lecture and skills lab, allowing assessment of the skills on a synthetic or tissue-based model
Level 4	Certifies the learner performed the procedure on a patient in a clinical setting with supervision (proctor or preceptor)
Level 5	Certifies the learner performed a series of clinical cases, the outcomes of which have been reviewed and verified. An example of level 5 learning may be submitting a series of video-recorded cases with outcomes to a review committee for verification

Adapted from Blackmon et al. [9]

to existing therapy. There may be an established procedure that has been performed for years in the field but involves a technology that has been granted a humanitarian device exemption (HDE) by the FDA like the gastric electrical stimulator, for example. IRB approval is needed for HDEs. When an FDA-approved device is used off-label, IRB approval is not usually needed unless the use is novel and there exists a lack of safety data. Of note, not only informed consent but proper disclosure to patients is also recommended in these circumstances as will be discussed later in the chapter.

Last but not least, since the highest priority needs to be given to patient safety in any adoption of new technology, all aspects have to be considered. The entire procedure team plays a very important role in adoption and has to be involved in the implementation. The team's education has to be planned out, including the equipment needed, number of personnel to perform the procedure, failure scenarios, and trouble shooting. Getting the procedure suite leadership involved is key as well to making it all happen. Accounting for all the various important aspects in getting started with a new procedure, the STS has developed a checklist to use as a guide for privileging as shown in Table 27.3 [9].

What Supervisory Options Are Available to Surgeons Adopting NT&T: Preceptoring vs Proctoring vs Telementoring?

Industry, institutions, and specialty societies are all stakeholders in having programs for preceptorship and proctorship to help surgeons learn new procedures. It is important to clarify the differences between them. Preceptors are usually experts in the procedures being taught and their role is to help a trainee acquire new skills. They usually assist in the procedures and provide feedback to the learners to help achieve learning objectives. They can take over the

TABLE 27.3 STS committee checklist for privileging

Verification of knowledge and skills assessment

ABTS-eligible or ABTS-certified surgeon

Documented completion of a course or didactic session

For recent graduates of an accredited program, case logs and a program director letter attesting to competence

Team management

Draft of implementation program complete

Education plan for team members complete

Crisis management plan complete

Institutional collaboration

IRB and/or institutional innovative care/new technology committee approval

Monitoring of outcomes

Participation in a continuous quality improvement committee and/or morbidity/mortality conference

Participation in an auditable database (e.g., National Surgical Quality Improvement Program, STS National Database, Michigan Society of Thoracic and Cardiovascular Surgeons Quality Collaborative) or registry or shared database that is accessible by the host institution

Demonstration of ability to present accurate and detailed morbidity and mortality rates to administration upon request

Patient-centered transparency

Provide appropriate consent forms for IRB and/or innovative committee approval

Provide the patient information on the risks and benefits of the new procedure, alternative treatments, general costs (i.e., to the patient or payer, or both), and comparative effectiveness of the new technology vs existing treatment options

(continued)

TABLE 27.3 (continued)

Provide the patient with information on the surgeons training and experience to date

Adapted from Blackmon et al. [9]

ABTS American Board of Thoracic Surgery, *IRB* Institutional Review Board, *STS* The Society of Thoracic Surgeons

care/surgery of the patient and carry more legal responsibility. An extended example of a preceptorship is a fellowship or a mini-fellowship.

Proctors also play an important role in the implementation of new procedures. They are involved in assessment and verification of knowledge and skills of the learner. They can provide feedback to the learner, but they generally do not teach the learner. They also usually don't scrub in the case and thus can't take over. The proctor reports their assessment to the accreditation body, such as the hospital credentialing committee. They are commonly used in assessment of surgeons starting new procedures in their practice as the logistical constraints are less, as is the legal risk for the proctor. These differences are highlighted in Table 27.4.

Telementoring

Telementoring is a further development in this field. This is especially relevant now since the COVID-19 pandemic. The definition of telementoring is "a relationship, facilitated by telecommunication technology, in which an expert (Mentor) provides guidance to a less-experienced learner (Mentee) from a remote location" [10]. Published systematic reviews on this topic showed no difference in clinical or educational outcomes for trainees that received on telementoring vs on-site mentoring [11, 12]. Some of the studies (four studies or 33% of them), in the most recent review, showed telementoring to be inferior to on-site mentoring, for example, with increased

TABLE 27.4 Principal differences between the roles and responsibilities of a preceptor and proctor

Preceptor

Principal role is to help the surgeon learner acquire new surgical knowledge and skills during the steep portion of the learning curve

Assesses and verifies the knowledge and skills of the surgeon learner to ensure achievement of learning objectives

Always provides feedback to the learner

Must be an expert in the performance of the new procedure or use of the new technology; such expertise is necessary for effective preceptoring

Generally assists in the operation and is readily available to take charge if the need arises

Associated with greater legal risk

Logistics more complex

Proctor

Principal role is to assess the knowledge and skills of the surgeon learner during the steep portion of the learning curve

Assesses and verifies the knowledge and skills of the surgeon learner to report the results to the Chief of Surgery or the institutional credentialing committee

May provide feedback to the learner

Does not always need to be an expert in the performance of a new procedure or use of a new technology; such expertise is desirable but not always necessary for effective proctoring

Generally serves as an observer

Associated with lesser legal risk

Logistics less complex

Adapted from Sacheva and Russell [6]

operative time; however, the majority showed telementoring to be as effective as on-site mentoring [12]. Telementoring was also thought to superior to no mentoring at all, but as the authors admit to in the limitations in their study, the data available has significant heterogeneity of the outcome measures and procedures [12]. Better designed studies are needed to draw more meaningful conclusions about telementoring, but it seems to be better than no mentoring, and maybe as good as on-site mentoring. Due to the logistical and financial challenges of on-site mentoring including its usually short time span, telementoring may have the ability to be superior as a training platform due to its ability to provide longitudinal training and follow-up with less logistical strain on the system. This recognition was the impetus for SAGES to convene the "Project 6 Summit" and publish a white paper [10]. They described the concerns regarding rapid adoption, using the example of laparoscopic cholecystectomies and the increase of common bile duct injuries by almost threefold initially. This technique was mostly adopted after attending weekend-type short courses without much longitudinal guidance. In contrast, there continue to be concerns about the very slow adoption of laparoscopy for colectomies [10]. The "Project 6" name was inspired by the military term "I got your six," meaning I got your back, describing the mentor and mentee relationship. One of the main barriers identified was availability of adequate training for surgeons in practice so they can feel comfortable to offer it to their patients. It may be that for more complex minimally invasive procedures, with a longer and steeper learning curve, more continued guidance may be needed. Due to the evolving field of surgery, with increased use of technology and new devices, surgeons may be required to undergo additional training several times in their career. A discussion of the details regarding the challenges and opportunities in telementoring is beyond the scope of this chapter, but they laid out the various areas that require work. These included legal and regulatory challenges of medical licensing, credentialing, liability, privacy, and consent. Business and value propositions for all the stakeholders like the surgeon (trainee), the hospital, industry, health insurance, and government are key areas as well. This would require a coordinated effort by all the stakeholders for success. They also include establishing appropriate communication and education requirements for the trainees so the training episodes can be efficient and effective. They also discussed technology limitations, logistics, and requirements to advance the field forward [12].

What Is the Role of Surgical Societies in NT&T?

Expert consensus from the SAGES guidelines suggested that health technology assessments for new procedures should be done by medical societies while keeping the patient's interests as a priority. Keeping this as an active committee that works to provide timely information regarding new procedures can help surgeons and hospital credentialing committees to make appropriate decisions regarding adoption of new procedures. Surgical societies can also play a role in helping follow outcomes. Database management can be quite challenging when left completely on a voluntary basis at and the individual or local level. National databases like NSQIP from the ACS can provide an important framework for data collection and monitoring.

To date, the most common way of learning a new procedure after postgraduate training is through a hands-on course. This is typically a 1-day or weekend course, with a cognitive portion and a skills portion, usually on a simulated model like a cadaver or porcine model [13]. The concern is that the return on investment in such courses is very low, as most practitioners fail to adopt in their practice what they have learned at these courses [13, 14]. With rapid advances in most surgical fields, nearly all surgeons will have to learn a new or modified procedure at some point in their career. The surgical societies, as advocates of surgeons and the surgical field itself, do and can play an even more important role in ensuring safe and timely adoption of new procedure, for the benefit of patients, surgeons, and society in general. With these concerns in mind, SAGES, through its Continuing Education Committee and its Quality, Outcomes, and Safety Committee, developed a hands-on course that employed standardized teaching techniques at the annual meeting and included a subsequent yearlong mentorship program. This was called the Acquisition of Data for Outcomes and Procedure Transfer (ADOPT) program.

The course participants were paired with a faculty member with whom they could communicate throughout the year to help them with case selection, preparation, etc. for starting new procedures in their practice. They were encouraged to participate in web meetings and submit videos for critique if needed. The timeline of training is shown in Fig. 27.2 [13]. The participants' experience was then compared to a standard hands-on course at the same meeting. The ADOPT participants performed significantly more procedures over the course of the first 3 months following the course compared to the stand hands-on course as shown in Fig. 27.3 [13].

Based on the positive results from the initial ADOPT course in 2015, all participants enrolled in the SAGES 2016 Annual Meeting Hands-on Hernia course were included in the ADOPT course (Fig. 27.3). This again demonstrated that adoption rates of the learned procedures were higher than before with increased confidence in participants as well [14].

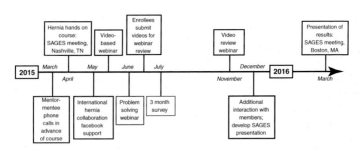

FIGURE 27.2 SAGES ADOPT program timeline 2015–2016. (Adapted from Dort et al. [13])

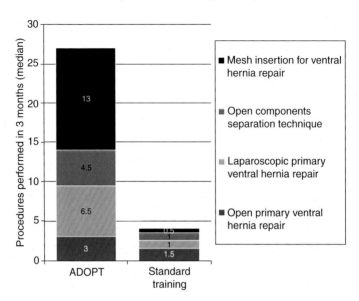

FIGURE 27.3 Median number of procedures performed over 3 months following training for ADOPT and standard training learners. (Adapted from Dort et al. [13])

This is thought to be in large part due to ongoing engagement and mentorship. Several barriers to mentorship have been described. These include time constraints, limited qualified mentors, lack of mentorship training and differences related to culture, and gender and generation gap between mentor and mentee [14, 15]. The SAGES ADOPT program enabled good mentorship by facilitating leaders in the field of hernia surgery to be available through a structured program. The program also mitigated potential barriers to good mentorship by standardizing instruction and feedback delivery and by selecting faculty from diverse backgrounds. As stated by Dort et al., the ADOPT program "...underscores the importance of standardized instruction by trained faculty, longitudinal mentorship, and the creation of a community of practice/ learners as a forum for discussion and learning" [14].

The surgical societies have an obligation not just to their members and sponsors but also to the patients and society at large. They can play a very important role in not just dissemination of the current "state of the science" information but also providing structured programs, backed by science, to increase adoption of new procedures. The surgeons/members have trust and confidence in these societies to do the vetting of appropriate programs and courses that they can then use to learn new procedures. As with the program described earlier where one of the authors went to India for additional training or with the ADOPT program, they would not be possible without the leadership and guidance of the national and international societies.

Ethics of Patient Disclosure

Patient safety is of utmost importance every time the decision is made to proceed with surgery. "*Primum non nocere*," the famous Hippocrates oath that guides our principal role as physicians, translates to "First, do no harm." As surgeons, we bear the foremost responsibility of effectively detailing the risks and benefits of a particular procedure to our patient including a discussion of alternatives, and thus obtaining "informed consent." In the era of surgical innovation, this is a delicate task for modern surgeons to balance, and we need to be well equipped to handle the ethical questions that arise especially as we deploy such new techniques and technology.

New surgical techniques and procedures fall outside the regulatory purview of the US Food and Drug Administration (FDA). Consequently, innovative procedures that are not performed under the supervision of IRB-approved research protocols are regulated at the local institutional level, and as a result, no uniform standards exist. Ultimately for patients, this translates to variability in timing and access to new surgical techniques and procedures based on practice patterns in their local community.

In 2014, SAGES released a detailed document outlining important ethical questions that are relevant to the implementation of new surgical techniques and technology in surgery [16]. In their manuscript, the authors pose six critical ethical questions that currently exist:

1. How is the safety of a new technology or technique ensured?
2. What are the timing and process by which a new technology or technique is implemented at a hospital?
3. How are patients informed before undergoing a new technology or technique?
4. How are surgeons trained and credentialed in a new technology or technique?
5. How are the outcomes of a new technology or technique tracked and evaluated?
6. How are the responsibilities to individual patients and society at large balanced?

This is followed by a thoughtful reflection on how best institutional strategies and cohesive efforts can be made to provide optimal execution of new surgical techniques in clinical practice. While the nuances of their manuscript are outside the scope of this discussion, we do want to highlight one of the key ethical and common questions that surgeons might encounter as they integrate novel surgical technique into their practice: How do we consent patients? This is an introspective question that reflects the important underlying theme of patient safety. When a patient is selected for a novel procedure or technique, in reality we are accepting potential morbidity and mortality that could very well befall patients that are exposed to so-called early adopters of new techniques and technology that is not present compared to the standard of care. In the 1990s, before laparoscopic cholecystectomy became standard of care, the learning curve associated with the operation most likely contributed to the prevalence of common bile duct injuries [16, 17].

The learning curve associated with the adoption of new surgical technique into clinical practice poses a serious ethical dilemma for the surgeon-patient relationship. In surgical innovation, the inability of the surgeon-innovator to flatten the learning curve without gaining experience from patients in clinical practice compounds this ethical dilemma. Of note, this dilemma is not entirely akin to the situation that exists with trainees in surgical residency programs specifically in two distinct ways. Firstly, residents are ultimately subject to oversight from credentialed surgeons as mandated by ACGME clinical competency guidelines [18]. Secondly, surgeon-innovators are typically experienced physicians with demonstrated proficiency in their field of practice seeking out a new skill set. Thus, surgical innovation portends a different ethical entity.

In 2014, Bracken-Roche et al. published a systematic review regarding patient disclosure and autonomy in surgical innovation [19]. In their manuscript, they highlight "four central tension points" identified in the literature that impact the patient disclosure process and autonomy. One of these points is the "misconception" that patients might construe "new or innovative" to mean better care for their surgical disease. They also describe the notion of the skewed surgeon-innovator and patient relationship with its inherent asymmetric power differential that exists – "patients feel they owe a certain deference to surgeon." This could be further exacerbated by the fact that "surgeons may lack objectivity when they themselves are the innovator or strong supporters of the innovation." All of these contribute to a complicated disclosure process that preserves patient autonomy and legal determination.

Against this backdrop, surgeons must understand and develop equitable inclusion-exclusion criteria of patient selection for novel procedures and techniques. At the crux of this selection algorithm is patient-centered transparency. Clear communication of known risks, benefits, long-term outcomes if available, and how this novel technique compares to the standard of care should be provided to the patient. Conflicts of interests that exist, for example, any financial relationships with medical industry sponsoring proposed technique or device, must also be disclosed to the patient [17].

Additionally, in our increasingly litigious society, the learning curve should be addressed as part of the disclosure process [20]. In their manuscript, Healy and Samanta tackle the ethical and legal implications of this learning curve in clinical practice. As alluded to earlier, the "drive to … enhance (clinical) outcomes places surgical innovation as pivotal to clinical progress." However, as the authors point out, this comes with a learning curve that poses "material risk" to patients and therefore subject to disclosure in law. Therefore, given this legal precedence, the "performance data of a surgeon may be a material factor for a patient in the consent process" and ideally should be disclosed. An important final point to highlight is that the decision to proceed or not is a shared decision process between the surgeon and patient after weighing both merits and risks of the proposed technique or technology.

Finally, as surgeons, we must recognize biases inherent in our role as physician. In essence, our duty is not just to our individual patients at a single point in time. We also hold a larger responsibility to society in our role as stewards of surgical innovation in order to advance the fields of science and surgery. We also ought to weigh the financial cost of implementing new technology in today's economy of ballooning healthcare costs and be cognizant of our role in providing cost-effective care to patients. Against this milieu of competing interests, we must always strive to provide high-quality care to our patients as we make strides in surgical innovation and technology.

References

1. Hutchinson K, Rogers W, Eyers A, et al. Getting clearer about surgical innovation: a new definition and a new tool to support responsible practice. Ann Surg. 2015;262:949–54.
2. SAGES. Guidelines for the introduction of new technology and techniques. Available at: https://www.sages.org/publications/guidelines/guidelines-introduction-new-technology-techniques/. Accessed 8 Aug 2020.

3. Maddern GJ. Introduction of new surgical techniques and technologies. ANZ J Surg. 2019;89:625–7.
4. Khachane A, et al. Appraising the uptake and use of the IDEAL framework and recommendations: a review of the literature. Int J Surg. 2018;57:84–90.
5. Hirst A, et al. No surgical innovation without evaluation: evolution and further development of the IDEAL framework and recommendations. Ann Surg. 2019;269(2):211–20.
6. Sacheva AK, Russell TR. Safe introduction of new procedures and emerging technologies in surgery: education, credentialing, and privileging. Surg Clin North Am. 2007;87(4):853–66, vi–vii.
7. Murnaghan JJ. The learning curve and the practicing surgeon: Integrating a new skill and procedure into your practice. **2013.
8. Herron DM, Marohn M, SMRSC Group. A consensus document on robotic surgery. Surg Endosc. 2008;22(2):313–25; discussion 311–2.
9. Blackmon SH, Cooke DT, Whyte R, et al. The Society of Thoracic Surgeons expert consensus statement: a tool kit to assist thoracic surgeons seeking privileging to use new technology and perform advanced procedures in general thoracic surgery. Ann Thorac Surg. 2016;101(3):1230–7. https://doi.org/10.1016/j.athoracsur.2016.01.061. PMID: 27124326.
10. Schlachta CM, Nguyen NT, Ponsky T, et al. Project 6 summit: SAGES telementoring initiative. Surg Endosc. 2016;30(9):3665–72. https://doi.org/10.1007/s00464-016-4988-5. Epub 2016 Jun 6. PMID: 27270593.
11. Erridge S, Yeung DKT, Patel HRH, et al. Telementoring of surgeons: a systematic review. Surg Innov. 2019;26(1):95–111. https://doi.org/10.1177/1553350618813250. Epub 2018 Nov 22. PMID: 30465477.
12. Bilgic E, Turkdogan S, Watanabe Y, et al. Effectiveness of telementoring in surgery compared with on-site mentoring: a systematic review. Surg Innov. 2017;24(4):379–85. https://doi.org/10.1177/1553350617708725. Epub 2017 May 11. PMID: 28494684.
13. Dort J, Trickey A, Paige J, et al. Hands-on 2.0: improving transfer of training via the Society of American Gastrointestinal and Endoscopic Surgeons (SAGES) Acquisition of Data for Outcomes and Procedure Transfer (ADOPT) program. Surg Endosc. 2017;31(8):3326–32. https://doi.org/10.1007/s00464-016-5366-z. Epub 2016 Dec 30. PMID: 28039640.

14. Dort J, Trickey A, Paige J, et al. All in: expansion of the acquisition of data for outcomes and procedure transfer (ADOPT) program to an entire SAGES annual meeting hands-on hernia course. Surg Endosc. 2018;32(11):4491–7. https://doi.org/10.1007/s00464-018-6196-y. Epub 2018 May 1. PMID: 29717374.

15. Entezami P, Franzblau LE, Chung KC. Mentorship in surgical training: a systematic review. Hand (N Y). 2012;7(1):30–6. https://doi.org/10.1007/s11552-011-9379-8. Epub 2011 Nov 29. PMID: 23448749; PMCID: PMC3280364.

16. SAGES. Ethical considerations regarding the implementation of new technologies and techniques in surgery. Available at: https://www.sages.org/publications/guidelines/ethical-considerations-regarding-implementation-new-technologies-techniques-surgery/. Accessed 15 Aug 2020.

17. Sudarshan M, Blackmon S. Best practices for training, educating and introducing new techniques and technology into practice. Thorac Surg Clin. 2018;28:573–8.

18. ACGME. Common Program Requirements (Residency). Available at: https://www.acgme.org/Portals/0/PFAssets/ProgramRequirements/CPRResidency2020.pdf. Accessed 7 Sept 2020.

19. Bracken-Roche D, Bell E, Karpowicz L, et al. Disclosure, consent, and the exercise of patient autonomy in surgical innovation: a systematic content analysis of the conceptual literature. Account Res. 2014;21(6):331–52.

20. Healey P, Samanta J. When does the 'learning curve' of innovative interventions become questionable practice? Eur J Vasc Endovasc Surg. 2008;36:253–7.

Part IV
Working Towards Surgical Quality, Outcomes, and Safety

Chapter 28
Team Training

John T. Paige

Introduction

"Do what you can, with what you have, where you are."
– Theodore Roosevelt

Roosevelt's words highlight the importance of functional teamwork in modern healthcare. Teams are the foundational component for the effective delivery of safe, quality patient care. This fact is especially true in the contemporary, dynamic clinical setting in which the sheer volume of annually introduced new knowledge and technology makes it impossible for an individual provider to care solely for a patient. Instead, distributed expertise across a team is necessary in which the members seamlessly coordinate and smoothly communicate with one another to achieve the common goal of optimizing patient outcomes. To Theodore Roosevelt, clinicians can do what they can to help a patient through optimization of the function of the teams on which they participate in the healthcare setting.

J. T. Paige (✉)
Department of Surgery, MedicineLouisiana State University (LSU) Health New Orleans School of Medicine, New Orleans, LA, USA
e-mail: jpaige@lsuhsc.edu

J. R. Romanelli et al. (eds.), *The SAGES Manual of Quality, Outcomes and Patient Safety*,
https://doi.org/10.1007/978-3-030-94610-4_28

537

Given the importance of teams in providing care to the patient, team development is a high priority within the healthcare industry in general and organizations and their institutions in particular. Team science provides many such interventions to improve team function [1]. Their successful application in healthcare would do much to address the many deficiencies in teamwork that currently exist. Key to achieving this goal is a knowledge of team dynamics as well as a familiarity of the useful strategies for optimizing them.

This chapter's goal is to aid in developing high-functioning teams in healthcare. It will accomplish this task in the following three ways: (1) reviewing the present status of teamwork in healthcare, (2) applying team science to develop effective healthcare teams, and (3) employing a framework for the successful implementation of team development initiatives.

Present Status of Teamwork in Healthcare

One of the best examples of the importance of team interaction in healthcare is Schmutz et al.'s meta-analysis of 1390 teams in acute care settings that demonstrated a positive, medium-sized effect between teamwork and clinical performance [2]. Their work showed that high team performance was 2.8 times more likely to occur in teams who used team processes. The fact that team training in healthcare improves care processes and outcomes in addition to team processes and behaviors is further proof of the power of teamwork in providing safe, quality care [3].

Teamwork is a crucial component in the delivery of effective healthcare. For more than a decade, however, investigators have demonstrated that it has been less than ideal. Moreover, deficiencies are not isolated to one specific competency or aspect of teamwork, but, instead, encompass elements across the entire spectrum of knowledge, skills, and abilities (KSAs) associated with it. Most salient is the cultural milieu in which the members of the healthcare team conduct their work. Early on, researchers recognized the pervasive silo mentality, best illustrated in the operating room (OR), that resulted in multi-professional interaction in lieu of true inter-professional collaboration [4, 5]. This attitude arises in part out of the episodic, specialty-centered structure of care [6]. In addition, it develops due to the cloistered nature of the educational and training processes for each profession [7]. Finally, it evolves from the differing value systems within each profession [5, 8] that leads to socialization favoring early and rigid differentiation between and hierarchical ordering among the different professions [9].

Not surprisingly, the healthcare work culture also promotes a professional tribalism fostering an "us" versus "them" mindset that facilitates blame shifting to other professions (i.e., "them") [10]. As a result, separate professions might harbor values and attitudes, use communication techniques, learn, and have expectations related to the progression of care that are diametrically opposed to one another [7, 8]. This situation reduces team cohesion, leading to tension and conflict [11]. Interestingly, the cultural context of the work environment, not the innate character of the individual team members themselves, seems to contribute to this tribalism [12]. Such a toxic clinical setting becomes self-perpetuating through the adoption of negative attitudes and behaviors by students who rotate through it as part of their educational experience, the so-called "hidden curriculum" [13].

The silo mentality and tribalism of the healthcare cultural environment negatively influence team processes and performance on multiple levels. Ineffective communication within the OR team is a prominent example. In the 2000s, research demonstrated that approximately one-third of communications within the OR failed in their intentions [14]. Almost a decade later, such communication failures persisted [15, 16]. Even today, OR team members might not know one another's name [17]. They may not communicate a clear understanding of the steps of a procedure to one another [18, 19]. Closed-loop communication may be lacking [20]. Trauma team communication is an additional example. Like the OR, closed-loop communication is also limited between the team members [21]. Furthermore, communication is often via so-called "mixed mode" methods in which a team member infers a task via a question; these mixed mode methods are ineffective in promoting team function [22].

Communication within healthcare teams is fraught with difficulties, including failure to translate requests into action, use of ineffective methods of communication, and an inability to convey basic pieces of information such as names and procedure steps. Similar deficiencies exist related to the lack of role clarity within healthcare teams [23], differing perceptions of interprofessional collaboration [24–27] and communication [28], and disparate hierarchical views [18, 29], and mental models [30]. These issues related to teamwork have negative consequences related to various professions' view of the safety culture [31, 32], discouraging individuals from speaking up regarding safety issues [33, 34]. In addition, they lead to disruptions, incivility, and bullying that undermine individual and team clinical performance and impede workflow [35, 36]. These altered team processes negatively impact clinical processes and outcomes [37–39].

Almost two decades ago, therefore, researchers knew that teamwork in healthcare had significant deficiencies and gaps that required interventions to improve them. Unfortunately, these issues have persisted to present day. Fortunately, a century's worth of team science research can lead to a better understanding of how teams work and the evidence-based interventions that can help them improve performance.

Team Science and Developing Healthcare Teams

Since its origins defining the Hawthorne effect [40], team science has grown into a field encompassing a wide variety of specialties ranging from social to applied psychology. This field has made major contributions to defining and delineating the intricacies of teams, teamwork, and team performance and ways to improve their function. One of its key foundational principles is that a team is more than the sum of its individual constituent members [41]. The expression "a team of experts does not necessarily make an expert team" encapsulates this concept in conveying the fact that even a group of experts can fail if they cannot coordinate and communicate well in order to cooperate [41]. Thus, a useful framework in which to view a team is as a *complex adaptive system (CAS)*. Within a CAS, interrelations within the system interact with influences outside the system in an iterative, nonlinear, interdependent manner to create evolving and emerging outcomes that are more than a cause-and-effect relationship [42]. At the team level, these interrelations arise from the fact that individual team members act autonomously according to their own internal motivations and rules of behaviors. An action on one member's part, however small, therefore, can have an outsized impact on team function. Additionally, as the team reacts to its past actions and environmental conditions, unpredictable and new team behaviors can arise. In this manner, the output of a team is greater than the cumulative sum of what its individual members could produce [43].

A further layer of complexity, seen in healthcare, is the fact that a team does not typically operate in a vacuum, but, instead, it interacts in an interdependent manner with other teams within an organization. Within such a multi-team system, each individual team has its own interactions and goals. These specialized goals are part of the "superordinate" goals of the system itself that require coordination, communication, and cooperation among the teams for their achievement [44]. The interaction of the multiple teams caring for a trauma victim is a good example of such a multi-team system. First, the emergency medical services (EMS) team must go to the scene, then assess, stabilize, and transport the patient to the emergency department, communicating and coordinating with the trauma resuscitation team there. Next, the trauma team must evaluate and resuscitate the patient, communicating and coordinating with the OR team for transfer to surgery or the critical care team for transfer to the intensive care unit. Finally, the OR and critical care teams must communicate and coordinate between each other for trips to the OR to care for the patient. Although each team may have a specialized goal, the overarching system goal is to provide safe, quality care to the trauma patient.

A useful definition of a team is as a group of two or more individuals working interdependently with defined roles to achieve a common goal [45]. In healthcare, teams vary considerably according to their skill differentiation, temporal stability, and authority differentiation, depending on their composition [46]. For example, a trauma resuscitation team that forms consisting of emergency physicians, trauma surgeons, emergency nurses, and respiratory therapists during a shift to treat a critically injured patient brought into the emergency department is a team having a high degree of skill differentiation and authority differentiation but temporal instability. Conversely, all the members of a team of oncologists working together to treat a cancer patient with chemotherapy have the same set of skills and equal hierarchical positions, making this team one with low skill differentiation and authority differentiation but temporal stability.

In order to achieve a team's common goal, team members perform both *taskwork* and *teamwork*. Taskwork consists of those processes that an individual performs that are *independent* of other team members' activities. Teamwork, on the other hand, are those processes of an individual that are *interdependent* with other team members' actions, requiring coordination among those individuals involved [47]. As such, teamwork consists of an interrelated set of team-level attitudinal (e.g., team cohesion and trust), behavioral (e.g., coordination, communication), and cognitive states (e.g., team learning, shared mental model) (the so-called ABCs of teamwork), which combine to influence team performance [48]. A team's effectiveness, therefore, is dependent on the quality of its teamwork.

The input-process-output (IPO) model of team effectiveness is a popular framework in which to conceptualize teamwork and its components ([49], Fig. 28.1). This model posits that inputs to the team influence team processes, thereby

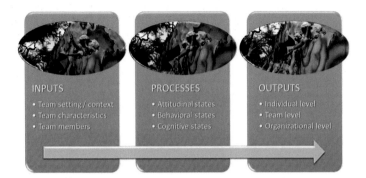

FIGURE 28.1 IPO model of team effectiveness

affecting team outcomes. Inputs can arise from the setting or context in which the team operates (e.g., the work environment, information available to the team), from the team characteristics themselves (e.g., the team composition, the difficulty of the assignment), or from the individuals who constitute the team (e.g., personality traits, KSAs). Team processes are those ABCs of teamwork that allow the team to coordinate, communicate, and cooperate. Finally, outputs consist of the team outcomes flowing from the processes they enact. In healthcare, these outputs fall into individual, team, and organizational categories [46]. Team member satisfaction, health, well-being, engagement, commitment, and performance are individual-level outcomes. At the team level, outcomes include the quality of healthcare the team provides and patient satisfaction. Organizational-level outcomes consist of overall patient satisfaction and quality of care as well as resource use, staff turnover and absenteeism, financial performance, and patient mortality and morbidity.

The IPO framework further subdivides teamwork into three additional processes: (1) transition, (2) action, and (3) interpersonal ([49], Fig. 28.2). The team's episodes of performance temporally situate these phases with transition processes occurring between episodes, action processes spanning the episodes, and interpersonal processes taking place both between and during episodes. Each process, in turn, has

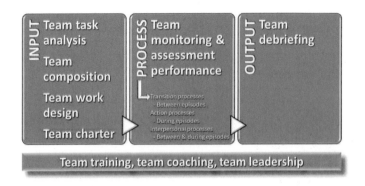

FIGURE 28.2 The input-process-output (IPO) model and team development interventions

discrete phases that can occur within it [50]. Mission analysis, goal specification, and strategy formation and planning comprise the transition process components. Monitoring progress toward goals, systems monitoring, team monitoring and backup behavior, and coordination make up the action process constituents. Finally, conflict management, motivating and confidence building, and affect management are the interpersonal process elements.

All three processes and their more narrowly defined components positively correlate with team performance and team member satisfaction. Once more, they also have a positive, strong relationship with team cohesion (i.e., team members' attraction and commitment to their team, team members, and team task) and team potency (i.e., the shared belief that the team can be effective). Finally, the correlation between these processes and team performance is stronger with increasing team size and greater task interdependence [50].

In addition to elucidating the dynamics of team interaction via the IPO model, team science has also identified which team processes help teams to achieve superior outcomes. Several frameworks exist delineating the critical process components that promote high team performance. One of these frameworks is healthcare-based. The Team Strategies & Tools to Enhance Performance and Patient Safety™ (TeamSTEPPS™) promotes team structure through a focus on leadership, communication, situation monitoring, and mutual support [51]. This program's framework arose from the Big Five Model of Teamwork that defined five key team-based competencies, team leadership, team orientation, backup behavior, mutual performance monitoring, and adaptability, moderated by three coordinating mechanisms, shared mental models, closed-loop communication, and mutual trust [52]. Finally, the 7C's framework posits five components: cooperation, coordination, communication, cognition, and coaching, with two influencing factors, competence and conditions [53].

Evidence-based team development interventions (TDIs), targeting one or more components of the IPO framework, can aid in teaching teams these recognized team processes that lead to superior team performance ([45], Fig. 28.2). TDIs targeting team inputs include team task analysis, which identifies key behaviors for success, and team composition, which selects team members based on their individual attributes. Team composition can influence team performance by shaping the ABCs of teamwork via team attributes, team operationalizations, the context in which the team is acting, and temporal considerations [48]. Thus, team composition can influence the emergence of particular team moods based on individual personality traits. Teams with members who value teamwork cooperate more and have greater confidence. Conscientious team members led to teams that self-regulate teamwork. Members who are sociable help teams perform the ABCs better and promote reciprocity among members. Finally, teams with high cognitive abilities tend to work well together. On the downside, team composition can create fault lines in which the creation of intra-team coalitions causes conflict and impedes performance [48]. The two final input-oriented TDIs are team-based work design, which attempts to structure roles and tasks within the broader team, and team charter, a process of clarifying team direction through the creation of a charter of team activity [45].

Team monitoring and assessment performance and team debriefing are process- and output-targeted TDIs, respectively [45]. The former attempts to assess the team's progress to its goal(s). The latter involves self-reflection and team reflexivity to identify gaps in performance and develop process improvements to advance outcomes. Team debriefing is a powerful method of TDI, since it engages team members in active experiential learning, makes them more open to new ideas and insights, and builds a team's shared mental model [1]. Its utility is illustrated by the fact that team debriefs alone increase team performance by an average of 20–25% [54].

Team training, team building, team coaching, and team leadership are four TDIs that can target inputs, processes, or outputs within the IPO framework [45]. Team training and team building target team-level processes with team training that teaches team-based competencies and team building that focuses on interpersonal interactions [1]. Team training improves specific KSAs related to high team performance. Knowledge-based competencies include situational awareness, transactive memory systems, and shared mental models. Skill-based competencies encompass coordination, communication, conflict resolution, shared leadership, and backup behavior. Attitude-based competencies involve team cohesion, commitment to teamwork, psychological safety, mutual trust, and collective efficacy. Team training as a TDI has demonstrated moderate, positive effects between interventions and team KSAs, processes, performances, and outcomes [47, 55]. Team building focuses on improving the dynamics of the team through goal setting, interpersonal-relationship management, role clarification, and problem solving [1].

Team leadership is the one of the few TDIs that focuses its activities at the individual team member level [1]. Such training can be as powerful as team debriefing, improving learning, transfer, and organizational outcomes by as much as 29% [56]. Additional benefits include that it improves outcomes related to the leader's subordinates (e.g., satisfaction levels, turnover) and it increases leadership capabilities, thereby improving team performance. Key to success of leadership training is using evidence-based recommendations in curricula development. In particular, quality training content, learner motivation, and organizational support are essential for transfer of learning [1]. Finally, team coaching is a TDI used to enhance behavior changes arising out of other TDIs through interaction with the team to help its members coordinate tasks and resources in order to achieve its goal(s) [45].

TDIs have value in healthcare. As stated earlier, teams that use team processes in healthcare are 2.8 times more likely to have high team performance [2]. Two of the most popular TDIs used in healthcare currently are team debriefing and team training [57]. Team debriefing leads to improved outcomes [58]. It accomplishes this improvement through active learning of the team members and the creation of a shared understanding of team priorities, strengths, and weaknesses [1]. Such team-level reflection of goals, processes, and strategies with adaptation to team function is the hallmark of team reflexivity, a characteristic especially useful in situations involving complex tasks and uncertainty of outcomes [59].

Team training is the most popular TDI currently used in healthcare. It leads to better clinical processes and outcomes by improving team processes and performance [3]. Additionally, it causes reductions in medical errors as well as improvements in safety climate [60]. Among team training modalities, simulation-based training (SBT) and the use of structured curricula focusing on team-based competencies, such as TeamSTEPPS™, are common approaches. Advantages of SBT that make it particularly attractive as a team training modality are several. First, it provides a team the opportunity to practice team-based KSAs in a safe learning environment without harm to a patient [61]. Second, it gives teams the ability to practice treating low-frequency, high-risk events in order to hone team response and efficiency of therapy [62]. When combined with curricula such as TeamSTEPPS™, SBT results in enhanced skill acquisition, decreased adverse outcomes, and retention of learning [63].

In addition to SBT, team training can occur via didactic lectures, tabletop exercises, web-based teaching, video-based activities, and role-play [64, 65]. Regardless of the approach taken, the training must rest on sound educational principles related to curriculum development, delivery, and evaluation. Adherence to an established curriculum development framework when putting such training together ensures optimal effectiveness. Kern's approach is popular in medical education. It involves employing the following six steps: (1) problem identification and general needs assessment, (2) targeted needs assessment, (3) creation of goals and objectives, (4) selection of educational strategies, (5) implementation of curriculum, and (6) curriculum evaluation and feedback [66]. Another framework uses the acronym ADDIE to delineate its key components: analysis, design, development, implementation, and evaluation [67].

Effective delivery of a curriculum also relies on using recognized methods. For example, in SBT, the scenario used has an important impact on the experiential learning. One useful methodology for its development is the event-based approach to training (EBAT) [68] that has had success in creating scenarios for trauma team training [69]. In addition, SBT requires skilled facilitators for after-action debriefing. They must foster a safe learning environment, guide learners through their emotional response to the scenario, assist in identifying gaps in performance and finding solutions to them, and encourage participants to commit to change in behavior. In short, their duties include making it safe, making it stick, and making it last [70].

Finally, curricula and training programs must undergo comprehensive evaluation in order to determine how well they work and to discover areas for improvement. Like curriculum development, curricula and program evaluation should follow an accepted, systematic approach to gauge its effectiveness. Kirkpatrick's framework for evaluating training effectiveness is a well-known one that assesses a program on four levels of potential change. The first level gauges participants' reaction to the training. The second level assesses the degree of learning of the participants resulting from the training. The third level measures the extent of participant behavioral change in the workplace arising from the training, and the fourth level evaluates the organizational impact in terms of outcomes due to the training [71]. Team training in healthcare demonstrates a clear progression from learning to behavior change to improvement in outcomes [60].

Like all TDIs, their utility is only as effective as the measurements used to assess their effectiveness. Thus, any teamwork or team performance instrument must be accurate and reliable and show validity for use in the population assessed. Due to the complexity of interaction among the affective states, behaviors, and cognitive components of teamwork, such tools require multiple items to address the multidimensional aspects of teamwork in order to assess it adequately [72]. In healthcare, this need has produced over 80 different rater-based assessments of teamwork and nontechnical skills, that combination of interpersonal and cognitive abilities [73]. Nearly all these instruments assess communication, teamwork, and leadership constructs, and up to 80% of them evaluate task management and situation awareness. All have undergone a degree of content validity and about two-thirds have compared the tool to various learner characteristics, such as expertise. Only about 15% have evidence of convergent validity. Eighty percent of these tools have measured inter-rater reliability. Only a little over half have evidence of internal consistency, and only about 15% have evaluated test-retest reliability [73]. A lack of comprehensive psychomotor evaluation also exists among the self-report surveys used to gauge participants' views of team interactions [74]. With these types of instruments, items related to team cohesion and perceived team effectiveness are common.

Successfully Implementing Team Development Interventions

Applying team science to enhancing teamwork in healthcare is insufficient without employing an implementation strategy that will foster its success. The field of implementation science has developed in order to ensure the systematic uptake of evidence-based research into clinical practice in healthcare. Its application can quintuple the effectiveness of an intervention and decrease the time it takes to implement it by one-sixth [75]. The World Health Organization delineates several critical components to implementation. These include having adequate resources, proper training and education, oversight and measurement of progress, effective communication strategies, and collaboration through cultural change [76].

Cultural change is quite challenging in any situation. It involves multiple steps that help change the prevailing attitudes and assumptions of an organization over time. John Kotter's eight-step model is promoted by TeamSTEPPS™ [51]. It begins with creating a sense of urgency for change. Next, it involves bringing together a guiding coalition of like-minded individuals who then help with the subsequent steps of developing a vision and strategy for change that they then communicate to others in the organization. The subsequent step empowers other individuals in the organization for broad-based action. These steps then allow the generation of short-term wins that are celebrated. Gains consolidate to encourage more change, and then, finally, the new approaches anchor themselves into the culture [77].

For team training in healthcare, Friscella et al. have recognized five key components to ensure its successful implementation [78]. First, a careful needs assessment helps determine the targeted gaps that one addresses. Second, the team training must occur in a safe, noncritical learning environment. Third, the training program's design must maximize availability, learning, and usability. Fourth, the training program must undergo an evaluation of its effectiveness. Finally, a means to sustain the learned team behaviors must develop [78].

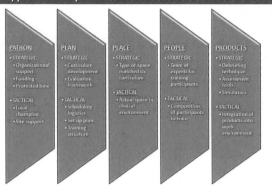

FIGURE 28.3 The 5P approach to implementation of simulation-based team training

An illustrative example of the successful implementation of a team training program is the NetworkZ SBT program to enhance communication and teamwork in the operating room across all of New Zealand [79]. The researchers used the Organizing for Quality framework in identifying and addressing challenges to adoption of the program. Through this process, they learned several key lessons. National backing of the program and local ownership of it were two such learning points. Multilevel support and the necessity of presenting evidence for training were another set of insights. The recognition of the difficulty of cultural change and the impact of quality on fostering acceptance of the program were also important lessons. Finally, ongoing communication was necessary to maintain support [79].

Another example is the successful creation of a point of care SBT program for OR team training [80]. In this situation, the researchers utilized a "5P" approach to guide them in recognizing and tackling barriers to implementation (Fig. 28.3) [81]. This framework divides such challenges into five broad categories of decreasing order of importance: (1) finding a *patron*, (2) developing a *plan*, (3) locating a *place*, (4) assembling your *people*, and (5) choosing your *products*.

Each category has tactical and strategic components that require consideration.

Conclusion

Teams remain the foundational unit in healthcare, and their effective function leads to safe, quality patient care. Current teamwork, however, continues to be less than ideal in clinical settings. Team science can help enhance team dynamics through proven TDIs that, when combined with sound educational and implementation science principles, can foster highly reliable team behavior to improve patient processes and outcomes.

References

1. Lacerenza CN, Marlow SL, Tannenbaum SI, Salas E. Team development interventions: evidence-based approaches for improving teamwork. Am Psychol. 2018;73(4):517–31.
2. Schmutz JB, Meier LL, Manser T. How effective is teamwork really? The relationship between teamwork and performance in healthcare teams: a systematic review and meta-analysis. BMJ Open. 2019;9(9):e028280. https://doi.org/10.1136/bmjopen-2018-028280.
3. Weaver SJ, Dy SM, Rosen MA. Team training in healthcare: a narrative synthesis of the literature. BMJ Qual Saf. 2014;23(5):359–72.
4. Bleakley A. You are who I say you are: the rhetorical construction of identity in the operating theatre. J Work Learn. 2006a;18(7):414–25.
5. Bleakley A, Boyden J, Hobbs A, Walsh L, Allard J. Improving teamwork climate in operating theatres: the shift from multiprofessionalism to interprofessionalism. J Interprof Care. 2006b;20(5):461–70.
6. Pepler EF, Pridie J, Brown S. Predicting and testing a silo-free delivery system. Healthc Manage Forum. 2018;31(5):200–5.

7. Weller J, Boyd M, Cumin D. Teams, tribes and patient safety: overcoming barriers to effective teamwork in healthcare. Postgrad Med J. 2014;90(1061):149–54.

8. Hall P. Interprofessional teamwork: professional cultures as barriers. J Interprof Care. 2005;19(Suppl 1):188–96.

9. Price S, Doucet S, Hall LM. The historical social positioning of nursing and medicine: implications for career choice, early socialization and interprofessional collaboration. J Interprof Care. 2014;28(2):103–9.

10. Mannix R, Nagler J. Tribalism in medicine-us vs them. JAMA Pediatr. 2017;171(9):831.

11. Gillespie BM, Chaboyer W, Wallis M, Fenwick C. Why isn't 'time out' being implemented? An exploratory study. Qual Saf Health Care. 2010;19(2):103–6.

12. Braithwaite J, Clay-Williams R, Vecellio E, Marks D, Hooper T, Westbrook M, Blakely B, Ludlow K. The basis of clinical tribalism, hierarchy and stereotyping: a laboratory-controlled teamwork experiment. BMJ Open. 2016;6(7):e012467-2016-012467.

13. Doja A, Bould MD, Clarkin C, Eady K, Sutherland S, Writer H. The hidden and informal curriculum across the continuum of training: a cross-sectional qualitative study. Med Teach. 2016;38(4):410–8.

14. Lingard L, Espin S, Whyte S, Regehr G, Baker GR, Reznick R, Bohnen J, Orser B, Doran D, Grober E. Communication failures in the operating room: an observational classification of recurrent types and effects. Qual Saf Health Care. 2004;13(5):330–4.

15. Halverson AL, Casey JT, Andersson J, Anderson K, Park C, Rademaker AW, Moorman D. Communication failure in the operating room. Surgery. 2011;149(3):305–10.

16. Sevdalis N, Wong HW, Arora S, Nagpal K, Healey A, Hanna GB, Vincent CA. Quantitative analysis of intraoperative communication in open and laparoscopic surgery. Surg Endosc. 2012;26(10):2931–8.

17. Bodor R, Nguyen BJ, Broder K. We are going to name names and call you out! Improving the team in the academic operating room environment. Ann Plast Surg. 2017;78(5 Suppl 4):S222–4.

18. Etherington N, Wu M, Cheng-Boivin O, Larrigan S, Boet S. Interprofessional communication in the operating room: a narrative review to advance research and practice. [Communication interprofessionnelle en salle d'operation: un compte rendu narratif pour faire avancer la recherche et la pratique]. Can J Anaesth. 2019;66(10):1251–60.

19. Kenawy D, Schwartz D. An evaluation of perioperative communication in the operating room. J Perioper Pract. 2018;28(10):267–72.
20. Davis WA, Jones S, Crowell-Kuhnberg AM, O'Keeffe D, Boyle KM, Klainer SB, Smink DS, Yule S. Operative team communication during simulated emergencies: too busy to respond? Surgery. 2017;161(5):1348–56.
21. El-Shafy IA, Delgado J, Akerman M, Bullaro F, Christopherson NAM, Prince JM. Closed-loop communication improves task completion in pediatric trauma resuscitation. J Surg Educ. 2018;75(1):58–64.
22. Jung HS, Warner-Hillard C, Thompson R, Haines K, Moungey B, LeGare A, Shaffer DW, Pugh C, Agarwal S, Sullivan S. Why saying what you mean matters: an analysis of trauma team communication. Am J Surg. 2018;215(2):250–4.
23. Lingard L, Reznick R, DeVito I, Espin S. Forming professional identities on the health care team: discursive constructions of the 'other' in the operating room. Med Educ. 2002;36(8):728–34.
24. Carney BT, West P, Neily J, Mills PD, Bagian JP. Differences in nurse and surgeon perceptions of teamwork: implications for use of a briefing checklist in the OR. AORN J. 2010;91(6):722–9.
25. Collette AE, Wann K, Nevin ML, Rique K, Tarrant G, Hickey LA, Stichler JF, Toole BM, Thomason T. An exploration of nurse-physician perceptions of collaborative behaviour. J Interprof Care. 2017;31(4):470–8.
26. House S, Havens D. Nurses' and physicians' perceptions of nurse-physician collaboration: a systematic review. J Nurs Adm. 2017;47(3):165–71.
27. Makary MA, Sexton JB, Freischlag JA, Holzmueller CG, Millman EA, Rowen L, Pronovost PJ. Operating room teamwork among physicians and nurses: teamwork in the eye of the beholder. J Am Coll Surg. 2006;202(5):746–52.
28. Cruz SA, Idowu O, Ho A, Lee MJ, Shi LL. Differing perceptions of preoperative communication among surgical team members. Am J Surg. 2019;217(1):1–6.
29. Undre S, Sevdalis N, Healey AN, Darzi S, Vincent CA. Teamwork in the operating theatre: cohesion or confusion? J Eval Clin Pract. 2006;12(2):182–9.
30. Nakarada-Kordic I, Weller JM, Webster CS, Cumin D, Frampton C, Boyd M, Merry AF. Assessing the similarity of mental models of operating room team members and implications for

patient safety: a prospective, replicated study. BMC Med Educ. 2016;16(1):229. https://doi.org/10.1186/s12909-016-0752-8.

31. Alzahrani N, Jones R, Rizwan A, Abdel-Latif ME. Safety attitudes in hospital emergency departments: a systematic review. Int J Health Care Qual Assur. 2019;32(7):1042–54.

32. Pimentel MPT, Choi S, Fiumara K, Kachalia A, Urman RD. Safety culture in the operating room: variability among perioperative healthcare workers. J Patient Saf. 2017;17(6):412–6. Jun 1 Epub ahead of print.

33. Etchegaray JM, Ottosen MJ, Dancsak T, Thomas EJ. Barriers to speaking up about patient safety concerns. J Patient Saf. 2020;16(4):e230–4.

34. Martinez W, Etchegaray JM, Thomas EJ, Hickson GB, Lehmann LS, Schleyer AM, Best JA, Shelburne JT, May NB, Bell SK. 'Speaking up' about patient safety concerns and unprofessional behaviour among residents: validation of two scales. BMJ Qual Saf. 2015;24(11):671–80.

35. Villafranca A, Fast I, Jacobsohn E. Disruptive behavior in the operating room: prevalence, consequences, prevention, and management. Curr Opin Anaesthesiol. 2018;31(3):366–74.

36. Villafranca A, Hamlin C, Enns S, Jacobsohn E. Disruptive behavior in the operating room: a contemporary review. Can J Anesthe. 2017;64(2):128–40.

37. Gjeraa K, Spanager L, Konge L, Petersen RH, Ostergaard D. Non-technical skills in minimally invasive surgery teams: a systematic review. Surg Endosc. 2016;30(12):5185–99.

38. Kurmann A, Keller S, Tschan-Semmer F, Seelandt J, Semmer NK, Candinas D, Beldi G. Impact of team familiarity in the operating room on surgical complications. World J Surg. 2014;38(12):3047–52.

39. Pucher PH, Aggarwal R, Batrick N, Jenkins M, Darzi A. Nontechnical skills performance and care processes in the management of the acute trauma patient. Surgery. 2014;155(5):902–9.

40. Macefield R. Usability studies and the Hawthorne effect. J Usability Stud. 2007;2(3):145–54.

41. Salas E, Reyes DL, McDaniel SH. The science of teamwork: Progress, reflections, and the road ahead. Am Psychol. 2018;73(4):593–600.

42. The Health Foundation. Evidence scan: complex adaptive systems. London; 2010. Retrieved from https://www.health.org.uk/sites/default/files/ComplexAdaptiveSystems.pdf.

43. Pype P, Mertens F, Helewaut F, Krystallidou D. Healthcare teams as complex adaptive systems: understanding team behaviour through team members' perception of interpersonal interaction. BMC Health Serv Res. 2018;18(1):570. https://doi.org/10.1186/s12913-018-3392-3.

44. Shuffler ML, Carter DR. Teamwork situated in multiteam systems: key lessons learned and future opportunities. Am Psychol. 2018;73(4):390–406.

45. Shuffler ML, Diazgranados D, Maynard MT, Salas E. Developing, sustaining, and maximizing team effectiveness: an integrative, dynamic perspective of team development interventions. Acad Manag Ann. 2018;12(2):688–724.

46. Lyubovnikova J, West MA. Why teamwork matters: enabling health care team effectiveness for the delivery of high-quality patient care. In: Salas E, Tannenbaum S, Cohen D, Latham G, editors. Developing and enhancing teamwork in organizations: evidence-based best practices and guidelines. San Francisco: Jossey-Bass; 2013. p. 313–47.

47. Salas E, Cooke NJ, Rosen MA. On teams, teamwork, and team performance: discoveries and developments. Hum Factors. 2008;50(3):540–7.

48. Bell ST, Brown SG, Colaneri A, Outland N. Team composition and the ABCs of teamwork. Am Psychol. 2018;73(4):349–62.

49. Driskell JE, Salas E, Driskell T. Foundations of teamwork and collaboration. Am Psychol. 2018;73(4):334–48.

50. LePine JA, Piccolo RF, Jackson CL, Mathieu JE, Saul JR. A meta-analysis of teamwork processes: tests of a multidimensional model and relationships with team effectiveness criteria. Pers Psychol. 2008;61(2):273–307.

51. Agency for Healthcare Research and Quality. About TeamSTEPPS™; 2019, June. Retrieved from https://www.ahrq.gov/teamstepps/about-teamstepps/index.html.

52. Salas E, Sims DE, Burke CS. Is there a big five in teamwork? Small Group Res. 2005;36:555–99.

53. Salas E, Shuffler ML, Thayer AL, Bedwell WL, Lazzara EH. Understanding and improving teamwork in organizations: a scientifically based practical guide. Hum Resour Manag. 2015;54(4):599–622.

54. Tannenbaum SI, Cerasoli CP. Do team and individual debriefs enhance performance? A meta-analysis. Hum Factors. 2013;55(1):231–45.

55. McEwan D, Ruissen GR, Eys MA, Zumbo BD, Beauchamp MR. The effectiveness of teamwork training on teamwork behaviors and team performance: a systematic review and meta-analysis of controlled interventions. PLoS One. 2017;12(1):e0169604.

56. Lacerenza CN, Reyes DL, Marlow SL, Joseph DL, Salas E. Leadership training design, delivery, and implementation: a meta-analysis. J Appl Psychol. 2017;102(12):1686–718.

57. Buljac-Samardzic M, Doekhie KD, van Wijngaarden JDH. Interventions to improve team effectiveness within health care: a systematic review of the past decade. Hum Resour Health. 2020;18(1):2. https://doi.org/10.1186/s12960-019-0411-3.

58. Couper K, Salman B, Soar J, Finn J, Perkins GD. Debriefing to improve outcomes from critical illness: a systematic review and meta-analysis. Intensive Care Med. 2013;39(9):1513–23.

59. Schmutz JB, Eppich WJ. Promoting learning and patient care through shared reflection: a conceptual framework for team reflexivity in health care. Academic medicine. J Assoc Am Med Coll. 2017;92(11):1555–63.

60. Hughes AM, Gregory ME, Joseph DL, Sonesh SC, Marlow SL, Lacerenza CN, Benishek LE, King HB, Salas E. Saving lives: a meta-analysis of team training in healthcare. J Appl Psychol. 2016;101(9):1266–304.

61. Paige JT, Garbee DD, Brown KM, Rojas JD. Using simulation in interprofessional education. Surg Clin N Am. 2015;95(4):751–66.

62. Beaubien JM, Baker DP. The use of simulation for training teamwork skills in health care: how low can you go? Qual Saf Health Care. 2004;13(Suppl 1):i51–6.

63. Fung L, Boet S, Bould MD, Qosa H, Perrier L, Tricco A, Tavares W, Reeves S. Impact of crisis resource management simulation-based training for interprofessional and interdisciplinary teams: a systematic review. J Interprof Care. 2015;29(5):433–44.

64. Hull L, Sevdalis N. Advances in the teaching and assessing of nontechnical skills. Surg Clin N Am. 2015;95(4):869–84.

65. Dedy NJ, Zevin B, Bonrath EM, Grantcharov TP. Current concepts of team training in surgical residency: a survey of north American program directors. J Surg Educ. 2013;70(5):578–84.

66. Kern DE. Overview: a six-step approach to curriculum development. In: Thomas PA, Kern DE, Hughes MT, Chen BY, editors. Curriculum development for medical education: a six-step approach. 3rd ed. Baltimore: Johns Hopkins University Press; 2016. p. 5–9.

67. Chauvin SW. Applying educational theory to simulation-based training and assessment in surgery. Surg Clin N Am. 2015;95(4):695–715.

68. Rosen MA, Salas E, Wu TS, Silvestri S, Lazzara EH, Lyons R, Weaver SJ, King HB. Promoting teamwork: an event-based approach to simulation-based teamwork training for emergency medicine residents. Acad Emerg Med. 2008;15:1190–8.

69. Nguyen N, Elliott JO, Watson WD, Dominguez E. Simulation improves nontechnical skills performance of residents during the perioperative and intraoperative phases of surgery. J Surg Educ. 2015;75(5):957–63.

70. Paige JT. Making it stick: keys to effective feedback and debriefing in surgical education. In: Stefanidis D, Kordorffer Jr JR, Sweet R, editors. Simulation for surgery and surgical subspecialties. New York: Springer; 2019. p. 131–41.

71. Kirkpatrick DL. Evaluating training programs: the four levels. San Francisco: Berrett-Koehler; 1994. p. 229.

72. Widaman KF. Objective measurement of subjective phenomena in (OBSSR), editor, OBSSR online resource for behavioral and social sciences research. In: OBSSR e-Source online, editor. Office of behavioral and social sciences research; 2020. Retrieved from http://www.esourceresearch.org/eSourceBook/ObjectiveMeasurementofSubjectivePhenomena/11AuthorBiography/tabid/722/Default.aspx.

73. Higham H, Greig PR, Rutherford J, Vincent L, Young D, Vincent C. Observer-based tools for non-technical skills assessment in simulated and real clinical environments in healthcare: a systematic review. BMJ Qual Saf. 2019;28(8):672–86.

74. Kash BA, Cheon O, Halzick NM, Miller TR. Measuring team effectiveness in the health care setting: an inventory of survey tools. Heal Serv Insight. 2018;11:1–18.

75. Hull L, Athanasiou T, Russ S. Implementation science: a neglected opportunity to accelerate improvements in the safety and quality of surgical care. Ann Surg. 2017;265(6):1104–12.

76. Weiser TG, Forrester JA, Negussie T. Implementation science and innovation in global surgery. Br J Surg. 2019;106:e20–3.

77. Kotter J, Rathgeber H, Johnson S. Our iceberg is melting: changing and succeeding under any conditions. New York: Portfolio; 2005.

78. Friscella K, Mauksch L, Bodenheimer T, Salas E. Improving care teams' functioning: recommendations from team science. Jt Comm J Qual Patient Saf. 2016;43(7):361–8.

79. Jowsey T, Beaver P, Long J, Civil I, Gardner AL, Henderson K, Merry A, Skilton C, Torri J, Weller J. Towards a safer culture: implementing multidisciplinary simulation-based team training in New Zealand operating theatres – a framework analysis. BMJ Open. 2019;9(10):e027122.

80. Paige JT, Kozmenko V, Yang T, Paragi Gururaja R, Hilton CW, Cohn I Jr, Chauvin SW. High-fidelity, simulation-based, interdisciplinary operating room team training at the point of care. Surgery. 2009;145(2):138–46.

81. Paige JT. Team training at the point of care. In: Tsuda S, Scott DJ, Jones DB, editors. Textbook of simulation, surgical skills, and team training. Woodbury: Ciné-Med, Inc.; 2012.

Further Reading

Villamane M, Larranaga M, Alvarez A. Rating monitoring as a means to mitigate rater effects and controversial evaluations. Paper presented at the proceedings of 5th international conference on technological ecosystems for enhancing multiculturality, Cadiz, Spain. 7 p. 2017. https://doi.org/10.1145/3144826.3145389

Paige JT, Sonesh SC, Garbee DD, Bonanno LS, editors. Comprehensive healthcare simulation: interprofessional team training and simulation. Springer Nature Switzerland AG; 2020.

Nestel D, Dalrymple K, Paige JT, Aggarwal R, editors. Advancing Surgical Education: Theory, Evidence, and Practice. Springer Nature Singapore Pte Ltd; 2019.

Chapter 29
Simulation and OR Team Performance

Jaisa Olasky and Daniel B. Jones

Unsafe surgery results from a combination of technical and nontechnical errors. These errors, when unrecognized or when combined with latent system failures, can lead to significant injury to the patient and even death. The recognition that human error is inevitable in complex tasks has been slow to reach the medical community. In early writings on the topic [1, 2], Leape describes the scope of the problem of medical errors and the difficulty of the culture of medicine in addressing these problems. Twenty percent of all hospitalized patients suffer an iatrogenic illness and 69% of medical errors are preventable. In the Harvard Medical School Institutions, for example, 44% of claims in the perioperative period are for technical reasons. The remainder of claims is from nontechnical reasons such as wrong-site surgery, retained objects, abnormal blood loss,

J. Olasky
Mount Auburn Hospital, Harvard Medical School,
Boston, MA, USA

D. B. Jones (✉)
Department of Surgery, Rutgers New Jersey Medical School,
Newark, NJ, USA
e-mail: djones1@bidmc.harvard.edu

561
J. R. Romanelli et al. (eds.), *The SAGES Manual of Quality, Outcomes and Patient Safety*,
https://doi.org/10.1007/978-3-030-94610-4_29

and hematoma, which may have had technical components to the error but were all associated with communication breakdown. In the analysis of these closed claims, the Harvard-affiliated insurance company, CRICO, recognized some common features of these communication gaps: they were verbal; there was status asymmetry; there was ambiguity as to responsibility; and there were multiple handoffs and transfers. To remedy these communication errors, CRICO proposed several solutions: a surgical safety checklist, closed-loop communication, and assertiveness in communication (i.e., speaking up). The following chapter will address the use of simulation and OR team training as a possible vehicle to train operation room teams, with the final goal being to reduce surgical error and improve the safety of surgical inpatients.

Adverse events occur when errors happen at an inopportune moment. Far more common than adverse events are near misses or slips – those examples of risky behavior that do not result in injury. If one million adverse events occur each year in the USA, it is estimated that the number of near misses would be five million. Therefore, any training of medical personnel should include careful review of performance to identify such risky behavior. In an observational study of operating room safety, Christian et al. [3] reviewed 63 h of surgery and had over 4500 observations. They observed a number of critical system failures that had impact on patient safety. All of these critical events involved either communication and information flow or workload and competing tasks. This group recognized at least one close call during each surgical procedure. All members of the OR team also had periods of decreased activity. A strategy to recognize times of task overload and share the workload was suggested. Thus, multidisciplinary teams that are performing complex tasks can be observed and assessed for specific parameters of patient safety and team performance.

Simulation

The advantage that simulation has over a performance review of actual surgeries is that comparison of time-adverse events can be generated with great frequency and the resultant discussion and intervention can be documented and reviewed in a timely fashion. The scenarios can be constructed from actual events that have occurred, can be taken from closed-claim archives, or can even be constructed to predict future operations. The tasks performed by the operating team can be reasonably realistic. For example, surgeons can sew anastomoses, control bleeding, and practice wound closures. Anesthesia personnel can intubate, transfuse, draw laboratory samples, and administer medications. Nurses can assemble and arrange equipment, facilitate communication, and count remaining sponges and needles. The tasks are both familiar and validated. While some "suspension of disbelief" is required, most operating room teams report substantial face validity and can adapt to the simulation environment to perform the operative plan and to participate in their usual role on the team. The Imperial College in London published their seminal experience with procedures in a simulated operating theater with a standardized OR team in 2005. Their group observed OR crisis and used a checklist and global assessment to record technical skills and communication during femoral arterial hemorrhage. All team members participated in a debriefing session after the scenario and rated the face validity of the simulated environment. Darzi et al. [4] sought a high degree of realism in order to better understand team interactions and performance (Figs. 29.1 and 29.2). The Carl J. Shapiro Simulation and Skills Center at Beth Israel Deaconess Medical Center expanded this concept and built a mock minimally invasive surgery endosuite for team simulation. Multiple camera mountings and directional microphones record all communication and activity. Models of intraabdominal organs that bleed were created and placed

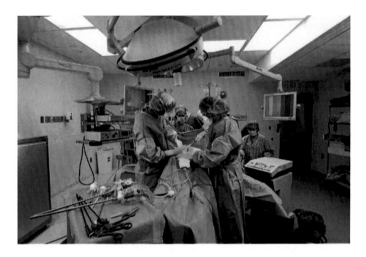

FIGURE 29.1 Carl J Shapiro simulation and skills center mock endosuite

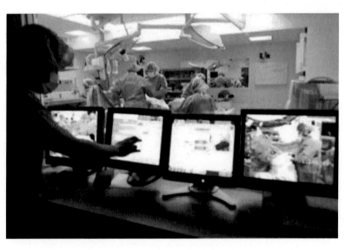

FIGURE 29.2 Control room for mock endosuite

behind a one-way mirror, while staff may control the simulation, including bleeding and vital signs, and they can signal confederates [5].

Powers et al. demonstrated face and construct validity of the mock operating endosuite with laparoscopic crisis scenarios [6]. Performances of Fundamentals of Laparoscopic Surgery (FLS)-certified and non-FLS-certified surgeons were placed in a laparoscopic crisis scenario and recorded the time to diagnose intraoperative bleeding following Veress needle entry, time to inform the operating team for the need to convert to an open procedure, and the actual time to conversion. Technical and nontechnical skills were assessed (Table 29.1). This scenario was recreated at the SAGES 2007 Annual Meeting Learning Center. The American College of Surgeons recognized the value of simulation with the release of the American College of Surgeons/Association of Program Directors in Surgery National Skills Curriculum (Table 29.2).

Team Training

Team training is an organizational approach that attempts to identify and practice the essential aspects of teamwork and communication in certain endeavors that by their nature show high activity, potential for disaster, or high stress. Therefore, much of the early team training efforts have focused on military operations, aviation, and the nuclear power industry. Effective teams adapt a "shared mental model" and work to balance the effort, anticipate problems, seek relevant data, resolve conflicts, and communicate effectively. In addition, such team training can identify stressors such as fatigue, work overload, and crises that can test any team. Most team training performance reviews include a comprehensive debriefing. Several validated assessment tools have been developed to help with the debriefing and maximize the value of these activities.

TABLE 29.1 Nontechnical skills

Category	Question
Communication and interaction	Instructions to assistant/scrub nurse; clear and polite
	Awaits acknowledgment from the assistant/scrub nurse
	Assistance sought from team members
Vigilance/situation awareness	Monitored patient's parameters throughout procedures
	Awareness of anesthetist
	Actively initiates communication with anesthetist during crisis periods
Team skills	Maintains a positive rapport with the whole team
	Open to opinions from other team members
	Acknowledges the contribution made by other team members
	Supportive of other team members
Leadership and management skills	Adherence to best practice during the procedure, e.g., does not permit corner cutting by self or team
	Time management, e.g., appropriate time allocation without being too slow or rushing team members
	Resource utilization, i.e., appropriate task-load distribution and delegation of responsibilities
	Authority/assertiveness
Decision-making crisis	Prompt identification of the problem
	Informed team members; promptly, clearly, and to all team members

TABLE 29.1 (continued)

Category	Question
	Outlines strategy/institutes a plan, i.e., asks scrub nurse for suction, instruments, suture materials
	Anticipates potential problems and prepares a contingency plan, e.g., asks to order blood, calls for help
	Option generation; takes the help of the team (seeks team opinion)

TABLE 29.2 ACS-APDS simulation modules

Teamwork in the trauma bay

Postoperative pneumonia (hypoxia, septic shock)

Postoperative hypotension

Laparoscopic crisis

The preoperative briefing

Laparoscopic troubleshooting

Postoperative pulmonary embolus

Postoperative myocardial infarction (cardiogenic shock)

Latex allergy anaphylaxis

Abdominal compartment syndrome (hypotension)

Patient handoff

Retained sponge on postoperative chest radiograph

A number of assessment tools have been developed to measure the performance of operating teams in a simulated OR environment. Most of these tools utilize the taxonomy of crisis management principles and have a graded assessment of each item in the taxonomy. Assessment of leadership, delegation, workload distribution, data collection, avoidance of fixation, utilization of resources, and recognition of limitations are included in most assessment tools. All of these tools suffer from time constraints during the scenario, the use of clipped phrases during crises, undeclared thoughts or concerns, and the performance anxieties of being in the spotlighted, videotaped, artificial environment of a simulation.

In addition to trained rater evaluations of team training performance, there have also been descriptions of self-assessments that use a Likert-type scale rating to evaluate the effectiveness of team training exercises using simulated operating room scenarios. One report [7] cited significant improvements in role clarity, anticipation, cross monitoring, and team cohesion/interaction. Thus, self-assessment tools exist to demonstrate a perceived improvement in the cognition and interpersonal skills required for successful team training.

The use of simulation to teach effective team training has been demonstrated in a number of medical disciplines. All of these disciplines have a high acuity environment and require the use and interpretation of complex and technical monitors and instruments. One example is a program that simulates high-risk pediatric trauma events. Pediatric trauma teams are complex, often including many members such as pediatric surgeons, emergency medicine physicians, nurses, paramedics, respiratory therapists, residents, and critical care fellows. The team training exercise using simulation was able to demonstrate an improvement over time of the performances of the pediatric trauma team, who appropriately completed tasks 65% of the time before the program and 75% of the time 1 year after the program [8].

Another example is from a multicenter study [9] involving emergency medicine clinicians, in which high-fidelity simulation was used to construct a team training course that improved clinical performance, increased patient safety, and decreased liability. The emergency room team was asked to care for two patients who presented with significant acuity and hemodynamic instability (anaphylaxis and splenic rupture). The tasks were appropriate and time critical (vital sign assessment, abdominal ultrasound), and the treatments were monitored not only for timeliness and efficiency but also for appropriate safety checks (identification of patient, labeling of tubes, checking blood). In an area of medicine where the cost of teamwork failure is high, such team training was shown to improve outcomes and reduce liability.

The use of simulation is also becoming routine in preparing the OR team for robotic surgery cases. These "dress rehearsals" allow the team to simulate high-risk scenarios, such as an emergency conversion to open for sudden major bleeding, which requires excellent team communication in order to rapidly undock the robot. In addition to case-specific team training, best practice guidelines for new robotics programs published by Dr. Estes et al. in 2017 [10] recommended that trainees experience a minimum of 8 h of hands-on training, including inanimate models.

At Harvard Medical School, a malpractice insurer [The Risk Management Foundation of the Harvard Medical Institutions ("CRICO/RMF")] developed a unique program with leaders from the medical school, as part of a Harvard Surgical Safety Collaborative. In this program, surgical education leaders at each of the four major teaching hospitals helped design and coordinate ten patient safety team training scenarios using simulation, and organized a systematic evaluation of this program. Each team contained at least one attending surgeon, one attending anesthesiologist, and one operating room nurse. The participants had a debriefing at the end and 99% filled out a survey about their experience. Participants found the scenarios realistic, challenging, and relevant. The research group concluded that a standardized, realistic, multicenter full operative team training program is feasible and would have a significant impact on patient safety in the future. While the initial ratings were very high, Hung et al. [11] preformed a follow-up survey 1 year after the initial study period ended. The respondents who had experienced an adverse event in the interim, such as lost sponge/miscount or a bleeding crisis, reported higher satisfaction with the previous training. Overall, 67% of respondents reported that they still believed the simulation would improve patient care, but only 37% were receptive to more team training themselves. There are several limitations to team training that may account for this lower-than-expected rate of participants who would like to participate in more training in the future.

Limitations of Simulation for Training

Despite many studies showing the benefits of simulation, there are some limitations to universal adoption. Studies have shown that simulation centers are used more often if they are in close proximity to the intended user; however, not all medical institutions have space available near clinical centers. Surveys of trainees also show that a lack of mandatory protected simulation time limits their ability to participate in these programs. Ideally, all clinical sites with trainees will have simulation time built into the curriculum for learners. CME and hospital safety programs will be more successful if there is compensation available for the participants' time. In addition, centers that use simulation for team training do not always use validated assessment or debriefing tools, which potentially limits the benefit of the team training session. Therefore, OR team training safety programs should be organized by or with consultation from a simulation expert.

Future Directions

Some of the limitations of in-person OR team training simulations can be overcome with the use of a mock OR set in virtual reality (VR). De et al. [12] have developed and tested an immersive VR OR fire simulator (Fig. 29.3). Initial studies evaluated one provider (surgeon, anesthesiologist, surgical technician, or nurse) as they safely respond to an OR fire. Participants reported it felt real and provoked anxiety. Researchers are now funded by NIH to expand the simulation to include four participants at a time. This new version of

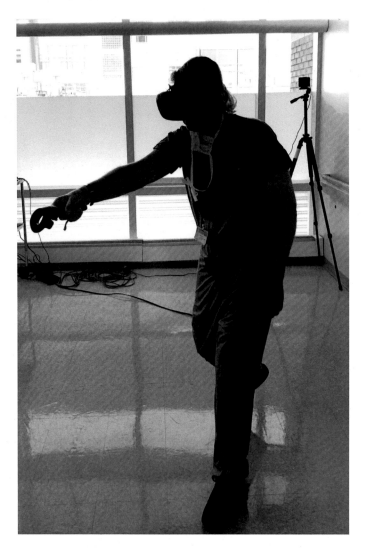

FIGURE 29.3 Virtual reality mock OR simulator

the immersive VR model will enable OR team training of high-risk scenarios to occur at any day or location that is convenient to the user.

Summary

Cognitive and interpersonal skills that are central to team training exercises include situational awareness, anticipation, and flexibility. The interpersonal skills focus on planning, advice, and feedback. In each category of skills, there are suggested behavioral markers that indicate both good and poor performance. The SAGES Masters Program [13] is a curriculum for the deliberate lifelong learning of surgery after residency. The current pathways include hernia, foregut, robotic, colorectal, bariatric, biliary, and endoscopy. In the future, a leadership development pathway will be made available to learners. OR team training using simulation and/or virtual reality would complement this curriculum perfectly.

In conclusion, OR team training using simulation has been shown to improve these skills of teamwork and communication that are so often deficient in episodes of patient injury. The simulated operation room provides a safe environment not only for the patient but also for the practitioner. The surgeon can rehearse necessary technical skills as well as prepare for rare but known complications. The current level of simulation has adequate face validity and provides sufficient challenges to engage the fully trained surgeon. Team training reinforces a set of cognitive and interpersonal skills that are essential to competent crisis management. Surgeons, surgical training programs, and professional societies should embrace the use of high-fidelity simulation to teach OR team training to its trainees, as a periodic refresher course to its graduates, and for continued medical education and leadership programs.

Selected References

1. Leape LL. Error in medicine. JAMA. 1994;272(23):1851–7.
2. Leape LL. Reporting of adverse events. NEJM. 2002;3(20):1633–8.
3. Christian CK, Gustafson ML, Roth EM, Sheridan TB, Gandhi TK, Dwyer KD, et al. A prospective study of patient safety in the operating room. Surgery. 2006;139:159–73.

4. Moorthy K, Munz Y, Adams S, Pandey V, Darzi A. A human factors analysis of technical and team skills among surgical trainees during procedural simulations in a simulated operating theatre. Ann Surg. 2005;242:631–9.

5. Arriaga AF, Gawande AA, Raemer DB, Jones DB, Smink DS, Weinstock P, Dwyer K, Lipsitz SR, Peyre S, Pawlowski JB, Muret-Wagstaff S, Gee D, Gordon JA, Cooper JA, Berry WR. Pilot testing of a model for insurance-driven, large scale multicenter simulation training for operating room teams. Ann Surg. 2013;259(3):403–10. PMID:24263327.

6. Powers KA, Rehrig ST, Irias N, Albano HA, Feinstein DM, Johansson AC, et al. Simulated laparoscopic operating room crisis: approach to enhance the surgical team performance. Surg Endosc. 2008;22(4):885–900.

7. Paige JT, Kozmenko V, Yang T, Gururaja RP, Hilton CW, Cohn I Jr, et al. High-fidelity simulation-based interdisciplinary operating room team training at the point of care. Surgery. 2009;145:138–46.

8. Falcone RA, Daughterty M, Schweer L, Patterson M, Brown RL, Garcia VF. Multidisciplinary pediatric trauma team training using high-fidelity trauma simulation. J Pediatr Surg. 2008;43:1065–71.

9. Small SD, Wuerz RC, Simon R, Shapiro N, Conn A, Setnik G. Demonstration of high fidelity simulation team training for emergency medicine. Acad Emerg Med. 1999;6(4):312–23.

10. Estes SJ, Goldenberg D, Winder JS, et al. Best practices for robotic surgery programs. JSLS. 2017;21(2):e2016.00102.

11. Hung T, Nuwar RM, Therrien S, Sullivan AM, Jones SB, Pawlowski J, Parra JM, Jones DB. OR team training using simulation: hope or hype? Am J Surg. 2020;222:1146–53. submitted. Oral at ASE 2020.

12. Truong H, Qi D, Ryason A, Cudmore J, Alfred S, Jones SB, Sullivan AM, Parra JM, De S, Jones DB. Does your team know how to respond safely to an operating room fire? Outcomes of a virtual reality, AI-enhanced simulation training. Ann Surg. 2020; Submitted. https://www.youtube.com/watch?v=T0tp-8sDSBE.

13. Jones DB, Stefandidis D, Korndorffer JR, Dimick JB, Schultz L, Scott DJ. SAGES University MASTERS Program: a structured curriculum for deliberate, lifelong learning. Surg Endosc. 2017;31(8):3061–71. 28634631.

14. Anderson M, Leflore J. Playing it safe: simulated team training in the OR. AORN J. 2008;87(4):772–9.

15. Blum RH, Raemer DB, Carroll JS, Dufresne RL, Cooper JB. A method for measuring the effectiveness of simulation-based team training for improving communication skills. Anesth Analg. 2005;100:1375–80.

16. Cooper JD, Clayman RV, Krummel TM, Schauer PR, Thompson C, Moreno JD. Inside the operating room – balancing the risks and benefits of new surgical procedures: a collection of perspectives and panel discussion. Cleve Clin J Med. 2008;75(6):S37–54.

17. Nestel D, van Herzeele I, Aggarwal R, O'Donoghue K, Choong A, Clough R, et al. Evaluating training for a simulated team in complex whole procedure simulations in the endovascular suite. Med Teach. 2009;31:e18–23.

18. Powers K, Rehrig S, Schwaitzberg SD, Callery MP, Jones DB. Seasoned surgeons assessed in a laparoscopic crisis. J Gastrointest Surg. 2009;13:994–1003.

19. Sundar E, Sundar S, Pawlowski J, Blum R, Feinstein D, Pratt S. Crew resource management and team training. Anesthesiol Clin. 2007;25:283–300.

20. Tsuda S, Scott D, Doyle J, Jones DB. Surgical skills training and simulation. Curr Probl Surg. 2009;46(4):261–372.

21. Tsuda S, Scott DJ, Jones DB, editors. ASE textbook of simulation: technical skills and team training. Woodbury: Cine-Med Inc; 2010.

22. Yule S, Flin R, Paterson-Brown S, Maran N. Non-technical skill for surgeons in the operating room: a review of the literature. Surgery. 2006;139:140–9.

23. Shohan S, Zevin B, Grantcharov TP, Roberts KE, Duffy AJ. Perceptions, training experiences, and preferences of surgical residents toward laparoscopic simulation training: a resident survey. J Surg Educ. 2014;71(5):727–33.

24. Robertson JM, Dias RD, Yule S, Smink DS. Operating room team training with simulation: a systematic review. J Laparoendosc Adv Surg Tech. 2017;27(5):475–80.

25. Qi D, Ryason A, Milef N, Alfred S, Abu-Nuwar R, Kappus M, De S, Jones DB. Virtual reality operating room with AI guidance: design and validation of fire scenario. Surg Endosc. 2021;(2):35, 779–786. PMID: 32072293.

Chapter 30
Debriefing After Simulation

Brandon W. Smith and Neal E. Seymour

The term "debriefing" generally describes a process to elicit information pertaining to an experienced event from the event's participants in order to gain a better understanding of it. Systematic debriefing models are employed as educational tools to enhance learning in numerous fields. This process of learning may also provide therapeutic benefits which might occur with debriefings after traumatic events [1]. In medical education, debriefings are a critical component in both simulation and clinical surgical training. The goals of debriefing in these settings are ultimately to stimulate reflection on individual and team performance in order to gain insights that improve the quality of clinical practice. This is especially true of debriefing after simulated patient care in healthcare team contexts. All such simulation scenarios ought to be debriefed, focusing on things that went well, things did not go well, and opportunities for improvement.

In order to appreciate the essential nature of debriefing in medical education, it is helpful to consider it in the context of

B. W. Smith · N. E. Seymour (✉)
Baystate Medical Center, Department of Surgery,
Springfield, MA, USA
e-mail: brandon.smithmd@baystatehealth.org;
neal.seymour@bhs.org

J. R. Romanelli et al. (eds.), *The SAGES Manual of Quality, Outcomes and Patient Safety*,
https://doi.org/10.1007/978-3-030-94610-4_30

basic human pedagogical models. Learning in simulation is experiential in the same way it would be for real-world experiences. Several taxonomies, most notably Kolb's learning cycle [2], describe cognitive consolidation of recent experiences by a process of reflection (Fig. 30.1) in the timeframe immediately following the experience. This process is a personal one and can involve cognitive and perceptual challenges that might color a participant's reflective account of the experience. Participants new to simulation or to the experience being simulated, who have little or no prior experience with debriefings, may find this especially challenging. They may require significant help and support to initiate the reflec-

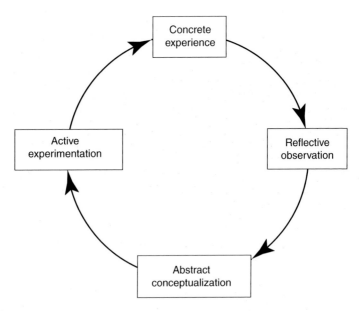

FIGURE 30.1 Kolb's learning cycle is one way to view the process of experiential learning such as might occur in a simulation training environment. The reflection-conceptualization components describe the principal opportunities offered during debriefing. Irrespective of the pedagogical model by which learning might be thought to occur during a session of simulated patient care, the importance of a high-quality debriefing cannot be overemphasized

tive process. The best post-simulation debriefing models call for a skilled debriefer to help compensate for this. This person does not behave as a traditional teacher in post-simulation debriefing. Rather, it is his or her responsibility to serve (a) as a prompter when reflective process stalls or stops and (b) as an objective contributor to help define the record of actual events when it is appropriate to do so and (c) to guide the process in an ongoing fashion toward achievement of the stated educational goals. For these reasons, this role is more commonly described as "facilitator," given the nature of responsibilities. There are numerous commentaries on these basic requirements that provide a generally consistent view of the facilitator's role [3–7].

In clinical medical education, the concept of the prototypical "teacher-learner" relationship is not conducive to efficient performance improvement. Over time, the paradigm in medical education has shifted from "teaching" to "coaching." Teaching implies a unidirectional flow of information that is not dependent on conversation or observation. Coaching is more than just providing feedback to learners; it involves providing practical suggestions for improvement with the aim of enhancing learner performance at a specific activity. Successful coaching involves identification of individualized goals with performance-based feedback in light of these goals. Feedback can be provided in a variety of forms, including debriefing. For these reasons, the role of a facilitator is better aligned with coaching than teaching [8].

Many standard and situation-specific prompts are available to a facilitator; these may be particularly helpful for novice facilitators with minimal experience. This can be demonstrated by the EXPRESS trial, which demonstrated improved learner outcomes with novice instructors using a scripted debriefing tool compared to those educators who did not use a script [9]. These prompts take the form of questions (Table 30.1) that are open-ended and stimulate learner engagement in reflective process. The process should not become facilitator-centric, however, and must remain focused on the participant(s) and develop an understanding of their

TABLE 30.1 Example facilitator open-ended questions

1. How did you feel when you noticed that?
2. What were your other options at that point?
3. How did you think things went during….?
4. What do you think was right/not right about that decision?

role in the simulation event in order to be effective. Although the term "structured" is often used to describe high-quality debriefing methods, this does not suggest the need for rigidity in either facilitator prompting or sequencing of questions. One debriefing expert stated that "our belief in the importance of debriefing and in the utility of the structured variety led us to the construction of various debriefing protocols. This approach frequently resulted in undesirable rigidity on the part of the facilitator and unmitigated boredom on the part of the participants" [10]. An analysis of interviews with peer-nominated debriefing experts revealed that as facilitators gained experience with debriefings, they tended to use "blended debriefing" approaches, acknowledging that no single debriefing model is a perfect fit for every scenario. Additionally, expert facilitators emphasized the ability to fluidly navigate the dynamic nature of these debriefing interactions. Summarized as "thinking on your feet," one expert stated the need to be flexible enough to address learners' needs rather than rigid learning objectives as one component of a successful debriefing [7]. Structure in the form of general strategies, goal-directed phases, and a systematic plan for assessment [4] are all compatible with effective debriefing.

In the final analysis, debriefing is a tool of fundamental importance to stimulate reflection as an aid to experiential learning. There are several options to ensure that learner reflection occurs. Debriefings can take the form of discussion among participants in the course of reviewing the simulation, with the facilitator taking steps to direct discussion only if the process stalls or deviates from an educationally valuable direction. Alternatively, the facilitator can specifically direct individual participants to present aspects of their performance, working toward an understanding of good (or bad) performance. The degree of comfort and prior experience of the learners can be a major determinant of the degree of input made by the facilitator. Ideally, reflection would be spontaneous and complete, and no facilitator would be required. This is rarely the case with student or resident learners in medical simulation, although there are numerous examples of self-debriefing and written debriefing models that do not involve external facilitation. Irrespective of the degree of direction provided, participants are given the opportunity to critically analyze and to discuss their actions, decisions, and emotional states.

In addition to traditional debriefing at the end of a case scenario, many debriefing experts utilize "reflection-in-action" or so-called reflective pauses. This form of debriefing takes place in the midst of the simulated scenario and may be initiated by the facilitator or the learner. The concept of reflective pauses takes advantage of the continuous internal monologue of the learner(s). As learners navigate scenarios, they may be internally debriefing their own decision-making, technical skills, or performance as a team leader. Reflective pauses take advantage of this internal monologue as a springboard to further capture learner engagement, and offers opportunity to address elements of learner performance that otherwise may be missed at the formal end of scenario debrief. Another advantage of the reflective pause is the ability of the facilitator to gain insight into the learner's thought process. This allows the facilitator to evaluate not only the learner's actions, but the reasoning yielding that action. One can imagine a scenario during which the learner performs the correct action, such as intubating the patient, but under the pretense of an incorrect diagnosis. If the facilitator only observes the outcome (the decision to intubate), they may miss the learner's knowledge gap. Missing these opportunities in simulation can lead learners to develop a false sense of understanding. Another advantage of reflective pauses is to celebrate and reinforce high performance during the scenario.

This can build confidence appropriately in the learner and thus augment learning [11].

Rudolph et al. [12] used a phasic description of debriefing in order to better define how it fits into a formative assessment methodology (Table 30.2). Of particular interest is the "analysis" phase, which provides the critical information for assessment by defining the gap between actual and desired performance during the simulation. This performance gap is revealed through facilitated discussion of the simulation, which is also the principal means to ensure a good reflective learning experience. An opportunity to address knowledge gaps with "brief didactics targeted to immediate learning needs" is also defined. Although it is important not to allow this to preempt other debriefing dialogue, overall learning objectives ought to accommodate this type of information flow.

Ensuring learner engagement during debriefing is arguably the most difficult challenge facing the facilitator [5]. An actively engaged participant has the best opportunity for a solid learning experience and presumably the best opportunity for retention and transfer of what is learned to clinical care. The common facilitator pitfalls are all detriments to effective learner engagement (Table 30.3). In addition to facilitator "lecturing," ineffective use of audiovisual (A-V) recordings can be problematic. Systems to deliver recorded video represent significant investments for simulation facilities and are now widely available. A-V records of the simulated event may be used as an aid to the debriefing process, provided there are appropriate annotations to guide access to relevant sites in oftentimes lengthy recordings. Excessive

TABLE 30.2 Phases of debriefing [12]

Reactions phase	Learner expresses initial emotional reactions to simulation
Analysis phase	Discussion process directed to close performance gap between actual and desired performance
Summary phase	Distill lessons learned into discrete concepts that can be used in practice

TABLE 30.3 Pitfalls of debriefing

1. Facilitator lecturing
2. Close-ended questions
3. Inadequate emotional safety (recriminations, accusations)
4. Interruptions to find relevant video segments

time spent scanning videos for segments that are worth reviewing can be a significant distraction and break the flow of the debriefing. If the video is not well annotated, it is probably more effective to use participant recall than to risk losing participant engagement. When systematically studied, many reports suggest that video-assisted and non-video-assisted debriefing methods offer similar outcomes [13, 14].

Most simulation training events occur in a training lab, a simulation suite, or an actual clinical environment (in situ simulation). There is no single successful formula for the site of debriefing, and issues of convenience and feasibility often help determine where the debriefing takes place. It is important that the timing of debriefing be as soon after the completion of the simulated scenario as possible to take advantage of the learner's experience while it is fresh in their minds. The site should be quiet, distraction-free, and should accommodate all participants in the simulation session in a way that permits face-to-face discussion. Sometimes access to the simulation environment can be helpful for focused reenactment, but most debriefings occur outside the simulation suite in a classroom setting with access to A-V recordings of the simulation event, which can be referred to as an aid in the reflective process.

Irrespective of the physical site in which debriefings occur, the environment must be one that ensures emotional safety for the learner [2, 5]. A variety of factors pertinent to the learners, the simulation, and/or the facilitator may potentially compromise this sense of safety and cause a debriefing situation to become emotionally charged to the detriment of effective education [15]. The learner may be new to clinical care or to the specific problem being managed and may become defensive, especially if they feel that their performance might be viewed by others as inadequate. The learner's sense of vulnerability may be increased by the impression of having been "deceived" by the manner in which a difficult simulation problem was presented [16]. If other participants are critical or even overbearing, this problem may be accentuated. An unskilled facilitator may provoke the same response by either being excessively critical or expounding their knowledge of good performance at the cost of good learner reflection. The facilitator essentially adjusts the level of supportiveness that a learner encounters in the debriefing environment.

Improving the effectiveness of debriefing may require careful observation of the process by experienced personnel and then a second debriefing for the facilitator. The Center for Medical Simulation developed the Debriefing Assessment for Simulation in Healthcare (DASH©), a tool to assess the effectiveness of debriefing using global ratings applicable to any medical discipline [17]. This is an example of systematic quality improvement in simulation, focusing on development of the educator's skills. Ultimately, experience through repeated trials coupled with feedback from both learners and expert debriefers is the best formula for improvement of debriefing skills. The degree to which debriefing can be made a positive learning experience may very well be the most important single determinant of the success of a simulation training effort. As educators improve their debriefing skill, this may translate to successful coaching outside of the simulation environment.

In the final analysis, the goal of medical simulation is to improve clinical performance with the hope that this results in improved quality of patient care and improved patient outcomes. Truly effective debriefing as an educational intervention and adjunct to the effectiveness of simulation methods can make the difference between a high and a low impact experience for simulation learners. There are no compelling studies showing where this intervention falls in Kirkpatrick's four-level model of training evaluation [18], but our goal as surgical educators ought to ultimately be to improve clinical outcomes (Kirkpatrick Level 4). Over the last two decades, the value of simulation in improving surgical learner technical and nontechnical performance in clinical settings (Kirkpatrick Level 3) has been well established [19–21] with some tantalizing suggestion that there are outcomes benefits. Mounting evidence suggests that if teaching faculty members adopt coaching models and utilize more organized, structured approaches to educate in the perioperative setting, trainees can be expected to perform better than they would in response to traditional teaching [22–24]. One such model offering a structured approach incorporating formalized debriefings into intraoperative teaching is the "Briefing, Intraoperative Teaching, Debriefing" (B-I-D) model proposed by Roberts and colleagues [25]. The consolidation of information acquired at each of the B-I-D experiential stages culminates with the debriefing and offers the best opportunity to close the learning loop and extract the maximum benefit from the coaching model of teaching. This structured model has recently been put before SAGES membership, suggesting that it represents a "best practice" to maximize opportunities for effective learning from experiences in the operating room [26]. Building on this, we propose that expanded adaptation of routine high-quality debriefings into surgical simulation events of all types, in conjunction with effective preparation and teaching, will produce superior educational results. However, even considering it in isolation from other important educational methods, the importance of debriefing in simulation and medical education cannot be overstated.

References

1. Tuckey MR, Scott JE. Group critical incident stress debriefing with emergency services personnel: a randomized controlled trial. Anxiety Stress Coping. 2014;27(1):38–54.

2. Kolb D. Experiential learning: experience as the source of learning and development. Englewood Cliffs: Prentice-Hall; 1984.
3. Salas E, Klein C, King H, et al. Debriefing medical teams: 12 evidence-based best practices and tips. Jt Comm J Qual Patient Saf. 2008;34(9):518–27.
4. Lederman LC. Debriefing: toward a systematic assessment of theory and practice. Simul Gaming. 1992;23(2):145–60.
5. Petranek C. A maturation in experiential learning: principles of simulation and gaming. Simul Gaming. 1994;25(4):513–22.
6. Fanning RM, Gaba DM. The role of debriefing in simulation-based learning. Simul Healthc. 2007;2(2):115–25.
7. Krogh K, Bearman M, Nestel D. "Thinking on your feet"—a qualitative study of debriefing practice. Adv Simul. 2016;1:12.
8. Landerville J, Cheung W, Frank J, Richardson D. A definition for coaching in medical education. Can Med Educ J. 2019;10(4):e109–10.
9. Cheng A, Hunt EA, Donoghue A, Nelson-McMillan K, Nishisaki A, Leflore J, Eppich W, Moyer M, Brett-Fleegler M, Kleinman M, Anderson J, Adler M, Braga M, Kost S, Stryjewski G, Min S, Podraza J, Lopreiato J, Hamilton MF, Stone K, Reid J, Hopkins J, Manos J, Duff J, Richard M, Nadkarni VM, EXPRESS Investigators. Examining pediatric resuscitation education using simulation and scripted debriefing: a multicenter randomized trial. JAMA Pediatr. 2013;167(6):528–36.
10. Thiagarajan S, Thiagi Gameletter. Seriously fun activities for trainers, facilitators, performance consultants, and managers; 2008. http://thiagi.net/archive/www/pfp/IE4H/august2008.html#ToolKit. Accessed 22 Dec 2020.
11. Clapper TC, Leighton K. Incorporating the reflective pause in simulation: a practical guide. J Contin Educ Nurs. 2020;51(1):32–8.
12. Rudolph JW, Simon R, Raemer DB, Eppich WJ. Debriefing as formative assessment: closing performance gaps in medical education. Acad Emerg Med. 2008;15(11):1010–6.
13. Cheng A, Eppich W, Grant V, Sherbino J, Zendejas B, Cook D. Debriefing for technology-enhanced simulation: a systematic review and meta-analysis. Med Educ. 2014;48(7):657–66.
14. Savoldelli GL, Naik VN, Park J, Joo HS, Chow R, Hamstra SJ. Value of debriefing during simulated crisis management: oral versus video-assisted oral feedback. Anesthesiology. 2006;105(2):279–85.
15. Savoldelli GL, Naik VN, Hamstra SJ, Morgan PJ. Barriers to the use of simulation-based education. Can J Anesth. 2005;52(9):944–50.

16. Stewart L. Ethical issues in postexperimental and postexperiential debriefing. Simul Gaming. 1992;23(2):196–211.
17. Simon R, Raemer DB, Rudolph JW. Debriefing assessment for simulation in healthcare (DASH)© Rater's handbook. Boston: Center for Medical Simulation; 2010. https://harvardmedsim. org/wp-content/uploads/2017/01/DASH.handbook.2010.Final. Rev.2.pdf.
18. Kirkpatrick D, Kirkpatrick J, editors. Evaluating training programs. The four levels. 3rd ed. San Francisco: Berrett-Koehler; 2006.
19. Capella J, Smith S, Philp A, Putnam T, Gilbert C, Fry W, Harvey E, Wright A, Henderson K, Baker D, Ranson S, Remine S. Teamwork training improves the clinical care of trauma patients. J Surg Educ. 2010;67(6):439–43.
20. Seymour NE, Gallagher AG, Roman SA, O'Brien MK, Bansal VK, Andersen DK, Satava RM. Virtual reality training improves operating room performance: results of a randomized, double-blinded study. Ann Surg. 2002;236(4):458–63.
21. Zendejas B, Cook DA, Bingener J, Huebner M, Dunn WF, Sarr MG, Farley DR. Simulation-based mastery learning improves patient outcomes in laparoscopic inguinal hernia repair: a randomized controlled trial. Ann Surg. 2011;254(3):502–11.
22. Yule S, Henrickson Parker S, Wilkinson J, McKinley A, MacDonald J, Neill A, McAdam T. Coaching non-technical skills improves surgical residents' performance in a simulated operating room. J Surg Educ. 2015;72(6):1124–30.
23. Bonrath EM, Dedy NJ, Gordon LE, Grantcharov TP. Comprehensive surgical coaching enhances surgical skill in the operating room: a randomized controlled trial. Ann Surg. 2015;262(2):205–12.
24. Gagnon LH, Abbasi N. Systematic review of randomized controlled trials on the role of coaching in surgery to improve learner outcomes. Am J Surg. 2018;216(1):140–6.
25. Roberts NK, Williams RG, Kim MJ, Dunnington GL. The briefing, intraoperative teaching, debriefing model for teaching in the operating room. J Am Coll Surg. 2009;208(2):299–303.
26. Gardner AK. The Briefing: Intra-Op Teaching-Debriefing (B-I-D) Model [Podium Presentation]. SAGES Annual Meeting 2017. Houston; 2017 Mar 2. https://www.sages.org/video/the-briefing-intra-op-teaching-debriefing-b-i-d-model/.

Chapter 31
Using Simulation for Disclosure of Bad News

Limaris Barrios

Educating the medical community with regard to disclosure of medical errors, unanticipated outcomes, and/or bad news has become a priority for physician educators, and a popular topic over the last two decades [1–6]. Unfortunately, physicians and surgeons are not well equipped to deliver difficult news due to inadequate training. It is not surprising that litigation, humiliation, and stress burden those charged with this responsibility [1, 3–6].

Today, patients, accreditation standards, laws, and hospital policies require explicit and candid communication after such events are recognized [1–3, 6, 7]. Training of physicians in this field has become critical. Seven states have passed laws that mandate notification of patients after an adverse event – Nevada, Florida, New Jersey, Pennsylvania, Vermont, Oregon, and California [1, 8], and the Joint Commission on Accreditation of Healthcare Organizations (JCAHO) and National Quality Forum (NQF) have created standards that

L. Barrios (✉)
Dr. Kiran C. Patel College of Allopathic Medicine (NSU MD),
Nova Southeastern University in Florida,
Fort Lauderdale, FL, USA
e-mail: limaris.barrios@hcahealthcare.com

© The Author(s), under exclusive license to Springer Nature Switzerland AG 2022
J. R. Romanelli et al. (eds.), *The SAGES Manual of Quality, Outcomes and Patient Safety*,
https://doi.org/10.1007/978-3-030-94610-4_31

require disclosure [1, 7, 9–15]. Similarly, Australia and the UK have launched pilot programs which promote full disclosure after an adverse event has occurred [3].

Moreover, aggressive disclosure policies developed by healthcare organizations aim to improve patient satisfaction, decrease litigation costs, and create safe practice protocols [1]. The University of Michigan Health System Program, the Dana-Farber Cancer Institute in Massachusetts, and the Johns Hopkins Hospital in Maryland are among others who have created disclosure policies with positive results thus far [1–3, 5, 9, 10, 12–14, 16]. Since the implementation of these programs, a number of claims and lawsuits have diminished, and the annual litigation costs were noted to be decreased as well.

"Full apology laws" whereby admission to fault is inadmissible in court have been passed in several states, including Georgia, Colorado, Arizona, and South Carolina, to name a few, and are under development in others [1, 4, 5, 13, 14, 17]. Thirty-nine states and the District of Columbia have "apology laws" which prohibit certain statements, expressions, or other evidence related to disclosure from being admissible in a lawsuit [18]. More importantly, patients are demanding full disclosure during adverse events. They want to understand how the adverse event occurred and want to ensure that future events will be prevented [1, 14].

Medical students and resident physicians are also required to prove competency in disclosure of adverse events. The United States Medical Licensing Examination (USMLE), sponsored by the Federation of State Medical Boards (FSMB) and the National Board of Medical Examiners (NBME), includes questions focused on full disclosure and public reporting under the topics of medical ethics, jurisprudence, and physician/patient relationship [19]. Medical students need to pass the USMLE, and therefore correctly answer questions regarding disclosure of adverse events, before qualifying for a medical license to practice in the USA.

The Accreditation Council for Graduate Medical Education (ACGME) has taken similar steps, whereby physician residents need to prove competency in this area before graduating from accredited residency programs in the USA. Unfortunately, many residents do not get an opportunity to lead or even witness such disclosures during their training [1, 19–21]. Most surgeons have learned this difficult task by observing their mentors, and have not had an opportunity to practice and improve this skill before using it in their professional career. This limited training will likely result in poor communication between the surgeon and patient, patient dissatisfaction, and perhaps a greater number of malpractice claims and lawsuits [21].

Simulation-based training is an integral and essential part of surgical residency training in this era. No one will deny its effectiveness in the acquisition of technical and nontechnical skills [22–26]. Different scenarios are recreated to assess and improve communication, team skills, and the ability to react under stress, providing the opportunity to practice and develop a variety of skills in a controlled, risk-free environment [22–26]. The simulated environment is the modern tool whereby learners acquire the skills required for real medical practice, decreasing potential injury to the patient [23, 24]. Simulation-based training has been studied and applied for the training of surgical residents in the disclosure of bad news [1].

One such study was conducted at Beth Israel Deaconess Medical Center in Boston from June of 2007 to March of 2008 [1]. The study aimed to use simulation to evaluate disclosure of bad news among surgical residents who performed a laparoscopic cholecystectomy on a virtual reality simulator in a mock operating room. The surgical residents were randomized into two different scenarios: one in which there was bile duct injury during the procedure and the other included incidental findings of metastatic gallbladder cancer. The residents were asked to deliver the bad news to a scripted family member after the procedure. The disclosure encounters were videotaped, and the residents were rated by independent reviewers using a modified SPIKES protocol as an assessment tool [27].

The study found that in general, trainees are ill-prepared for conversations that involve disclosure of adverse or unexpected outcomes. Senior residents were more comfortable with disclosure of bad news and obtained better ratings with the modified SPIKES protocol, likely secondary to their increased exposure to these difficult conversations. However, a minority of residents had led or even observed disclosures of iatrogenic injury or incidental operative findings during any portion of their training [1]. This study illustrates how simulation can be applied to the disclosure of bad news, and incorporated into medical school, residency, or physician training. Using a simulation-based module, the learner's responses during difficult conversations can be evaluated, and feedback provided to improve future disclosure encounters.

The American College of Surgeons and the Association of Program Directors in Surgery (ACS/APDS) have recognized the importance of training in disclosure of bad news and have incorporated simulation into a new training module. The surgical skills curriculum for residents (Phase III), developed in the summer of 2008, includes an Apology Module which integrates simulation for the practice and acquisition of skills required in disclosure of bad news [6]. In this module, the surgical resident goes through a scenario where a sponge is inadvertently left in the patient's abdomen during surgery. The resident is asked to disclose the bad news to the patient's husband, who is a confederate (trained actor). The disclosure is videotaped and debriefed, mainly evaluating the quality of the disclosure and the resident's communication skills [6].

One useful component to a successful simulation includes video-recording the experience; this technique has been used for years on many robust simulation scenarios to enhance the learning experience [1, 27–29]. The use of checklists has also been identified as another functional tool which improves the learning experience [28]. A study performed out of Vanderbilt University studied the use of a checklist to help faculty assess ACGME Milestones for Anesthesiology residents in an Objective Structured Clinical Examination

(OSCE). They concluded that the use of the checklist assisted in correct assessments of the learners [28]. Other key components to simulation in healthcare education include feedback debriefing, deliberate practice, and curriculum integration [30]. These components have been studied extensively and identified as having a positive impact on the learner's experience [30].

According to The Joint Commission Journal on Quality and Patient Safety, eight factors are the most critical elements necessary for successful simulation programs —*science, staff, supplies, space, support, systems, success, and sustainability* [31]. *Science* includes utilization of clinicians and training designers, checklists, training location, publicly announcing desired behaviors, and providing drills to offer trainees more opportunities to practice [31]. For *staff*, the recommendation is recruit champions to promote the use of simulation for training [31]. Procuring *supplies* from surplus or expired equipment available in other units [31] has been proposed. *Space* is the location where the simulation will take place. It is advisable to create *support* from leadership and staff for the simulation project. *Systems* includes matching the fidelity of the training system with desired training objectives, encouraging sharing *success* stories. Finally, *sustainability* includes accruing new simulation champions and instructors.

On the other hand, it is important to discuss some of the challenges and limitations of simulation training. Learner and faculty time constraints can limit the availability of simulation programs and dissemination. Additionally, resource intensive requirements may not allow for generalization and adoption across the board. As a result, simulation courses may be performed infrequently. As such, it may be difficult to achieve mastery due to lack of repetition. It has also been pointed out that simulation training may require adjustments to account for innovation along the learning pathway, in order to stay current and not stagnant or obsolete. These challenges may impede achievement of expertise in the subject at hand [32].

To summarize, policies, standards, and laws have been implemented in the USA and abroad which require open disclosure of adverse events and unanticipated outcomes to patients. It is evident that both physicians in training and practice are not prepared or adequately trained for these difficult conversations. Simulation provides the learner with a venue to practice and perfect their skills, including the disclosure of bad news.

Selected Reading

1. Barrios L, Tsuda S, Derevianko A, et al. Framing family conversation after early diagnosis of iatrogenic injury and incidental findings. Surg Endosc. 2009;23:2535–42.
2. Gallagher TH, Levinson W. Disclosing harmful medical errors to patients: a time for professional action. Arch Intern Med. 2005;165(16):1819–24.
3. Gallagher TH, Studdert D, Levinson W. Disclosing harmful medical errors to patients. N Engl J Med. 2007;356(26):2713–9.
4. Kowalczyk L. Doctors say they need protection to apologize. Boston: The Boston Globe; 2007.
5. Lazare A. Apology in medical practice: an emerging clinical skill. JAMA. 2006;296(11):1401–4.
6. ACS/APDS Skills Curriculum for Residents: Phase 3, Module 10-retained sponge on a postop chest X ray. http://elearning.facs.org/course/view.php?id=10&topic=12 (2008). Accessed 29 June 2009.
7. Joint Commission Resources. Hospital accreditation standards. Oakbrook Terrace: Joint Commission Resources; 2007.
8. http://www.aon.com/risk_management/default.jsp. Accessed 21 Jan 2008.
9. Kraman SS, Hamm G. Risk management: extreme honesty may be the best policy. Ann Intern Med. 1999;131(12):963–7.
10. Gallagher TH, Waterman AD, Garbutt JM, et al. US and Canadian physicians' attitudes and experiences regarding disclosing errors to patients. Arch Intern Med. 2006;166(15):1605–11.
11. The Leapfrog Group: The National Quality Forum safe practices leap. http://www.leapfroggroup.org/media/file/Leapfrog-National_Quality_Forum_Safe_Practices_Leap.pdf (2007). Accessed 18 Jan 2008.

12. Joint Commission on Accreditation of Healthcare Organizations. Health care at the crossroads: strategies for improving the medical liability system and preventing patient injury. http://www.jointcommission.org/NR/rdonlyres/3F1B626C-CB65-468B-A871-488D1DA66B06/0/medical_liability_exec_summary.pdf (2005). Accessed 18 Jan 2008.
13. Clinton HR, Obama B. Making patient safety the centerpiece of medical liability reform. N Engl J Med. 2006;354(21):2205–8.
14. Wojcieszak D, Banja J, Houk C. The sorry works! Coalition: making the case for full disclosure. Jt Comm J Qual Patient Saf. 2006;32(6):344–50.
15. National Quality Forum. National Quality Forum updates endorsement of serious reportable events in healthcare. http://www.qualityforum.org/pdf/news/prSeriousReportableEvents10-15-06.pdf (2006). Accessed 18 Jan 2008.
16. Lamb RM, Studdert DM, Bohmer RM, Berwick DM, Brennan TA. Hospital disclosure practices: results of a national survey. Health Aff (Millwood). 2003;22(2):73–83.
17. McMichael BJ. The failure of "sorry": an empirical evaluation of apology laws, health care and medical malpractice. Lewis & Clark Law Review, Forthcoming 73 Pages Posted: 21 Aug 2017. Last revised: 4 Jun 2018. https://papers.ssrn.com/sol3/papers.cfm?abstract_id=3020352. Accessed 18 Nov 2020.
18. McMichael BJ, Van Horn RL, Viscusi K. 'Sorry' is never enough, how state apology laws fail to reduce medical malpractice liability risk. Stanford Law Rev. 2019;71(2):341–409.
19. United States Medical Licensing Examination. http://www.usmle.org. Accessed 29 Jun 2009.
20. Hutul OA, Carpenter RO, Tarpley JL, Lomis KD. Missed opportunities: a descriptive assessment of teaching and attitudes regarding communication skills in a surgical residency. Curr Surg. 2006;63(6):401.
21. Rider EA, Hinrichs MM, Lown BA. A model for communication skills assessment across the undergraduate curriculum. Med Teach. 2006;28(5):e127–34.
22. Chang L, Petros J, Hess DT, Rotondi C, Babineau TJ. Integrating simulation into a surgical residency program: is voluntary participation effective? Surg Endosc. 2007;21(3):418–21.
23. Dunkin B, Adrales GL, Apelgren K, Mellinger JD. Surgical simulation: a current review. Surg Endosc. 2007;21(3):357–66.

24. Park J, MacRae H, Musselman LJ, et al. Randomized controlled trial of virtual reality simulator training: transfer to live patients. Am J Surg. 2007;194(2):205–11.
25. Passman MA, Fleser PS, Dattilo JB, Guzman RJ, Naslund TC. Should simulator-based endovascular training be integrated into general surgery residency programs? Am J Surg. 2007;194(2):212–9.
26. Powers KA, Rehrig ST, Irias N, et al. Simulated laparoscopic operating room crisis: an approach to enhance the surgical team performance. Surg Endosc. 2007;22(4):885–900.
27. Baile WF, Buckman R, Lenzi R, Glober G, Beale EA, Kudelka AP. SPIKES-A six-step protocol for delivering bad news: application to the patient with cancer. Oncologist. 2000;5(4):302–11.
28. Easdown LJ, Wakefield ML, Shotwell MS, Sandison MR. A checklist to help faculty assess ACGME milestones in a video-recorded OSCE. J Grad Med Educ. 2017;9(5):605–10.
29. Poirier TI, Pailden J, Jhala R, Ronald K, Wilhelm M, Fan J. Student self-assessment and faculty assessment of performance in an interprofessional error disclosure simulation training program. Am J Pharm Educ. 2017;81(3):54.
30. Motola I, Devine LA, Chung HS, Sullivan JE, Issenberg SB. Simulation in healthcare education: a best evidence practical guide. AMEE guide no. 82. Med Teach. 2013;35(10):e1511–30.
31. Lazzara EH, Benishek LE, Dietz AS, Salas E, Adriansen DJ. Eight critical factors in creating and implementing a successful simulation program. Jt Comm J Qual Patient Saf. 2014;40(1):21–9.
32. Using simulations for learning - advantages & disadvantages. https://www.designingdigitally.com/blog/2018/10/advantages-and-disadvantages-using-simulations-learning. Accessed 18 Nov 2020.

Chapter 32
Teleproctoring in Surgery

Julio Santiago Perez and Shawn Tsuda

Introduction

The Society of American Gastrointestinal and Endoscopic Surgeons (SAGES) previously established guidelines for the use of telecommunications technology for postgraduate surgical training and practice [1, 2]. It is necessary to continue developing and refining how telemedicine is incorporated in surgery as technology and paradigms evolve. The goal of this chapter is to establish a compendium of current knowledge on telemedicine to encourage efficiency, safety, and collaboration in promoting the best patient care possible.

Telemedicine has been used in some form for enhancing the health of patients and the quality of providers for over 50 years [3]. The medical-industrial complex has made prodigious strides with the development of technologies in radiology, minimally invasive surgery (MIS), emergency medicine,

J. S. Perez · S. Tsuda (✉)
Valley Health System General Surgery Department,
Las Vegas, NV, USA
e-mail: drshawntsuda@vipsurg.com

© The Author(s), under exclusive license to Springer Nature   595
Switzerland AG 2022
J. R. Romanelli et al. (eds.), *The SAGES Manual of Quality,*
Outcomes and Patient Safety,
https://doi.org/10.1007/978-3-030-94610-4_32

general medicine, and medical informatics. Such technologies have connected with advances in broadband communications to make telemedicine, in some cases, a seamless component of medical training and patient care [4–6]. Brought to the forefront with the 2020 COVID-19 pandemic, the medical community has been stimulated to expand and innovate ways to provide high-quality care to address a shortage of physicians, gaps in access, travel restrictions, and social-distancing requirements [7, 8]. In this document, we will address discourse and evolving guidelines regarding the increasing relevance of telemedicine in the current medical landscape, obstacles and possible solutions, practical benefits, reliability, learning curves, and recommendations for safe and efficacious telemedicine applications [9, 10].

Definitions

Previous guidelines by SAGES established definitions for concepts related to telemedicine and education [1, 2]. With evolving technology and concepts in telemedicine have come changes to the basic framework of this field, as well as its vernacular. The following are updated definitions related specifically to surgical training that should reflect a common language that is essential to instructors, learners, clinicians, and researchers in the area of telemedicine.

Telecommunications Telecommunications is communication over any distance using several means or modalities including, but not limited to, electrical signals, optical signals, or electromagnetic waves, over a number of mediums such as wire, optical fiber, or radio waves as wireless transmissions. "5G," or fifth-generation broadband technology, currently provides up to a gigabit per second of wireless transmission with almost imperceptible latency. Key elements of telecommunication are a *transmitter*, which takes information and transfers it to a signal; a *medium*, which can be a physical or over-the-air channel by which the signal is transmitted; and a *receiver*, which captures the signal and converts it to readable and usable information for the recipient. Telecommunications can also be synchronous, where the information is sent, received, and processed in as close to real time as possible by the transmitter, medium, and receiver, or asynchronous, where the information is transmitted and processed later by the receiver. For the purposes of telecommunication applications to surgery, we will be assuming primarily synchronous applications, and two-way communication which involves both audio and video signals.

Central Site A course or clinical location where the core activity is being performed will be referred to as the central site and is the target of telecommunication input. This differs from the remote site, which is the source of the telecommunication input from the instructor, preceptor, or proctor. The site may be a hospital, ward, operating room, simulation center, classroom, or any other location where the physician(s) or learner(s) are located and receiving input from their instructors, preceptors, or proctors.

Remote Site The remote site is the source of telecommunication input from the instructor, preceptor, or proctor. There is no defined distance of the remote site to the central site, which can range from a few feet such as between one robotic console and another console in the same operating room, or across continents. The remote site and central site can also be described as the site of input origin (remote) and site of endpoint (central) [1].

Telemedicine Telemedicine traditionally refers to the practice of medicine at a distance using telecommunications technology. However, while the majority of telemedicine involves a physician or healthcare provider administering care to a patient, it can also involve practitioner-to-practitioner consultation, education, preceptorship, and proctorship.

Telehealth Telehealth is a broader application of telecommunications technology compared to telemedicine, which expands to health administration, public health, health surveillance, or population health. Telemedicine is considered a subset of telehealth, while telehealth itself is often referred to as a subset of the larger umbrella term, "E-health." While the content of this chapter falls under telehealth by this definition, we will refer primarily to telemedicine as the overarching category under which surgical applications fall under.

Telematics The World Health Organization (WHO) utilizes telematics as a composite term to include both telemedicine and telehealth, referring broadly to the communication of health information over a distance.

Telestration There may be two types of telestration: 2D and 3D. *2D telestration* is currently most widely applied for surgical training purposes. This consists of superimposing a two-dimensional graphic over the working field which is typically seen by the instructor, trainer, or proctor and the learner or examinee (Fig. 32.1). This can be applied as a digital drawing or superimposed icons or figures using a computer pad or computer mouse. *3D telestration* is where a superimposed graphic is displayed over the perceived working field of the learner or examinee using two separate images simulating a 3D object. This is commonly found in robotic consoles and in developing virtual reality platforms and is an example of *augmented reality*.

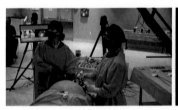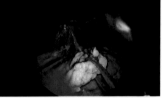

FIGURE 32.1 Simulated surgery on cadaver with simultaneous 2D telestration by an off-site telementor. Viticus Center, Las Vegas, NV

Telesurgery Telesurgery involves the use of telecommunications to facilitate all or parts of surgical procedures. It may also involve aided facilitation by an instructor or preceptor to a learner or mentee at the central site where the procedure is being performed. Teleproctorship would not be included in telesurgery since direct involvement of the proctor over the examinee or assessee would not be usual in proctorship except in emergency or unusual circumstances. Robotic-assisted surgery is an example of telesurgery or tele-assisted surgery since the surgeon communicates to the surgical platform from a console over wired communication, even though they may be only a few feet away. In 2002, a robotic-assisted cholecystectomy was performed trans-continentally from New York City to Strasbourg, France, using high-speed terrestrial networks [11]. Telestration may serve an integral role in telesurgery, where one surgeon is aiding another from a remote location.

When performing tele-assisted surgery or telesurgery in an experimental, novel, or unusual circumstance, having institutional board review (IRB) approval is a critical component. Vigilance must be taken to assure that at any time, a qualified surgeon or healthcare provider can intervene in an immediate capacity should technical or clinical difficulties arise during direct patient care.

Telepreceptorship A telepreceptorship is a period of instruction, usually for a limited time that can range from days to years, where a physician or learner acquires clinical knowledge and skills to improve their performance of specific surgical evaluations, management of diseases, techniques, or procedures using telecommunications technology.

Telepreceptor A telepreceptor is an expert surgeon, defined as a surgeon who has comprehensive and authoritative knowledge and skill in their area of precepting, who imparts their knowledge and skills in a defined setting and for a defined period of instruction to a preceptee using telemedicine.

Teleceptee A telepreceptee is a physician or learner with a gap in knowledge or skills seeking specific and individualized training under telemedical modalities to supplement or expand knowledge and skills acquired during their formal training.

Teleproctorship A teleproctorship is a supervised examination or assessment, involving either a real clinical or simulated evaluation or procedure, using telemedicine. There may be a checklist, pass/fail grading, or global rating scale applied by an observer or evaluator (proctor) to a physician or learner.

Teleproctor A teleproctor is a person, not always an expert in the area of proctorship, who is nonetheless trained on appropriate evaluation or assessment in the specific area of proctorship, who monitors and evaluates a physician or learner either in a real or simulated environment using telemedicine. A proctor differs from a preceptor in that they function as a passive observer and evaluator, and do not directly involve themselves in patient care or procedural execution as the context is an examination or assessment. In the real clinical environment, a proctor is usually a recognized expert in the area of assessment but may not be one in a simulated examination where the stakes are not critical. In the real clinical setting, there may be rare cases where the proctor may need to intervene on an emergency basis if patient safety becomes an issue. In those cases, however, it is important that the proctor be adequately licensed and credentialed in the institution, state, or region in which the proctoring is occurring.

Telementoring Mentoring is advising or training in a setting that is consensual and collaborative for the purpose of imparting knowledge and skills. In telementoring, synchronous and two-way interaction is usually an essential part of a meaningful mentoring experience, although asynchronous methods may be used. Telementoring can utilize verbal communication, telestration, or telesurgery as part of the educational model. Telementoring differs from telepreceptorship by scope: a mentorship is a broader cultivation of knowledge and skill, while a preceptorship usually is more focused and defined. An example of telementorship would be supervision of a laparoscopic expert over a laparoscopic novice for a period of cases to help foster the general skill set. Alternatively, a telepreceptorship would be more specific and goal-oriented: an example might be a 6-week supervision of laparoscopic cholecystectomies to remediate a surgeon on the safe performance of that specific procedure.

Telementor A telementor is an expert surgeon, at a remote site, who imparts their clinical knowledge and skills in a defined setting and for a defined time to a learner or student (mentee), who resides in a central site as previously described. The telementor must be appropriately credentialed in the site, and ideally be an expert in the area of mentoring. The telementor may intervene in the clinical or simulated activities using the telecommunications interface.

Telementee A telementee is the learner or student who, at the central site, is the recipient of the teaching of the telementor. The telementee will ideally be able to interact in real time with the telementor to allow for immediate feedback and adjustments to feedback, although asynchronous sharing of information may also be used (such as the telementee sending videos of procedures for evaluation by the telementor later).

Telemonitoring Telemonitoring is either one-way or two-way monitoring (evaluation) of behaviors, functions, or procedures performed by physicians or other healthcare providers. Telemonitors may not necessarily be content experts in the field of practice being monitored but may be authorized or trained in some capacity to provide surveillance from a credentialing, licensing, or regulatory standpoint. Telemonitoring may fall under a greater umbrella of *telemanagement*, which in the healthcare setting would refer to the use of telecommunications to facilitate administration of a healthcare organization's functions.

Telemonitor A telemonitor is a person who supervises or monitors learners or subjects using telecommunications technologies. A telemonitor is a general term for an observer who does not directly participate in patient care, as they are serving in an observatory manner only. An example of a telemonitor would be an agent of a privileging committee or oversight organization. There have been emerging conversations of having specialists from fields outside of medicine observe and critique surgical techniques – for example, in a crowd-sourcing capacity. Obstacles to telemonitoring in this way must still be addressed in terms of its validity, and in regard to patient privacy.

Teleconsulting Teleconsulting is evaluation of patient(s), patient data, or consultation regarding patient management from a remote site using telecommunications technology. On one level, teleconsulting has been used since the inception of basic technologies such as the telephone. The teleconsultant, by definition, does not have the ability to physically interact with the patient, except through the telecommunications interface. Improvements in technology have allowed teleconsulting through combined, two-way audio-visual communication as with inhospital mobile interfaces (robots that move from room to room) that allow physicians to evaluate and speak with patients from any distance. In the radiology field, asynchronous teleconsulting has been prominent with remote readings of radiographic images.

Teleconsultant A teleconsultant is a physician or healthcare provider at a remote site who evaluates a patient, and/or patient data, and who presents an opinion of his or her findings and/or recommendations for further evaluation or treatment to the patient or other healthcare provider at the remote site, using a telecommunications interface.

Remote Patient Management Remote patient management is a subset of telehealth that allows for the supervision and evaluation of patients in a nonoperative setting, using a telecommunications interface. This may include mobile applications that allow physicians or healthcare providers to monitor patient labs, weight, vitals, diet, activity, or other information important to a number of chronic diseases and conditions.

Current Landscape of Telemedicine

Rapidly evolving technology has allowed practitioners to participate in patient care from remote locations with increasing frequency, and with less latency. The impact to learners such as medical students and residents has allowed access to a wide range of mentors. For practicing physicians, telementoring and teleproctoring fulfill a goal of exposing a higher number of providers to newer knowledge and techniques that may be more efficacious, safe, or cost-effective compared to the status quo. Telemedicine also aids in minimizing the delay of current training in areas or institutions with lower funding, infrastructure, environmental resources, or proximity to such resources. Telecommunications technology has been used to deliver patient care in austere and socially difficult environments such as the military, prisons, disaster relief sites, search and rescue scenarios, and remote locations such as Antarctica.

Advantages for remote technology have become increasingly evident with COVID-19 and its associated challenges due to provider scarcity, personal protective equipment shortages, and need for physical distancing. In response to the 2020 COVID-19 pandemic, the Centers for Medicare & Medicaid Services (CMS) relaxed regulations to telehealth allowing for appropriate reimbursement and cross-state delivery of care. Technological and privacy improvements by over 200 vendors of telehealth software and hardware further facilitated the use of telehealth, not just with patient care, but with telementoring, teleproctorship, teleconsultation, and other modalities of remote collaboration.

Obstacles

Learning Curves

Discourse surrounding technology-assisted medicine often involves the learning curve of users. The coronavirus pandemic has likely led to a burst of use and delivery of telecommunications technology out of necessity. However, both technical learning curves and those involved in adapting to the limitations of remote collaboration require specific attention. Shortening the pathway to proficiency with telemedical applications will be best addressed through directly addressing the technology-naive physician, integrating physician and healthcare provider input into development of platforms and protocols, and forming best practices for the rules of engagement regarding various telemedicine applications. More data is required to develop a language and common behavior for communication during telemedicine applications. An example would be the verbal cues for speaking in turn, without the benefit of observing body language. Another example would be a common nomenclature for directions, establishing if "up," for example, means "screen up," or toward the head of a patient.

Technological Limitations

While Internet, server, and infrastructure reliability has improved with time, there are still several limitations that can serve as barriers to adoption. Without addressing these issues, frustration by early adoptees may in some cases lead to abandonment of telemedicine altogether. *Time delays* can be due to transmitter, medium, or receiver limitations. Institutional firewalls often serve to slow transmittal of real-time data, and in some situations, may prohibit them without administrative approval. While some applications of telemedicine may not require immediate, real-time feedback, those involving direct patient care, especially in procedural settings, may increase risk of injury to patients. Collaboration with information technology personnel is essential. Improvements in transmittal methods and mediums have made time delays in ideal settings almost minimal, however, with the advent of 5G information transfer, expansion of broadband fiber-optic networks, and improvements in the compression and unpacking of data on the transmitter and receiver endpoints. *Cybersecurity* and risk of cyberattacks pose an additional layer of technological and regulatory complexity to telemedicine. The 2020 widespread ransomware attack on the Universal Health Services hospital system was an example of how vulnerable institutional digital infrastructure can be.

Telementoring and Teleproctoring in Surgery

Advancements in surgical telemedicine, specifically telementoring and teleproctoring, have had significant growth due to intentional efforts to assess and improve the need for remote medicine [9]. Recently, there has been a push to improve the safety, reliability, transmission quality, ease of use, and cost of telementoring and teleproctoring technology [12].

The surgical field has progressively seen benefits associated with minimally invasive surgery (MIS). However, situations arise with training gaps that fail to produce enough safe and capable surgeons to meet the growing demand for MIS. Attempts have been made to establish surgical telementoring programs (STMPs) to help alleviate this gap [13]. Telementoring via STMPs has been proposed by the SAGES Project 6 for developing competencies in trauma, laparoscopic surgery, orthopedics, pediatrics, and transplant surgery. The primary goal of the initiative is to provide a software-based space where mentors and mentees could collaborate to eliminate the gap between advancements in new surgical technology and the number of qualified surgeons to perform them.

Utilizing benefits of telementoring and teleproctoring globally requires innovative solutions that address problems both around the world and those specific to individual communities. First, ongoing efforts are made to evaluate and consider solutions for the financial burden of telementoring [14]. This is particularly true in low resource countries. The median cost of establishing a professional system can reach $80,000 USD or more without accounting for annual maintenance fees, which have been reported to be approximately $10,000–$20,000 per year, depending on the type of telecommunications systems used. Additionally, administrative hurdles with manufactured telementoring systems can include latency or broadband deficiencies, and legal, ethical, or privacy considerations [15].

Traditional, in-person mentoring may be preferred by most mentees, but studies have demonstrated that telementoring and teleproctoring are not just beneficial in conferring targeted competencies but show no difference between in-person mentoring and telementoring with regard to complication rates and operative times [16]. Teleproctoring, as discussed earlier, differs from telementoring in that it assesses an examination or evaluation for credentialing or certification. As such, teleproctoring can be an ideal modality to administer high-stakes certification programs like the Society of American Gastrointestinal and Endoscopic Surgeons (SAGES)/American College of Surgeons (ACS)/American Board of Surgery (ABS)-endorsed Fundamentals of Laparoscopic Surgery (FLS) and Fundamentals of Endoscopic Surgery (FES) programs when distance for proctors and assessees is an issue [17]. Costs associated with FLS exams have prompted the evaluation and validation of teleproctoring as a potential value solution while maintaining testing reliability and validity. One study found no significant score differences between in-person and remote proctoring of the FLS exam [18].

While efforts to ensure the quality of training is maintained during both telementoring and teleproctoring to account for the lack of in-person interaction, there can be potential pitfalls secondary to the deficiencies in medium. A study by Okrainec et al. showed great improvement of Fundamentals of Laparoscopic Surgery (FLS) competencies as measured through improvement of posttest and pretest scores via telementoring over 3 days of training; however, of the participants, only 2 out of 20 did well enough to pass the skills test. These findings suggest that a curriculum should be designed to have an appropriate duration for the baseline skill sets of the assessees, adequate mentor training, and pre-activity evaluation of the duration required for adequate transfer of competencies [19]. These factors may be dependent on the esoteric nature of the skills being transferred. In another study, participants were guided by telementoring through damage-control and emergent field procedures with no previous formal surgical training, as they were non-surgeon military personnel. These procedures consisted of surgical airways, chest tube placements, and resuscitative thoracotomies which were done with 100% effectiveness and without complications as assessed by their proctors [20].

Telementoring, telepreceptorship, or teleproctorship may be resource intense, but varying levels of technological fidelity can be applied to help curtail costs [21]. Levels of technology and complexity range from simple verbal communication via telephonic or simple radio means, off-the-shelf mobile phone, tablet, or computer technologies, or preexisting infrastructures available in the institution for nonmedical teleconferencing. Healthcare providers can use this principle to incrementally improve their telecommunications hardware and software as their experience with the technology progresses. One study found a financial solution by utilizing a novel, low-cost setup with readily available equipment including personal computers, a laparoscopic stack, a video-capturing system, and free video-conferencing software totaling $2750 USD [15]. Another recent study showed how residents were able to engage in effective mentoring during the COVID-19 pandemic using messaging software on smart phones to train in laparoscopic surgery from the safety of their homes [22]. Limiting factors such as transmittal speed will become less inhibiting as high-speed Internet becomes widely available. Networks such as 5G have been shown to be equivalent, or superior, to fiber-optic transmission with latency as little as 1–2 milliseconds and data transfer speeds as high as a gigabit per second [15]. Consumer products continue to evolve to include wearables with augmented reality technology. These products have shown benefit in multiple settings to facilitate telementoring in rural and resource-poor settings, with benefits including mentee procedural confidence, decreasing errors, achieving better performance scores, and shortening learning curve duration [23–25].

Discussion and Recommendations

Telemedicine has traditionally been hampered by barriers that were both financial and cultural. Fear of technology or the unwillingness to learn and adapt to new technologies provides hurdles on the individual level, and financial or legal constraints on the institutional level. Despite this, it appears telemedicine is here to stay. The COVID-19 pandemic has provided a setting for telemedicine to thrive out of necessity. The advantages of utilizing these modalities include improvements in physician accountability, adaptation of new procedural skills, and overall healthcare quality.

Best Practice Recommendations

As with any emerging field, the dynamic nature and variability of new data, opinions, guidelines and standards can make adoption with institutional confidence challenging. Our goal is to provide a framework for the safe and effective use of telecommunications technology to implement telementoring, telepreceptorship, teleproctoring, telesurgery, and other remote applications.

1. *Quality*: The quality of various telemedicine applications will only be as good and effective as the core training principles which it supplements. Both trainees and trainers should have shared expectations of their educational experience. The SAGES ADOPT (Acquisition of Data Outcomes for Procedure Transfer) program is an example of a framework on which to build the telemedicine experience. Instructors, mentors, preceptors, and proctors should be trained in their educational or evaluator modalities with in-person activities in a standardized way prior to commencing in telemedicine applications. Once trainers demonstrate competence in the in-person program, specific training for the telemedical modality should be undertaken.

2. *Simulation*: Whether applying telementoring, telepreceptorship, or teleproctoring to a simulated or real clinical environment, simulating (practicing) the activity using all the remote technologies will help to avoid pitfalls, delays, confusion, or poor transfer of knowledge and skills. This also provides a dry run opportunity to identify and troubleshoot any technical or personnel issues that may arise during the planned activity (Fig. 32.2).

3. *Security*: Intentional cyberattacks or unintentional lapses in security can lead to a loss of patient privacy, or the privacy of participants in telemedicine activities (i.e., the examination scores of assessees for a teleproctored examination). Solutions include utilization of dedicated information technology personnel, robust firewalls, data encryption, closed-circuit channels when possible, and industry-standard or industry-exceeding non-digital patient privacy practices (i.e., assuring that screens containing protected information are not readily viewed by passers-by). Cybersecurity insurance may be a consideration when institutional exposure warrants it.

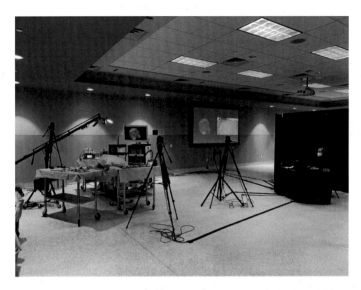

FIGURE 32.2 Dry run setup for telementoring, central site, with IT personnel. Viticus Center, Las Vegas, NV

4. *Contingency planning*: Almost inherent to the complexities of telecommunications is the expectation of systems failures. These failures often derive from connection failures between transmitter and receiver. A robust, layered approach of engineering can attenuate the effects of a lost connection, regardless of duration. This may include overlapping or contingency Internet connections, backup power supplies, the ability to enter a "safe default mode," and a plan for "on-the-fly" diagnostics to help maintain endpoint communication, or to circumvent the main channels to communicate issues to the endpoint users. Contingencies also include clinical protocols, especially with telesurgery or telementoring, where a trained provider can intervene effectively if (1) a connection is disrupted, (2) endpoint users are providing inadequate or unsafe care, or (3) telecommunications appear to be hampering quality care.

References

1. Guidelines for the surgical practice of telemedicine. Society of American Gastrointestinal Endoscopic Surgeons. Surg Endosc. 2000;14(10):975–9.
2. Framework for post-residency surgical education and training. The Society of American Gastrointestinal Endoscopic Surgeons. Surg Endosc. 1994;8(9):1137–42.
3. DeBackey M. Telemedicine has now come of age. Telemed J. 1995;1:3–4.
4. Bashshur RL. On the definition and evaluation of telemedicine. Telemed J. 1995;1(1):19–30.
5. Houtchens BA, Allen A, Clemmer TP, Lindberg DA, Pedersen S. Telemedicine protocols and standards: development and implementation. J Med Syst. 1995;19(2):93–119.
6. Sanders JH, Bashshur RL. Challenges to the implementation of telemedicine. Telemed J. 1995;1(2):115–23.
7. McElroy JA, Day TM, Becevic M. The influence of tele-health for better health across communities. Prev Chronic Dis. 2020;17:200254.
8. Jin MX, Kim S, Miller LJ, et al. Telemedicine: current impact on the future. Cureus. 2020;12(8):e9891.
9. Huang EY, Knight S, Guetter CR, et al. Telemedicine and tele-mentoring in the surgical specialties: a narrative review. Am J Surg. 2019;218(4):760–6.
10. Lesher AP, Shah SR. Telemedicine in the perioperative experience. Semin Pediatr Surg. 2018;27(2):102–6.
11. Marescaux J, Leroy J, Rubino F, Smith M, Vix M, Simone M, Mutter D. Transcontinental robot-assisted remote telesurgery: feasibility and potential applications. Ann Surg. 2002;235(4):487–92.
12. Bogen EM, Schlachta CM, Ponsky T. White paper: technology for surgical telementoring-SAGES Project 6 Technology Working Group. Surg Endosc. 2019;33(3):684–90.
13. Camacho DR, Schlachta CM, Serrano OK, Nguyen NT. Logistical considerations for establishing reliable surgical telementoring programs: a report of the SAGES Project 6 Logistics Working Group. Surg Endosc. 2018;32(8):3630–3.
14. Erridge S, Yeung DKT, Patel HRH, Purkayastha S. Telementoring of surgeons: a systematic review. Surg Innov. 2019;26(1):95–111.

15. Singh S, Sharma V, Patel P, Anuragi G, Sharma RG. Telementoring: an overview and our preliminary experience in the setting up of a cost-effective telementoring facility. Indian J Surg. 2016;78(1):70–3.

16. Bilgic E, Turkdogan S, Watanabe Y, et al. Effectiveness of tele-mentoring in surgery compared with on-site mentoring: a systematic review. Surg Innov. 2017;24(4):379–85.

17. Mizota T, Kurashima Y, Poudel S, Watanabe Y, Shichinohe T, Hirano S. Step-by-step training in basic laparoscopic skills using two-way web conferencing software for remote coaching: a multicenter randomized controlled study. Am J Surg. 2018;216(1):88–92.

18. Okrainec A, Vassiliou M, Jimenez MC, Henao O, Kaneva P, Matt RE. Remote FLS testing in the real world: ready for "prime time". Surg Endosc. 2016;30(7):2697–702.

19. Okrainec A, Smith L, Azzie G. Surgical simulation in Africa: the feasibility and impact of a 3-day fundamentals of laparoscopic surgery course. Surg Endosc. 2009;23(11):2493–8.

20. Dawe P, Kirkpatrick A, Talbot M, et al. Tele-mentored damage-control and emergency trauma surgery: a feasibility study using live-tissue models. Am J Surg. 2018;215(5):927–9.

21. Hung AJ, Chen J, Shah A, Gill IS. Telementoring and telesurgery for minimally invasive procedures. J Urol. 2018;199(2):355–69.

22. Trujillo Loli Y, D'Carlo Trejo Huamán M, Campos MS. Telementoring of in-home real-time laparoscopy using whatsapp messenger: an innovative teaching tool during the COVID-19 pandemic. A cohort study. Ann Med Surg (Lond). 2021;62:481–4.

23. Rojas-Muñoz E, Cabrera ME, Lin C, et al. The System for Telementoring with Augmented Reality (STAR): a head-mounted display to improve surgical coaching and confidence in remote areas. Surgery. 2020;167(4):724–31.

24. Datta N, MacQueen IT, Schroeder AD, et al. Wearable technology for global surgical teleproctoring. J Surg Educ. 2015;72(6):1290–5.

25. Nguyen NT, Okrainec A, Anvari M, et al. Sleeve gastrectomy telementoring: a SAGES multi-institutional quality improvement initiative. Surg Endosc. 2018;32(2):682–7.

Chapter 33
Training for Quality: Fundamentals Program

Sofia Valanci and Gerald M. Fried

Introduction

Over the years, our priority to protect patient safety has influenced the way we teach medicine. We have evolved from case numbers toward more competency-based programs to ensure the proficiency of our trainees. Tasked with the goal to improve quality and safety for patients undergoing laparoscopic surgery, the Society of American Gastrointestinal and Endoscopic Surgeons (SAGES) launched the fundamentals program in 2004 with the funda-

S. Valanci
Doctoral student in Experimental Surgery, Education
Concentration, McGill University, Montreal, QC, Canada
e-mail: sofia.valanci@mail.mcgill.ca

G. M. Fried (✉)
Professor of Surgery and Associate Dean for Education Technology
and Innovation, Montreal, QC, Canada

Faculty of Medicine and Health Sciences, McGill University,
Montreal, QC, Canada

Director, Steinberg Centre for Simulation and Interactive Learning,
Faculty of Medicine and Health Sciences, McGill University,
Montreal, QC, Canada
e-mail: gerald.fried@mcgill.ca

© The Author(s), under exclusive license to Springer Nature   613
Switzerland AG 2022
J. R. Romanelli et al. (eds.), *The SAGES Manual of Quality,*
Outcomes and Patient Safety,
https://doi.org/10.1007/978-3-030-94610-4_33

mentals of laparoscopic surgery program. This initiative, designed to teach the knowledge, judgment, and skills that form the foundation for performance of laparoscopic surgery, was a game-changer by presenting not only a robust educational curriculum but also an assessment component that had metrics that were validated to the level of a high-stakes examination. The success of the FLS program led the way to subsequent development of analogous programs to teach flexible endoscopy and safe use of surgical energy. All three programs were developed jointly by surgeons and educators. Whether it be the fundamentals of laparoscopic surgery (FLS), the fundamentals of endoscopic surgery (FES), or the fundamental use of surgical energy (FUSE), the end goal, albeit in different but related areas, is to achieve *and verify* competency and improve patient safety.

Fundamentals of Laparoscopic Surgery

Development

Laparoscopic surgery was introduced into general surgical practice in the late 1980s. Its potential to benefit patients was immediately apparent. There were great pressures on practicing surgeons to adopt minimally invasive techniques in their practices or risk becoming rapidly obsolete. As a result, weekend courses popped up everywhere, but they were inconsistent in their structure and content, and were often run by industry, who was highly motivated to expand the market. Armed with a diploma from a weekend course, surgeons returned to their hospitals, received privileges to practice laparoscopy, and then introduced laparoscopy in their practices. Although many surgeons were skillful laparoscopists, others were not and a spate of serious complications occurred, such as bile duct and major vascular injuries. SAGES saw the responsibility, as a major specialty society in this field, to take a leadership role to provide surgeons with a high-quality educational curriculum of didactic and simulation-based technical skills training. By including a didactic and hands-on test in this program, the verification that the learners had acquired the minimal acceptable knowledge and skills to practice safely would provide an additional measure of safety.

The development of a training curriculum covering basic skills and knowledge to perform laparoscopic surgery safely was led by a SAGES task force. Four major principles guided FLS development including:

- Assessment of the cognitive and psychomotor domains that are fundamental to the practice of laparoscopic surgery (i.e., the foundational knowledge and skills to build on).
- Focus only on those aspects that are *specific to* laparoscopic surgery, assuming the learner is trained in the fundamentals of open surgical practice and perioperative care (not to teach all aspects of surgery).
- Be agnostic to specific procedures or specialties by being relevant to all laparoscopic surgery and surgeons.
- Include a reproducible, reliable, and validated assessment that can be administered securely through a series of regional test centers by trained proctors with the standards of a high-stakes examination.

A further aspiration was to have FLS incorporated as part of certification of all surgeons at the level of the American Board of Surgery. This was accomplished. The American College of Surgeons (ACS) partnered with SAGES during the development phase and is a full and equal partner in the program now.

Components and Validation

The FLS end goals are to establish proficiency criteria and ensure a minimal standard of care for all patients undergoing laparoscopic surgery. As stated on the FLS program web site, FLS was developed "to provide surgical residents, fellows and practicing physicians an opportunity to learn the fundamentals of laparoscopic surgery in a consistent, scientifically accepted format; and to test cognitive, surgical decision-making, and technical skills, all with the goal of improving the quality of patient care" [1].

The program is not procedure, discipline, or anatomic location specific. It includes didactic and manual skills components provided online through a highly visual interface rich with multimedia content. The didactic part consists of a web-based study guide including theory modules, patient scenarios, and explanations of fundamental technical skills. The modules describe equipment and tools of laparoscopic surgery, energy sources, patient considerations, anesthesia, patient positioning, establishment and physiology of pneumoperitoneum, abdominal access and trocar placement, tissue handling, exposure and examination of the abdomen and pelvis, biopsy techniques, hemorrhage and hemostasis, tissue approximation, exiting the abdomen, and postoperative care [2] (Table 33.1). Each module ends with practice questions. Study material is presented in a self-paced curriculum [3], supported by references and self-assessment. The formal evaluation of the didactic knowledge is through a 90-minute multiple-choice proctored exam taken at a certified test site.

The manual skills test consists of five tasks: peg transfer, pattern cut, ligating loop, extracorporeal suturing and knot tying, and intracorporeal suturing and knot tying (Table 33.2). A curriculum has been developed to guide practice with quantitative proficiency goals. Individuals who reach these proficiency levels on self-assessment are highly likely to pass the proctored test. This hands-on training and assessment is performed in a box trainer with a built-in camera connected to a monitor. Tasks are scored for efficiency and precision; penalties are assigned for errors. To develop the tasks, experts reviewed a variety of laparoscopic procedures and listed those skills that would be required to perform laparoscopic surgery. These included working with a monocular optical system, through trocars, using both the dominant and non-dominant hands to manipulate tissue, provide optimal exposure for dissection, secure a tubular structure, suture, and tie knots. These skills were modeled into tasks and metrics were developed [4].

TABLE 33.1 Didactive FLS content [1]

Preoperative considerations	Laparoscopic equipment Energy sources OR setup Patient selection Preoperative assessment
Intraoperative considerations	Anesthesia Patient positioning Pneumoperitoneum establishment Trocar placement Physiology of pneumoperitoneum Exiting the abdomen
Basic laparoscopic procedures	Current laparoscopic procedures Diagnostic laparoscopy Biopsy Laparoscopic suturing Hemorrhage and hemostasis
Postoperative care and complications	
Manual skills training	Practice FLS trainer assembly 5 tasks

Self-Assessment Curriculum and Proficiency Targets

Both components of the FLS test have been extensively validated. The knowledge-based assessment was developed through an iterative process by expert surgeons and educators with expertise in development of high-stakes examinations. Questions were screened for relevance by surgeons and then reviewed by the committee. Questions that performed poorly were either revised or eliminated, and two examinations were prepared for beta testing. The test measures laparoscopic-specific knowledge. Self-rating of competence and experience correlated with test scores [5]. The internal consistency of the cognitive test items was 0.81 [4, 6].

TABLE 33.2 Performance-based proficiency levels FLS tasks [1]

Task name	Errors (penalties assigned)	Repetitions	Time allowed (seconds)
Peg transfer	No drops outside field of view	2 consecutives +10 nonconsecutive	48
Pattern cut	Cuts within 2 mm of line	2 consecutives	98
Ligating loop	Up to 1 mm accuracy error allowed	2 consecutives	53
Extracorporeal suture		2 consecutives	136
Intracorporeal suture		2 consecutives +10 nonconsecutive	112

The manual skills component shows evidence of both face and content validity. Laparoscopic surgeons developed a list of 14 skills required to perform safe laparoscopic surgery, and 11 of those skills are represented in the 5 tasks of the test. The rest (safe use of the electrosurgical unit, cannulation, and trocar placement) are part of the didactic program [5]. The FLS metrics showed significant differences between novice, intermediate, and expert surgeons, providing evidence for construct validity. FLS pass scores were set to differentiate competent from incompetent surgeons in the basic skills required for laparoscopy [4]. Predictive validity was established by first assessing operative performance in the clinical setting using the Global Operative Assessment of Laparoscopic Skills (GOALS); the correlation between FLS and GOALS scored within 2 weeks of each other was 0.81 [7].

Outcomes

In 2007, Ritter and Scott established benchmarks for practice. Using the FLS box, both authors, who are fellowship-trained laparoscopic surgeons, performed the five tasks for a total of five repetitions. They defined target performance, errors, and time for each of the tasks (Table 33.2). The metrics are simplified to facilitate self-scoring by trainees [8]. They then applied this curriculum to medical students (novices) with access to the manual skills videos and a proctor. Students achieved 96% proficiency levels of all tasks after a mean time of 9.7 h of practice and 119 mean repetitions, and 100% achieved a passing score on the FLS examination [9]. Other studies have expanded on the benchmarks, to provide for adequate resident preparation for more complex laparoscopic cases. By using real FLS scores from previous residents, a group established PGY-specific benchmarks by averaging the total time to complete each task. Some of the PGY-specific benchmarks were faster than the proficiency times that have been used previously. After the PGY-specific benchmarks were implemented, resident performance significantly improved compared to residents that were given the expert proficiency goals. Time to reach the expert goals was shorter, giving senior residents more time to practice more advanced tasks [10]. A previous study had also demonstrated that setting more attainable goals improved performance in the FLS [11].

Because FLS is a self-paced curriculum, studies have suggested guidelines for skills practice; participants have an 84% chance of passing the exam on their first try if they achieve a mean of 53 s for peg transfer, 50 s for pattern cut, 87 s for endoloop, 99 s for extracorporeal suturing, and 96 s for intracorporeal suturing [3]. Following the FLS curriculum has resulted not only in higher rates of passing the test, but the improvement has been found to be durable. One study found a 91% retention of skills at 13 months for all 5 skills without retraining [12], and 90% for intracorporeal suturing at 6 months [13]. Another study found that students who completed the FLS curriculum achieved 86–87% pass rate at 6.5 months without retraining, improving to 96% at 12.5 months with a refresher program [14], demonstrating that ongoing training in the FLS simulator is beneficial and minimizes skill loss over time.

Studies have provided evidence that performance in FLS correlates with intraoperative laparoscopic performance ($r = 0.77$). An FLS score of 70 predicted a GOALS score of 20 (experienced surgeon) [15]. In a randomized controlled trial, residents training to proficiency using FLS had a significant improvement in laparoscopic skills in the operating room as measured by GOALS scores (increase of 6.1 ± 1.3 vs 1.8 ± 2.1). This required a mean of 7.5 h (2.5 h supervised and 5 h of individual practice). The increase in GOALS scores is equivalent to the difference in performance between a first year and a third year resident [16].

Through didactic coursework based on the FLS curriculum, the introduction of FLS skills training, proctored hands-on surgery, feedback, and support from industry and governments, FLS has been a cornerstone for training surgeons in remote areas or developing countries. In Ghana, for example, laparoscopic surgery had not been widely performed before 2017. Using the FLS curriculum and box trainer tasks, an expatriate laparoscopic surgeon trained 78 surgeons in a 3-year span. Only 5% had ever been the primary surgeon for a laparoscopic case before, 22% had assisted on a laparoscopic case, and the rest had only observed or had some previous theoretical knowledge. Before the introduction of the FLS curriculum, laparoscopic surgery in this hospital was not available; during the time of the study, a total of 82 laparoscopic surgeries were performed. During the first year, the laparoscopic surgeon was the primary operator in 100% of the cases; during the second and third year, local newly trained surgeons became the primary operators in 41% and 79% of the cases, respectively [17].

In Mongolia, only 2% of gallbladders were removed laparoscopically in 2005. One team used the didactic portion of the FLS to teach surgeons. In a 9-year span, the team created sustainable laparoscopic surgery for all of the country. Now cholecystectomy is performed nearly 80% of the time in 19 of the 21 states with over 315 healthcare workers trained. The first cohort study showed improved overall outcomes, with lower infection rates, shorter hospitalization stays, shorter recovery time, and lower overall cost. Complication rates were 0.7% with a conversion rate of 2% for the first 4 years of training. Laparoscopic adoption benefited women in Mongolia, where the rate of gallbladder disease is 70%. One study has reported that, even though mean laparoscopic surgery cost is higher, its adoption has been cost-effective for both the patient and the payers' perspectives, because of the cost-related savings related to shorter time to return to work, improved quality of life, and fewer complications [18–22].

In Botswana, laparoscopy was introduced in 2004, but not widely adopted. With the support of the Ministry of Health, a program to teach laparoscopic cholecystectomy was established. After having taught the skills, the workshops transitioned to the operating room, and programs such as FLS were used. Dr. Allan Okrainec from Toronto telementored surgeons weekly and showed that they achieved higher scores than non-telementored surgeons in the same area. Telementoring surgeons achieved 100% FLS pass scores compared with only 38% of non-telementored surgeons [23]. The number of laparoscopic cases increased, and the proportion of cases completed by local surgeons increased from 31% to 98%. Seven years after the program was established, better patient outcomes were observed, with fewer complications, shorter hospital stays, and a conversion rate within standards (5.2%) [24].

Fundamentals of Endoscopic Surgery

Development

According to the American Board of Surgery (ABS), endoscopy accounts for up to 40% of the general surgeon's case volume [25], and, as reported in 2010, 39.8% of the practice of general surgeons in rural areas is made up of endoscopic procedures [26]. However, even when documenting a reasonable volume of flexible gastrointestinal (GI) endoscopy procedures, graduates may have a challenging time obtaining privileges to perform endoscopy at their hospital. Although case numbers are one surrogate that has been used to determine competence, variability of cases, quality of coaching, individual learning curves, and quality of the educational experience also contribute to the development of flexible endoscopy skill. Current guidelines require general surgery residents to complete at least 35 upper and 50 lower GI endoscopies [25, 27]. However, the literature suggests that procedural numbers are poor predictors of skill, which is why an objective, validated assessment of knowledge and skill was needed [28, 29]. The FES was the second fundamentals program developed by SAGES, and was modeled on the experience developing the FLS program [27, 30].

Components and Validation

The goal of the FES program is to establish a standard by which all endoscopists can be measured. Passing FES would establish that the candidate demonstrated the knowledge and skills required, at a minimum, to perform flexible GI endoscopy [29].

Like FLS, FES is a validated high-stakes examination of endoscopic cognitive and manual skills. It is comprised of a multiple-choice test of knowledge and a hands-on virtual reality skills test. The program also provides extensive didactic online material, presented in a highly visual manner. Topics include technology and equipment, patient preparation, anesthesia monitoring and recovery, upper endoscopy, lower GI endoscopy, ERCP, and endoscopic therapies (Table 33.3). The didactic part of FES is available free of charge and can be accessed through a web-based study guide; it contains printable material and practice questions. Each chapter was reviewed by a panel of expert endoscopists (surgeons and gastroenterologists) to ensure that the content is clearly presented, accurate, and up-to-date [31].

The skills test includes five modules designed to assess scope navigation, loop reduction, retroflexion, traversing a sphincter, management of insufflation, mucosal evaluation, and targeting (Table 33.4) [1]. The high-stakes skills assessment is conducted using the GI Mentor II, GI Bronch Mentor, or GI Mentor Express from Simbionix [1, 32].

TABLE 33.3 Didactive FES content [1]

Technology and equipment	Characteristics of endoscopes Setup Troubleshooting Equipment care
Patient preparation	Informed consent Anesthesia risk assessment Bowel preparation Prophylactic antibiotic therapy Management of anticoagulation
Sedation and analgesia	Monitoring Moderate sedation Medications Recovery Alternative sedation Small-caliber endoscopy
Upper gastrointestinal endoscopy	Indications Preparation Diagnostic EGD Complications
Lower endoscopy	Indications Preparation
Performing lower GI procedures	Diagnostic colonoscopy Rigid endoscopy Lower GI endoscopy Important considerations
Lower GI anatomy, pathology and complications	Pathology recognition Complications

(continued)

TABLE 33.3 (continued)

Didactic ERCP	Indications
	Preparation
	Performance of ERCP
	Complications
	Pathology recognition
Hemostasis	Nonthermal techniques
	Thermal techniques
Tissue removal	Resective techniques
	Sampling techniques
	Ablative techniques
Enteral access	Preparation
	Indications
	PEG
	Procedures with PEJ
	Replacement
	Complications
Endoscopic therapies	Dilation
	Foreign body removal
	Transgastric laparoendoscopy
	Choledochoscopy
	Intraoperative endoscopy
	Tumor localization

TABLE 33.4 FES tasks [33]	Scope navigation
	Loop reduction
	Retroflexion
	Mucosal evaluation
	Targeting

FES has been validated with the goal of setting a passing score that must be achieved by an endoscopist with a minimum level of competency [31, 34, 35]. The FES cognitive evaluation was developed by SAGES in consultation with

Kryterion Inc., a company dedicated to developing high-stakes examinations [31]. High-volume clinicians in the field of endoscopy (both surgeons and gastroenterologists) were tasked with developing multiple-choice questions for the cognitive component. Beta testing was then carried out on 393 participants [31]. Items were analyzed for validity evidence. Items with unusual performance were reviewed by the task force, and the decision was then made to retain, delete, or rework each question. A pool of 220 final questions was then used to create 2 parallel test forms with 75 questions each [31]. A panel of 11 experts discussed what the "minimally qualified" or "just acceptable" candidate should be expected to know and do. The items were then correlated with level of experience, demonstrating that years of training and experience were strongly correlated with higher cognitive scores [31].

For the hands-on test, the fundamental skills were identified by a group of expert endoscopists using an iterative process until a final list was developed. The original skills included scope navigation, loop reduction, retroflexion, traversing a sphincter, management of insufflation, mucosal evaluation, and targeting [34]. Multiple simulators were considered, but no commercially available VR system met all the needs required for FES. Thus, after proposals were considered, a virtual reality simulator was selected, and tasks and metrics were constructed to evaluate the fundamental skills identified by the expert panel. Simbionix and SAGES forged a partnership and the hands-on skills component of FES was created. Although the specific details of the assessment metrics of FES are confidential, the hands-on component has been tested for both reliability and validity. Internal consistency reliability for all tasks was >0.70, and test-retest reliability and the intraclass correlation coefficient (ICC) was 0.85 [34]. As for validity, the total FES score correlated (0.73) with the experience of the participants [34]. Also, as an additional measure, a final verification of validity was made with 25 experienced endoscopists who obtained a pass rate of 92% [34].

Outcomes

Since the FES manual skills component was not designed as a training system, test-takers have no previous access to these specific simulation modules prior to testing. Commercially available practice modules, however, are commercially available on the GI Mentor and other simulators. The commercially available GI Mentor simulator module scores have been noted to correlate well with prior endoscopy experience, and authors have suggested it may be a valuable tool to prepare for the FES evaluation [36]. Other simulation training curricula and practice in the clinical setting have also proven to be valuable preparation for FES certification.

FES has provided a validated standard by which endoscopists from different training pathways can be assessed for competence. Experience in residency training varies from one program to another. One study showed that endoscopy exposure in surgical training, without supplemental study, resulted in a 79.5% pass rate [37]. Thus, in order to achieve higher pass rates in FES, curricula have to be improved. To support this, SAGES developed a Fundamentals of Endoscopy Curriculum, which can be used by all training programs [30]. Studies have found that the incorporation of proficiency-based curricula in training programs is effective and efficient in preparing residents for the FES skills test [33, 38]. Additional simulation training, beyond reaching the minimum proficiency level, is very useful for trainees in preparation for the test, regardless of prior experience [33]. After the formal curriculum training, 84% residents passed the manual portion of the exam, significantly higher than without the curriculum [39].

Studies have shown that the total score on FES correlates highly with lower endoscopic experience. For example, 77% of participants with an experience of 0–24 lower endoscopy cases pass on the first try, while 97% of those with experience of >200 cases pass on their first attempt [34, 40]. Another study showed that it takes an average of 103 global clinical endoscopy cases to pass the technical exam [37].

To our knowledge only one study has correlated FES scores and evaluation of endoscopy performance in the clinical setting. In this study, a score of 15 or greater on the Global Assessment of Gastrointestinal Endoscopic Score (GAGES) clinically was associated with a higher initial passing score on the FES exam; further, FES manual skills scores correlated positively with clinical performance, providing evidence of validity for the FES hands-on test [41]. Like FLS, FES has been also adopted as a requirement for certification by the American Board of Surgery.

Additional research is required to correlate FES scores with clinical outcomes, e.g., polyp detection rate.

Fundamental Use of Surgical Energy (FUSE)

Development

The FUSE program was established to address an unmet need in educating surgeons, nurses, and other OR personnel on the safe use of energy in surgery, FUSE emerged as the third SAGES fundamentals program [42]. Historically, heat has been applied to control hemorrhage for centuries. The widely known monopolar electrosurgical generator was developed in the 1920s by Drs. William Bovie and Harvey Cushing [43]. Based on the physics of electrosurgery, a wide variety of energy devices have been developed to control bleeding and divide tissues in the operating room and other interventional suites.

Despite their presence in virtually every operating suite, these energy devices remain poorly understood. If not used correctly, they can result in severe complications. For example, operating room fires were ranked as one of the top ten health technology hazards [44]. Also, unrecognized injuries from energy devices can be highly morbid, with an estimated 25.2% complications rate; 18% of surgeons have personally experienced a burn during laparoscopy [45–49]. In 2011

SAGES assessed their members and found that 31% did not know how to handle an operating room fire, 31% could not identify the device least likely to interfere with a pacemaker, 13% did not know that a thermal injury could extend beyond the jaws of the bipolar instrument and 10% thought that a dispersive pad could be cut to fit a child [50]. No standardized curriculum or textbook information was available to understand the principles of surgical energy, which is why the FUSE curriculum was conceived as an effort to promote patient safety [42].

Components and Validation

The premise of the FUSE program is that, by understanding the underlying principles of each device, users can use energy devices to their fullest potential, prevent complications, and improve the outcomes and safety of surgery [51].

The FUSE program provides a free online course to disseminate knowledge [52]. In the beginning both didactic lectures and hands-on stations were included, but subsequently the hands-on station was eliminated when it became clear that the content could be more practically disseminated by an online or text program. A simulation-based workshop can be added to vividly demonstrate the principles of the FUSE program, but is not a part of the course [53]. An assessment test is available to verify that the learner has acquired the knowledge provided in the FUSE program. To date, this is a voluntary self-evaluation. Passing this test provides verification that the participant is proficient in the safe use of energy-based devices in the OR or other procedural settings.

Topics included in the curriculum are fundamental physics of each energy device, principles of safe use of the currently available and soon to be introduced forms of energy and electrical tools in the OR (as well as some on the horizon), recognition of faulty equipment, troubleshooting, application of correct settings, and appropriate indications of specific energy tools and technology in the OR [51] (Table 33.5).

The FUSE program was developed by SAGES and Kryterion Inc. The FUSE examination has been validated using established psychometric processes, and two forms of the examination have been beta tested. Each exam started with 160 questions measuring 62 test objectives. Following beta testing, the performance of each question was evaluated, and 72 questions were selected in alignment with the content blueprint. The individual expert ratings for each question were averaged to establish a passing score [54].

Outcomes

Evidence has demonstrated that FUSE is useful for both surgeons and trainees. A study has shown that studying the didactic material for a minimum of 2 h is associated with a much improved probability of passing the test [54]. The first study in which FUSE was piloted demonstrated an increase in median correct answers from 55% to 90% in the posttest.

TABLE 33.5 Didactic FUSE content [51]

Fundamentals of electrosurgery
Mechanisms and prevention of adverse effects
Monopolar instruments
Bipolar devices
Radiofrequency for soft tissue ablations
Endoscopic devices
Ultrasonic energy devices
Microwave energy devices
Energy devices in pediatric surgery
Integration of energy systems with other medical devices

Another study of the durability of the FUSE course training found, at 3 months, the examination score was 71% [53]. Although there are not many studies focusing on outcomes of FUSE with respect to clinical events (e.g., burns, fires, etc.), some studies have commented on the clinical impact and the improved safety when using energy instruments by understanding the fundamentals [55].

Current Uses of Fundamentals Programs

Currently both FLS and FES certifications are required of graduating general surgery residents prior to certification by the American Board of Surgery [27, 30]. Recently, the American Board of Obstetrics and Gynecology has also mandated FLS certification for all graduating residents [30]. FLS is encouraged, but not mandatory, around the world, with more than 30 countries having incorporated the FLS program in some way. According to public access data, as of 2015, more than 10,000 FLS certifications have been issued [1]; this has risen to 25,000 as of 2020.

Even though the need for FUSE has been acknowledged widely, it is still underutilized. However, FUSE is highly rated among participants [56, 57]. FUSE France went live in 2015 as a mandatory program to be taken every 3 years by all surgeons and trainees and is, to this date, the only mandatory program. To encourage dissemination and implementation of the FUSE program, it has been translated into Spanish, French, and Chinese [51]. Currently several surgical societies around the world are considering adopting the FUSE program for their country.

Conclusion

Passing the fundamentals programs means that participants have shown the minimum competence required to perform the procedures assessed in a safe manner. The final goal of the fundamentals program is to enhance patient safety and improve education and quality.

References

1. SAGES The Fundamentals of Laparoscopic Surgery.
2. Choy I, Okrainec A. Fundamentals of laparoscopic surgery-FLS. In: The SAGES manual of quality, outcomes and patient safety. Cham: Springer; 2012. p. 461–71.
3. Cassera MA, Zheng B, Swanström LL. Data-based self-study guidelines for the fundamentals of laparoscopic surgery examination. Surg Endosc. 2012;26:3426–9.
4. Vassiliou MC, Dunkin BJ, Marks JM, Fried GM. FLS and FES: comprehensive models of training and assessment. Surg Clin North Am. 2010;90:535–58.
5. Peters JH, Fried GM, Swanstrom LL, Soper NJ, Sillin LF, Schirmer B, Hoffman K, Committee SF. Development and validation of a comprehensive program of education and assessment of the basic fundamentals of laparoscopic surgery. Surgery. 2004;135:21–7.
6. Swanstrom LL, Fried GM, Hoffman KI, Soper NJ. Beta test results of a new system assessing competence in laparoscopic surgery. J Am Coll Surg. 2006;202:62–9.
7. Fried GM, Feldman LS, Vassiliou MC, Fraser SA, Stanbridge D, Ghitulescu G, Andrew CG. Proving the value of simulation in laparoscopic surgery. Ann Surg. 2004;240:518.
8. Ritter EM, Scott DJ. Design of a proficiency-based skills training curriculum for the fundamentals of laparoscopic surgery. Surg Innov. 2007;14:107–12.
9. Scott DJ, Ritter EM, Tesfay ST, Pimentel EA, Nagji A, Fried GM. Certification pass rate of 100% for fundamentals of laparoscopic surgery skills after proficiency-based training. Surg Endosc. 2008;22:1887–93.
10. Hoops HE, Haley C, Kiraly LN, An E, Brasel KJ, Spight D. PGY-specific benchmarks improve resident performance on Fundamentals of Laparoscopic Surgery tasks. Am J Surg. 2018;215:880–5.
11. Kishiki T, Lapin B, Tanaka R, Francis T, Hughes K, Carbray J, Ujiki MB. Goal setting results in improvement in surgical skills: a randomized controlled trial. Surgery. 2016;160:1028–37.

12. Rosenthal ME, Ritter EM, Goova MT, Castellvi AO, Tesfay ST, Pimentel EA, Hartzler R, Scott DJ. Proficiency-based fundamentals of laparoscopic surgery skills training results in durable performance improvement and a uniform certification pass rate. Surg Endosc. 2010;24:2453–7.

13. Stefanidis D, Korndorffer JR Jr, Markley S, Sierra R, Scott DJ. Proficiency maintenance: impact of ongoing simulator training on laparoscopic skill retention. J Am Coll Surg. 2006;202:599–603.

14. Castellvi AO, Hollett LA, Minhajuddin A, Hogg DC, Tesfay ST, Scott DJ. Maintaining proficiency after fundamentals of laparoscopic surgery training: a 1-year analysis of skill retention for surgery residents. Surgery. 2009;146:387–93.

15. McCluney A, Vassiliou M, Kaneva P, Cao J, Stanbridge D, Feldman L, Fried G. FLS simulator performance predicts intraoperative laparoscopic skill. Surg Endosc. 2007;21:1991–5.

16. Sroka G, Feldman LS, Vassiliou MC, Kaneva PA, Fayez R, Fried GM. Fundamentals of laparoscopic surgery simulator training to proficiency improves laparoscopic performance in the operating room—a randomized controlled trial. Am J Surg. 2010;199:115–20.

17. Kang MJ, Apea-Kubi KB, Apea-Kubi KAK, Adoula N-G, Odonkor JNN, Ogoe AK. Establishing a sustainable training program for laparoscopy in resource-limited settings: experience in Ghana. Ann Glob Health. 2020;86:89.

18. Price R, Sergelen O, Unursaikhan C. Improving surgical care in Mongolia: a model for sustainable development. World J Surg. 2013;37:1492–9.

19. Wells KM, Lee Y-J, Erdene S, Erdene S, Sanchin U, Sergelen O, Zhang C, Rodriguez BP, deVries CR, Price RR. Building operative care capacity in a resource limited setting: the Mongolian model of the expansion of sustainable laparoscopic cholecystectomy. Surgery. 2016;160:509–17.

20. Vargas G, Price RR, Sergelen O, Lkhagvabayar B, Batcholuun P, Enkhamagalan T. A successful model for laparoscopic training in Mongolia. Int Surg. 2013;97:363–71.

21. Lombardo S, Rosenberg JS, Kim J, Erdene S, Sergelen O, Nellermoe J, Finlayson SR, Price RR. Cost and outcomes of open versus laparoscopic cholecystectomy in Mongolia. J Surg Res. 2018;229:186–91.

22. Laparoscopy Mongolia Model.

23. Okrainec A, Henao O, Azzie G. Telesimulation: an effective method for teaching the fundamentals of laparoscopic surgery in resource-restricted countries. Surg Endosc. 2010;24:417–22.

24. Bedada AG, Hsiao M, Bakanisi B, Motsumi M, Azzie G. Establishing a contextually appropriate laparoscopic program in resource-restricted environments: experience in Botswana. Ann Surg. 2015;261:807–11.

25. Decker MR, Dodgion CM, Kwok AC, Hu Y-Y, Havlena JA, Jiang W, Lipsitz SR, Kent KC, Greenberg CC. Specialization and the current practices of general surgeons. J Am Coll Surg. 2014;218:8–15.

26. Harris JD, Hosford CC, Sticca RP. A comprehensive analysis of surgical procedures in rural surgery practices. Am J Surg. 2010;200:820–6.

27. Hazey JW, Marks JM, Mellinger JD, Trus TL, Chand B, Delaney CP, Dunkin BJ, Fanelli RD, Fried GM, Martinez JM. Why fundamentals of endoscopic surgery (FES)? Surg Endosc. 2014;28(3):701–3. Springer.

28. Barsuk JH, Cohen ER, Feinglass J, McGaghie WC, Wayne DB. Residents' procedural experience does not ensure competence: a research synthesis. J Grad Med Educ. 2017;9:201–8.

29. Dunkin BJ. Fundamentals of endoscopic surgery. In: The SAGES manual of quality, outcomes and patient safety. Cham: Springer; 2012. p. 473–84.

30. American Board of Surgery.

31. Poulose BK, Vassiliou MC, Dunkin BJ, Mellinger JD, Fanelli RD, Martinez JM, Hazey JW, Sillin LF, Delaney CP, Velanovich V. Fundamentals of endoscopic surgery cognitive examination: development and validity evidence. Surg Endosc. 2014;28:631–8.

32. Mueller CL, Kaneva P, Fried GM, Mellinger JD, Marks JM, Dunkin BJ, Van Sickle K, Vassiliou MC. Validity evidence for a new portable, lower-cost platform for the fundamentals of endoscopic surgery skills test. Surg Endosc. 2016;30:1107–12.

33. Gearhart S, Marohn M, Ngamruengphong S, Adrales G, Owodunni O, Duncan K, Petrusa E, Lipsett P. Development of a train-to-proficiency curriculum for the technical skills component of the fundamentals of endoscopic surgery exam. Surg Endosc. 2018;32:3070–5.

34. Vassiliou MC, Dunkin BJ, Fried GM, Mellinger JD, Trus T, Kaneva P, Lyons C, Korndorffer JR, Ujiki M, Velanovich V. Fundamentals of endoscopic surgery: creation and validation of the hands-on test. Surg Endosc. 2014;28:704–11.

35. Lineberry M, Ritter EM. Psychometric properties of the Fundamentals of Endoscopic Surgery (FES) skills examination. Surg Endosc. 2017;31:5219–27.

36. Byrne RM, Hoops HE, Herzig DO, Diamond SJ, Lu KC, Brasel KJ, Tsikitis VL. Assessing the value of endoscopy simulator modules designed to prepare residents for the fundamentals of endoscopic surgery examination. Dis Colon Rectum. 2019;62:211–6.

37. Gardner AK, Ujiki MB, Dunkin BJ. Passing the fundamentals of endoscopic surgery (FES) exam: linking specialty choice and attitudes about endoscopic surgery to success. Surg Endosc. 2018;32:225–8.

38. Hashimoto DA, Petrusa E, Phitayakorn R, Valle C, Casey B, Gee D. A proficiency-based virtual reality endoscopy curriculum improves performance on the fundamentals of endoscopic surgery examination. Surg Endosc. 2018;32:1397–404.

39. Mizota T, Anton NE, Huffman EM, Guzman MJ, Lane F, Choi JN, Stefanidis D. Development of a fundamentals of endoscopic surgery proficiency-based skills curriculum for general surgery residents. Surg Endosc. 2020;34:771–8.

40. Lineberry M, Park YS, Hennessy SA, Ritter EM. The Fundamentals of Endoscopic Surgery (FES) skills test: factors associated with first-attempt scores and pass rate. Surg Endosc. 2020;34(8):3633–43.

41. Mueller C, Kaneva P, Fried G, Feldman L, Vassiliou M. Colonoscopy performance correlates with scores on the FES™ manual skills test. Surg Endosc. 2014;28:3081–5.

42. Feldman LS, Jones DB, Schwaitzberg SD. Fundamentals for use of safe energy. In: The SAGES manual of quality, outcomes and patient safety. Cham: Springer; 2012. p. 485–8.

43. Pollack SV, Carruthers A, Grekin RC. The history of electrosurgery. Dermatol Surg. 2000;26:904–8.

44. ECR Institute. Top 10 health technology hazards for 2011; 2010. p. 12.

45. Nduka CC, Super PA, Monson J, Darzi AW. Cause and prevention of electrosurgical injuries in laparoscopy. J Am Coll Surg. 1994;179:161–70.

46. Madani A, Jones DB, Fuchshuber P, Robinson TN, Feldman LS. Fundamental Use of Surgical Energy™(FUSE): a curriculum on surgical energy-based devices. New York: Springer; 2014.

47. Van der Voort M, Heijnsdijk E, Gouma D. Bowel injury as a complication of laparoscopy. Br J Surg. 2004;91:1253–8.

48. Tucker RD. Laparoscopic electrosurgical injuries: survey results and their implications. Surg Laparosc Endosc. 1995;5:311–7.
49. Ha A, Richards C, Criman E, Piaggione J, Yheulon C, Lim R. The safe use of surgical energy devices by surgeons may be overestimated. Surg Endosc. 2018;32:3861–7.
50. Feldman LS, Fuchshuber P, Jones DB, Mischna J, Schwaitzberg SD. Surgeons don't know what they don't know about the safe use of energy in surgery. Surg Endosc. 2012;26:2735–9.
51. SAGES Fundamental Use of Surgical Energy.
52. Jones SB, Munro MG, Feldman LS, Robinson TN, Brunt LM, Schwaitzberg SD, Jones DB, Fuchshuber PR. Fundamental use of surgical energy (FUSE): an essential educational program for operating room safety. Perm J. 2017;21:16–050.
53. Madani A, Watanabe Y, Vassiliou MC, Fuchshuber P, Jones DB, Schwaitzberg SD, Fried GM, Feldman LS. Impact of a hands-on component on learning in the Fundamental Use of Surgical Energy™(FUSE) curriculum: a randomized-controlled trial in surgical trainees. Surg Endosc. 2014;28:2772–82.
54. Robinson TN, Olasky J, Young P, Feldman LS, Fuchshuber PR, Jones SB, Madani A, Brunt M, Mikami D, Jackson GP. Fundamental Use of Surgical Energy (FUSE) certification: validation and predictors of success. Surg Endosc. 2016;30:916–24.
55. Vizzielli G, Conte C, Romano M, Fagotti A, Costantini B, Lodoli C, Alletti SG, Gaballah K, Pacelli F, Ercoli A. Clinical impact of a surgical energy device in advanced ovarian cancer surgery including bowel resection. In Vivo. 2018;32:359–64.
56. Fuchshuber PR, Robinson TN, Feldman LS, Brunt LM, Madani A, Jones SB, Rozner MA, Munro MG, Mishna J, Schwaitzberg SD. Fundamental use of surgical energy (FUSE)–closing a gap in medical education. Ann Surg. 2015;262:20.
57. Jones DB, Brunt M, Feldman LS, Mikami DJ, Robinson TN, Jones SB. Safe energy use in the operating room. Curr Probl Surg. 2015;52:447–68.

Chapter 34
Training to Proficiency

Madhuri B. Nagaraj and Daniel J. Scott

Introduction

"See one, do one, teach one." William Stewart Halsted, a renowned surgeon and first chief of general surgery at Johns Hopkins, was also the first to have created the surgical residency. His goal, with the mantra above, was to create a system of learners who transformed into teachers allowing for a formal self-sustaining training system for surgeons [1]. While this ideology continues to be a guiding principle of modern surgeons, many aspects of surgical training have evolved considerably. The question now is twofold: (1) "how to train a surgeon both efficiently and reliably to a desired level of proficiency?", (2) "how to maintain proficiency in practice?"

M. B. Nagaraj
University of Texas Southwestern, Department of Surgery, Dallas, TX, USA
e-mail: madhuri.nagaraj@utsouthwestern.edu

D. J. Scott (✉)
University of Texas Southwestern, Department of Surgery and Simulation Center, Dallas, TX, USA
e-mail: daniel.scott@utsouthwestern.edu

J. R. Romanelli et al. (eds.), *The SAGES Manual of Quality, Outcomes and Patient Safety*,
https://doi.org/10.1007/978-3-030-94610-4_34

The Historical Perspective

Until Halsted's transformation of surgical education, the majority of surgeons were born from an apprenticeship model. Training would last anywhere from 5 to 7 years under a single mentor starting at age 12 or 13 without any discrete guidelines or educational objectives. Halsted, who drew from his experience in Europe and particularly his German training, later came to America where he founded the first surgical residency at Johns Hopkins University. His landmark address in 1904 at Yale University documented the tenets of his training process including (1) intense supervised repetitive opportunities for care, (2) incorporation of basic science understanding, and (3) complex training with graded responsibility over time. His training methodology persisted for decades until change began in the mid-twentieth century [2]. Various bodies such as the American Medical Association (AMA) and American Board of Surgery (ABS) created the Committee on Graduate Training in Surgery. In 1950 this led to the formation of a Residency Review Committee in Surgery (RRC-S), the first review committee in any specialty to oversee the certification and accreditation of training programs. Finally, in 1982 the Accreditation Council for Graduate Medical Education (ACGME) was established, and with it came several changes in surgical education including the restriction of work hours, and two decades later came the focus on six required core competencies prior to graduation. This also represented a shift to outcome-based practice – a revolutionary aspiration to change training from time-based graded independence to a focus on outcomes and competency as the basis for adequate training [3].

Through all these organizational changes, the world of surgery continued to adapt. Advancements in disease management and technological development (e.g., minimally invasive surgery, novel devices, and robotic surgery) have now expanded the expected knowledge base and requisite skills immensely, creating new challenges for how to adapt our training and evaluation processes. Gone now is the era of purely apprenticeship training with solely intraoperative learning, which became prohibitive due to cost and patient safety concerns. Modern training now also consists of inanimate models, animal/cadaver training, and simulation training with validated benchmark assessments. These adjuncts allow a trainee to gain dexterity both physically and mentally with objectivity, but in a manner less constrained by time limits and fixed operating room schedules.

Simulation as a Training Tool

Surgical simulation has lagged far behind military and aviation technology, but has made substantial progress over the past 30–40 years [4, 5]. The explosive growth of minimally invasive surgery in the 1990s led to an increased demand for skill acquisition [6, 7]. It was quickly recognized that using operating room time to gain familiarity and practice with these tools was expensive and time-consuming [8]. In response, surgical educators began developing laparoscopic simulators to foster the development and practice of skills such as laparoscopic hand-eye coordination, depth perception, diminished tactile feedback, and restricted range of motion [9–11]. For these novel training methods to gain acceptance, it was pivotal to generate scientific proof that simulation-based training resulted in improvements in operative ability, i.e., that skills were transferable to the operating room environment. In 2000, Scott et al. performed the first study documenting skill transferability where PGY2 and PGY3 residents were randomized to 5 hours of basic laparoscopic skills training (box-trainer drills) compared to a control group that received only traditional clinical training. Using the validated Objective Structured Assessment of Technical Skills (OSATS) tool, raters blinded to the training group assignments detected a significant improvement in operative performance of the simulation-based training group during laparoscopic cholecystectomies performed on actual patients [9]. In 2002, Seymour et al. documented similar evidence for a virtual reality (VR) training curriculum [12]. In this study, 16 surgical residents PGY1–4 were evaluated at baseline and then randomized to a VR training or non-VR arm after which they performed a laparoscopic cholecystectomy with independent review. This double-blinded, randomized controlled trial showed that VR-trained residents operated 29% faster and made 6 times fewer errors while non-VR-trained residents injured structures 5 times more frequently and failed to make progress in dissection 9 times more frequently [12]. Numerous additional studies were subsequently published; collectively these data helped significantly advance the field [13–20].

These revolutionary studies were paralleled by similar efforts in the world of simulator-based endoscopy training. Like laparoscopic surgery, training learners during actual endoscopic procedures posed potential time and cost burdens [21]. Early studies to promote the use of endoscopic simulators showed promising results but were limited in their ability to document skill transferability [22, 23]. Since then, prospective trials have shown that endoscopic simulation results in a positive impact on technical skill acquisition as well as transferability to real patient care [24–26]. Thus, many carefully performed studies have provided much-needed support regarding the efficacy of simulation-based training for laparoscopy and endoscopy training; in aggregate, this body of evidence has helped simulation become a standard part of proficiency-based training.

Performance Goals for Training and Their Impact

Early simulation training focused on a "one-size-fits-all" approach. Arbitrary endpoints such a predetermined duration or number of repetitions were used out of convenience and in hopes of ensuring adequate training. However, studies showed that the rate of skill acquisition varied among trainees, even when the learners had similar prior surgical experience. Additional studies documented that some learners required extended periods of training and their training would be prematurely truncated due to endpoints that were not linked to performance [27–30]. It became readily apparent that using time or repetitions was not an ideal design for curricula, as some individuals may require additional practice whereas others may need less practice and therefore could spend less time than required.

A paradigm shift happened in 2002 when Seymour et al. introduced the concept of proficiency-based training, which allowed trainees to use as much time or repetitions as individually needed to achieve an expert-derived endpoint [12]. In this study, residents assigned to VR training were required to practice until they reached a performance criterion derived from four expert surgeons. This investigative team selected practicing surgeons who were known to have the requisite skills in laparoscopy, and these surgeons performed ten repetitions on the VR trainer. Their mean performance was used as the proficiency level that resident trainees were required to achieve. This curriculum proved feasible, with all residents completing training; moreover, the time required was quite variable, ranging from three to eight 1-hour sessions. As mentioned above, this proficiency-based training resulted in significantly better outcomes on actual patients during laparoscopic cholecystectomy compared to the control group [12].

Subsequently, this methodology was successfully applied to other laparoscopic curricula (e.g., camera navigation, suturing), box trainers, and VR simulators [6, 7, 16–19, 31, 32]. Following the introduction of Fundamentals of Laparoscopic Surgery (FLS) in 2004, a proficiency-based curriculum was developed and documented to result in a 100% pass rate on the FLS technical skills examination; this curriculum became adopted nationally and has been in use since that time [31, 32]. Similar proficiency-based curricula have since been developed in robotics and endoscopy. Multiple papers cite evidence for improved skill acquisition after the development of proficiency-based robotic curricula [33–36]. One of these entitled Fundamentals of Robotic Surgery (FRS) was a large grant-funded initiative that accrued multi-institutional validity evidence [36]. Debates regarding training requirements for endoscopy also fueled the development of robust endoscopic curricula [37, 38]. Proficiency-based endoscopic curricula have since been shown to have evidence of validity, be affordable, and increase skill acquisition in both upper and lower endoscopies [39–43]. Adoption of these curricula has further shown direct correlation to improved performance on the Fundamentals of Endoscopy Surgery (FES) examination [41, 43, 44]. Thus, as evidence grew for proficiency-based curriculum development, it was soon being adopted into all modalities of surgical training.

It must be recognized that the responsibility of determining appropriate performance goals then is a vital part of curriculum design. First, the metrics applied must be accurate. While the original concept of construct validity remains relevant, it is important to acknowledge that a newer framework for validity science was introduced in 1999. This framework states that validity is a unitary concept to describe the results of a simulator, rather than the simulator itself. Therefore, there may be various types of validity evidence, not types of validity [45–47].

According to early papers in surgical education, construct validity refers to the "ability of an assessment method to measure the trait it purports to measure" [48, 49]. For example, a laparoscopic simulator should measure specific laparoscopic skills and not other factors, such as open surgical skills or other unrelated domains of performance. Construct validity is often evaluated by discerning differences in tested individuals known to have varying levels of experience [34, 48, 50–52]. When significant performance differences are detected between such groups, evidence is generated in support of validity for the metrics used. For example, a study performed by Korndorffer in 2005 tested 142 different individuals of varying laparoscopic experience – novice, intermediate, and advanced – on the Southwestern video trainer and showed significant statistical differences in performance on 5 various tasks [50]. This concept is fundamental to the use of performance criteria as training endpoints since it is critical that an expert-derived score accurately reflects the level of expertise that is desired. While some simulators may generate numerous metrics, especially for VR simulators, only a subset of these metrics may be associated with construct validity [53, 54].

Once construct validity evidence is established for the metrics being used, it is still important to tailor the performance goals to the level of learners and the tasks involved. For example, the FLS training curriculum documented construct validity for all task metrics (time and errors) and used performance levels derived from experts; the mean performance was used for simple exercises (e.g., peg transfer), while a slighter easier level (mean plus two standard deviations) was used for more difficult tasks (e.g., intracorporeal knot tying) to avoid learner frustration [55, 56]. It is important to recognize that curricula should be designed for the learners to meet an acceptable level of performance and not necessarily the high level possessed by true experts. As Gallagher et al. described, in their work they specifically defined "expert" not as a group of physicians that were in the top 1–5% but rather as a representative sample of proficient surgeons [7].

The concepts of reliability and fidelity are also relevant. Reliability refers to the concept that metrics are reproducible when assessments are performed by different proctors (inter-rater reliability) and when performed repeatedly (test-retest reliability). Additionally, fidelity refers to the concept of how much a simulator reflects reality [57–59]. Various laparoscopic trainers range from low-fidelity models such as the simple box trainers to high-fidelity virtual reality models that replicate entire procedures with realistic anatomical features. Similarly, endoscopic trainers range from rudimentary-appearing models using tubes, boxes, targets, and foam all the way to procedure-specific VR equipment with variations in anatomy and pathology. Of note, despite the increased cost, studies have shown no statistical advantage in skill acquisition for high-fidelity models [59, 60]. Both low- and high-fidelity simulators have proven effective, and selection should be based on the learning objectives [61–63].

As we continue down this pathway of training to proficiency, there is a new reform happening. Griswold-Theodorson et al. used translational science criteria as a framework for documenting outcomes following simulation-based mastery learning (SBML), which is a more modern term for proficiency-based training [64–66]. This structure defines outcomes by T1–T4 (Fig. 34.1). Historically, most studies documented T1 outcomes with improvement of skills measured in the simulation environment, or T2 outcomes with improvement of skills measured in the clinical environment. Increasingly, there are studies that document improved T3 and T4 (patient and clinical) outcomes following SBML. In fact, studies document improved patient comfort, operative or procedural time, task success, and reduction in complication rates and cost in a variety of fields such as colonoscopy,

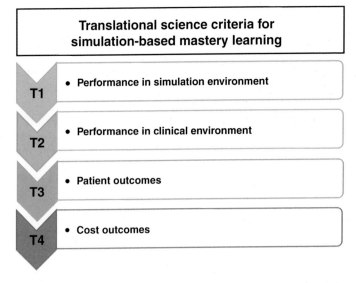

FIGURE 34.1 SMBL translation science criteria developed by Dougherty and Conway and in 2008 and adapted by Griswold-Theodorson et al. in 2015

central line insertion, and urologic procedures [64]. Specific to laparoscopy, Zendejas et al. performed a single-blinded randomized control trial with surgical residents performing a laparoscopic total extraperitoneal (TEP) inguinal hernia repair. Compared to a standard practice group, the SBML group had statistically significant shorter operative times, participated more as the operating surgeon, and had higher performance scores on the Global Operative Assessment of Laparoscopic Skills (GOALS) assessment, and their patients had fewer overnight hospital stays [67].

Lessons from Psychology

The work of Ericsson revolutionized our understanding of expert performance. He noted that traditional theories of skill acquisition focused on an innate plateau of ability that people reached after a certain time period of experience. He also noted that a level of automation that makes intentional change difficult tempers the amount of skill acquisition. Instead, he proposed the theory of "deliberate practice." In extensive studies of experts in numerous fields – such as music, sports, chess, and surgery – he identified the components of training which were unique to experts who showed consistent improvement in any given field [68]. From this work, he determined that deliberate practice has three key components: (1) learning well-defined tasks, (2) receiving detailed immediate feedback, and (3) being afforded discrete, focused opportunities for practice [68]. Part of this learning process is breaking up tasks into smaller pieces, providing the learner with an assessment of their baseline performance level, setting expectations for a higher level of performance, and coaching the learner to correct mistakes and achieve the predetermined performance goals after ample practice. These concepts make sense, as learners continuously push themselves to improve and avoid prematurely plateauing in their level of performance.

Indeed, learners do best in acquiring new skills with guidance as they are pushed outside of their comfort zone. Conceptualized by psychologist Lev Vygotsky, the zone of proximal development (ZPD) is the learning space that occurs between two levels, which are benchmarked by what a learner can do independently and what a learner cannot do even with guidance (Fig. 34.2). Essentially, it states that learners do best when they are encouraged by a mentor to obtain new skills that are beyond their current abilities but are not so difficult as to be unachievable [69–71]. By steadily increasing their abilities, expert assistance can be tapered off (a concept known as scaffolding), and learners can work toward acquiring more complex skills [72–74]. By keeping learners in the area beyond their core abilities, this process results in a gradual increase in what learners can do independently.

Additionally, having opportunities for practice over time is important. Distributed practice refers to acquiring skills over numerous sessions spread out over time. Compared to

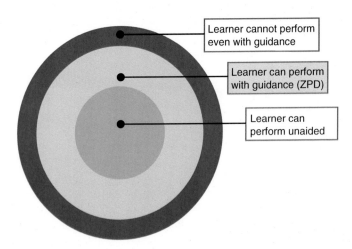

Figure 34.2 The theory of Zone of Proximal Development (ZPD) as developed by psychologist Lev Vygotsky

massed practice, where longer sessions are conducted in a condensed fashion, distributed practice avoids mental and physical fatigue and is associated with better initial skill acquisition and long-term skill retention [75]. Moreover, consolidation occurs between practice sessions, allowing integration of concepts via neural processing for "more efficient and faster retrieval and processing" and thereby improved skill execution during subsequent practice sessions [76, 77]. Ultimately, repetitive, goal-oriented practice results in diminishing the attention resource capacity required to perform the skill of interest (primary task), such that mental capacity is available for other demands (secondary tasks) [78–80]. Many of these lessons from psychology have been applied to surgical skill acquisition and substantially enhance the associated learning opportunities, especially when using simulation.

Integrating Simulation into Residency Training

As recently as two decades ago, simulation-based training and assessment did not have wide adoption in surgery. For instance, a 2004 survey found that 55% of residency programs had skills labs but only about half of these had required participation [81]. FLS was one of the first national programs to be introduced. The initial desire to create FLS began in the 1990s in parallel with the growth of laparoscopy and the subsequent rise in simulation as a way to acquire skills in a safe environment and measure proficiency. In 2004, the Society of American Gastrointestinal and Endoscopic Surgeons (SAGES) introduced the FLS program and subsequently joined with the American College of Surgery (ACS) to oversee the program [82]. The examination consists of two parts, a written multiple-choice examination and a skills section made up of five box-trainer tasks. Content validity was confirmed by finding that 11/14 (79%) of skills required for safe operating as deemed by 44 content experts in the field of laparoscopic surgery were represented in these tasks [13]. Pass/fail thresholds were carefully determined by comparing frequency distribution curves for participants known to be competent or noncompetent based on their clinical experience [83]. Later studies showed that FLS score correlated highly with the validated GOALS scale and was a predictor of operative performance [56]. A proficiency-based curriculum was developed then that allowed trainees self-practice in a distributed fashion until expert-derived performance goals were achieved; this curriculum was associated with a 100% pass rate on the FLS technical skills examination [31, 55]. With the success of FLS and the need for a similar method of training and assessment for endoscopy, SAGES developed the FES program, which launched in 2010. Content experts helped determine the skills components, validity testing was undertaken, and the Global Assessment of Gastrointestinal Endoscopic Skills (GAGES) tool was created [82, 84, 85]. Importantly, passing the FES examination correlated to satisfactory performance in the clinical arena; specifically, a GAGES colonoscopy score above 15 showed a significant correlation to passing FES [43]. Given this strong validity evidence, the ABS incorporated FLS and FES certification as requirements for initial board certification in 2010 and 2014, respectively [86]. Additionally, the American Board of Obstetrics and Gynecology (ABOG) incorporated FLS certification as a requirement in 2020 [87].

It is worth noting the considerable evolution of competency frameworks for graduate medical education shown within this discussion. The ACGME introduced the six core competencies in 1999, which are well known; of note, technical skills were considered part of the patient care competency. In 2014, more granular milestones were widely adopted which aimed to assess performance according to 16 subdomains of the original competencies; a scale defining critical deficiency and four levels of performance was used to afford a more objective assessment of the learner [88, 89]. The education community became quite excited about a potentially more practical framework called *entrustable professional activities or* EPAs [90]. In 2005, Dr. Olle Ten Cate first proposed the adoption of these discrete proficiency achievements for medical school and residency. He defined EPAs as "tasks or responsibilities that can be entrusted to a trainee once sufficient, specific competence is reached to allow for unsupervised execution" [90]. Like the method of Halsted's graded independence and responsibility, he proposes that as competency is verified, graded independence can be given. The difference is rather than time and general concepts; his EPAs reference discrete clinical practice with proficiency-based assessments. And rather than replace competencies, an EPA such as "the workup for right lower quadrant pain" incorporates a variety of competencies such as "communication," "focused physical examination," and "differential formation," in addition to performing the appendectomy, managing complications, and rendering postoperative care. Importantly, EPAs rely on multiple assessments performed frequently by numerous raters using discrete anchors, such that a robust evaluation process is afforded. The expectation is that it becomes readily apparent when a learner has sufficiently mastered all judgment, knowledge, and skill aspects required for a given clinical situation. Having gained traction in numerous fields and in several countries, EPAs are now similarly findings themselves incorporated into modern surgical training. In 2018, the ABS created a pilot residency study with 28 programs and 5 core EPAs dealing with common clinical situations [91, 92]. This has been paralleled by a concurrent effort to implement EPAs in fellowship training through the Fellowship Council (FC), which oversees the accreditation process for Minimally Invasive Surgery, Bariatric, Hepatopancreaticobiliary (HPB), Endoscopy, and other gastrointestinal surgical fellowships [6, 93]. Ultimately, incorporating EPAs into the assessment process may provide useful verification of all competency aspects, including technical skill performance in the clinical arena.

Beyond Residency Training

While many efforts have been made to optimize graduate medical education by incorporating proficiency-based training, arguably few meaningful programs exist for surgeons in practice. It is well recognized that lifelong learning is critically important to provide high-quality patient care. In keeping with Ericsson's model of deliberate practice, surgeons who do not continuously push themselves to improve are at risk for suboptimal performance. Importantly, sufficient data exist which directly link patient outcomes to surgeon performance. For example, in 2013, Birkmeyer et al. reported a landmark study which documented outcomes following bariatric surgery [94]. Each surgeon submitted a non-edited video of a laparoscopic gastric bypass operation. Each video was then edited to the critical portions of the operation and rated by ten blinded peers using the validated OSATS instrument. The technical skill ratings were correlated with surgeon-specific patient outcomes from 10,343 operations obtained from a statewide bariatric surgery registry. Out of the 20 surgeons enrolled, 5 had video-based skill ratings in the lowest quartile. Compared the other quartiles, this group's skill rating correlated with significantly higher frequency of complications, mortality, reoperations, and readmissions and longer case times [94]. Several other studies have since supported these findings [95–100]. One of the most robust studies was published in 2020 by Stulberg et al. and focused on the relationship of surgeon skill according to video-based performance during a laparoscopic right hemicolectomy and patient outcomes from the National Surgical Quality Improvement Program (NSQIP) database. In a 2-year span, the 17 surgeons performed 1120 colectomies. These were reviewed by at least ten peer reviewers and two expert raters and given a score of up to five based on technical skills. Those with higher technical skills scores had a lower rate of complications, morbidity, mortality, and unplanned reoperation. Furthermore technical skill accounted for an impressive 25.8–27.5% of the variation in complication rates after various operations [101].

Given the growing awareness and evidence indicating that surgeon performance has a direct impact on patient outcomes, innovative national efforts have been developed to implement proficiency training and verification in practice. One of the most comprehensive frameworks is the SAGES Masters Program [102]. This effort was conceptualized in 2014 and ambitiously aims to organize the wealth of educational resources within SAGES into discrete curricula for eight content domains: acute care, biliary, bariatric, colorectal, hernia, foregut, flexible endoscopy, and robotic surgery. Within each domain, three levels of performance are identified and rely on the Dreyfus educational model: competency (the level of a graduating resident or fellow), proficiency (the level of a practicing surgeon early in their career), and mastery (the level of an expert surgeon in practice for at least several years). Each domain contains cognitive materials, technical skill requirements, and anchoring procedures associated with each level of performance. For example, a laparoscopic fundoplication is the anchoring procedure for the foregut domain at the competency level. Essential to this effort is the video-based assessment (VBA) program being pursued by SAGES. Within the Masters Program, surgeons who voluntarily enroll are required to submit a video documenting their performance of the anchoring procedure to be evaluated according to the VBA protocol. While this work is still in development, substantial progress has been made in both the overarching Masters Program and validation of the VBA methodology [103, 104]. This work, employing novel methods of coaching, has the potential to effectively provide practicing surgeons with objective feedback on their performance and ample opportunities for knowledge and skill acquisition. It is expected that this framework will positively impact patient outcomes.

The Future of Proficiency Verification

Much of the groundwork that has been developed and is currently being pursued will likely be transformed further by rapid advancements in technology to come. It is conceivable that all operations will be video recorded in the near future and linked to patient outcomes using automated algorithms. One impressive advancement in this area is the black box technology created by Teodor Grantcharov at the University of Toronto [105]. After many years of development, a nonprofit university-based company, Surgical Safety Technologies, launched installation of self-contained units within operating rooms at multiple institutions (Surgical Safety Technologies Inc., Toronto, ON, Canada). This system records not only operative video footage but also audio feed and numerous data from the operative environment, including patient vitals, personnel interactions, and equipment usage. A variety of analyses are then performed which include validated methods for surgeon performance assessment and measures of operating room efficiency. Investigative teams examine data for meaningful correlations to desired outcomes and iteratively incorporate these findings into their reports to facilitate quality improvement. For example, when analyzing 132 cases with the black box, 64% of cases showed evidence of at least one type of cognitive distraction; there was an auditory distraction once every 40 seconds, and errors occurred at a median rate of 13 per hour although only approximately 5 per hour were detected [106]. Moreover, this group develops automated algorithms to detect such events and the associated operating room factors. Indeed, there is much interest in the surgical community regarding machine learning and the use of artificial intelligence (AI). It is anticipated that such technology may facilitate surgeon performance assessment in a real-time fashion with targeted feedback provided through the establishment of normative data sets and the identification of specific areas for improvement. This technology may even eventually facilitate the creation of AI systems designed to aid surgeons intraoperatively. For example, the SAGES

Safe Cholecystectomy Program has highlighted the need for surgeons to obtain a critical view of safety as part of their strategy to minimize the risk of common bile duct injury [107]. This group has documented the effectiveness of photo and video documentation to verify the adequacy of obtaining a critical view [108, 109]. In the future, AI systems may be able to provide decision-making assistance in a real-time fashion for anatomic identification during laparoscopic cholecystectomy and many other procedures. Exciting work is being pursued by the SAGES AI Task Force, and the team is making progress in many of these areas [110]. Given these extraordinary advancements, proficiency-based education is expected to remain a core part of surgical training and expand further into surgical practice.

References

1. Kotsis SV, Chung KC. Application of the "see one, do one, teach one" concept in surgical training. Plast Reconstr Surg. 2013;131(5):1194–201.
2. Halstead WS. The training of the surgeon. Bull Johns Hopkins Hospital. 1904;xv:267–75.
3. Polavarapu H, Kulaylat A, Sun S, Hamed O. 100 years of surgical education: the past, present, and future. Bull Am Coll Surg. 2013;98(7):22–7.
4. Satava RM. Virtual reality surgical simulator. The first steps. Surg Endosc. 1993;7(3):203–5.
5. Martin J, Regehr G, Reznick R, MacRae H, Murnaghan J, Hutchison C, Brown M. Objective structured assessment of technical skill (OSATS) for surgical residents. Br J Surg. 1997;84:273–8.
6. Scott DJ. Proficiency-based training for surgical skills. Semin Colon Rectal Surg. 2008;19(2):72–80.
7. Gallagher AG, Ritter EM, Champion H, Higgins G, Fried MP, Moses G, Smith CD, Satava RM. Virtual reality simulation for the operating room: proficiency-based training as a paradigm shift in surgical skills training. Ann Surg. 2005;241(2):364–72.
8. Bridges M, Diamond D. The financial impact of teaching surgical residents in the operating room. Am J Surg. 1999;177(1):28–32.

9. Scott D, Bergen P, Rege R, Laycock R, Tesfay S, Valentine RJ, Euhus D, Jeyarajah DR, Thompson W, Jones D. Laparoscopic training on bench models: better and more cost effective than operating room experience? J Am Coll Surg. 2000;191(3):272–83.

10. Rosser J, Rosser L, Savalgi R. Skill acquisition and assessment for laparoscopic surgery. Arch Surg. 1997;132(2):200–4.

11. Derossis A, Fried G, Abrahamowicz M, Sigman H, Barkun J, Meakins J. Development of a model for training and evaluation of laparoscopic skills. Am J Surg. 1998;175(6):482–7.

12. Seymour NE, Gallagher AG, Roman SA, O'Brien MK, Bansal VK, Andersen DK, Satava RM. Virtual reality training improves operating room performance: results of a randomized, double-blinded study. Ann Surg. 2002;236(4):458–63; discussion 463–454.

13. Peters J, Fried G, Swanstrom L, Soper N, Sillin L, Schirmer B, Hoffman K, Committee TSF. Development and validation of a comprehensive program of education and assessment of the basic fundamentals of laparoscopic surgery. Surgery. 2004;135(1):21–7.

14. Grantcharov T, Kristiansen V, Bendix J, Bardram L, Rosenberg J, Funch-Jensen P. Randomized clinical trial of virtual reality simulation for laparoscopic skills training. Br J Surg. 2004;91(2):146–50.

15. Hamilton E, Scott D, Kapoor A, Nwariaku F, Bergen P, Rege R, Tesfay S, Jones D. Improving operative performance using a laparoscopic hernia simulator. Am J Surg. 2001;182(6):725–8.

16. Korndorffer J, Dunne B, Sierra R, Stefanidis D, Touchard C, Scott D. Simulator training for laparoscopic suturing using performance goals translates to the operating room. J Am Coll Surg. 2005;201(1):23–9.

17. Korndorffer J, Hayes D, Dunne JB, Sierra R, Touchard C, Markert R, Scott D. Development and transferability of a cost-effective laparoscopic camera navigation simulator. Surg Endosc. 2005;19:161–7.

18. Andreatta P, Woodrum D, Birkmeyer J, Yellamanchilli R, Doherty G, Gauger P, Minter R. Laparoscopic skills are improved with LapMentor™ training results of a randomized, double-blinded study. Ann Surg. 2006;243(6):854–63.

19. Ahlberg G, Enochsson L, Gallagher A, Hedman L, Hogman C, McClusky D III, Ramel S, Smith D, Arvidsson D. Proficiency-based virtual reality training significantly reduces the error rate for residents during their first 10 laparoscopic cholecystectomies. Am J Surg. 2007;193(6):797–804.

20. Hyltander A, Lilijegren E, Rhodin P, Lonroth H. The transfer of basic skills learned in a laparoscopic simulator to the operating room. Surg Endosc. 2002;16:1324–8.
21. McCashland T, Brand R, Lyden E, de Garmo, P.a. The time and financial impact of training fellows in endoscopy. CORI research project. Clinical outcomes research initiative. Am J Gastroenterol. 2002;95(11):3129–32.
22. Ferlitsch A, Glauninger P, Gupper A, Schillinger M, Haefner M, Gangl A, Schoefl R. Evaluation of a virtual endoscopy simulator for training in gastrointestinal endoscopy. Endoscopy. 2002;34(9):698–702.
23. Moorthy K, Munz Y, Jiwanji M, Bann S, Chang A, Darzi A. Validity and reliability of a virtual reality upper gastrointestinal simulator and cross validation using structured assessment of individual performance with video playback. Surg Endosc. 2004;18(2):328–33.
24. Cohen J, Cohen S, Vora K, Xue Xi, Burdick JS, Bank S, Bini EJ, Bodenheimer H, Cerulli M, Gerdes H, Greenwald D, Gress F, Grosman I, Hawes R, Mullin G, Schnoll-Sussman F, Starpoli A, Stevens P, Tenner S, Villanueva G. Multicenter, randomized, controlled trial of virtual-reality simulator training in acquisition of competency in colonoscopy. Gastrointest Endosc. 2006;64(3):361–8.
25. Hochberger J, Matthes K, Maiss J, Koebnick C, Hahn E, Cohen J. Training with the compact EASIE biologic endoscopy simulator significantly improves hemostatic technical skill of gastroenterology fellows: a randomized controlled comparison with clinical endoscopy training alone. Gastrointest Endosc. 2005;61(2):204–15.
26. Gerson L. Evidence-based assessment of endoscopic simulators for training. Gastrointest Endosc Clin N Am. 2006;16:489–509.
27. Brunner WC, Korndorffer JR Jr, Sierra R, Massarweh NN, Dunne JB, Yau CL, Scott DJ. Laparoscopic virtual reality training: are 30 repetitions enough? J Surg Res. 2004;122(2):150–6.
28. Scott D, Young W, Tesfay S, Frawley W, Rege R, Jones D. Laparoscopic skills training. Am J Surg. 2001;181(2):137–42.
29. Brunner W, Korndorffer J, Sierra R, Dunne JB, Yau CL, Corsetti R, Slakey D, Townsend M, Scott D. Determining standards for laparoscopic proficiency using virtual reality. Am Surg. 2005;71(1):29–35.

656   M. B. Nagaraj and D. J. Scott

30. Korndorffer J, Scott D, Sierra R, Brunner W, Dunne JB, Slakey D, Townsend M, Hewitt R. Developing and testing competency levels for laparoscopic skills training. JAMA. 2005;140(1):80–4.
31. Scott D, Ritter EM, Tesfy S, Pimentel E, Nagji A, Fried G. Certification pass rate of 100% for fundamentals of laparoscopic surgery skills after proficiency-based training. Surg Endosc. 2008;22(8):1887–93.
32. Satava R, Gallagher A, Pellegrini C. Surgical competence and surgical proficiency: definitions, taxonomy, and metrics. J Am Coll Surg. 2003;196(6):933–7.
33. Dulan D, Rege R, Hogg D, Gilberg-Fisher K, Arain N, Tesfay S, Scott D. Developing a comprehensive, proficiency-based training program for robotic surgery. Surgery. 2012;152(3):477–88.
34. Dulan G, Rege R, Hogg D, Gilberg-Fisher K, Arain N, Tesfay S, Scott D. Proficiency-based training for robotic surgery: construct validity, workload, and expert levels for nine inanimate exercises. Surg Endosc. 2012;26(6):1516–21.
35. Martin J, Stefanidis D, Dorin R, Goh A, Satava R, Levy J. Demonstrating the effectiveness of the fundamentals of robotic surgery (FRS) curriculum on the RobotiX mentor virtual reality simulation platform. J Robot Surg. 2020. https://doi.org/10.1007/s11701-020-01085-4.
36. Satava R, Stefanidis D, Levy J, Smith R, Martin J, Monfared S, Timsina L, Darzi AW, Moglia A, Brand T, Dorin R, Dumon K, Francone T, Georgiou E, Goh A, Marcet J, Martino M, Sudan R, Vale J, Gallagher A. Proving the effectiveness of the fundamentals of robotic surgery (FRS) skills curriculum: a single-blinded, multispecialty, multi-institutional randomized control trial. Ann Surg. 2019;272(2):384–92.
37. Bittner J, Coverdill J, Imam T, Deladisma A, Edwards M, Mellinger J. Do increased training requirements in gastrointestinal endoscopy and advanced laparoscopy necessitate a paradigm shift? A survey of program directors in surgery. J Surg Educ. 2008;65(6):418–30.
38. Vassiliou M, Kaneva P, Poulose B, Dunkin B, Marks J, Sadik R, Sroka G, Anvari M, Thaler K, Adrales G, Hazey J, Lightdale J, Velanovich V, Swanstrom L, Mellinger J, Fried G. How should we establish the clinical case numbers required to achieve proficiency in flexible endoscopy? Am J Surg. 2010;191(1):121–5.
39. Van Sickle K, Buck L, Willis R, Mangram A, Truitt M, Shabahang M, Thomas S, Trombetta L, Dunkin B, Scott D. A multicenter, simulation-based skills training collaborative using shared

GI Mentor II systems: results from the Texas Association of Surgical Skills Laboratories (TASSL) flexible endoscopy curriculum. Surg Endosc. 2011;25(9):2980–6.

40. Weis J, Grubbs J, Scott D, Abdelfattah K, Abdelnaby A, Farr D, Hennessy S. Are we better off than we were 4 years ago? Measuring the impact of the ABS flexible endoscopy curriculum. Surg Endosc. 2020;34(9):4110–4.

41. Guzzetta A, Weis J, Hennessy S, Willis R, Wilcox V Jr, Dunkin B, Hogg D, Scott D. Proficiency-based preparation significantly improves FES certification performance. Surg Endosc. 2018;32(11):4451–7.

42. Ritter EM, Taylor Z, Wold K, Franklin B, Placek S, Korndorffer J, Gardner A. Simulation-based mastery learning for endoscopy using the endoscopy training system: a strategy to improve endoscopic skills and prepare for the fundamentals of endoscopic surgery (FES) manual skills exam. Surg Endosc. 2018;32(1):413–20.

43. Mueller C, Kaneva P, Fried G, Feldman L, Vassiliou M. Colonoscopy performance correlates with scores on the FES™ manual skills test. Surg Endosc. 2014;28(11):3081–5.

44. Weis J, Scott D, Busato L, Hennessy S. FES exam outcomes in year two of a proficiency-based endoscopic skills curriculum. Surg Endosc. 2020;34(3):961–6.

45. Korndorffer J, Kasten S, Downing S. A call for the utilization of consensus standards in the surgical education literature. Am J Surg. 2010;199(1):99–104.

46. Kane M. Validation. In: Educational measurement. New York: American Council on Education and Greenwood; 2006. p. 17–64.

47. Testing, J.C.o.S.f.E.a.P., APA, A.E.R.A.a.N.C.o., Education, M.i. The standards for educational and psychological testing. Washington, DC: APA; 1999.

48. Winckel C, Reznick R, Cohen R, Taylor B. Reliability and construct validity of a structured technical skills assessment form. Am J Surg. 1994;167(4):423–7.

49. Cohen R, Reznick R, Taylor B, Provan J, Rothma A. Reliability and validity of the objective structured clinical examination in assessing surgical residents. Am J Surg. 1990;160(3):302–5.

50. Korndorffer JR Jr, Clayton JL, Tesfay ST, Brunner WC, Sierra R, Dunne JB, Jones DB, Rege RV, Touchard CL, Scott DJ. Multicenter construct validity for southwestern laparoscopic videotrainer stations. J Surg Res. 2005;128(1):114–9.

51. McDougall EM, Corica FA, Boker JR, Sala LG, Stoliar G, Borin JF, Chu FT, Clayman RV. Construct validity testing of a laparoscopic surgical simulator. J Am Coll Surg. 2006;202(5):779–87.

52. Woodrum DT, Andreatta PB, Yellamanchilli RK, Feryus L, Gauger PG, Minter RM. Construct validity of the LapSim laparoscopic surgical simulator. Am J Surg. 2006;191(1):28–32.

53. Koch A, Buzink S, Heemskerk J, Botden S, Veenendaal R, Jakimowicz J, Schoon E. Expert and construct validity of the Simbionix GI Mentor II endoscopy simulator for colonoscopy. Surg Endosc. 2008;22(1):158–62.

54. Duffy A, Hoghle N, McCarthy H, Lew J, Egan A, Christos P, Fowler D. Construct validity for the LAPSIM laparoscopic surgical simulator. Surg Endosc. 2005;19:401–5.

55. Ritter EM, Scott D. Design of a proficiency-based skills training curriculum for the fundamentals of laparoscopic surgery. Surg Innov. 2007;14(2):107–12.

56. Fried G, Feldman L, Vassiliou M, Fraser S, Stanbridge D, Ghitulescu G, Andrew C. Proving the value of simulation in laparoscopic surgery. Ann Surg. 2004;240(3):518–25.

57. Alessi S. Fidelity in the design of instructional simulations. J Comput Based Instruct. 1988;15(2):40–7.

58. Brydges R, Carnahan H, Rose D, Rose L, Dubrowski A. Coordinating progressive levels of simulation fidelity to maximize educational benefit. Acad Med. 2010;85(5):806–12.

59. Lefor AK, Harada K, Kawahira H, Mitsuishi M. The effect of simulator fidelity on procedure skill training: a literature review. Int J Med Educ. 2020;11:97–106.

60. Nguyen T, Braga LH, Hoogenes J, Matsumoto ED. Commercial video laparoscopic trainers versus less expensive, simple laparoscopic trainers: a systematic review and meta-analysis. J Urol. 2013;190(3):894–9.

61. Ritter EM, Lineberry M, Hashimoto D, Gee D, Guzzetta A, Scott D, Gardner A. Simulation-based mastery learning significantly reduces gender differences on the fundamentals of endoscopic surgery performance exam. Surg Endosc. 2018;32:5006–11.

62. Preisler L, Svendsen M, Nerup N, Svendsen L, Konge L. Simulation-based training for colonoscopy. Establishing criteria for competency. Medicine. 2015;94(4):e440.

63. Wilcox V Jr, Trus T, Salas N, Martinez J, Dunkin B. A proficiency-based skills training curriculum for the SAGES surgical training for endoscopic proficiency (STEP) program. J Surg Educ. 2014;71(3):282–8.

64. Griswold-Theodorson S, Ponnuru S, Dong C, Szyld D, Reed T, McGaghie W. Beyond the simulation laboratory: a realist synthesis review of clinical outcomes of simulation-based mastery learning. Acad Med. 2015;90(11):1553–60.

65. McGaghie W, Barsuk J, Wayne D. Comprehensive healthcare simulation: mastery learning in health professions education. Evanston: Springer Nature; 2020.

66. Dougherty D, Conway P. The "3Ts" road map to transform US health care. J Am Med Assoc. 2008;299:2319–21.

67. Zendejas B, Cook D, Bingener J, Huebner M, Dunn W, Sarr M, Farley D. Simulation-based mastery learning improves patient outcomes in laparoscopic inguinal hernia repair: a randomized controlled trial. Ann Surg. 2011;254(3):502–9.

68. Ericsson KA. Deliberate practice and the acquisition and maintenance of expert performance in medicine and related domains. Acad Med. 2004;79(10 Suppl):S70–81.

69. Vygotsky L. Mind in society: the development of higher psychological processes. Cambridge, MA: Harvard University Press; 1978.

70. Burkitt E. Zone of proximal development. In: Encyclopaedic dictionary of psychology; 2006.

71. Zone of proximal development. In: Penguin dictionary of psychology; 2009.

72. Wells G. Dialogic inquiry: towards a sociocultural practice and theory of education. Learning in doing: social, cognitive and computational perspectives. Jessup: Cambridge University Press; 1999.

73. Wood D, Bruner J, Ross G. The role of tutoring in problem solving. J Child Psychol Psychiatry. 1976;17:89–100.

74. Kurt S. Vygotsky's zone of proximal development and scaffolding. 2020. https://educationaltechnology.net/vygotskys-zone-of-proximal-development-and-scaffolding/. Accessed 28 Aug 2020.

75. Moulton C-A, Dubrowski A, MacRae H, Graham B, Grober E, Reznick R. Teaching surgical skills: what kind of practice makes perfect? A randomized, controlled. Trial Ann Surg. 2006;244(3):400–9.

76. Ericsson KA, Charness N, Hoffman R, Feltovich P. Consolidation and integration. In: Ericsson KA, Charness N, Hoffman R, Feltovich P, editors. The Cambridge handbook of expertise and expert performance. New York: Cambridge University Press; 2006. p. 180–1.

77. Brashers-Krug T, Shadmehr R, Bizzi E. Consolidation in human motor memory. Nature. 1996;382(6588):252–5.

78. Stefanidis D, Scerbo M, Sechrist C, Mostafavi A, Heniford BT. Do novices display automaticity during simulator training? Am J Surg. 2008;195(2):210–3.

79. Stefanidis D, Scerbo M, Korndorffer J, Scott D. Redefining simulator proficiency using automaticity theory. Am J Surg. 2007;193(4):502–6.

80. Meneghetti A, Pachev G, Zheng B, Panton O, Qayumi K. Objective assessment of laparoscopic skills: dual-task approach. Surg Innov. 2012;19(4):452–9.

81. Korndorffer J, Stefanidis D, Scott D. Laparoscopic skills laboratories: current assessment and a call for resident training standards. Am J Surg. 2006;191(1):17–22.

82. Vassiliou M, Dunkin B, Marks J, Fried G. FLS and FES: comprehensive models of training and assessment. Surg Clin N Am. 2010;90(3):535–58.

83. Fraser S, Klassen D, Feldman L, Ghitulescu G, Stanbridge D, Fried G. Evaluating laparoscopic skills: setting the pass/fail score for the MISTELS system. Surg Endosc. 2003;17(6):964–7.

84. Vassiliou M, Kaneva P, Poulose B, Dunkin B, Marks J, Sadik R, Sroka G, Anvari M, Thaler K, Adrales G, Hazey J, Lightdale J, Velanovich V, Swanstrom L, Mellinger J, Fried G. Global assessment of gastrointestinal endoscopic skills (GAGES): a valid measurement tool for technical skills in flexible endoscopy. Surg Endosc. 2010;24:1834–41.

85. Vassiliou M, Dunkin B, Fried G, Mellinger J, Trus T, Kaneva P, Lyons C, Korndorffer J, Ujiki M, Velanovich V, Kochman M, Tsuda S, Martinez J, Scott D, Korus G, Park A, Marks J. Fundamentals of endoscopic surgery: creation and validation of the hands-on test. Surg Endosc. 2014;28(3):704–11.

86. Training requirements. https://www.absurgery.org/default.jsp?certgsqe_training. Accessed 2 Sept 2020.

87. Brissman I. ABOG announces new eligibility requirement for board certification. 2018. https://www.flsprogram.org/news/abog-announces-new-eligibility-requirement-board-certification/. Accessed 2 Sept 2020.

88. Nasca T, Philibert I, Brigham T, Flynn T. The next GME accreditation system — rationale and benefits. N Engl J Med. 2012;366:1051–6.

89. Cogbill TH, Swing SR. Development of the educational milestones for surgery. J Grad Med Educ. 2014;6(1):317–9.

90. Ten Cate O. Competency-based education, entrustable professional activities, and the power of language. J Grad Med Educ. 2013;5(1):6–7.
91. Englander R, Flynn T, Call S, Carraccio C, Cleary L, Fulton TB, Garrity MJ, Lieberman SA, Lindeman B, Lypson ML, Minter RM, Rosenfield J, Thomas J, Wilson MC, Aschenbrener CA. Toward defining the foundation of the MD degree: core entrustable professional activities for entering residency. Acad Med. 2016;91(10):1352–8.
92. Lindeman B, Petrusa E, Phitayakorn R. Entrustable professional activities (EPAs) and applications to surgical training. Resources in Surgical Education; 2017.
93. Scott D. About the fellowship council: creating a bright future for fellowship training. 2018. https://fellowshipcouncil.org/about/. Accessed 8 Jul 2020.
94. Birkmeyer JD, Finks JF, O'Reilly A, Oerline M, Carlin AM, Nunn AR, Dimick J, Banerjee M, Birkmeyer NJ, Michigan Bariatric Surgery Collaborative. Surgical skill and complication rates after bariatric surgery. N Engl J Med. 2013;369(15):1434–42.
95. Keller DS, Delaney CP, Hashemi L, Haas EM. A national evaluation of clinical and economic outcomes in open versus laparoscopic colorectal surgery. Surg Endosc. 2016;30(10):4220–8.
96. Archampong D, Borowski D, Wille-Jørgensen P, Iversen L. Workload and surgeon's specialty for outcome after colorectal cancer surgery. Cochrane Database Syst Rev. 2012;14(3):CD005391.
97. Hall BL, Huffman KM, Hamilton BH, Paruch JL, Zhou L, Richards KE, Cohen ME, Ko CY. Profiling individual surgeon performance using information from a high-quality clinical registry: opportunities and limitations. J Am Coll Surg. 2015;221(5):901–13.
98. Quinn CM, Bilimoria KY, Chung JW, Ko CY, Cohen ME, Stulberg JJ. Creating individual surgeon performance assessments in a statewide hospital surgical quality improvement collaborative. J Am Coll Surg. 2018;227(3):303–12.
99. Varban OA, Greenberg CC, Schram J, Ghaferi AA, Thumma JR, Carlin AM, Dimick JB, Collaborative MBS. Surgical skill in bariatric surgery: does skill in one procedure predict outcomes for another? Surgery. 2016;160(5):1172–81.
100. Fecso AB, Szasz P, Kerezov G, Grantcharov TP. The effect of technical performance on patient outcomes in surgery: a systematic review. Ann Surg. 2017;265(3):492–501.

101. Stulberg JJ, Huang R, Kreutzer L, Ban K, Champagne BJ, Steele SE, Johnson JK, Holl JL, Greenberg CC, Bilimoria KY. Association between surgeon technical skills and patient outcomes. JAMA. 2020;155(10):960–8.
102. Jones DB, Stefanidis D, Korndorffer JR Jr, Dimick JB, Jacob BP, Schultz L, Scott DJ. SAGES University MASTERS program: a structured curriculum for deliberate, lifelong learning. Surg Endosc. 2017;31(8):3061–71.
103. Feldman LS, Pryor AD, Gardner AK, Dunkin BJ, Schultz L, Awad MM, Ritter EM. SAGES video-based assessment (VBA) program: a vision for life-long learning for surgeons. Surg Endosc. 2020;34(8):3285–8.
104. Ritter EM, Gardner AK, Dunkin BJ, Schultz L, Pryor AD, Feldman L. Video-based assessment for laparoscopic fundoplication: initial development of a robust tool for operative performance assessment. Surg Endosc. 2020;34(7):3176–83.
105. Goldenberg MG, Jung J, Grantcharov TP. Using data to enhance performance and improve quality and safety in surgery. JAMA. 2017;152(10):972–3.
106. Jung J, Juni P, Lebovic G, Grantcharov T. First-year analysis of the operating room black box study. Ann Surg. 2020;271(1):122–7.
107. The SAGES Safe Cholecystectomy Program. Strategies for minimizing bile duct injuries: adopting a universal culture of safety in cholecystectomy. https://www.sages.org/safe-cholecystectomy-program/. Accessed 10 Sept 2020.
108. Mascagni P, Fiorillo C, Urade T, Emre T, Yu T, Wakabayashi T, Felli E, Perretta S, Swanstrom L, Mutter D, Marescaux J, Pessaux P, Costamagna G, Padoy N, Dallemagne B. Formalizing video documentation of the critical view of safety in laparoscopic cholecystectomy: a step towards artificial intelligence assistance to improve surgical safety. Surg Endosc. 2020;34:2709–14.
109. Tokuyasu T, Iwashita Y, Matsunobu Y, Kamiyama T, Ishikake M, Sakaguchi S, Ebe K, Tada K, Endo Y, Etoh T, Nakashima M, Inomata M. Development of an artificial intelligence system using deep learning to indicate anatomical landmarks during laparoscopic cholecystectomy. Surg Endosc. 2020. https://doi.org/10.1007/s00464-020-07548-x.
110. Hashimoto DA, Rosman G, Rus D, Meireles OR. Artificial intelligence in surgery: promises and perils. Ann Surg. 2018;268(1):70–6.

Chapter 35
The Critical View of Safety: Creating Procedural Safety Benchmarks

William C. Sherrill III and L. Michael Brunt

Introduction and Background

Laparoscopic cholecystectomy (LC) remains one of the most common procedures performed by surgeons in the United States. According to recent literature, an estimated 750,000–1000,000 cholecystectomies are completed on an annual basis [1]. In 2010 it was estimated that 90% of these procedures were performed laparoscopically, and this percentage has only continued to increase as it has become gold standard treatment for treatment of biliary gallstone disease [2]. Though this change initially came with improvement in cosmetics, hospital stay, decreased pain scores, and increased patient satisfaction, there was the unintended consequence of an increase in bile duct injuries (BDIs) [3]. Several studies

W. C. Sherrill III · L. M. Brunt (✉)
Department of Surgery and Section of Minimally Invasive Surgery, Washington University School of Medicine, St. Louis, MO, USA
e-mail: bruntm@wustl.edu

J. R. Romanelli et al. (eds.), *The SAGES Manual of Quality, Outcomes and Patient Safety*, https://doi.org/10.1007/978-3-030-94610-4_35

published in the 1990s showed laparoscopic associated BDI rates higher than the reported rate of 0.1–0.2% from open cholecystectomies [4].

With increased training and experience, these numbers appear to have trended downward. However, the incidence may be underreported since most studies from the United States use administrative coding data, where the estimated incidence of major BDI ranged between 0.15% and 0.4% [5, 6]. One study of large payor claims database that looked at 319,184 patients who underwent a cholecystectomy between 2011 and 2014 found that the rate of BDI had plateaued and remained at 0.23% in the patient populations examined [5]. Despite the low incidence of BDI overall, given the frequency with which this procedure is performed, it is estimated that approximately 2300–3000 injuries occur in the United States annually [6].

In 2014, the Society of American Gastrointestinal and Endoscopic Surgeons (SAGES) formed the Safe Cholecystectomy Task Force with the goal to enhance a universal culture of safety around cholecystectomy to reduce the incidence of bile duct injuries. Using a Delphi consensus process, this group established a six-step program for safe cholecystectomy [7] and developed a series of educational modules on this topic. More recently, a multi-society consensus conference was held sponsored by SAGES, the Americas Hepato-Pancreato-Biliary Association, the International Hepato-Pancreato-Biliary Association, the Society for Surgery of the Alimentary Tract, and the European Association for Endoscopic Surgery, and guidelines were subsequently published that addressed 18 key questions around reduction of BDI [6]. This review will discuss both the six-step program and will highlight some of the consensus guideline recommendations.

SAGES Six-Step Program

The SAGES six-step program comprises procedural strategies from the SAGES safe cholecystectomy initiative that surgeons can employ to enhance the safe performance of cholecystectomy and reduce the risk of bile duct injury. There should be few barriers for surgeons to embrace these steps once they understand the principles and rationale behind these as reviewed below.

- *Step 1. Use the critical view of safety (cvs) method of iden-tification of the cystic duct and cystic artery during laparo-scopic cholecystectomy [8]*

The critical view of safety was first described in 1995 as a protective method against misidentification of the cystic artery and cystic duct [9]. In order to obtain the CVS, meticu-lous dissection along with appropriate traction must be applied to isolate the two cystic structures. The first criterion required is the removal of fat and fibrous tissue from the hepatocystic triangle. This step is carried out with a combina-tion of blunt dissection and electrosurgical energy per the surgeon's preference. The hepatocystic triangle is bordered by the cystic duct laterally, the common hepatic duct medially, and the inferior edge of the liver. Of note, exposure of the common hepatic duct and common bile duct is not a part of the CVS, and one should *not* attempt to do so, although these can, in many cases, be seen without any added dissection. Regardless, one should always maintain vigilance and aware-ness of their possible location.

The second criterion of the CVS is separation of the lower one-third of gallbladder from the liver to expose the cystic plate. This component of the CVS is based on the principles of safety in open cholecystectomy where the cystic duct and artery were isolated, and then the gallbladder was completely disconnected from the liver bed before these structures were ligated and divided [8]. With laparoscopic cholecystectomy, it is technically challenging to completely disconnect the gall-bladder, so separating the lower 1/3 of the gallbladder is used instead. This step is critically important to minimize the risk of injuring aberrant anatomy of the right hepatic duct or artery, to avoid misidentification of the cystic duct for the bile duct in the initial part of the dissection, and to prevent clipping or division of the bile duct of hepatic duct. The sequence of the dissection to achieve this step of the CVS is shown in Fig. 35.1.

Completing components one and two of the CVS allows for greater lateral retraction of the gallbladder neck which helps to expose the cystic duct from the gallbladder, and allows for a more complete and safe dissection. The final criterion is to ensure that only two individual structures (cystic artery and cystic duct) are seen entering the gallbladder as shown in Fig. 35.2.

In some cases, more than two structures can be seen, which is due to the presence of an anterior and posterior cystic artery with early bifurcation. In such cases, it should be possible to trace the artery branches well up onto the gallbladder. However, this should raise one's awareness to ensure the dissection was not being carried out too low and an additional unintended structure has become involved.

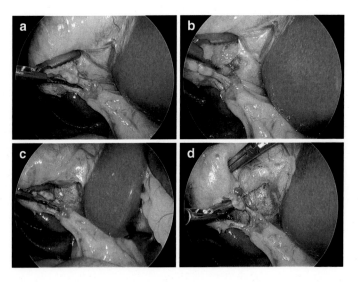

FIGURE 35.1 (**a**) Small window between cystic duct and artery; (**b**) initial window between cystic artery and liver bed; (**c**), further opening of the cystic plate; (**d**), completion of separation of 1/3 of lower GB off the liver bed

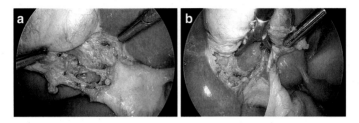

FIGURE 35.2 Completion of the CVS with doublet photographic documentation from the anterior (**a**) and posterior (**b**) perspective

The consensus guidelines examined whether use of the CVS can help mitigate the risk of bile duct injuries. To date there have been no controlled, randomized control trials to support the usage of CVS over any other methods of identification as such a study would require more than 10,000 patients and would be too costly and impractical to perform. The panel did perform a retrospective pooled BDI incidence analysis when comparing studies that use the CVS versus the infundibular identification technique and found an incidence of 2 in one million cases when the CVS was used versus 1.5 BDIs in 1000 cases when it was not [6]. Additionally, the guideline panel also reviewed multiple single-institutional case series which found that when BDIs occurred, they were in cases in which the CVS was not obtained [10]. As a result, the panel made a *strong recommendation for use of the CVS* as the preferred method of ductal identification.

Incorporation of proper education on the critical view safety and its components are essential for its implementation into daily practice. A study performed at Thomas Jefferson University of 43 general surgery residents examined the impact of proper education in this regard [11]. All surgical residents were required to attend a comprehensive education course on preforming safe cholecystectomy. Fifty-one cases were recorded pre-education, and another 50 cases were recorded post-education. The videos from the resident cases were given a CVS score ranging from 1 to 6 using the Sanford-Strasberg scoring method [12]. Pre-intervention, the average CVS score was 2.3, which dramatically increased to a mean of 4.3 after the educational intervention. Furthermore, the number of procedures that were found to have a CVS score ≥4 increased from 15.7% to 52%.

The guideline panel also investigated whether the usage of CVS coaching of surgeons limited the risk or severity of BDI. Though the quality of evidence was low, in a study in which ten practicing surgeons submitted intraoperative videos, it was found that only 20% obtained the CVS prior to clipping any structures [13]. After the surgeons received coaching about the CVS, a measurable increase in their CVS scores from 1.75 to 3.75 was seen. These studies suggest that both practicing surgeons and trainees have an incomplete understanding of the CVS or ability to clearly demonstrate it via video and that directed educational interventions can improve its attainment.

- *Step 2. understand the potential for aberrant anatomy in all cases*

The majority of biliary injuries are a result of misidentification of anatomy, mistaking the common bile duct for the cystic duct; this risk is increased in the setting of aberrant anatomy [9]. The most common biliary abnormalities involve a short cystic duct or a deviation in the normal insertion of the cystic duct into the common hepatic duct. Additionally, the other common anomaly is an aberrant right hepatic duct or right posterior sectoral duct onto which the cystic duct may insert and which may run very proximate to the hepatocystic triangle (Fig. 35.3). Cholangiography may be useful in helping identify an aberrant duct and, thereby, avoiding injury.

A recent study from Natsume and colleagues examined 1289 patients in which they reviewed MR cholangiography for both thickening of the gallbladder wall and aberrant anatomy and compared the incidence of bile duct injury [14]. They found that aberrant anatomy was an independent predictor for possible BDI with an OR of 10.96. Radiological

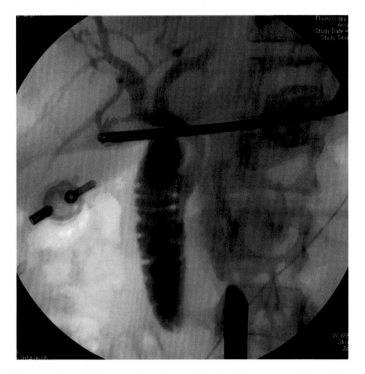

FIGURE 35.3 Cholangiogram demonstrating aberrant anatomy with cystic duct that enters the right hepatic duct

studies have also examined the incidence of cystic duct variation. One study that examined MRCPs in 198 patients, a normal lateral insertion of the cystic duct into the middle third of the common hepatic duct occurred in only 51% of cases [15].

Mastering biliary anatomy should consist of not only operative findings but also preoperative and intraoperative imaging. Aberrant biliary anatomy may be seen on imaging tests such as ERCP which if done should always be reviewed preoperatively by the surgeon, and abnormal arterial anatomy may be occasionally seen on preoperative CT scans (done more commonly in patients with acute cholecystitis). Recognition of aberrant ducts on intraoperative cholangiography or other intraoperative imaging modalities (ultrasound, near-infrared cholangiography) is also an essential skill that all surgeons should have in their armamentarium.

- *Step 3. make liberal usage of cholangiography or other methods to image the biliary tree intraoperatively.*

The consensus guideline panel examined the use of intra-operative cholangiography (IOC) vs no IOC in mitigating the risk of BDI. Fourteen studies were pooled by the panel for a combination of 2.5 million patients to look into the benefit of IOC in mitigation of bile duct injury [6]. Overall the pooled data showed a reduced incidence of BDI when using IOC with an OR 0.78 and when risk-adjusted an OR of 0.81, both which were found to be statistically significant [6]. In a study from the Swedish Gallriks inpatient registry database that examined the rate of BDI, out of the 152,776 cholecystecto-mies performed, a total of 613 BDIs were reported [16]. Overall, IOC was used in 94,569 of these patients and showed a 34% risk reduction in BDI when compared to no IOC. Also from the Gallriks database, in patients with acute cholecysti-tis (AC) or a history of acute cholecystitis, IOC use was asso-ciated with a reduced risk of BDI OR 0.59 (95% CI 0.30–0.63) and OR 0.59 (95% CI 0.35–1.00), respectively [17]. An asso-ciation was not found in patients who did not have AC of a history of AC (OR 1.06, 95% CI 0.75–1.49). Given these find-ings, the consensus panel recommended liberal usage of intra-operative cholangiography in patients with acute cholecystitis (AC) or with a history of AC to help decrease the risk of BDI [6]. Due to the uncertainty of the evidence, no recommenda-tion was made regarding IOC for LC in elective non-acute cholecystitis. However, surgeons should consider other fac-tors that may favor the use of IOC including a history of abnormal liver function tests, gallstone pancreatitis, a difficult dissection, or history of prior gastric bypass, which would make subsequent ERCP challenging.

Additionally, the panel made a strong recommendation that surgeons incorporate intraoperative biliary imaging in the setting of an uncertain biliary anatomy or if there is a concern for a possible BDI. A meta-analysis was performed using 8 independent studies that included a total of 1256 BDIs and compared the usage of IOC or not [6]. The usage of IOC was associated with increased operative recognition of BDI with an OR of 2.92 when compared to no IOC.

Other intraoperative imaging modalities: Laparoscopic intraoperative ultrasound (LUS) has not been as extensively studied when compared to IOC. One meta-analysis that compared usage of LUS versus IOC for successful visualization of biliary anatomy demonstrated similar rates of ductal identification [18]. Recently, near-infrared (NIR) light technology has been investigated as an adjunct for ductal identification use during cholecystectomy. A prospective, randomized trial reported by Dip et al. compared the detection rate for biliary anatomy using white light ($N = 318$) vs white light plus NIR cholangiography ($N = 321$) during LC [19]. The seven biliary structures examined were the cystic duct, right hepatic duct, common hepatic duct, common bile duct, cystic common bile duct junction, cystic gallbladder junction, and accessory bile ducts, before and after surgical dissection. Detection rates of these structures were found to be statistically higher in the NIR group when compared to the white light group prior to any surgical dissection with an OR ranging from 2.3 to 3.6. Similar results were found after dissection excluding the common duct and cystic common bile duct junction. Two patients from the study sustained "mild" biliary duct injuries, both in the white light group. Currently a second randomized control trial (FALCON Trial, NCT02558556) is underway that compares NIR to white light with results pending.

As a result of the Dip study, the consensus panel recommended that the use of NIR imaging may be considered as an adjunct to white light alone for identification of biliary anatomy during cholecystectomy [6]. This was a conditional recommendation with a very low certainty of evidence. No recommendation was made in regard to use of NIR vs IOC because of insufficient evidence to answer the question. It is important to note that the panel emphasized that NIR should not be a substitute for a complete dissection and identification of the critical view of safety.

- *Step 4. Consider an intraoperative momentary pause prior to clipping, cutting, or transecting any ductal structures*

As a general operating room safety measure, the use of a time-out prior to starting the case has been implemented broadly to reduce wrong site surgery and surgical errors and to enhance communication between team members. The original Step 4 of the safe chole program used the term "time-out" before clipping or cutting ductal structures. The guideline panel included this question in its deliberations, but at the consensus meeting, there was considerable pushback from both the expert panel and surgeons in attendance because of the potential medicolegal implications of the term "time-out." As a result, the recommendation was revised and subsequently approved that "as a best practice, it is suggested that surgeons conduct a momentary pause before clipping/cutting the cystic duct and cystic artery." The purpose of this recommendation is to serve as a stop point for the surgeon to step back, pause, and verify that the anatomy is correct and that an adequate CVS has been obtained before committing to clipping and dividing the critical structures. This approach may help mitigate against the heuristic unconscious assumptions that can occur with visual perception [20]; it should be easy to integrate into each operation, does not involve any significant delay, and requires minimal additional effort.

Another question addressed by the panel was whether two surgeons versus one surgeon should be considered to lower the risk of BDI. Ultimately, no literature was found to address this question, and it would be impractical to apply in many practice settings. Nonetheless, in cases in which there is difficulty with the dissection, a lack of progression, or uncertainty of anatomy, intraoperative consultation with a surgical colleague or a hepatobiliary surgeon (a second set of eyes) where feasible should be considered.

Since the intraoperative physical presence of an additional surgeon is not as easily established, Sobba et al. at Wake Forest University investigated the usage of a secure multimedia message system (MMS) to grade intraoperative CVS images [21]. In this study, 193 laparoscopic cholecystectomies were performed which involved 14 surgeons. Once the operating team had "obtained" the CVS, both anterior and posterior images of it were taken and sent via MMS for grading by another surgeon remotely. The average response time was found to be under 5 min, and images were graded on a scale of 0–6. The authors suggested that this approach could be used for providing real time for feedback of achievement of the CVS to surgeons during the course of an operation. While there were a number of limitations of the study, this is valid proof of concept for having a second surgeon to evaluate and validate the CVS without having to be physically present in the operating room.

An area of controversy in the use of the CVS is to whether to obtain photo documentation of it. This question was addressed by the guideline panel, but no recommendation was made because of concerns regarding feasibility, acceptability, and medicolegal implications. It should be noted that the accuracy of documentation of obtaining the CVS with operative notes is generally poor. For surgeons who choose to document, doublet photographs (of the anterior and posterior views) are considered to be superior to single photographs, as described by Sanford et al. [12]. Video is also generally superior to still photographic documentation. Each surgeon should consider their own practice and, alternatively, whether photo documentation may be utilized as a quality improvement measure across their hospital.

Another potentially intriguing application to enhancing operative safety is artificial intelligence (AI) and machine learning which are being studied across the field of medicine. Though this is not ready for implementation to evaluate the critical view of safety, studies have begun to address this around laparoscopic cholecystectomy. Tokuyasu and colleagues looked at artificial intelligence for identification of surgical landmarks during laparoscopic cholecystectomy [22]. In their study, the cystic duct, common bile duct, lower edge of the left medial liver segment, and Rouviere's sulcus were selected. After a learning period, the computer software was tested using 23 unique images. The software was able to successfully determine all 4 landmarks in 22 of 23 cases after being confirmed with 2 expert surgeons. Future applications of AI could include verifying identification of the CVS and/or areas of potential danger for the dissection. Madani et al. recently analyzed 308 LC videos and was able to segment them into safe (GO) and dangerous (NO GO) zones using AI following expert annotation with a high degree of reliability [23].

• *Step 5. Recognize when the dissection is approaching a zone of significant risk, and halt the dissection before entering that zone. The operation should be finished by a safe method other than cholecystectomy if conditions around the gallbladder are too dangerous.*

A number of preoperative risk factors have been identified that are associated with increased difficulty of cholecystectomy. Accordingly, the guideline panel asked the question whether surgical risk/complexity stratification should be done or not prior to undertaking cholecystectomy. For reference, the two most commonly used models for acute cholecystitis (AC) are the Tokyo guidelines and the American Association for the Surgery of Trauma (AAST) severity grading classification [24, 25]. The Tokyo guidelines were recently updated in 2018 (TG 18). Although there were limitations in the evidence in the literature, it was felt that since more severe grades of cholecystitis are associated with greater risk of BDI, that utilization of a risk stratification system could potentially mitigate the risk of BDI. TG 18 goes an additional step by providing a recommend algorithm for the care of each grade of AC. Both the TG 13 and TG 18 produced strong evidence to suggest that the risk of BDI increased with the severity of inflammation. A summary of the T18 and AAST grading classifications is shown in Table 35.1.

TABLE 35.1 Grading classification systems for acute cholecystitis

Tokyo grade	Criteria
I	1. Local signs of inflammation (Murphy sign, right upper quadrant mass/pain/tenderness)
	2. Systemic signs of inflammation (fever, elevated CRP and/or WBC)
	3. Imaging findings consistent with acute cholecystitis
	4. Absence of Grade II or II criteria
II	Elevated WBC >18,000/mm^3
	Palpable tender RUQ mass
	Symptom duration >72 h
	Marked local inflammation (gangrenous or emphysematous cholecystitis, peri-cholecystic abscess, biliary peritonitis)
III	Dysfunction of cardiovascular (hypotension on pressors), neurological (altered LOC), respiratory (PaO2/FiO$_2$ < 300), renal (oliguria, Cr > 2.0), hepatic (INR > 1.5), or hematologic (Plts <100,000/mm^3) systems

AAST grade	Description (imaging/operative)
I	Localized gallbladder inflammation, wall thickening, peri-cholecystic fluid
II	Distended gallbladder with purulence or hydrops, necrosis/gangrene of wall without perforation/air in GB wall or biliary tree
III	Perforation with bile localized to RUQ
IV	Peri-cholecystic abscess, bilioenteric fistula, gallstone ileus
V	Grade IV disease but with generalized peritonitis/free intraperitoneal fluid

Modified from Yokoe et al. [25] and Hernandez et al. [35]
CRP C-reactive protein, WBC white blood cell count, LOC loss of consciousness, Cr creatinine, Plts platelets

For patients who present with TG Grade I AC, the panel recommended surgical intervention within 72 h of symptom onset [6]. No recommendations were made in regard to timing of surgery for those with TG II or Grade III AC because the evidence was insufficient. The TG 18 guidelines also support surgical intervention for Grade I acute cholecystitis; however, advise antibiotics and medical management for those with Grade II and Grade III without emergent surgical indications [25].

A 2016 case-control study performed by Tornqvist et al. [26] examined data from all iatrogenic bile duct injuries within the Swedish inpatient registry, and compared these to a control group from the same registry who underwent uneventful cholecystectomy. Patients with TG 1 AC did not have an increased risk of bile duct injury (OR 0.96); however, patients with TG Grade II AC had over double the risk of BDI (OR 2.41), and those with Tokyo Grade III had almost eight times increased odds of BDI (OR 8.43). Overall, the adjusted risk of BDI was almost double in patients with moderate to severe AC (OR 1.97). Additionally, as stated previously, the use of intraoperative cholangiography reduced BDI injury risk by 52% (OR 0.48).

In addition to acute cholecystitis, it is important to recognize other risk factors that portend a more difficult gallbladder. In one literature review of 91 studies that included a total of 324,553 patients, several risk factors were identified as shown in Table 35.2 [27]. Strasberg has described the presence of biliary inflammatory fusion when there is severe fibrosis and contraction in the area of the hepatocystic triangle [28]. This situation poses an increased risk of injury and should lead to consideration of a bailout option.

A number of different bailout techniques have been described for when dissection of the gallbladder, specifically the hepatocystic triangle, becomes too difficult due to severe inflammation or other factors. They include the fundus-first approach (top-down) and subtotal cholecystectomy, either by the fenestrating or reconstituting technique [29]. No direct randomized control trial has been performed to compare

TABLE 35.2 Risk factors for difficult cholecystectomy

Male gender	Increased age
Chronic cholecystitis with fibrosis	Obesity
Liver cirrhosis	Previous upper abdominal surgery
Emergent cholecystectomy	Cystic duct stones
Hepatomegaly	Biliary malignancy
Bilioenteric fistula	Anatomic abnormalities
Inexperience	

these two techniques and their impact on BDI. However, it was the opinion of the guideline panel that avoiding entry into the hepatocystic triangle would be preferable in such cases, which would be more readily accomplished by subtotal cholecystectomy than a top-down approach. Moreover, the top-down approach has been associated with severe vascular-biliary injuries [30].

Subtotal cholecystectomy may be performed either laparoscopically or open depending on the surgeon's experience instead of attempting a total cholecystectomy. A fenestrating subtotal cholecystectomy is generally preferred over the reconstituting type in order to avoid a remnant gallbladder. In the uncommon situation in which the neck of the gallbladder cannot be exposed, one should consider placement of a surgical cholecystostomy tube in the fundus of the gallbladder and abort attempts at further dissection. Oftentimes, open cholecystectomy has been the preferred bailout option. It should be noted, however, that biliary injuries may still occur after conversion of a laparoscopic to open procedure [31], and most recent surgical graduates and trainees have little operative experience with difficult open cholecystectomies.

- *Step 6. Get help from another surgeon (when the dissection or conditions are difficult).*

As previously discussed, engagement of another surgeon can be extremely valuable when there is difficulty with the dissection and lack of progression, and especially if there is concern that a complication or biliary injury has occurred. There is some evidence in the literature to support the notion that more experienced surgeons have a lower rate of BDI. A 2014 observational study examined 52,632 LCs from an insurance claims database which was linked to surgeons who had completed the Fundamental of Laparoscopic Surgery course or not [32]. Overall, they found that more experienced surgeons (20.7 mean years in practice) had a significantly lower BDI rate (0.14%) compared to less experienced surgeons (6.1 mean years in practice) who had a BDI rate of 0.47%. The recommendation on this issue by the guideline panel was conditional due to concerns regarding feasibility and acceptability, especially in smaller hospitals with limited surgical support. One strategy in such cases would be telephone or video consultation with a senior or HPB surgeon in a referral center when local expertise is not available.

Importance of Avoiding BDI

Although BDI is not the most common complication after LC, it is the most common consequential complication. Compared to the initial intended procedure that is typically outpatient with an expected rapid recovery and full return to health, it is highly morbid; requires additional surgical, radiologic, and endoscopic interventions; significantly increases the cost of care; is associated with a several-fold increase in mortality rate; and often results in medicolegal consequences. Bile duct injury is, in fact, the most common reason for litigation against general surgeons. Further interventions can occur over weeks to months leading to a significant harm to the patient's quality of life (QOL) and trust in the healthcare system.

Multiple studies in regard to quality of life (QOL) after BDI have been performed. Some show no differences, while others show significant differences in multiple realms. Halbert et al. investigated the long-term outcomes of patients with common bile duct injury following surgical treatment for cholelithiasis between 2005 and 2010 in a New York State administrative database [33]. Of 156,958 LCs, 125 patients with CBD injuries were identified with follow-up ranging from 4 to 9 years. They found that all-cause mortality was approximately 20.8% with a mean time to death of 1.64 years for those who required operative intervention. They determined that patients who sustained injuries had an increase of 8.8% above the cohort's expected age-adjusted death rate.

Despite the potential consequences of a BDI, outcomes have improved over the years in regard to success of surgical treatment. In a combined analysis between Indiana University and the Massachusetts General Hospital, a multidisciplinary team managed a total of 528 patients over an 18-year period [34]. Outcomes were examined from patients with all types of Strasberg level injuries. The vast majority of bile leaks, Type A, were managed by endoscopic interventions alone (96%). The other bile duct injuries were managed by a multidisciplinary team of interventional endoscopists (40%), experienced HPB surgeons (36%), and interventional radiologists (24%). The success rates were highest for surgery at 88% and lowest for interventional radiology at 50%. They also found that the subset of patients with surgery in more recent years had an even higher overall success rate of 95%.

The issue of who should manage a BDI when it occurs was also addressed at the consensus conference. A strong recommendation was made that the patient be referred promptly to a surgeon with experience in biliary reconstruction and to a center with a hepatobiliary multidisciplinary team [6]. One must also consider that when a BDI does occur, the emotional and psychologic impact on the surgeon can be considerable, and the importance of having an independent perspective cannot be overstated.

Implementation Considerations

Overall, the six steps listed above provide procedural guidance to enhance the safety of cholecystectomy with evidence to support each step. None of these has significant associated barriers to implementation (with the exception in some centers of obtaining direct intraoperative help) beyond lack of education, awareness, and acceptance. Unfortunately, nationwide standardization is difficult due to the varying circumstances and situations surgeons may face, meaning resources at a large tertiary care center with multiple surgeons will not be the same as a solo surgeon practicing in a rural setting.

Our aim here is to offer awareness of different approaches and techniques in order to achieve these six steps. Greater detail is available in the SAGES safe cholecystectomy modules which are available on line at http://fesdidactic.org/. We also recommend that the consensus conference guideline be read in depth by all surgeons who perform cholecystectomy to understand both the panel recommendations and the rationale and justification behind each of these principles [6]. We strongly believe that adherence to these principles, and, in particular, to use of the critical view of safety on every case and altering to a bailout option when the CVS cannot be safely obtained, has the greatest potential to lower BDI rates.

Future Directions

The final recommendation from the consensus meeting was that national initiatives should be undertaken for prevention of BDI and tracking of outcomes [6]. Studies to date have been limited by the lack of a system in the United States for monitoring the incidence and severity of BDIs. Instead, data are obtained mostly from administrative insurance claims-type databases, which inherently lack the details for accurately measuring not only the incidence but also the underlying circumstances under which BDI occurs.

One strategy going forward would be to develop ICD codes along with procedural codes to specifically register when a BDI occurred, categorize it by standardized approach (e.g., Strasberg classification), and determine interventions required for management. Unlike NSQIP which measures 30-day outcomes, longer-term results would need to be a part of any such system (minimum 1-year outcomes). A collective effort that involved multiple surgical societies and engaged regulatory and payor systems in the United States would likely be needed to accomplish this goal.

Additionally, the creation of regional and nationally recognized institutions for BDI injury repair would provide an avenue for fast-tracking of referrals and transfers of patients to facilities where there is expertise in management. As stated previously, high-volume surgeons and hospital systems have better outcomes for BDI repair, and this approach could help lower the morbidity and mortality of BDI when it occurs.

The ultimate goal should be to push the incidence of BDI to as close to zero as possible. We believe this can be accomplished through awareness of guidelines, careful and meticulous surgical approaches, and enhanced education for surgeons at all levels, starting with trainees throughout our general surgery residency programs.

References

1. Duncan CB, Riall TS. Evidence-based current surgical practice: calculous gallbladder disease. J Gastrointest Surg. 2012;16:2011–25. https://doi.org/10.1007/s11605-012-2024-1.
2. Csikesz NG, Singla A, Murphy MM, Tseng JF, Shah SA. Surgeon volume metrics in laparoscopic cholecystectomy. Dig Dis Sci. 2010;55:2398–405. https://doi.org/10.1007/s10620-009-1035-6.
3. Archer SB, Brown DW, Smith CD, Branum GD, Hunter JG. Bile duct injury during laparoscopic cholecystectomy: a prospective nationwide series. J Am Coll Surg. 1997;184:571–8.

4. Roslyn JJ, Binns GS, Hughes EFX, Saunders-Kirkwood K, Zinner MJ, et al. Open cholecystectomy: a contemporary analysis of 42,474 patients. Ann Surg. 1993;218:129–37. https://doi.org/10.1097/00000658-199308000-00003.

5. Barrett M, Asbun HJ, Chien HL, Brunt LM, Telem DA. Bile duct injury and morbidity following cholecystectomy: a need for improvement. Surg Endosc. 2018;32:1683–8. https://doi.org/10.1007/s00464-017-5847-8.

6. Brunt LM, Deziel DJ, Telem DA, Strasberg SM, Aggarwal R, et al. Safe cholecystectomy multi-society practice guideline and state of the art consensus conference on prevention of bile duct injury during cholecystectomy. Ann Surg. 2020;272:3–23. https://doi.org/10.1097/SLA.0000000000003791.

7. Pucher PH, Brunt LM, Fanelli RD, Asbun HJ, Aggarwal R. SAGES expert Delphi consensus: critical factors for safe surgical practice in laparoscopic cholecystectomy. Surg Endosc. 2015;29:3074–85. https://doi.org/10.1007/s00464-015-4079-z.

8. Strasberg SM, Brunt M. Rationale and use of the critical view of safety in laparoscopic cholecystectomy. 2010. https://doi.org/10.1016/j.jamcollsurg.2010.02.053.

9. Strasberg SM, Hertl M, Soper NJ. An analysis of the problem of biliary injury during laparoscopic cholecystectomy. J Am Coll Surg. 1995;180:101–25.

10. Booij KAC, De Reuver PR, Nijsse B, Busch ORC, Van Gulik TM, et al. Insufficient safety measures reported in operation notes of complicated laparoscopic cholecystectomies. Surg (United States). 2014;155:384–9. https://doi.org/10.1016/j.surg.2013.10.010.

11. Chen CB, Palazzo F, Doane SM, Winter JM, Lavu H, et al. Increasing resident utilization and recognition of the critical view of safety during laparoscopic cholecystectomy: a pilot study from an academic medical center. Surg Endosc. 2017;31:1627–35. https://doi.org/10.1007/s00464-016-5150-0.

12. Sanford DE, Strasberg SM. A simple effective method for generation of a permanent record of the critical view of safety during laparoscopic cholecystectomy by intraoperative "doublet" photography. J Am Coll Surg. 2014;218:170–8. https://doi.org/10.1016/j.jamcollsurg.2013.11.003.

13. Stefanidis D, Chintalapudi N, Anderson-Montoya B, Oommen B, Tobben D, et al. How often do surgeons obtain the critical view of safety during laparoscopic cholecystectomy? Surg Endosc. 2017;31:142–6. https://doi.org/10.1007/s00464-016-4943-5.

14. Natsume S, Kato T, Hiramatsu K, Shibata Y, Yoshihara M, et al. Presence of aberrant anatomy is an independent predictor of bile duct injury during cholecystectomy. Int Surg. 2017;102:250–7. https://doi.org/10.9738/INTSURG-D-15-00049.

15. Sarawagi R, Sundar S, Gupta SK, Raghuwanshi S. Anatomical variations of cystic ducts in magnetic resonance cholangio-pancreatography and clinical implications. Radiol Res Pract. 2016;2016:1–6. https://doi.org/10.1155/2016/3021484.

16. Waage A, Nilsson M. Iatrogenic bile duct injury: a population-based study of 152 776 cholecystectomies in the Swedish inpatient registry. Arch Surg. 2006;141:1207–13. https://doi.org/10.1001/archsurg.141.12.1207.

17. Törnqvist B, Strömberg C, Akre O, Enochsson L, Nilsson M. Selective intraoperative cholangiography and risk of bile duct injury during cholecystectomy. Br J Surg. 2015;102:952–8. https://doi.org/10.1002/bjs.9832.

18. Aziz O, Ashrafian H, Jones C, Harling L, Kumar S, et al. Laparoscopic ultrasonography versus intra-operative cholan-giogram for the detection of common bile duct stones during laparoscopic cholecystectomy: a meta-analysis of diagnostic accuracy. Int J Surg. 2014;12:712–9. https://doi.org/10.1016/j.ijsu.2014.05.038.

19. Dip F, LoMenzo E, Sarotto L, Phillips E, Todeschini H, et al. Randomized trial of near-infrared incisionless fluorescent chol-angiography. Ann Surg. 2019;270:992–9. https://doi.org/10.1097/SLA.0000000000003178.

20. Way LW, Stewart L, Gantert W, Liu K, Lee CM, et al. Causes and prevention of laparoscopic bile duct injuries. Ann Surg. 2003;237:460–9. https://doi.org/10.1097/01.sla.0000060680.92690.e9.

21. Sobba KB, Fernandez AZ, Mcnatt SS, Powell MS, Nunn AM, et al. Live quality assurance: using a multimedia messaging ser-vice group chat to instantly grade intraoperative images. 2020. https://doi.org/10.1016/j.jamcollsurg.2019.09.022.

22. Tokuyasu T, Iwashita Y, Matsunobu Y, Kamiyama T, Ishikake M, et al. Development of an artificial intelligence system using deep learning to indicate anatomical landmarks during laparoscopic cholecystectomy. Surg Endosc. 2020. https://doi.org/10.1007/s00464-020-07548-x.

23. Madani A, Namazi B, Altieri MS, Hashimoto DA, Rivera AM, et al. Artificial Intelligence for Intraoperative Guidance. Ann Surg. 2020. https://doi.org/10.1097/sla.0000000000004594.

24. Vera K, Pei KY, Schuster KM, Davis KA. Validation of a new American Association for the Surgery of Trauma (AAST) anatomic severity grading system for acute cholecystitis. J Trauma Acute Care Surg. 2018;84:650–4. https://doi.org/10.1097/TA.0000000000001762.

25. Okamoto K, Suzuki K, Takada T, Strasberg SM, Asbun HJ, et al. Tokyo guidelines 2018: flowchart for the management of acute cholecystitis. J Hepatobiliary Pancreat Sci. 2018;25:55–72. https://doi.org/10.1002/jhbp.516.

26. Törnqvist B, Waage A, Zheng Z, Ye W, Nilsson M. Severity of acute cholecystitis and risk of iatrogenic bile duct injury during cholecystectomy, a population-based case-control study. World J Surg. 2016;40:1060–7. https://doi.org/10.1007/s00268-015-3365-1.

27. Hussain A. Difficult laparoscopic cholecystectomy: current evidence and strategies of management. Surg Laparosc Endosc Percutan Tech. 2011;21:211–7.

28. Strasberg SM. A teaching program for the "culture of safety in cholecystectomy" and avoidance of bile duct injury. J Am Coll Surg. 2013;217:751. https://doi.org/10.1016/j.jamcollsurg.2013.05.001.

29. Strasberg SM, Pucci MJ, Brunt LM, Deziel DJ. Subtotal cholecystectomy-"Fenestrating" vs "reconstituting" subtypes and the prevention of bile duct injury: definition of the optimal procedure in difficult operative conditions. J Am Coll Surg. 2016;222:89–96. https://doi.org/10.1016/j.jamcollsurg.2015.09.019.

30. Strasberg SM, Gouma DJ. "Extreme" vasculobiliary injuries: association with fundus-down cholecystectomy in severely inflamed gallbladders. HPB. 2012;14:1–8. https://doi.org/10.1111/j.1477-2574.2011.00393.x.

31. Navez B, Ungureanu F, Michiels M, Claeys D, Muysoms F, et al. Surgical management of acute cholecystitis: results of a 2-year prospective multicenter survey in Belgium. Surg Endosc. 2012;26:2436–45. https://doi.org/10.1007/s00464-012-2206-7.

32. Schwaitzberg SD, Scott DJ, Jones DB, McKinley SK, Castrillion J, et al. Threefold increased bile duct injury rate is associated with less surgeon experience in an insurance claims database: more rigorous training in biliary surgery may be needed. Surg Endosc. 2014;28:3068–73. https://doi.org/10.1007/s00464-014-3580-0.

33. Halbert C, Altieri MS, Yang J, Meng Z, Chen H, et al. Long-term outcomes of patients with common bile duct injury following laparoscopic cholecystectomy. Surg Endosc. 2016;30:4294–9. https://doi.org/10.1007/s00464-016-4745-9.

34. Pitt HA, Sherman S, Johnson MS, Hollenbeck AN, Lee J, et al. Improved outcomes of bile duct injuries in the 21st century. Ann Surg. 2013;258:490–7.
35. Hernandez M, Murphy B, Aho JM, Haddad NN, Saleem H, et al. Validation of the AAST EGS acute cholecystitis grade and comparison with the Tokyo guidelines. Surgery. 2018;163:739–46. https://doi.org/10.1016/j.surg.2017.10.041.

Chapter 36
Mentorship and Quality in Surgery

Dina Tabello and Jonathan M. Dort

Mentor was the name of the advisor of the young Telemachus in Homer's Odyssey. The word mentor is both a noun and a verb, the noun defined as "an experienced and trusted advisor" and the verb defined as "to advise or train (someone, especially a younger colleague)." As surgical education moved from the pure apprenticeship model to an increasingly formalized and regulated structure, the necessity to define optimal mentorship has become increasingly important. Equally, as the focus on evaluating quality care and optimizing patient outcomes becomes more resolute and the focus on individual surgeons more intense, the requirement of the surgical community to identify best practices in mentorship has become paramount. In its purest form, a mentor is a senior member of a field who guides a trainee in personal, professional, and educational matters. Mentoring differs from coaching in that coaching is more performance driven, designed to improve on-the-job perfor-

D. Tabello
Inova Fairfax Medical Campus, Falls Church, VA, USA
e-mail: Dina.tabello@inova.org

J. M. Dort (✉)
Department of Surgery, Inova Fairfax Medical Campus,
Falls Church, VA, USA
e-mail: Jonathan.dort@inova.org

© The Author(s), under exclusive license to Springer Nature   687
Switzerland AG 2022
J. R. Romanelli et al. (eds.), *The SAGES Manual of Quality, Outcomes and Patient Safety*,
https://doi.org/10.1007/978-3-030-94610-4_36

mance, while mentoring is more development driven, focused more on long-term goals and career development. In this chapter, the current state of mentorship and coaching will be discussed, specifically covering the qualities that best define optimal mentorship, the structure of how it is best delivered, and finally the assessments of how well-executed mentorship can positively impact surgical outcomes, patient safety, and surgeon performance. SAGES programs aimed at evaluating current mentorship practices and proposing innovative ways to provide optimal mentorship will also be presented. At the end of the Odyssey, Telemachus achieves immortality. Fortunately, the current assessment metrics around successful mentorship outcomes are not that severe.

Surgical trainees (be they residents, medical students, or junior faculty) need high-quality mentors to learn from. The surgical environment is unique; it consists of several distinct characteristics that set it apart from other professional settings even within the healthcare system. The expectations and personalities of surgical staff and attending surgeons, combined with the stresses associated with the operating room, often present a challenging learning environment for surgical trainees of all disciplines [1]. As a result, mentors have been an integral part of surgical training since William Halsted; influenced by the Socratic teaching method, he incorporated them into his design for surgical education. Halsted's own mentee, Harvey Cushing, who went on to develop the specialty of neurosurgery, exemplifies the fruitfulness of good mentorship [2]. The importance of surgical mentors is still recognized, and many surgical training programs assign a faculty mentor to support and guide their less experienced colleagues. However, as Rohrich noted in his commentary on mentoring in medicine, he is "fearful that mentoring is becoming a lost art in medicine..." [3].

In a systematic review of surgical mentorship, Entezami et al. found the most frequent topic written on mentorship focused on mentor qualities. The most commonly discussed mentor qualities deemed to be essential for an effective mentor were (in order of importance) acting as a professional role model, staying involved (specifically in terms of time and effort), being compassionate/kind/supportive, acting as a critic/evaluator/assessor, being a leader in the field, and challenging the surgical student. Additional topics found in their meta-analysis included the structure of mentor-mentee relationships, and advice for overcoming barriers to mentoring. They also point out the relative scarcity of literature related to surgical mentoring, and that there is not a standard or consensus on how to address these questions [1].

As Entezami et al. pointed out, several of the barriers to effective surgical mentoring were time constraints and a lack of female mentors. These barriers can be overcome, and effective mentor-mentee relationships can be built. By developing formal programs to alleviate time constraints, some authors suggested formally adding time to meet with mentees to the mentor's schedule. Others encouraged mentors to meet with mentees in a nonmedical setting, which would also allow for discussions regarding personal aspects of life. Due to this shortage of female mentors, the vast majority of female mentees are paired with male mentors. Although gender may not directly affect mentorships in the professional setting, men and women may encounter different decisions and barriers throughout their careers and personal lives [1]. Nevertheless, Gurgel et al. found that only about 8% of residents (both male and female) prefer a mentor of the same gender [4].

The mentoring of surgical students is an art that has evolved considerably since Halsted's apprenticeship model, and has helped the field expand into new disciplines. What differentiates mentoring from other professional relationships is its emphasis on teaching. The role of the mentor is to define professional or academic goals, and then serve as a guide toward the achievement of those goals. Learning from a mentor should be via active teaching, and not just observational [5]. Mentoring has been identified by some learners as the single most important aspect of training [6]. In addition, positive surgical role models have been shown to increase the likelihood of medical students pursuing surgical careers. Conversely, negative role models and negative behavior of superiors were major deterrents from a career in surgery [7].

Mentoring is also directly associated with improved professional satisfaction. Sambunjak et al. demonstrated that junior attendings with mentors were more likely to be promoted [6], and Steele et al. showed that the experience of a mentor relationship led to faculty retention [8]. Additional studies have addressed the link between surgical coaching and surgeon outcomes. Greenberg et al. identified three domains that effective coaching could target: technical skill, cognitive skill, and nontechnical skill [9]. They point out that although these domains are considered separate, they are interrelated, and that coaching interventions may target any or all three. They conclude with identifying four questions which need to be addressed in optimizing surgical coaching. These questions include identifying which surgical skills are amenable to coaching, how to best identify and train effective coaches, how to deliver the most effective coaching experience, and if and how effective coaching can improve surgical performance and patient outcomes.

While studies identifying direct links between mentorship and surgical outcomes are lacking, there are many publications starting to address the connection. Berian et al. set up a mentor program for 27 surgeons, paired with surgeon mentors to help improve hospital quality through a statewide QI initiative [10]. The survey-based study showed satisfaction among the participants with the agreement of the importance of mentorship to achieve the objective, and also identified four key themes from the responses of the mentors and mentees: nuances of data management, culture of quality and safety, mentor-mentee relationship, and logistics. While identifying strategies for the initiative, they state that the mentor's role required sharing experiences and acting as a resource, and the mentee's role required raising questions and identifying barriers. Wolter et al. reported on a mentorship program in bariatric surgery, where 12 emerging bariatric centers were coached by 5 experienced bariatric centers by providing guidance on pre- and postsurgical management of their patients and proctoring of the first interventions. They found comparable outcomes in experienced and emerging centers under this coaching arrangement, with no differences seen in complication rates or resolution of obesity-related comorbidities [11]. Bonrath et al. published a randomized controlled trial evaluating the effect of a structured coaching plan on the operative skill level of trainees. In the study, they randomized residents undergoing a minimally invasive surgery rotation either to the standard rotation didactics and feedback or to a structured coaching plan including performance analysis, debriefing, feedback, and behavior modeling. They found significant improvements in procedure-specific skill ratings and decreased technical errors in the coaching group than the conventional training group. Given these results and others, it is fair to ask why this level of coaching is not more universal [12]. Mutabdzic et al. attempted to evaluate that question with a qualitative interview-based study examining the barriers to the widespread acceptance of coaching. They found three main concerns among the queried surgeons: questioning the value of technical improvement, worry about appearing incompetent, and concern about losing autonomy. Their conclusion was that the perception of the values of competency and autonomy deters the full applicability of coaching, and actually limits the ways in which surgeons can improve their practice [13]. In an analysis of these two studies, Greenberg and Klingensmith point out that the goal of surgical coaching is "to provide a structured approach to teach self-reflection through facilitated analysis, feedback, and debriefing." They also recognize that this type of coaching not only improves current performance but confers the long-term skill set of ongoing performance improvement and the ability and desire to seek and perform self-assessment. Additionally, they offer approaches to address the stated concerns about and potential barriers to the widespread acceptance of surgical coaching. While surgeons may feel they have sufficient technical skill for the procedures in their practice, coaching offers approaches that are more effective, and are applicable to both technical and nontechnical skills. To combat the worry of loss of appearance of competence and expertise, they suggest moving coaching to a more private setting, away from the clinical setting, as well as assuring it is offered in a nonpunitive way. Finally, to offset the perceived loss of autonomy, the coaching should be aimed at self-directed learning and self-assessment [14].

A mandatory, structured mentorship program with senior surgeons benefits most junior faculty members in terms of academic career planning and becoming more involved with surgical organizations, according to Phitayakorn et al. [15]. Here, a departmental faculty mentoring program was implemented that consisted of both structured and informal meetings between junior faculty mentees and assigned senior faculty mentors. All senior faculty mentors attended a brief mentor training session. They developed an evidence-based mentorship instrument that featured standardized metrics of academic success. This instrument was completed by each mentee, and then reviewed at the junior faculty's annual career conference with their division chief. A survey was distributed to assess junior faculty satisfaction with the new mentorship program. Over 75% of junior faculty members were very or somewhat satisfied with the mentorship program and would like to continue in the program. In terms of program outcomes, junior faculty members agreed that the mentorship program improved their overall career plans and enhanced their involvement in professional organizations but has not yet helped with academic productivity, home and/or work balance, and overall job satisfaction. A survey by Kibbe et al. showed that only half of the departments of surgery in the United States have an established mentorship program and that most are unstructured and informal [16].

Dutta et al. completed a study that looked at the mechanisms by which mentoring may support professional development in underrepresented groups. They compared various health-related and attitudinal measures in mentees at baseline, 6 months, and 1 year into the mentoring relationship and compared pre-mentoring expectations to outcomes at 6 months and 1-year follow-up for mentees and mentors. Job-related well-being (anxiety-contentment), self-esteem, and self-efficacy all improved significantly, and work-family conflict diminished at 1 year. Highest expectations were career progression (89%), increased confidence (87%), development of networking skills (75%), better time management (66%), and better work-life balance (64%). For mentees, expectations at baseline were higher than perceived achievements at 6 months or 1-year follow-up. This uncontrolled pilot study suggests that mentoring can improve aspects of job-related well-being, self-esteem, and self-efficacy over 6 months, with further improvements seen after 1 year for female academics. Work-family conflict can also diminish. Despite these gains, mentees' prior expectations were shown to be unrealistically high, but mentors' expectations were exceeded [17]. In medicine, an increasing number of women are pursuing academic careers, but available senior mentors to provide career guidance are often lacking. Levinson et al. reported the results of a national survey of 558 full-time faculty women, aged 50 years and younger, in departments of medicine in the United States, regarding their experience with role models and mentors. Women with mentors report more publications and more time spent on research activity than those without mentors. Women with a role model reported higher overall career satisfaction [15].

Another study by DeCastro et al. did demonstrate that women acknowledged the importance of at least one female mentor. This group surveyed 100 former National Institutes of Health-mentored career development award winners and 28 of their mentors. Three important themes emerged from this survey: that mentors serve in numerous and varied roles in academic medicine; that a single mentor is unlikely to fulfill the diverse needs of a mentee; and that a network of mentors is typically more helpful overall [18].

SAGES has long sought, and continues to strive for, best practices as it relates to improving quality care and patient outcomes through robust mentorship. The SAGES ADOPT program has shown that the duration of mentorship can affect mentee performance when learning new procedures. The program, developed by the SAGES Continuing Education Committee, examined the effect of longitudinal mentorship on the qualitative and quantitative benefits of procedure adoption by mentees. By standardizing the approach to mentorship through a train-the-trainers course and by expanding the single hands-on course to a yearlong longitudinal mentorship, both the qualitative confidence levels of the mentees and the number of new procedures performed by the mentees were both shown to significantly increase [19]. Originally studied for the hands-on hernia course, these findings have been confirmed over multiple specialty areas, including foregut and colorectal surgery [20]. Nguyen et al. studied the feasibility, effectiveness, and satisfaction of a telementoring program for laparoscopic sleeve gastrectomy as part of a SAGES multi-institutional quality improvement initiative. They showed that the program was well received by the mentees and mentors and found to be feasible, practical, and successful [21]. The Project 6 SAGES telementoring initiative was created to address the current state of telementoring and detail the challenges and opportunities of the future. They identified five opportunity areas that would require review and evaluation: legal and regulatory, business development and proving value, effective communication and education requirements, technology requirements, and logistics. The value of placing the mentor and mentee in the same operating room on a large scale was recognized, but the work necessary to push this grand-scale vision forward was explored [22].

The story of surgical mentorship is both ancient and still in its infancy. The best way to provide mentorship, the qualities that make it more or less successful, and ultimately the positive effect on both surgeons and the patients they care for, are all metrics that are still being evaluated and recognized. While the science of best practices to produce optimal mentorship is still being researched, there are elements for success we know to be true. The success of mentorship is two-sided, with responsibilities for both the mentor and the mentee. The benefits of this relationship must be bidirectional in order for it to succeed. It is the responsibility of both the student and the mentor to assure this bidirectional exchange of benefit. This relationship requires time, patience, dedication, and to some degree selflessness. This mentorship will ultimately be the best tool for mastering complex professional skills and maturing through various learning curves. There is little doubt that surgeons require strong mentorship as part of their training. After all, the life of a surgeon is unique and often challenging, and an effective mentor can be the difference between a surgeon who is skilled and fulfilled, as opposed to one who is simply competent. This passage of wisdom, skills, and support from mentor to mentee, which is then passed through many generations, achieves its own type of immortality. And that is no myth.

References

1. Entezami P, Franzblau L, Chung K. Mentorship in surgical training: a systemic review. Hand. 2012;7:30–6.
2. Assael LA. Every surgeon needs mentors: a Halsteadian/Socratic model in the modern age. J Oral Maxillofac Surg. 2010;68(6):1217–8.
3. Rohrich RJ. Mentors in medicine. Plast Reconstr Surg. 2003;112(4):1087–8.
4. Gurgel RK, Schiff BA, Flint JH, et al. Mentoring in otolaryngology training programs. Otolaryngol Head Neck Surg. 2010;142(4):487–92.
5. Platz J, Hyman N. Mentorship. Clin Colon Rectal Surg. 2013;26(4):218–23. https://doi.org/10.1055/s-0033-1356720.
6. Sambunjak D, Straus SE, Marusić A. Mentoring in academic medicine: a systematic review. JAMA. 2006;296(9):1103.
7. Healy NA, Glynn RW, Malone C, Cantillon P, Kerin MJ. Surgical mentors and role models: prevalence, importance and associated traits. J Surg Educ. 2012;69(5):633–7.
8. Steele MM, Fisman S, Davidson B. Mentoring and role models in recruitment and retention: a study of junior medical faculty perceptions. Med Teach. 2013;35(5):e1130–8.
9. Greenberg CC, Ghousseini HN, Pavuluri Quamme SR, et al. Surgical coaching for individual performance improvement. Ann Surg. 2015;261:32–4.

10. Berian JR, Thomas JM, Minami CA, et al. Evaluation of a novel mentor program to improve surgical care for US hospitals. Int J Qual Health Care. 2017;29(2):234–42.
11. Wolter S, Dupree A, El Gammal A, et al. Mentorship programs in bariatric surgery reduce peri-operative complication rate and equal short-term outcome- results from the OPTIMIZE trial. Obes Surg. 2019;29(1):127–36.
12. Bonrath EM, Dedy NJ, Gordon LE, et al. Comprehensive surgical coaching enhances surgical skill in the operating room: a randomized controlled trial. Ann Surg. 2015;262(2):205–12.
13. Mutabdzic D, Mylopoulos M, Murnaghan ML, et al. Coaching surgeons: is culture limiting our ability to improve? Ann Surg. 2015;262(2):213–6.
14. Greenberg CC, Klingensmith ME. The continuum of coaching: opportunities for surgical improvement at all levels. Ann Surg. 2015;262(2):217–9.
15. Levinson W, Kaufman K, Clark B, Tolle SW. Mentors and role models for women in academic medicine. West J Med. 1991;154(4):423–6.
16. Kibbe MR, Pellegrini CA, Townsend CM, Helenowski IB, Patti MG. Characterization of mentorship programs in departments of surgery in the United States. JAMA Surg. 2016;151:900–6.
17. Dutta R, Hawkes SL, Kuipers E, Guest D, Fear NT, Iversen AC. One year outcomes of a mentoring scheme for female academics: a pilot study at the Institute of Psychiatry, King's College London. BMC Med Educ. 2011;11:13. Published 7 Apr 2011. https://doi.org/10.1186/1472-6920-11-13.
18. DeCastro R, Sambuco D, Ubel PA, Stewart A, Jagsi R. Mentor networks in academic medicine: moving beyond a dyadic conception of mentoring for junior faculty researchers. Acad Med. 2013;88(4):488–96.
19. Dort J, Trickey A, Paige J, Schwarz E, Dunkin B. Hands-on 2.0: improving transfer of training via the Society of American Gastrointestinal and Endoscopic Surgeons (SAGES) Acquisition of Data for Outcomes and Procedure Transfer (ADOPT) program. Surg Endosc. 2017;31(8):3326–32.
20. Dort J, Trickey A, Schwarz E, Paige J. Something for everyone: the benefits of longitudinal mentorship with the application of the acquisition of data for outcomes and procedure transfer (ADOPT) program to a SAGES hands-on colectomy course. Surg Endosc. 2019;33(9):3062–8.

21. Nguyen NT, Okrainec A, Anvari M, et al. Sleeve gastrectomy telementoring: a SAGES multi-institutional quality improvement initiative. Surg Endosc. 2018;32(2):682–7.
22. Schlachta CM, Nguyen NT, Ponsky T, Dunkin B. Project 6 summit: SAGES telementoring initiative. Surg Endosc. 2016;30(9):3665–72.

Part V
Threats to Surgical Quality, Outcomes, and Safety

Chapter 37
Disparities in Healthcare: The Effect on Surgical Quality

Valeria S. M. Valbuena and Dana A. Telem

Introduction

Disparities in healthcare, defined as "differences in health status that result from the social disadvantage that is itself associated with characteristics such as race or ethnicity and socioeconomic status" [1], have a critical role in determining the health and wellness of individual patients and communities alike. In surgical practice, differential access to basic healthcare and surgical providers' specialized services is deeply affected by the modifiable and non-modifiable characteristics of patients and communities. Surgical quality and the standard post-care and post-procedural outcome measures we defined it by have often failed to account for the

V. S. M. Valbuena
University of Michigan, Department of Surgery,
Ann Arbor, MI, USA
e-mail: vvaleria@med.umich.edu

D. A. Telem (✉)
National Clinician Scholars Program, University of Michigan,
Ann Arbor, MI, USA
e-mail: dtelem@med.umich.edu

© The Author(s), under exclusive license to Springer Nature   701
Switzerland AG 2022
J. R. Romanelli et al. (eds.), *The SAGES Manual of Quality, Outcomes and Patient Safety*,
https://doi.org/10.1007/978-3-030-94610-4_37

ecological and systemic influences exerted on the patients for whom we care. Dedicated surgeons delivering quality care in both community and academic healthcare systems face the challenge of recognizing and addressing disparities in healthcare access and delivery to ensure quality care for patients of all backgrounds.

Disparities in surgical care affect the health of patients, the effectiveness of surgeons, and the bottom line of healthcare systems. No surgeon or surgical practice is immune to the effects of inequity; hence, it is imperative to (1) learn about health disparities in surgical care and (2) invest in both surgeon-facing and system-wide solutions. In this chapter, we will describe how disparities in healthcare access and delivery affect surgical outcomes. We will provide the reader with strategies that can be employed to eliminate or reduce outcome differences in the surgical patient.

Healthcare Access and the Surgical Patient

To illustrate how healthcare disparities affect the quality of care of surgical patients, we will discuss differential access to healthcare resources, which is a significant factor driving healthcare disparities. Access to healthcare means having the opportunity to timely obtain healthcare services to achieve the best health outcomes [2]. Access to healthcare has been historically influenced by patient factors, including gender, socioeconomic status, race, ethnicity, employment, and insurance status [3]. Although each one of these patient factors has been independently associated with disparities in access to almost every aspect of modern healthcare, their compounded effect and close relationships (especially as it pertains to racial identity and socioeconomic status) make it difficult to tell them apart when investigating the role of healthcare access as a driver of healthcare disparities.

Patients living in poverty, patients who belong to minoritized racial and ethnic communities, and patients who belong to gender minorities have been shown to have more limited access to both well-resourced primary care [4] and quality surgical services [5]. Safety net hospitals that serve higher proportions of minoritized patients have fewer resources and worse outcomes than hospitals who serve more socially secure patients [6]. Similarly, a patient's geographical location, independent of race or gender, plays a large role in access disparities [7]. For example, geographical disparities have been reported in the patterns of utilization of surgical therapy for the management of hepatocellular carcinoma [8].

When equal access to healthcare services is provided, this has a positive effect on healthcare disparities. A recent evaluation of TRICARE insurance data, which represents a large population with universal insurance, found no risk-adjusted differences in outcomes between Black and White patients following coronary artery bypass grafting (CABG). This was a notable finding given the well-documented racial disparities in outcomes among patients undergoing the same procedure in settings without universal coverage [9]. When thinking about surgical quality, concentrating strictly on access to surgical services it is a logical first step, but extending the discussion beyond the initial surgical encounter is paramount. For example, a lack of access to basic primary care and screening services affects the natural history of many diseases in the surgical spectrum. The current body of evidence demonstrates patients presenting with advanced oncologic disease at the time of diagnosis are more likely to be members of minoritized groups and have lower socioeconomic status [10, 11]. Despite the major role that healthcare access plays in surgical quality, having equal access on its own does not translate into quality care. The delivery of such services, the systems that support patients, and the providers play a similarly important role in the larger framework of healthcare equity.

Healthcare Delivery and the Surgical Patient

"A healthcare delivery system is an organization of people, institutions, and resources to deliver the health needs of a target population" [12]. In the field of surgery, this encompasses the care delivery systems and surgical providers. It also includes when and why we provide surgical services to a population. Similar to surgical care access, delivery of surgical care is not equal across different groups. Disparities in patient perceptions, as well as short- and long-term surgical outcomes, are well documented. Perioperative racial and ethnic disparities have been described in patients undergoing major cancer and non-cancer procedures at American College of Surgeons National Surgical Quality Improvement Program institutions [13]. Significant racial disparities are reported in limb-salvage revascularization, with Black patients comprising 29% of patients undergoing a major lower extremity amputation, but only 10% of those undergoing a procedure for limb salvage when compared to White patients [14]. In inflammatory bowel disease (IBD) patients, Black patients with IBD had 37% greater risk of death and serious morbidity after surgery compared to White patients [15].

From urologic cancer surgery, to surgical readmission rates across specialties, wound complications, and reoperations, minoritized patients receiving similar care to White patients have poorer outcomes and worse prognosis [16, 17]. When we control for race, ethnicity, and gender and evaluate the delivery of surgical care based solely on the type of insurance used by the patient, uninsured patients and patients using primary Medicaid insurance (the national public health insurance in the United States for low-income citizens) have similar trends toward worse outcomes [18]. For example, both Medicaid and Medicare primary payer status have been shown to be associated with worse postoperative outcomes for patients with gynecologic malignancies, with Medicare and Medicaid patients being more likely to require ICU admission and longer lengths of stay compared to privately insured patients [19].

The stark reality of our surgical care delivery problem can be overwhelming. The existing evidence may indicate that operating on patients with certain modifiable and non-modifiable characteristics may lead to worse outcomes; however, this narrative is incorrect. Being Black and Hispanic/Latinx and belonging to a low socioeconomic status are not in themselves the root causes of why the care delivered to these patients does not translate in similar outcomes to White patients. The larger system in which care is delivered is one that was not initially designed for the benefit of these groups. And so, hospital systems and surgeons alike face a larger challenge than just personal change, the challenge to recognize and address the effects of bias and systemic racism in surgical quality [17].

Systemic Racism and the Differential Access and Delivery of Surgical Care

Systemic racism, also known as institutional racism, is a form of racism that is embedded as normal practice within society or an organization. It can lead to such issues as discrimination in criminal justice, employment, housing, healthcare, political power, and education [20]. In simpler words, systemic racism as it pertains to healthcare represents the insidious way both society and the system of care access and delivery have been designed to underserve non-White patients. Although specific provider factors (e.g., referral patterns, cultural competency, awareness of inequities) and system of care delivery characteristics (e.g., hospital quality and location) have been shown to account in part for health disparity trends [1], a large part of the association between non-modifiable patient characteristics such as race and healthcare disparities remains unaccounted for. The long-standing use of race as a risk factor for worse clinical outcomes may give us a clue as to where this association's real culprit resides [21]. As it pertains to race specifically, systems of care are inherently biased against patients of color. It is racism, and not race, that drives the disparate outcomes in surgical patients and the variation in quality surgical care documented in the literature. Race is not a biological trait, but a social construct that has been medicalized to explain away the effects injustice and racism have on a patient's health and well-being with no scientific evidence to base these claims on [22].

Although not direct culprits, hospital quality and "who gets care where" also contribute to this phenomenon. Minoritized and vulnerable patients have been shown to access care at lower-quality hospitals and receive interventions by less experienced surgeons compared to White patients [23, 24]. For example, in a 2014 study of hospital quality and its relationship with racial disparity outcomes in cardiac surgery, hospital quality alone impacted the mortality rates of patients undergoing CABG, with non-White patients having a 33% higher risk-adjusted mortality rate after the procedure compared to White patients, with hospital quality driving 35% of the observed disparity in mortality rates [25]. Turning our attention away from "patient risk factors" and redirecting it to social determinants of health (i.e., availability of safe housing, access to healthy food, educational opportunities, job safety, transportation, social support, exposure to crime, literacy) and the other modifiable aspects of surgical care playing a role in surgical disparities is a promising conceptual framework for the hospital and surgeon hoping to make a change [1]. Changing the narrative of surgical disparities by shifting the responsibility away from patients and onto the systems of oppression dominating the professional environments where we work and provide care is the first step toward addressing these issues and starting the journey toward surgical equity.

Surgical Equity

A solution framework to address healthcare disparities and their effect in surgical quality is one that has as its primary goal-achieving surgical equity. The interplay between access, delivery, and patient factors on surgical outcomes is best illustrated by Haider et al. in their comprehensive review of racial disparities in surgical outcomes [17]. Within their proposed framework, one can recognize the contribution of patient characteristics, system limitations, and provider factors to healthcare disparities in surgery. Their framework also provides one way to think about the complex issues of healthcare disparities within the lens of surgical care delivery systems where the multiple components interact with each other. It can be used to evaluate the independent role of stakeholders in the phenomenon and as a roadmap for thinking critically about actionable strategies for improvement. Although some of the strategies proposed as part of their thesis are larger tasks than others, there is a role for every surgeon, surgical department, and healthcare system in the journey toward making care accessible and delivery equal for all patients.

Strategies to Reduce Outcome Disparities in Surgical Care

Much of the academic work in healthcare disparities has concentrated on describing the phenomena of differential healthcare access and outcomes for minoritized patients over the last three decades. Less evidence exists for effective interventions to address these disparities, especially in surgical practice. Progress in this area has been led by social scientists and primary care specialists who are regularly confronted with the realities of differential access in their practices. In their 2000 publication, "Inequality in Quality: Addressing Socioeconomic, Racial, and Ethnic Disparities in Health Care," Fiscella et al. outlined five principles for addressing disparities in healthcare quality. These principles included:

1. Recognizing that disparities are a significant quality problem
2. Changing clinical and outcome data collection too inadequate to identify and address disparities

3. Stratifying performance measures to reflect race/ethnicity
4. Incorporating adjustment for race/ethnicity and socioeconomic status in population-wide monitoring
5. Developing strategies to adjust financial incentives and payments for race/ethnicity and socioeconomic status given the role these factors have in access and outcomes [26]

More recently, Bonner et al. proposed an actionable "center-department-surgeon" model to address the worsening surgical disparities unveiled by the COVID-19 pandemic [27]. It included similar principles of individual awareness of health disparities, pertinent data collection for surgical equity, and development of community partnerships for surgical needs assessment. Considering these works, we outline four succinct ways how individual surgeons and surgical care delivery systems can modify their practice models to strive for surgical equity.

1. *Surgeon Awareness: Recognize Disparities as a Surgical Quality Problem*

Some of the information presented earlier in the chapter might seem like common knowledge in surgical practice, but there are profound misinformation and disbelief regarding surgical disparities [28]. In a 2016 survey of 536 general surgeon members of the American College of Surgeons, only 37% of participants agreed that racial/ethnic disparities exist in healthcare, and 5% reported witnessing disparities in their practice [29]. Commitment to reducing health disparities starts with an increased state of awareness [30]. Hence, the first step toward improving health disparities in surgery is for surgeons to learn about the phenomena by engaging with the wealth of literature about the topic. Once a baseline level of knowledge has been established, individual surgeons can progress toward committing to recognize and address the disparities within their practice. This strategy is particularly important for surgeons who do not personally identify with minoritized groups. Understanding the problem of surgical disparities will make the surgical workforce more motivated to address them [28].

2. *Collection of Relevant and Reliable Data Is Needed to Address Surgical Quality Disparities*

Every care delivery ecosystem is different. Effective interventions to address healthcare disparities and, in this case, surgical outcome and quality disparities need to be tailored to the needs of the community. Quality reporting needs to address disparities in healthcare [31]. The lack of baseline data for surgical access is a large problem. Strategies for surgical access disparities detecting process have been discussed in the literature [3]. Outcomes, complications, and readmission data need to be stratified by race, and socioeconomic status needs to be accounted for when performing risk stratification. For example, take a quality improvement intervention to decrease readmissions secondary to surgical site infections. If the complications are not stratified by race/ethnicity or socioeconomic status, interventions that do not account for the specific challenges of these patient populations and adequately design interventions aimed to address root causes (i.e., ability to complete postoperative recovery plan, access time off from work to recover, appropriate nutrition, transportation to be evaluated when the signs of the complication started, financial ability to afford dressing supplies) will be less likely to succeed.

3. *Quality and Performance Measures Need to Be Stratified and Adjusted for Socioeconomic Position, Race, and Ethnicity*

Metrics used to assess quality and healthcare delivery have historically not comprehensively accounted for disparities in access to care and the differential outcomes experienced by minoritized communities [32]. Quality has been defined by the ideal outcomes experienced by the dominant patient group in healthcare; however, a line of service cannot claim to be high quality if this high quality is only experienced by some patients. Equity in quality should be the goal. In a systematic review of surgical access as part of the American College of Surgeons MEASUR initiative (Metrics for Equitable Access and Care in SURgery), the authors proposed a conceptual model for classifying surgical access disparity measures in the United States [33]. Surgical detection, progression to surgery, and optimal care receipt were identified as concrete areas where incorporating new reporting measures and quality metrics both at the surgeon level and the healthcare system level would be necessary.

4. *Interventions Need to Be Designed to Specifically Target the Surgical Outcomes of Minoritized/Marginalized Groups*

Given the profound disparities in surgical access and quality experienced by minoritized patients, the relative lack of policy and programmatic interventions to improve the access and quality of surgical care for these patients is a large area for improvement. Individualized interventions that go beyond attempting to allocate responsibility for poor outcomes to the social phenotype of each patient and rather recognize the ways how society has placed an undue burden in large fractions of a population in ways that can significantly affect the way they receive care and remain healthy are very important. Paying specific attention to how health disparities affect surgical outcomes and addressing these factors directly can change the narrative of care for patients in need. There are several types of interventions to address surgical disparities. A recent research review identified four themes that dominated surgical disparities interventions: (1) condition-specific targeted efforts; (2) increased reliance on quantitative factors; (3) doctor-patient communication; and (4) cultural humility [34]. Examples of these interventions span from regional collaboratives to reduce health disparities in access to kidney transplantation among Black patients with ESRD [35] to the Enhanced Recovery After Surgery (ERAS) initiative, which has improved the racial disparities in postoperative length of stay after major colorectal surgery [36]. Adapting successful disparity-reducing interventions from other disciplines, such as the formation of a regional quality improvement collaborative to reduce racial disparities in severe maternal morbidity from postpartum hemorrhage [37], is another promising strategy. Organizational commitment, engagement of experts outside of surgery and patient groups who have unique and key perspectives on what their barriers to accessing care are, and comprehensive engagement of local and national regulatory and policy mechanisms are key elements of designing interventions targeting the access and quality of surgical care of minoritized groups, and making progress in health disparities as a whole [30].

Conclusions

Surgical quality and outcomes are impacted by disparities in surgical access and delivery. Individual and system-wide interventions are needed, starting with recognizing the problem. Data collection, stratified quality measures, and interventions targeted toward differential allocation of resources to those who need them the most are important strategies to ensure quality surgical care is available for all.

References

1. Perez NP, Pernat CA, Chang DC. Surgical disparities: beyond non-modifiable patient factors. In: Dimick JB, Lubitz CC, editors. Health services research. Cham: Springer; 2020. p. 57–69.
2. Gulliford M, et al. What does 'access to health care' mean? J Health Serv Res Policy. 2002;7(3):186–8.
3. Wong JH, et al. Development and assessment of a systematic approach for detecting disparities in surgical access. JAMA Surg. 2020;156(3):239–45.
4. Varkey AB, et al. Separate and unequal: clinics where minority and nonminority patients receive primary care. Arch Intern Med. 2009;169(3):243–50.
5. Rothenberg BM, et al. Explaining disparities in access to high-quality cardiac surgeons. Ann Thorac Surg. 2004;78(1):18–24; discussion 24–5.

6. Hoehn RS, et al. Effect of hospital safety-net burden on cost and outcomes after surgery. JAMA Surg. 2016;151(2):120–8.

7. Horev T, Pesis-Katz I, Mukamel DB. Trends in geographic disparities in allocation of health care resources in the US. Health Policy. 2004;68(2):223–32.

8. Sonnenday CJ, et al. Racial and geographic disparities in the utilization of surgical therapy for hepatocellular carcinoma. J Gastrointest Surg. 2007;11(12):1636–46. discussion 1646

9. Chaudhary MA, et al. No racial disparities in surgical care quality observed after coronary artery bypass grafting in TRICARE patients. Health Aff (Millwood). 2019;38(8):1307–12.

10. Lannin DR, et al. Influence of socioeconomic and cultural factors on racial differences in late-stage presentation of breast cancer. JAMA. 1998;279(22):1801–7.

11. Chornokur G, et al. Disparities at presentation, diagnosis, treatment, and survival in African American men, affected by prostate cancer. Prostate. 2011;71(9):985–97.

12. Piña IL, et al. A framework for describing health care delivery organizations and systems. Am J Public Health. 2015;105(4):670–9.

13. Ravi P, et al. Racial/ethnic disparities in perioperative outcomes of major procedures: results from the National Surgical Quality Improvement Program. Ann Surg. 2015;262(6):955–64.

14. Hughes K, et al. Racial/ethnic disparities in revascularization for limb salvage: an analysis of the National Surgical Quality Improvement Program database. Vasc Endovasc Surg. 2014;48(5–6):402–5.

15. Montgomery SR Jr, et al. Racial disparities in surgical outcomes of patients with inflammatory bowel disease. Am J Surg. 2018;215(6):1046–50.

16. Sathianathen NJ, et al. Racial disparities in surgical outcomes among males following major urologic cancer surgery. Am J Prev Med. 2018;55(5 Suppl 1):S14–s21.

17. Haider AH, et al. Racial disparities in surgical care and outcomes in the United States: a comprehensive review of patient, provider, and systemic factors. J Am Coll Surg. 2013;216(3):482–92.e12.

18. LaPar DJ, et al. Primary payer status affects mortality for major surgical operations. Ann Surg. 2010;252(3):544–50; discussion 550–1.

19. Ahmad TR, et al. Medicaid and medicare payer status are associated with worse surgical outcomes in gynecologic oncology. Gynecol Oncol. 2019;155(1):93–7.

20. Griffith DM, et al. Dismantling institutional racism: theory and action. Am J Community Psychol. 2007;39(3–4):381–92.
21. Lim GHT, et al. Students' perceptions on race in medical education and healthcare. Perspect Med Educ. 2021;10(2):1–5.
22. Witzig R. The medicalization of race: scientific legitimization of a flawed social construct. Ann Intern Med. 1996;125(8):675–9.
23. Dimick J, et al. Black patients more likely than Whites to undergo surgery at low-quality hospitals in segregated regions. Health Aff (Millwood). 2013;32(6):1046–53.
24. Regenbogen SE, et al. Do differences in hospital and surgeon quality explain racial disparities in lower-extremity vascular amputations? Ann Surg. 2009;250(3):424–31.
25. Rangrass G, Ghaferi AA, Dimick JB. Explaining racial disparities in outcomes after cardiac surgery: the role of hospital quality. JAMA Surg. 2014;149(3):223–7.
26. Fiscella K, et al. Inequality in quality addressing socioeconomic, racial, and ethnic disparities in health care. JAMA. 2000;283(19):2579–84.
27. Bonner SN, et al. Covid-19 and racial disparities: moving towards surgical equity. Ann Surg. 2020;272(3):e224–5.
28. Britton BV, et al. Awareness of racial/ethnic disparities in surgical outcomes and care: factors affecting acknowledgment and action. Am J Surg. 2016;212(1):102–108.e2.
29. Britton BV, et al. US Surgeons' perceptions of racial/ethnic disparities in health care: a cross-sectional study. JAMA Surg. 2016;151(6):582–4.
30. Chin MH, et al. A roadmap and best practices for organizations to reduce racial and ethnic disparities in health care. J Gen Intern Med. 2012;27(8):992–1000.
31. Jha AK, Zaslavsky AM. Quality reporting that addresses disparities in health care. JAMA. 2014;312(3):225–6.
32. DeMeester RH, Xu LJ, Nocon RS, Cook SC, Ducas AM, Chin MH. Solving disparities through payment and delivery system reform: a program to achieve health equity. Health Aff. 2017;36(6):1133–9.
33. de Jager E, et al. Disparities in surgical access: a systematic literature review, conceptual model, and evidence map. J Am Coll Surg. 2019;228(3):276–98.
34. Hisam B, et al. From understanding to action: interventions for surgical disparities. J Surg Res. 2016;200(2):560–78.

35. Patzer RE, et al. A randomized trial to reduce disparities in referral for transplant evaluation. J Am Soc Nephrol. 2017;28(3):935–42.
36. Wahl TS, et al. Enhanced recovery after surgery (ERAS) eliminates racial disparities in postoperative length of stay after colorectal surgery. Ann Surg. 2018;268(6):1026–35.
37. Main EK, et al. Reduction in racial disparities in severe maternal morbidity from hemorrhage in a large-scale quality improvement collaborative. Am J Obstet Gynecol. 2020;223(1):123. e1–123.e14.

Chapter 38
Surgeon Wellness: Scope of the Problem and Strategies to Avoid Burnout

John R. Romanelli

Introduction

> "Physician wellness is on a spectrum, and where physicians reside on the spectrum can change due to the influence of acute and chronic stressors... burnout is the extreme pejorative end of the spectrum from which recovery is not thought to be possible...."

It is tempting today to frame a difficult problem as a crisis, but it is easy to argue that the decline in physician wellness is approaching crisis levels in the United States. The recent (and, as of the time of this writing, ongoing) pandemic has only served to exacerbate underlying problems that lead to physician wellness decline, or, worse, burnout. Population growth trends already forecast a shortage of surgeons in the coming decades [1] as caps on trainees per year are rendering the additions to the surgical workforce short. Further, the percentage of procedures needed is likely to increase as the

J. R. Romanelli (✉)
Department of Surgery, University of Massachusetts Chan Medical School - Baystate Medical Center, Springfield, MA, USA
e-mail: John.Romanelli@baystatehealth.org

© The Author(s), under exclusive license to Springer Nature Switzerland AG 2022
J. R. Romanelli et al. (eds.), *The SAGES Manual of Quality, Outcomes and Patient Safety*,
https://doi.org/10.1007/978-3-030-94610-4_38

population age increases due to medical advancements, yet this is superimposed with an overall decline in medical school graduates seeking surgical residencies [1]. Seeing the workforce decline further in numbers by deletions due to surgeons retiring or leaving the field would likely worsen this problem.

It is well known that physician wellness decline leads to adverse outcomes [2–4]. This problem, if left unaddressed, may present an existential threat to the quality of care delivered by healthcare practitioners. Like many negative behavioral drivers, the first step in addressing a critical problem is acceptance of the issue, and recognition that change is required. Many healthcare administrators fail to acknowledge the scope of the crisis and prefer to adopt a "see no evil, hear no evil" approach. Victim blaming is common and has become part of the current healthcare environment (e.g., "physicians need to be more resilient"). That said, we surgeons are not blameless, either. In fact, many of us during residency training were subjected to arduous and often nonsensical work hours, demeaning treatment from attendings and senior trainees, and an unrealistic work burden, and have modeled similar behavior toward our trainees and successors and have maintained expectations of a similarly unrealistic work burden. In fact, when mandatory work hour limits were imposed upon resident training in the early 2000s, many surgeons reacted with negativity or even scorn, rather than seeing this change as a much-needed improvement in the training culture. Nor was this seen as an opportunity to reform surgical residency to attract better candidates to the workforce by humanizing the rigorous training and, in so doing, accepting that we were a part of creating the decline in physician wellness.

This chapter will attempt to take a "30,000-foot view" of the entire problem. First, one will note the use of the term "physician wellness decline." The wellness of healthcare providers can wax and wane on a spectrum, with acute and chronic stressors pushing people to and fro on the spectrum. Therefore, we define "burnout" as the end stage of the wellness spectrum, from which recovery is not possible. Too often, this term is used interchangeably with a decline in wellness, but this distinction is important. Burnout is most commonly defined as the triad of emotional exhaustion (overextension), depersonalization (negative, callous, and detached responses to others), and reduced personal accomplishment (feelings of competence and achievement in one's work) [5]. This is known as the Maslach definition, and this appears frequently in writings on this subject. Another recent description from a surgical journal defines surgeon wellness as "...a multidimensional commitment that encompasses occupational, mental, physical, emotional, and social domains. Loss of professional control, autonomy, and flexibility; inefficient processes; disjointed workplace relationships and goals; excessive administrative burdens; poor work-life balance; and frustrations with (electronic) medical record systems have all been associated with burnout" [6].

A new version of a previously administered survey [7] has revealing and troubling statistics regarding physician burnout. The respondents were divided into generations such that "Millennials" were listed as age 40 and under (born 1980 or after); "Generation X" was defined as age 40–55 (born 1965–1980); and "Baby Boomers" were defined as aged 55–73 (born before 1965). 42% of physicians in this survey – offered to physicians of all specialties – felt burned out. This was worst among Generation X physicians, who reported a 48% rate of burnout. General surgeons reported a 35% rate of burnout. There were multiple causes listed, with bureaucratic tasks being the largest culprit (55%). Other causes, some of which will be delved into in this chapter, included the amount of work hours (33%), lack of respect from colleagues/administration (32%), electronic medical records (EMRs) (30%), compensation issues (29%), and a lack of control of autonomy (24%). These factors varied widely among generations; for example, EMRs were a much more common cause of burnout symptoms among Baby Boomers than among Millennials. Nonetheless, these results show that the driving factors of wellness decline are multifactorial.

The survey [7] also examined coping mechanisms for physicians suffering from wellness issues. Happily – many of these were positive behavioral maneuvers: exercise (45%), talking with family/friends (42%), sleep (40%), and listening or playing music (32%). Negative behaviors such as isolation (45%), eating junk food (33%), using/abusing alcohol (24%), and binge eating (20%) were also reported, however. Surprisingly, use of tobacco and marijuana and the abuse of prescription drugs were listed at 3% or less; while this survey could suffer from dishonesty in responses, smoking and/or drug use clearly does not appear to be a large factor in coping with professional or personal stressors, which is somewhat encouraging.

Burnout is frequently measured quantitatively by the Maslach Burnout Index [8]. In this index, emotional exhaustion is measured with nine questions; the depersonalization domain is measured with five questions; and the personal accomplishment domain is measured with eight questions. These are scored from 0 to 6 and are based on self-reported frequency of the item in question. Emotional exhaustion scores of 27 or greater, depersonalization scores of 10 or greater, and personal accomplishment scores of 33 or less are associated with high levels of burnout for physicians. Interestingly, the personal accomplishment domain does not tend to correlate with patient outcomes; but emotional exhaustion and depersonalization do. Although many assume that emotional exhaustion tends to drive physicians to burnout, depersonalization seems to more strongly align with the negative consequences of burnout [9].

It does not take a leap of logic to associate physicians who decline in wellness with poor patient outcomes. A large national survey of American physicians conducted in 2014 [9] demonstrated that physicians reporting errors were more likely to have symptoms of burnout (77.6% vs 51.5%; $P < 0.001$), fatigue (46.6% vs 31.2%; $P < 0.001$), and recent suicidal ideation (12.7% vs 5.8%; $P < 0.001$). Furthermore, in multivariate modeling, perceived errors were independently more likely to be reported by physicians with burnout. The reverse seems to be true as well: self-perceived medical errors were found to predict subsequent burnout [10]. Thus, there is a direct link between patient outcomes and physician wellness.

Studies have looked specifically at the surgeon population in examining these questions of wellness. One study determined that the following six factors led to increased burnout in surgeons: having children <21 years of age; being compensated purely by incentive-based pay; having a spouse as a healthcare professional; increases in call responsibilities; increasing years in practice; and increased number of hours per week [11]. While having 50% or greater of time protected was found to be protective against burnout, paradoxically, having children of any age and increased age were also found to be protective [11]. The survey, which had nearly 8000 respondents, reported that only 36% of surgeons felt that their work schedule left enough time for family or personal life, and disconcertingly, only 51% felt that they would recommend the profession to their children.

One aspect of physician wellness decline that tends to be overlooked is when the process begins. A recent survey of over 3500 PGY-2 residents of all specialties revealed that 45.2% reported burnout symptoms [12]. 14.1% expressed regret with regard to their career choice. Burnout symptoms varied by subspecialty, but general surgery, urology, and ophthalmology were among the surgical subspecialties that were associated with a higher rate of burnout. Most alarmingly, 14% would "definitely not" or "probably not" choose to become a physician again. Perhaps we are inoculating our trainees with wellness decline, or maybe physicians who are exhibiting signs of burnout are modeling the behavior. Nonetheless, attacking the problem likely requires meaningful steps to intervene during residency or even medical school, before the decline leads to depression, leaving the profession, or, even worse, self-harm, substance abuse, or suicide.

In fact, a new survey of surgical residents assessed at the time of the 2019 ABSITE examination reveals just how prevalent wellness decline is among trainees [13]. Granted, asking these questions at the conclusion of taking a high-stakes yearly examination may skew the results somewhat. Nonetheless, the incidence of emotional exhaustion at least once per week was 38.6%; the incidence of weekly depersonalization was 23.1%. Overall, 2607 general surgery residents (43.2% of respondents) reported weekly burnout symptoms on either of those two subscales. Worse, upon multivariate analysis, those scoring higher on burnout scales were associated with thoughts of attrition and suicidal thoughts [13]. These data alone illuminate the crisis level of concern for surgeon wellness decline: this is coming from our future workforce.

Further, we may be exacerbating the problem with a lack of preparedness for residency. A survey done during the 2017 ABSITE examination demonstrated that 48.1% of PGY-1 and PGY-2 respondents felt unprepared for surgical residency [14]. Residents who took overnight call during their third (51.6%) or fourth year (43.3%) of medical school were more likely to feel prepared for residency. Feeling prepared for residency resulted in a nearly twofold reduction in the risk of burnout symptoms. The study concluded that feeling unprepared for residency was related to inadequate exposure to resident responsibilities as medical students and that considering a change to more effective preparedness may help reduce burnout symptoms among surgical residents [14].

In this chapter, we will attempt to look at several sentinel causes of the decline of a physician's wellness. We will examine topics such as unreasonable work burden, cognitive overload, community, victim blaming/shaming, moral injury, the effects of medical malpractice, autonomy, resilience, the role of leadership in responding to concerns of burnout, and EMRs, and how they contribute to the crisis of surgeon wellness decline and burnout. We will also attempt to make suggestions to address the problem.

Moral Injury and Victim Blaming

"Moral injury describes the challenge of simultaneously knowing what care patients need but being unable to provide it due to constraints that are beyond our control [15]."

The concept of moral injury has taken root to describe the feeling that doctors are unable to provide the care they feel their patients need. A moral injury would be an act that transgresses our deeply held moral beliefs; as healthcare providers, that belief is putting the needs of our patients first [15]. Clinicians are forced to consider the needs of other stakeholders: the healthcare system at large; the hospital and its attendant administrators; the insurance companies; the EMR and its vendor; etc. When those needs trump those of our patients, physicians "feel a sting of moral injustice. Over time, these repetitive insults amass into moral injury" [15].

There is not necessarily a semantic difference between moral injury and physician burnout. As we define burnout as the end stage of physician wellness decline, think of moral injury as the stimulus that pushes us out of emotional inertia and into decline. A recent publication [15] makes this distinction for another reason entirely: it reframes the problem away from victim blaming. For example, the definitions of burnout tend to "suggest that the problem resides within the individual... It implies that the individual lacks the resources or resilience to withstand the work environment." That is why there is so much written about mindfulness, meditation, yoga, and wellness retreats as solutions to physician wellness decline: it serves as methods to force the individual to adapt to the work culture. Rather, the concept of moral injury points to system drivers of wellness decline, burnout, and even loss of physicians from the workplace. Thus, solutions to the problem of moral injury demand long-term changes to the culture in which healthcare is practiced. One such example is the reduced need for documentation in E&M coding that began in 2021; although there was a financial impetus to these changes, it was clear that reducing the documentation burden on the physician was a desirable side effect.

A recent blog by the same authors [16] expands upon this concept. They challenge healthcare administrators to own the problem – leaders that are willing to confront the problem and minimize competing demands for physicians' work time. "Physicians must be treated with respect, autonomy, and the authority to make rational, safe, evidence-based, and financially responsible decisions. Top-down authoritarian mandates on medical practice are degrading and ultimately ineffective. We need leaders who recognize that caring for their physicians results in thoughtful, compassionate care for patients, which ultimately is good business…" [16]. Investing in the wellness of physicians ultimately leads to retention of workforce, increased productivity, and, potentially, improved patient outcomes.

One problem is that there is no current accepted threshold to identify cases of moral injury [17]. Certainly, identifying physicians who are suffering in wellness decline and a conversation about identifying sources of moral injury should be part of crafting solutions to help these physicians. Whether that falls on departmental leaders or mental health professionals remains a question, however. These authors also express concern that "burnout (should) not become the catchall term for emotional distress experienced by physicians."

Another recent and much-viewed blog [18] argues that using the term "burnout" is not just victim blaming but victim *shaming*. The author argues that using the term "burnout" implies that physicians are "not resourceful enough, not resilient enough, not strong enough, to adapt to a system…." Further, moral injury is the result of what happens when "we cannot give our patients the care we know that we could give if we had the tools, and the resources, and the autonomy to do it" [18]. He argues that moral injury is the result when our ideals as healthcare providers clash with real-world constraints to medical practice. Once again, the implication is that system changes are needed to address the crisis of physician wellness decline, rather than focusing on the victims of the problem, and holding them accountable to adapt to the broken culture within which they are expected to practice.

Work Burden

"Physicians have no problem going the extra mile on behalf of their patients as long as they know they will benefit from these activities.... However, we now spend an incredible amount of time doing things not actually related to improving patient care..." [19]

It should come as no surprise that an overwhelming work burden can lead to physician burnout. For example, among intensivists, workload is independently associated with the intensity of burnout – and it is also correlated with the intention to leave one's job [20]. Further, as we develop physician shortages from early retirement – one study showed age greater than 55 was a significant factor in leaving academic medicine [21] – job change, and failing to train physicians commensurate with population growth, resources can become strained, adding to the feeling of an unmanageable work burden. Projected nursing shortages may also push care delivery back into the hands of physicians and advanced practice providers (APPs), adding to their daily work burden. A decrease in available workforce can require more overnight shifts or consecutive days or nights on call, which has also been shown to increase burnout [20, 22]. With this opening statement in mind, it is worth reviewing how efforts around physician work time have changed over the last three decades.

Resident work hours were unrestricted until the 1990s and were, frankly, abusive. There was an expectation of in-house overnight call responsibilities – often with a list of scores of patients unfamiliar to the resident – and this typically occurred once per however many same-level residents there were at that hospital at the time. For some, this meant being on-call every other night – typically 40 consecutive work hours followed by 8 hours of rest, only to repeat the process for a month or more. While change organically occurred by the mid-1990s, with call requirements "reduced" to every third or fourth night on-call, there was still an expectation of normal work hours and performance "post-call." The famous Libby Zion case in New York City did force mandatory changes. Libby Zion was a patient in New York Hospital in

1984, who died from a fatal reaction of Nardil and Demerol [23]. This fatal interaction was scarcely known at the time, and it is critical to note that the providers had no electronic aids to understand such an interaction – all care delivery at the time was conducted on paper. Although there was scant evidence to make the case, the family of the deceased blamed the error on resident overwork and lack of attending supervision of the residents involved in the case. (Of note, criminal charges against many involved were all dropped, and the Board of Medical Examiners in New York found that there was no negligence involved in the case and that fatigue and supervision were unlikely to have been involved in the case.) [23] The State of New York did, however, mandate that residents be restricted to work "only" 80 hours per week and no longer than 24 continuous hours. This was adopted nationwide in July 2003 by the ACGME, but sadly change of this magnitude did not come from within – it came from political pressure and lawyers. In fact, many attending surgeons scoffed at this change, despite the fact that a limitation of 80 hours per week spread over 5 years of training would result in 20,000 hours of training time – double what is described as necessary by Ericsson [24] in his seminal work on deliberate practice. Is it any wonder why many feel the leading cause of burnout are the physicians themselves?

Today, residents are carefully monitored for fatigue and steps are taken to watch closely for wellness decline. Work hour limitations are rigorously enforced. And medicine as a whole has recognized that "working harder, not smarter," is a recipe for non-wellness. But what other factors have developed that add to this problem, and increase the physician work burden? And how is that affecting surgeons who are well beyond their training?

One development over the latter part of the last decade was the shift of complex care to larger hospitals. Gone are the days where the mentality was "keep the patient here at all costs." A wide variety of complex general surgical care was delivered – with varying rates of quality – and it was rare and practically unheard of to recognize the need to transfer a patient to a tertiary care center. Nowadays, a recognized bile duct injury, for example, is considered a reason to transfer to a hepatobiliary center. Twenty years ago, this would have been unheard of – and in fact medicolegal issues might have hampered such a transfer despite medical appropriateness. Further, surgeons at smaller hospitals were expected to deliver 24-hour, 365-day-per year coverage of unassigned emergency consultation. But envision a hospital with only three full-time surgeons (and the workload to support that size workforce). How sustainable is call every third night? What about when one of them is on vacation? Surgeons began to push back against hospital bylaws requiring such coverage in the early 2000s, leaving these hospitals uncovered for some nights per month. This began with requests for transfers of simple surgical problems such as appendicitis and cholecystitis and has morphed over the last decade and a half into tertiary care centers often being the only night and weekend surgical coverage for a geographic region. As one might imagine, this has significantly impacted the work burden at these centers – and it is directly leading to physician wellness decline. Having to cover multiple hospitals at the same time while on-call can be overwhelming, and with time used as a critical factor in determining "delays in care" (something used against physicians in malpractice cases), there exists an urgency to handle transfers as timely as possible. This, too, adds to the work burden.

Further, the expectation of normal work performance after an overnight and weekend call shift has become patently unrealistic, yet administrators – so protective of financial productivity – often push back on a reduced work schedule for surgeons after their call shift. Surgeons are often faced with maintaining a normal elective schedule after working the previous night, with ill-regard to outcomes. While it is undeniable that fatigue is a threat to patient safety, administrators and surgical leaders have been loath to reduce schedules and provide appropriate time for rest after off-hour shifts. Surgeons are beginning to rethink the necessity of overnight or weekend operating – but system issues (operating time, length of stay issues forcing pressure for early discharge) represent an opposing force. Add to this the expectation of additional work time without compensation, and one begins to see how burdensome night or weekend shifts can become for surgeons over time. (To wit, try calling a plumber or a lawyer in the middle of the night. Do you think they will be responsive, and do so for free?) Perhaps it is time for a cultural change regarding the expectations of off-hour shifts, and surgeons ought to be granted appropriate time for rest after their shifts, without the guilt implied by reducing an elective schedule to do so.

The other consideration about work burden is the number of administrative tasks physicians are faced with to provide clinical care. A recent blog noted [19] "...the real damage to us from the volume and nature of the administrative work currently associated with patient care lies in the emotional responses it can trigger. It can create a deeply visceral conflict between the inherent desire and drive to do the right thing for patients and the personal sacrifice that doing so now involves." It is simply astounding that as our technological tools increase, the amount of time spent doing nonclinical tasks has also increased, not decreased. In fact, the blog notes that "for every hour spent on patient interaction, a physician has an added one-to-two hours of finishing progress notes, ordering labs, reviewing study results, prescribing medications, and completing additional documentation." This often bleeds into personal or family time, so much so that this phenomenon is known as "pajama time" [19]. Is it any wonder that work-life balance continues to be a struggle for physicians, when patient documentation is often occurring after hours or on weekends at home? The Center for Medicare and Medicaid Services has recognized this and is simplifying the amount of documentation needed to achieve certain evaluation and management codes. But much work remains to reduce the administrative burden on physicians.

Another example that surgeons face administratively is the need to have peer-to-peer reviews to get certain patients approved for procedures that in many instances have defined

CPT codes and that some payors routinely cover. Given that there is no governance of private insurance companies with regard to what cases they will and will not cover, surgeons are often left to fight for the ability to perform the procedures that they feel their patients need. These conversations, allegedly with a "peer," are to ostensibly argue the case for allowing the procedure. Yet, almost universally, the "peer" concludes with the statement that they are not empowered to overturn the decision. Although the time was spent by the surgeon advocating for their patient, it typically ends up as time wasted, leading to frustration and anger. As the same blog [19] notes: "It is increasingly difficult to see the benefit to patients in needing physician approval for a wide range of routine medical products and services for which the intended purpose is seemingly only to manage utilization, recording an increased volume of patient metrics that are not clearly associated with improved clinical outcomes, and spending huge amounts of time on insurance-related activities such as pre-authorizations that feel more like 'rationing by hassle' than a meaningful review of medical necessity."

The work burden surgeons face fall into two general categories: too much or unmanageable clinical work and administrative work that does not result in any meaningful supplementation to clinical care. While the former can result in chronic fatigue, leading to exhaustion and wellness decline, the latter has become a more insidious "mission creep" adding time to already-long hours, creating frustration and anger, and leading to significant wellness decline.

Cognitive Overload

"There are two kinds of residents – those that write things down, and those that forget." – William Sugarmann, MD, general surgeon, Somerset, NJ.

The amount of information a surgeon needs to know can be staggering. At any one given time, a surgeon is expected to know pertinent clinical details about their patients: laboratory results, radiology findings, inputs and outputs from the previous 24 hours, changes to the physical examination, medical history, medications, etc. Add to this having the technical "know-how" to perform the operations that they do in their clinical practice. Technical errors must be avoided, and understanding how to avoid them is also part of the surgeon's knowledge base. Although a surgeon's familiarity of key anatomic landmarks resides deep in the long-term memory bank, pattern recognition to detect aberrant anatomy is also necessary. Of course, many surgeons try to stay up to date on the latest literature that is most relevant to their clinical practice – a daunting task given the hundreds of thousands of journal articles written per year. So how is it possible that surgeons do not suffer from cognitive overload?

If we harken back to resident training, endless reams of rote learning and meaningless memorization are commonplace. Being on a team with several members – senior and junior residents, medical students, advanced practice providers, etc. – at least one team member is always supposed to know everything about every patient. Depending on the size of the "service" (the quotes emphasizing the imbalance between providing a service and receiving education) that one is serving on at the time, the near-impossible is expected, with scores of bits of information on dozens of patients with data changing in real time. Surgery residents are additionally tasked with learning everything there is to know about surgery (as required by the American Board of Surgery) in 5 years (or more) of a residency program; they typically start with an outlined curriculum such as SCORE, but some residency programs favor structured textbook review over a 1–2-year cycle. So in between treating hundreds of patients, there is an expectation of an in-depth understanding of thousands of pages of didactic information. The very structure of surgical resident training is laden with cognitive overload.

With that backdrop of thought, it is worthwhile to consider cognitive load theory [25]. In this theory, task completion relies on the complex interplay between sensory inputs, long-term memory acting as a repository of acquired knowledge and skills (with working memory as the intermediate stage), acting to attribute meanings to the sensory information, and deposit new learned information into the long-term memory. Although sensory and long-term memories can deal with large volumes of information, the capacity of working memory is comparatively very limited [26]. Cognitive overload is presumed to occur when this capacity is exceeded, requiring the individual to coordinate a larger than possible number of elements to accomplish tasks successfully [27]. Directing the working memory is called the metacognitive capacity of a person, which is functionally equivalent to an individual's attention [28]. This sorts through sensory inputs and long-term knowledge to manage the overall learning process. A physician approaching the point of cognitive overload may begin to exhibit symptoms like depressive symptoms, with the addition of deterioration in quality or quantity of work, relative to their own previous standard [27]. Given that, the phenomenon of burnout – or, more chronically, physician wellness decline – may be distinguished as a self-protective neuropsychological response to attempting to function beyond a fixed capacity [27]. This, as stated repeatedly in this chapter, leads to a decline in task performance acutely, or overall performance over a longer period. Further, an individual's capacity for cognitive load is fixed [27], but metacognition can be improved with training [29]; perhaps developing programs designed specifically for physicians to improve metacognition can help minimize the risk of cognitive overload.

Strategies to create supportive clinical practice environments would help physicians to reduce cognitive overload. The well-observed pattern of surgical practice that starts broadly and through time narrows in scope may be a self-protective mechanism against cognitive overload. Witness, for example, the development of breast surgery as its own subspecialty distinct from surgical oncology, which, in and of itself, became distinct from general surgery. Breast surgeons are faced with a rapidly changing treatment paradigm based on an overwhelming amount of literature that must be in consideration when considering options for breast patients.

One could surmise that attempting to practice breast surgery within the larger context of a surgical oncology practice could lead to cognitive overload solely from the cancer data about which they are expected to be knowledgeable. Further, some consideration with regard to future needs of maintenance of certification should be made with concerns of cognitive overload in mind. What value is there truly to study for a high-stakes examination asking questions about surgery well outside the scope of the examinee's clinical practice? And how does that imply competence? (Clearly, the ABS agrees given the recent development of focused-practice designation examinations.)

Further, the training of surgical residents should be filtered through the lens of concern about cognitive overload. While the days of requiring rotations in areas such as orthopedics, neurosurgery, urology, cardiac surgery, and burn surgery have passed, perhaps structuring learning objectives in a more nuanced way can steer trainees away from overload and wellness decline. Given that the problem of physician burnout can be traced back to medical school and residency, perhaps the burnout crisis should serve as a clarion call to rethink the dogmatic methodology though which we have passed down our knowledge to the next generation of surgical trainees.

Medical Malpractice and Physician Wellness

"There is significant research showing that coping with a medical malpractice suit can weigh heavily on a physician… Often physicians take the accusation of malpractice personally, and some are prone to symptoms of depression…." [30]

We will begin this section with some personal perspective. Early in my career, practicing in a private practice setting in a highly litigious area of the United States, I was sued multiple times in a short period of time. As a practitioner of bariatric surgery, I was performing complicated procedures in sicker patients, and at the time (early 2000s), medical malpractice attorneys sought bariatric cases with zeal. These early cases –

most of which were dropped – caused my malpractice rates to spike, making it financially untenable to remain practicing in the job and geographic area where I had been hired. The fear of being sued (again) caused me to become risk averse. I suffered from insomnia, was prone to unreasonable demonstrations of anger, and spent many months considering leaving clinical medicine altogether (despite hundreds of thousands of dollars of educational debt). Eventually, I moved to a hospital-employed job in a less litigious area, where I was able to thrive and triumph over this adverse beginning to my career. Put simply, the decline in my own wellness was visible and palpable to anyone paying attention to the issue. Fortunately, with counsel from trusted colleagues, support from family and friends, and faith in my training and ability, I was able to be rescued from this precarious position where I could have harmed patients and suffered untold personal costs.

A typical physician spends 11 percent of a 40-year career with an open malpractice claim against him or her [31]. Most claims, from letter of intent to file suit, through interrogatories, depositions, and expert testimony, to the actual court case itself, tend to last 5–7 years, depending on the jurisdiction. That means each case can last for almost 20% of a physician's career. Even though 90% of verdicts are in favor of the physician, being sued in a malpractice case is often a very stressful experience, and precious little about the tort system is beneficial or even fair to the physician. Sympathy for the plight of the defendant physician simply does not exist, and even victories at trial are pyrrhic at best; the doctor still stands as accused of malfeasance, as alleged by peers. Surgeons, as proceduralists, are more prone to lawsuit than other specialties. Facing malpractice is virtually an inevitability, and it can have a profound impact on surgeon wellness.

Consider this from a recent blog [32]: "The malpractice claim begins to affect all aspects of your life. You don't sleep well. You don't interact well with family members, friends, or colleagues. You remain dedicated to providing the best possible care, but you find yourself taking a more conservative approach with patients, asking yourself, 'How might this patient attempt to sue me?'" Does this sound like a prescription for physician wellness? Further, a doctor facing a lawsuit is instructed by counsel or a hospital risk management department not to discuss the case with colleagues – our typical sounding board – so we are forced to keep our feelings of concern, insecurity, sadness, and anxiety to ourselves. The case could be reviewed in a hospital mortality and morbidity conference or a peer review conference, which makes the surgeon re-live the complication or problem for which the lawsuit is based, furthering the symptoms. And worse, in some states, those conferences are discoverable, hampering their effectiveness in learning from error.

Medical malpractice comes with a significant cost to the healthcare system. This is not meant to defend or deny that medical errors kill nearly 100,000 of patients per year [33], and error prevention is the hallmark of any surgical quality program. But as physicians are under the constant threat of malpractice, we tend to over-order tests, radiology studies, and consultations. Defensive medicine, as it has been termed, adds tens of millions of dollars to the cost of delivering healthcare, and adds to a physician's already overwhelming work burden, which, as described elsewhere in this chapter, is a significant contributor to physician wellness decline. Further, risk-aversive behavior can develop, whereby surgeons decline to care for complicated patients or refer patients to tertiary care facilities to care for problems that do not in and of itself require their presence at such a facility. Since it is well-described that each procedure that we perform iteratively informs our future procedures, bad outcomes or experiences can negatively drive behavior away from repeating the same mistake, even if it is in the best interest of the patient. Such avoidant care can further increase healthcare costs, add to physician stress and dissatisfaction, and cause unintended harm or poor outcomes for patients.

There even exists a named syndrome for the litigation stress caused by a malpractice lawsuit: medical malpractice stress syndrome (MMSS) [34]. This syndrome is described as having symptoms like post-traumatic stress disorder (PTSD). Feelings of anger, despair, embarrassment, or stress are commonplace. It can manifest severe psychological symptoms, as well as physical symptoms, and can affect not just patient care delivery but personal life outside of the hospital. Furthermore, the anxiety generated by MMSS alone can lead to subsequent medical errors [34].

While avoiding medical malpractice is impossible in the delivery of surgical care, strategies to mitigate risk, avoid technical errors, manage complications, and continue lifelong learning can reduce the chances of being named in a lawsuit. Seeking professional support to cope with the stress of litigation is essential to preventing wellness decline. Building departmental systems such as peer support can also be a helpful adjunct to preventing MMSS or simply the personal stress generated by untoward patient outcomes.

Physician Autonomy and Wellness

"When doctors used to play golf on Wednesday afternoons, I didn't hear them talking about burnout." – Anonymous

One concept that is gaining attention is whether a loss of physician autonomy has become a factor in wellness decline. Certainly, the burden of administrative tasks – of which the physician has little control over and is required to complete – is a major factor in dissatisfaction, as has been well documented. But could the underlying reason really be a loss of control or autonomy? Consider how the scope of medicine has changed in recent decades and the parallel decline in physician wellness.

Decades ago, most physicians were in private practice. Surgeons booked as many cases as they wished to do. They saw patients in offices or clinics as needed to keep the OR schedule full. Time could be allocated to academic pursuit, education, or personal time as desired. Productivity was driven primarily by income and keeping referral pipelines flowing. While surgeons had to follow hospital bylaws and rules governing the operating room, there was very little oversight into the conduct of their medical practices. The private practice model allowed surgeons to work in competing healthcare systems, forcing the hospital administrative staff to cater to these physicians and curry favor with them or risk losing their business to the competition.

Fast forward to the modern era, where most surgeons are multispecialty group-employed or hospital-employed, and the private practice model is disappearing. Gone are the days whereby surgeons operated in competing hospitals in a community. Many compensation packages are based solely on productivity, with negative ramifications for failing to meet wRVU targets that are often not feasible. Time for academic pursuit and education is shrinking in the name of furthering productivity. Hospital administrative staff has a little role in helping the physicians achieve their goals. EMR use has become mandatory even on the outpatient side of patient care, and the many rules, inbox messages, laboratory, and X-ray results that must be addressed in the name of meeting medical record goals are often excessive. Physician time is completely controlled, and time for an afternoon of nonhospital social activity – even if it is done with referring physicians (i.e., helping to build a business relationship) – results in a deduction of hours from a personal time off bank. In short, in the name of practice stability and income guarantee, surgeons have forfeited autonomy, and this may have played a role in the general decline of physician wellness.

According to basic psychological needs theory [35], three innate human needs – autonomy, competence, and relatedness – should be supported by a work environment for individuals to experience optimal development, functioning, and well-being. A recent study by Walter and Kono [36] has shown that the need for autonomy had the largest positive effect on work satisfaction. In addition, the need for relatedness was also shown to be of importance, although the effect of competence was nonsignificant. This study was conducted outside of medicine but is relevant, nonetheless. A similar study [37] conducted with physicians in Canada determined relatedness to be the most important factor in professional well-being, although the physicians in this study had a high degree of autonomy and thus the author concluded that it played less of a role. Interestingly, one factor which has become a common buzzword for administrators is "engagement," and this study demonstrated that only relatedness had a positive effect on physician engagement. One way of framing this concept is to ask: is the work burden related to that which drives the physicians' well-being and satisfaction (i.e., patient care)? It can explain why overburdening physicians with administrative tasks (not related) can cause a loss of engagement and wellness decline.

A recent blog [38] listed five factors that have resulted in a loss of physician autonomy: insurance companies; middlemen such as pharmacy benefit managers (PBMs) or group purchasing organizations (GPOs); EMRs; government reporting and pay-for-performance; and physician replacement by lesser trained/qualified individuals. Insurance companies often dictate rules and regulations by which physicians must practice for them to cover a service or prescription. Consider what bariatric surgeons must do to gain authorization or how the concept of "mission creep" regarding prior authorization has been corrupted into nonevidence-based prescribing practices that take the decision out of the physicians' hands. The surgeon has little autonomy with regard to patient care decisions that are not filtered through the hands of a nonphysician at a third-party insurance company. PBMs and GPOs force surgeons into prescribing drugs that are "on formulary" and to use equipment in the operating room that is under contract, regardless of surgeon experience or comfort with the product. EMRs are covered in another section of this chapter. Quality reporting and the pressure of noncompensation for poor performance may take more clinical decision-making out of the hands of physicians, and greatly contribute to the loss of autonomy. Lastly, the explosion of advanced practice providers (APPs) may contribute to lower physician wages, as much of what a surgeon can do has recently been assumed by APPs, who typically are paid less than a physician. The blog [38] comments that administrators lump physicians and APPs together by calling all of us "providers," obscuring training and deceiving the public into the thinking that the care delivered is equivalent without any evidence that this is indeed the case. Nonetheless, an unintended consequence is stripping another layer of satisfaction away from physicians, and this too may contribute to wellness decline.

In 2011, 65% of physicians felt that the future of healthcare would see a decline in quality, largely due to a loss of autonomy [39]. Such was this concern that there were programs built into the Affordable Care Act designed to enhance physician autonomy… but at increased financial risk (and as such was born the concept of population health). While cost accountability should be part of any attempt at healthcare reform, dangling autonomy in exchange for financial risk leaves physicians in between two undesirable choices, leading to a decrease in satisfaction and reduced performance. While many initiatives with regard to technology, public quality reporting, increases in clinical volume, or new local standards are designed around patient safety and quality care delivery, the additional burdens placed on physicians lead to feelings of burnout and reduce the success of the initiatives [40].

Another recent example of loss of physician autonomy is the controversy over operating room attire, which is covered in detail in Chap. 49. While many decried the lack of evidence driving the AORN's 2015 recommendation to remove skullcaps from operating rooms (and newer evidence has led them to drop the recommendation altogether), surgeons also forcibly pushed back on the recommendations, seeing this as a loss of autonomy. As the American College of Surgeons stated in 2017, the skullcap is symbolic of the surgical profession. While the type of operating room head covering has never been associated specifically with surgeon wellness, the volume of the outcry and tone of the response spoke to the offense of the reduction in autonomy.

Loss of physician autonomy has clearly led to a decline in physician wellness, and considerations to large-scale change to address the burnout issue should focus on a meaningful restoration of physician autonomy.

Resilience

"Resilience is the collection of personal qualities that enable a person to adapt well and even thrive in the face of adversity and stress... Given the intensity of the (physician training process), resilience might be expected to be greater among practicing physicians than among workers in other careers...." [41].

Resilience is a topic often referred to in scholarly writing about physician burnout. While often defined as the collection of personal qualities that enable a person to adapt well and even thrive in the face of adversity and stress [41], the physical definition bears consideration: the capability of a strained body to recover its shape after deformation caused especially by stress. Recovery from stress, then, would be a way of framing how the concept of resilience applies to physician wellness. While it may seem sensible to associate the two ideas, the connection strains credibility when placed into the context of physician training.

Medical training is rigorous from the outset. It can begin in undergraduate studies with "weed out" courses such as organic chemistry, which often have endless memorization tasks and a near-unbearable knowledge load – all with the payoff that one may never utilize the information learned in their studies ever again. In medical school this can be multiplied, and this is among the reasons that many medical students report signs of burnout [42]. The learning burden is immense; and the hours spent studying, learning, and training can lead to social isolation, lack of meaningful relationships, and delay in starting families. Medical students are even taught to deny personal needs such as sleep and food, all in the name of service to patients [43] – and often disguised under the trope of "learning opportunities." (Witness the first two of the unofficial "rules of surgery": "Eat when you can," and "Sleep when you can.") Surgical residents are forced to learn an academic curriculum consisting of thousands of pages of textbook material; learn to read and critically appraise medical literature, which expands by thousands of scholarly articles per day; and perform well over a thousand operations in 5 or more years – all while taking care of scores of patients on "services" (note the use of the term again) on limited sleep, erratic and excessive work hours, and often unreasonable expectations of learning. One can make a very fair argument that physicians have well-developed resilience skills as they face difficulties daily and stress is near-constant in what they do. Thus, the argument that physicians need to improve their resilience to prevent wellness problems is neither credible nor particularly helpful.

Further, the concept of self-sacrifice in the name of service can lead to personal exhaustion – one of the hallmarks of burnout – and this expectation of sacrifice can be extended to the families of physicians [43]. Over time, this can lead to the struggle of work-life balance, that is, having to choose between patients and personal/family time. This can be additionally stressful for female physicians, who report higher rates of burnout than do their male colleagues [6, 41], and higher rates of divorce among physicians [44]. While many suggestions for physicians to avoid burnout speak of reserving professional time for family activities – e.g., canceling patient slots in one's schedule to attend a children's sporting event or artistic performance – this presumes that there exists enough professional autonomy to make such sacrifices. The author of this chapter personally witnessed this during fellowship training when his mentor would arrange surgical schedules around his son's hockey games; that mentor was the chair of an academic department of surgery and as such was granted the autonomy to control his schedule in such a manner. While he modeled an admirable work-life balance, most physicians do not have the autonomy to arrange their schedules in such a way. To wit, how much conversation was there about physician burnout in the era of "doctors playing golf on Wednesday afternoons"?

Additionally, in the practice of medicine, there exists the expectation of excellence and that our clinical results asymptotically approach perfection. Infinite reservoirs of knowledge and memory are demanded of our trainees, and zero tolerance for mistakes is commonplace [43]. While this concept leads to perfectionism, it leaves little room for acceptance of error, and learning from clinical mistakes. The omnipresent concern of sanction from internal or external bodies (in the name of "quality"), criticism from colleagues, and threat of malpractice hanging over physicians like a sword of Damocles leaves physicians with a fear of making a mistake that can lead to defensive medical practices, and feelings of inadequacy when mistakes inevitably occur. Further, our medical culture is still not comfortable with conversation (without repercussions) of error or patient harm as we often lack safe venues for meaningful discussion. Physicians are often forced to "move on to the next patient" without adequate time to heal from the painful feelings that arise from patient errors or deaths, and one can safely argue that they are highly dependent on resilience skills to do so.

A recent study looked at the association of resilience and burnout and reported important results to consider [41]. Not only do physicians exhibit higher levels of resilience than the general working population in the United States, but resilience was inversely associated with burnout symptoms. In other words, physicians with higher resilience scores scored lower in emotional exhaustion and depersonalization subdomains in the Maslach Burnout Index [5, 41]. So, while it would seem that resilience skills would be protective against burnout, the paper warns that "symptoms of burnout were common even among physicians with the highest possible resilience score" [41]. Further, "although efforts to maintain or strengthen resilience are appropriate... this approach aligns with evidence to date supporting equal or greater effectiveness of organizational solutions to reduce burnout" [41] rather than emphasis on the individual to improve skill sets in an effort to combat wellness decline.

Physicians are endowed with remarkable resilience skills – and one can argue from the rigor of training that surgeons are near the top in developing this skill. The suggestion that burnout is a result of resilience failure is not only lacking in credibility, but it tends toward blaming the victim, rather than focusing on system issues that are the true drivers of wellness decline.

EMRs and Wellness

"The average workday for its family physicians ha(s) grown to eleven and a half hours. The result has been epidemic levels of burnout among clinicians.... Something's gone terribly wrong."
– Atul Gawande [45]

The widespread adoption of EMRs into clinical practice is often blamed for a decline in physician wellness. And while it is true that dealing with the rigors of electronic documentation can be a frustrating experience – and a dissatisfier for patients, who often feel that their doctor is talking to a computer rather than talking to the patient – there can be no dispute that the technological advancement is a positive for the practice of clinical medicine. Gone are the days of illegible scribble being accepted as medical documentation or, worse, medical errors due to indecipherable order writing. And while many surgeons yearn for the days of yore with five-line progress notes inscribed in fluent abbreviation while stating nothing of consequence, there can be no dispute that electronic documentation had enhanced the readability of daily documentation in the patient's chart.

This is not to suggest that EMRs are a vast improvement. The notes that appear in charts are often several pages long, laden with automatically included data that clutters the note and makes the utility of the note decline. Medical records from lengthy hospitalizations have ballooned to thousands of pages simply with the "note diarrhea" that has become so prevalent. In many cases, the workload to create electronic documentation, especially in academic settings with trainees trying to document under time constraints, forces "copy-and-paste" behavior, which perpetuates information that can be inaccurate, is no longer timely, or may lead to false impressions about a patient's progress (not to mention that it is illegal per CMS guidelines). Many physicians complain that the EMR documentation system is subpar and that the EMR itself masquerades as a billing system. Others state, often correctly, that these systems were designed with minimal end-user input with the frustrating expectation that physicians would change their workflow to suit the program, rather than designing the program to suit physician needs while minimizing workflow changes. Is it any wonder that EMRs are blamed for the decline in physician wellness?

A recent survey that examined physician wellness in depth [7] did look at EMRs as a cause for burnout. There were important findings elucidated in this survey; regarding EMRs, there is a clear generational divide. Unsurprisingly, the group that reported the most difficulty with EMRs was the Baby Boomer group, which may imply less facility with computerized programs and technology in general. For example, 41% of Baby Boomers reported increasing computerization of practice as a contributor to a decline in wellness, but only 17% of Millennials did so. EMRs were the second *lowest* cited factor for burnout symptoms in the Millennial group. One can argue, then, that this problem should decline as a factor as Baby Boomers inch closer to retirement, and the younger workforce, already facile with technology, perhaps will view this less of an impediment to work completion. Overall, EMRs actually placed fourth overall in the survey [7] as a cause of burnout with 30% of physicians reporting it is a cause of wellness decline, behind other factors such as too many bureaucratic tasks (55%), total work hours (33%), and lack of respect from colleagues, administration, and staff (32%).

Numerous scholarly publications have ruminated on EMRs as a cause for physician burnout. One recent paper [46] has a quote that is informative: "[EMRs] contribute to burnout by turning physicians into unhappy data-entry clerks, and also by enabling 24-hour patient access without any system to provide compensation or coverage." A study by the RAND corporation [47] about physician professional satisfaction looked in depth at EMRs. Stating that EMRs were "a source of both promise and frustration," physicians in this survey did approve of EMRs in concept and appreciated the ability to remotely access patient information. Physicians also defined EMRs as an improvement in the quality of care. On the other hand, aspects of EMRs that routinely negatively affected satisfaction included "poor usability, time-consuming data entry, interference with face-to-face patient care, inefficient and less fulfilling work content, inability to exchange health information, and degradation of clinical documentation." Another recent study [48] ranked the usability (based on a standardized score to rank usability of software) of EMRs and found them to be rated a software usability score (SUS) of 45.9/100 – which is in the "not acceptable" range or a grade of "F." To compare, Excel, which is widely panned as difficult and unwieldy to use, scored a 57 (low marginal acceptability range but also a grade of F). This speaks to the drastic need to create future iterations of EMR technology with significant provider input to make them more usable. The authors state as such: "Given the association between EHR usability and physician burnout, improving EHR usability *may be an important approach* to help reduce health care professional burnout." This study also showed that older physicians were more likely to rate EMRs as less usable. It also demonstrated that physicians working in academic medical centers rated their EMR less favorably. Most concerningly, "EHR usability scores were strongly and independently associated with physician burnout in a dose-response relationship. The odds of burnout were lower for each 1 point more favorable SUS score, a finding that persisted after adjusting for an extensive array of other personal and professional characteristics." Data such as these should be sounding a clarion call to hospital administrators and software companies that physicians need better technology, but that has yet to occur. Even the Affordable Care Act includes a provision regarding interoperability of EMRs (another source of physician frustration), but in almost a decade since its passage, little tangible progress has been made on that front.

Famed author and surgeon Atul Gawande wrote an essay for the New Yorker [45] entitled "Why Doctors Hate Their Computers," which looks at the humanistic aspect of the EMR frustration for physicians. One quote stands out as a wonderful summation of the problem: "I've come to feel that a system that promised to increase my mastery over my work has, instead, increased my work's mastery over me." He also commented on a study [49] that demonstrated that physicians spent almost 2 hours doing computer work for every hour spent with a patient and that documentation tasks are often done after hours from home. "The result has been epidemic levels of burnout among clinicians," writes Gawande. One colleague of the author stated that the extra time spent documenting was not the concern – the pointlessness of doing the task in the ways required was what bothered her the most. Gawande also comments on how mundane but necessary tasks like medication refills or letters to patients – traditionally performed by office staff – often must be done by physicians, adding to the feeling of administrative overburden.

An article published in the *New England Journal of Medicine Catalyst* [50] examined the relationship between EMRs and burnout. There are revealing comments in this article that help to point toward the association with EMR design, physician workflow, and frustration. Once concept is alert fatigue – where physicians often see so many "alerts" that do not have clinical relevance that they miss alerts that are critically important. "Often, there are so many of these best practice alerts (requiring physician work to address them) that the clinicians just bypass them." Another comment summarizes the thoughts of many physicians: "What has happened over time is we have asked our clinicians to become sophisticated coders. They are clicking through screens that are cluttered, that are not designed with human factors in mind. They are filling out forms that at one time would have been triaged to a medical assistant or health assistant. They're having to respond in their inbox to messages that otherwise historically would not have come to their inbox, that would have been filtered away, and so it literally has added work to a busy day…." The authors conclude that a solution to the problem would be for "designers of EMRs to try and work to improve the user interface, the workflow, in a way similar to the way smartphones work or when you start a search on a search engine and it almost anticipates your needs. We're just behind. We're almost in generation one of that electronic medical record…."

One risk in blaming the EMRs as the main source of physician burnout is that administrators may focus on the physical concept of a "thing" causing the dissatisfaction, rather than the issue at hand: less-efficient workflow caused by electronic documentation requirements. In other words, blaming the computer for physician wellness decline misses the point entirely. We believe that EMRs are a *different* method to document and communicate, but that surgeons must strive to enhance their own personal workflow within the system to find efficiency. All systems are rife with inefficiency; the author of this chapter recalls clearly spending hours searching for patient charts on the floors during weekend rounds, as opposed to the current state of sitting at a computer and signing many notes all at once. It is unquestionably faster and more efficient now. **We believe the key to minimizing the frustration with EMRs is to become stakeholders – have input in design of templated notes, order sets, etc. – to make the computer conform to the workflow of a best practice standard.** The entire field of medical informatics is developing rapidly to marry the software coders and clinicians together to help make the use of the EMR less burdensome. Over time, this should minimize frustration and lessen the contribution toward physician burnout.

Leadership Perspective: How to Handle Burnout in a Department

"Choose a job that you love, and you will never a work a day in your life." – Confucius

The first and most obvious thought about a surgeon who has declining wellness is for others to be cognizant of the symptoms. Surgical department chairs, division chiefs, or even senior partners in private practices should be constantly on the lookout for the partner or colleague who is not doing well. External signs such as visible stigmata of fatigue, poor grooming, and a downward trajectory in attitude or overall happiness should be calls for attention to the situation. A pattern of surgical outcomes that deviates from the expected in a confined period of time should at least provoke the question of wellness. Downturns in productivity without a precipitating event should also prompt questions about whether or not the surgeon is exhibiting other signs of burnout. Of course, this responsibility should not only rely on surgical leadership but rather be the responsibility of everyone in a group as a whole. The trite expression "A rising tide rises all boats" certainly rings true in this instance.

Gaining an understanding of what the fears of surgeons are can be extraordinarily helpful to surgical leaders. In the Virtual SAGES Annual Meeting of 2020, there was a session entitled "Putting Out the Fire: Time to Burn the Burnout." In this session, Dr. Mark Talamini, a former SAGES president, who served as a department chair at multiple institutions, addressed this directly in his talk entitled: "The Principals of Burnout" [51]. Dr. Talamini stated that the job of the chair is to "create jobs that your faculty will love, and you can avoid some of the burnout/disruption/wellness issues that can arise." Further, he stresses that a critical goal of surgical leaders is to serve as a coach for the faculty – to assess his/her surgeons, learn their strengths and weakness, help to accentuate their strengths, try to address their weaknesses, and advise when "fixing" isn't possible and help them to move on to a position better suited to their talents. Also, in this lecture, Dr. Talamini refers to Marcus Buckingham's book, *The One Thing You Need to Know: About Great Managing, Great Leading, and Sustained Individual Success* [52]. Dr. Talamini discusses the five fears of surgeons in this talk, and the five solutions leaders need to address these fears. He states that the leader's role is to determine which of the fears applies to each surgeon under their command, and to work toward recognition of these issues. Namely, he discussed the fears of **death**, **being an outsider**, **the future**, **chaos**, and **insignificance**. Each of these fears has **corresponding needs** from leaders to address them. Fear of **death**, despite the melodramatic timbre, is really about the fear of having an inability to provide for oneself and their family. It raises questions of economic security. While not common among surgeons based on typical incomes, this can become an issue in productivity-driven compensation situations. The need from the leader is to provide **security**. Assuring surgeons that their employment is not threatened if certain financial goals are not met can reduce a stressor that could lead to burnout. Fear of **being an outsider** is often framed by an individual as "Am I part of this group?" The need for the leader to provide is a sense of **community**. Inclusiveness in a department or division can avoid corrosive relationships that can damage the psyche of a group and serves as a threat to overall success. It is important for all leaders to recognize the importance of developing a community so that common goals can be developed and shared. Fear of **the future** is often asked as "What is going to happen?" Certainly, during the COVID-19 pandemic, many of us have faced this fear, and it is frustrating for many to not have the answer to this question. The need for the leader is to provide **clarity** in their leadership style; clarity about where the department, division, or practice is going; where they hope to be in subsequent years; how growth will occur; and what needs to happen to achieve it. Mapping out what the future will look like for a surgeon helps to avoid wellness decline if she or he can see the path to accomplish what was mapped out. The fear of **chaos** is really rooted in questions of **authority**: "Whom do I answer to?" Many surgeons are pulled in several directions and the chain of command can become confusing. Do they only answer to the chairman? To the CEO or CMO? For surgical oncologists, do they answer to the director of the cancer center? Having a clear chain of command can avoid departmental chaos, and this can serve as an insidious cause of stress of surgeons. Lastly, the fear of **insignificance** can overwhelm physicians, although Dr. Talamini points out that surgeons are the least likely to suffer from this because each operation that we perform is a significant, tangible event in the care of a patient. One can imagine that emergency medicine providers, primary care physicians, or hospitalists struggle with this – with a never-ending list of patients, lengthy tasks to be completed in the EMRs, seeming like they are constantly behind in time, etc. The leader's role is to provide **respect**: assurance that what that physician does matters, reinforcing how important they are to the department, telling him or her that their job performance is excellent. In short, the "Attaboy!" comments make a difference.

The goal of the surgical leader is to sense when the colleague is straying from the clinical path that was created together, and this seems to be congruent with wellness decline. Understanding the drivers of stress and gaining the trust of the colleague to have open and honest discussion about their issues represents an important step toward wellness rescue. Of course, identifying concerns of mental illness is critical, and the use of the institution's employee assistance program can aid in helping the surgeon in wellness decline.

Putting out the Fire: Burning the Burnout

"The best defense is a good offense." – Jack Dempsey

So how does one move forward given the scope of this crisis of physician wellness? Obviously, solutions are far beyond the scope of a book chapter, but there are many items touched upon that can help lead us to a better understanding of the problem. It is incumbent upon physicians, especially physician leaders, administrators, and all concerned to recognize the magnitude of the problem and the threat that it serves to the physician workforce. Physician suicide is far too common, and tragic in every single instance. Attrition due to non-wellness and early retirements take talented, experienced physicians out of the workplace. And wellness decline can start very early in a physician's career, even as soon as medical school. So clearly, we at a minimum need to be attentive to the issue from the very beginning of training.

First, we as physicians need to better define the problem. As previously stated, burnout is the end stage of a spectrum of wellness; a better term that is both more descriptive and less judgmental than the term "burnout" is "physician wellness decline." Burnout implies a status from which one cannot recover; this is simply not the case in most physicians. Rather, appropriate intervention can produce wellness rescue, and this should be the singular goal in all situations of physician decline. Others prefer the concept of "moral injury," as "burnout" is a term that could be seen as blaming the victim as opposed to examining system issues that are driving the decline. Moral injury refers to the negative feelings that arise when physicians cannot care for their patients due to system issues. As discussed in this chapter, many system issues can lead to moral injury, be it limitations of electronic medical records, rules by third-party insurance companies, administrative burden, etc. So, clarity in definition is a necessary first step.

Second, a good baseline to move back to is to try and find the joy in surgery. Why did the physician become a surgeon in the first place? What drew her to the field? What makes him happy at work? What stressors are preventing them from finding joy? As discussed in a recent publication [53], "a paradigm shift in the profession of surgery would facilitate the rediscovery and reinvigoration of joy among surgeons and their family, friends, patients, and learners." This would require buy-in not only from surgeon leaders but all practicing surgeons. This could serve as an offensive maneuver to combat wellness decline – to shift surgeons in the positive direction on the wellness spectrum. The Institute for Healthcare Improvement published a white paper in 2017 focused on this topic [54]. They identified a four-step process to reintroduce joy to the work environment. The first step is to **ask surgeons what matters to them**. This gets at the heart of their internal motivation. But it can also help to identify what drives their wellness in the negative direction. For example, if colorectal surgeons are forced to take call for general surgery or trauma surgery, these surgeons might be forced to deliver care they are unaccustomed to providing or to perform operations they are not comfortable performing. What matters to them might be to stop taking such call and to focus on building their colorectal practices. The second step is to **identify unique impediments**. In the above example, it is achieving the desired result of not taking general/trauma call because of a lack of providers to cover the calls with enough time to rest and recover between calls. These colorectal surgeons might want to take call for colorectal surgery only but defining what would be "colorectal" could be contentious and fracture a department into subgroups with competing interests. The third step is to **commit to a systems approach**. This requires forming a multidisciplinary team to examine how to remove impediments to joy. For example, imagine a team where non-surgeons looked at the above issue; they examined how many patients are received on call, who else might be able to cover call (community surgeons?), how many colorectal patients would be expected per call, etc. Sometimes, working outside of the "silos" we tend to form in surgery can offer innovative solutions to difficult problems. The last step is to **use improvement science methodology to track, study, and share improvements with all key stakeholders** [53, 54]. Creating quality improvement projects around thorny issues that drive wellness in the negative direction could be a creative way of tackling the problems and finding a path back to joy in a surgical department.

Third, learning how to thrive in a constrained environment, while not necessarily a demonstration of resilience skills, is critical to not allowing limitations in care delivery to become drivers on non-wellness. As an example, look at the EMR. Rather than seeing the computer as the enemy, view it as a technological advance that helps to prevent medical errors. I chose to embrace electronic documentation by working with our informatics team to develop note templates that made my workflow faster and more efficient. I did so by automating anything that was repetitive in any way. As one might imagine, in a practice heavy on bariatrics, creating templates to cover preoperative and postoperative bariatric patients would go a long way toward aiding the surgeon with documentation. I view this as "making lemonade out of life's lemons," but it never moved my wellness negatively on the spectrum. It is true that we cannot force massive system changes such as the health insurance system, accreditation requirements, coding and billing rules, or hospital bylaws simply to provide improvement to physician wellness. But learning how to function within the boundaries – and then building and establishing a "comfort zone" – will go a long way toward not letting system issues induce feelings of burnout.

Fourth, I think a good faith attempt to balance productivity and appropriate rest is a prescription to financial health of a division or department and physical wellness of the workforce. It is without dispute that fatigue is a threat to patient care and overnight call can produce fatigue that can last for several days. As the surgical workforce ages in a department or group, recovery from disrupted sleep may take longer, and thus surgical leaders need to be cognizant of fatigue issues provoked by taking overnight call. For example, should elective work be scheduled the day after a 24-hour call shift? Are those surgeons best equipped to manage their patients safely? Are they as cognitively attuned to threats to patient safety as they would be if well-rested? How much productivity must be sacrificed to allow for time off – and wouldn't this be recaptured by a well-rested and thus more productive workforce? Gone are the days of the "suck it up" method of fatigue management. Emotional wellness is an impossible dream for surgeons if a lack of physical wellness permeates a department. Eating well, exercising, and other healthy endeavors to address stress in the workplace are difficult to achieve when chronically fatigued. So, an important strategy to combat physician wellness decline is to assure adequate rest and maintenance of physical wellness. Another strategy to consider would be to provide paid time off for each period of overnight or weekend call. This might allow surgeons to relax and refresh and come to work reinvigorated. Further, strategies to work smarter – and not harder – should be implemented. For example, is it necessary to perform all appendectomies immediately upon presentation? Should they still be performed in the middle of the night, when there is ample evidence that waiting until morning in the absence of peritonitis does not worsen outcomes? Wouldn't the outcomes theoretically improve if the surgeon was well-rested? Granted, system issues such as operating room availability and a clear schedule for the post-call surgeon would be necessary impediments to this process, but the dogmatic thought of "all appendectomies are surgical emergencies" should not only fall victim to evidence to the contrary but an effort to work smarter and gain valuable rest for the surgeon.

Last, we must remember that we are doctors committed to helping others. While in general that refers to patient care, we must not lose sight over the responsibility to care for one another. To extinguish burnout, we must strive to create a culture of accountability; part of our responsibility should be to make sure our partners, colleagues, and fellow caregivers are well. When one of our colleagues begins to slide in the negative direction on the wellness spectrum, we must take active steps to help. These could be small steps like recognizing fatigue in a colleague and offering to help offload the work burden by changing call assignments, scrubbing them out of a long operation, or being a friendly voice to listen when they need to vent their frustrations. A former colleague of mine, now retired, served that role for many years in my department, and he personally taught me how to listen to my colleagues – an important and often neglected skill for physicians. We must create a community that is inclusive, where everyone helps to get the work finished. That might mean creative solutions to handle the work burden that may represent a disruptive change – recognizing that some of those solutions might fail. Such a community must also beware of the negative power of inertia and acknowledge the natural resistance to change. We must be aware of implicit biases, even regarding how we interact with each other as colleagues, and to avoid microaggressions which quickly lead to feelings that produce a negative move on the wellness spectrum. Healthcare administrators should seek to be part of the solution by avoiding victim blaming, using multidisciplinary teams to creatively solve difficult system issues which drive non-wellness, and learning what problems are really plaguing physicians. They must be committed to implementing meaningful change to help improve wellness, and they should encourage department leaders to keep "wellness report cards" on its staff, so that there is attention to the problem on a regular basis with mechanisms to address those that are failing.

Conclusion

Surgeon burnout represents an existential threat to the delivery of high-quality surgical care. Although drivers of physician wellness decline are multifactorial, and certainly vary between different subspecialties of medicine, gaining an understanding as to how physicians begin to become unhappy in their jobs is crucial to addressing this crisis. We must begin by looking at drivers of non-wellness in our future workforce and strategize creative solutions to these issues with careful consideration of reform of surgical training. Leaders should be committed to building a pathway toward joy in their departments. We must recognize that physicians of all specialties are resilient enough – and that mindfulness and meditation are not realistic tools to address feelings of depersonalization, emotional exhaustion, or reduced personal accomplishment. We must grant physicians the autonomy necessary to improve their workflow, and we must audit their work burden and take meaningful steps to address it when it becomes overwhelming. This includes taking a careful look at how overnight and weekend call responsibilities are mitigated. Steps to prevent cognitive overload – either by overhauling surgical training for physicians new to the profession or reducing board accreditation requirements – need for continuing medical education, and the need to stay current in their area of surgery, perhaps with technological innovation, should be taken to ensure a healthy surgical workforce. Issues of medical malpractice should be handled with sensitivity of how they affect physicians emotionally, and risk management teams should incorporate systems to gauge physician wellness in the response to claims. The use and implementation of EMRs should be strategized with workflow improvements as the goal. And lastly, surgical leaders should strive to create a community whereby everyone takes care of one another, helps the colleague in need, and holds each other accountable for wellness.

References

1. Williams TE, Satiani B, Ellison EC. The coming shortage of surgeons: why they are disappearing and what that means for our health. Santa Barbara, CA: Praeger Publishing; 2009.
2. West CP, Dyrbye LN, Shanafelt TD. Physician burnout: contributors, consequences, and solutions. J Intern Med. 2018;283(6):516–29.
3. Garcia C, de Abreu LC, Ramos JLS, de Castro CFD, Smiderle FRN, et al. Influence of burnout on patient safety: systematic review and meta-analysis. Medicina. 2019;55(9):553.
4. Salyers MP, Bonfils KA, Luther L, Firmin RL, White DA, et al. The relationship between professional burnout and quality and safety in healthcare: a meta-analysis. J Gen Intern Med. 2017;32(4):475–82.
5. Maslach C, Schaufeli WB, Maslach C, Marek T. Professional burnout: recent developments in theory and research. Washington, DC: Taylor & Francis; 1993.
6. Senturk JC, Melnitchouk N. Surgeon burnout: defining, identifying, and addressing the new reality. Clin Colon Rectal Surg. 2019;32(6):407–14.
7. https://www.medscape.com/slideshow/2020-lifestyle-burnout-6012460. Accessed 17 Feb, 2020.
8. Maslach C, Jackson SE, Leiter MP. Maslach burnout inventory manual. 3rd ed. Palo Alto, CA: Consulting Psychologists Press; 1996.

754   J. R. Romanelli

9. West CP, Dyrbye LN, Shanafelt TD. Physician burnout: contributors, consequences and solutions. J Intern Med. 2018;283(6):516–29.
10. Tawfik DS, Profit J, Morganthaler TI, Satele DV, Sinsky CA, et al. Physician burnout, Well-being, and work unit safety grades in relationship to reported medical errors. May Clin Proc. 2018;93(11):1571–80.
11. Shanafelt TD, Balch CM, Bechamps GJ, Russell T, Dyrbye L, et al. Burnout and career satisfaction among American surgeons. Ann Surg. 2009;250(3):463–71.
12. Dyrbye LN, Burke SE, Hardeman RR, Herrin J, Wittlin NM, et al. Association of Clinical Specialty with Symptoms of burnout and career choice regret among US resident physicians. JAMA. 2018;320(11):1114–30.
13. Hewitt DB, Ellis RJ, Hu Y, Cheung EO, Moskovitz JT, et al. Evaluating the association of multiple burnout definitions and thresholds with prevalence and outcomes. JAMA Surg. 2020;155(11):1043–9.
14. Engelhardt KE, Bilimoria KY, Johnson JY. A national mixed-methods evaluation of preparedness for general surgery residency and the association with resident burnout. JAMA Surg. 2020;155(9):851–9.
15. Dean W, Talbot S, Dean A. Reframing clinical distress: moral injury, not burnout. Fed Pract. 2019;36(9):400–2.
16. https://www.statnews.com/2018/07/26/physicians-not-burning-out-they-are-suffering-moral-injury/. Accessed 10 Dec, 2020.
17. Kopacz MS, Ames D, Koenig HG. It's time to talk about physician burnout and moral injury. Lancet Psychiatry. 2019;6(11):e28.
18. https://zdoggmd.com/moral-injury. Accessed 10 Dec, 2020.
19. https://www.kevinmd.com/blog/2019/11/how-the-administrative-burden-contributes-to-physician-burnout.html. Accessed 3 Dec, 2020.
20. Embriaco N, Azoulay E, Barrau K, et al. High level of burnout in intensivists: prevalence and associated factors. Am J Respir Crit Care Med. 2007;175:686–92.
21. Dewa CS, Jacobs P, Thanh NX, et al. An estimate of the cost of burnout on early retirement and reduction in clinical hours of practicing physicians in Canada. BMC Health Serv Res. 2014;14:254.
22. Moss M, Good VS, Gozal D, et al. An official critical care societies collaborative statement: burnout syndrome in critical care healthcare professionals: a call for action. Crit Care Med. 2016;44:1414–21.

23. October 4, 1984 & Libby Zion: the day medicine changed forever. Accessed at https://conciergemedicinemd.com/october-4-1984-libby-zion-the-day-medicine-changed-forever/ on November 5, 2020.
24. Ericsson KA. Deliberate practice and the acquisition and maintenance of expert performance in medicine and related domains. Acad Med. 2004;79(10 Suppl):S70–81.
25. Sweller J. Cognitive load theory. Psychology of learning and motivation. Elsevier; 2011. p. 37–76.
26. Cowan N. Metatheory of storage capacity limits. Behav Brain Sci. 2001;24(1):154–76.
27. Iskander M. Burnout, Cognitive Overload and Metacognition in Medicine. MedSciEduc. 2019;29:325–8.
28. Kirschner PA. Cognitive load theory: implications of cognitive load theory on the design of learning. Learn Instr. 2002;12(1):1–10.
29. Scott BM, Schwartz NH. Navigational spatial displays: the role of metacognition as cognitive load. Learn Instr. 2007;17(1):89–105.
30. https://www.luc.edu/media/lucedu/law/centers/healthlaw/pdfs/advancedirective/pdfs/issue4/thomas.pdf. Accessed 3 Dec, 2020.
31. Seabury SA, Chandra A, Lakdawalla DN, Jena AB. On average, physicians spend nearly 11 percent of their 40-year careers with an open, unresolved malpractice claim. Health Aff. 2013;32(1):111–9.
32. https://www.thedoctors.com/articles/overcoming-the-stress-of-malpractice-litigation-solutions-to-help-physicians-stay-healthy-and-engaged/. Accessed 13 Oct, 2020.
33. Kohn LT, Corrigan J, Donaldson MS. To err is human: building a safer health system. Washington, DC: National Academies Press (US); 2000.
34. https://www.norcal-group.com/wellness/reduce-litigation-stress-to-help-prevent-physician-burnout. Accessed 13 Oct, 2020.
35. Ryan RM, Deci EL. Self-determination theory and the facilitation of intrinsic motivation, social development, and Well-being. Am Psychol. 2000;55:68–78.
36. Walter GJ, Kono S. The effects of basic psychological need satisfaction during leisure and paid work on global life satisfaction. J Posit Psychol. 2018;13:36–47.
37. Babenko O. Healthcare (Basel). 2018;6(1):12.
38. https://www.kevinmd.com/blog/2019/09/to-extinguish-burnout-bring-back-physician-autonomy.html. Accessed 10 Dec, 2020.
39. Emanuel EJ, Pearson SD. Physician autonomy and health care reform. J Am Med Assoc. 2012;307(4):367–8.
40. Dyrbye LN, Shanafelt TD. Physician burnout: a potential threat to successful health care reform. JAMA. 2011;305(19):2009–10.

41. West CP, Dyrybe LN, Sinsky C, et al. Resilience and burnout among physicians and the general US working population. JAMA Netw Open. 2020;3(7):e209385.
42. Dyrybe LN, Massie FS, Eacker A, et al. Relationship between burnout and professional conduct and attitudes among US medical students. JAMA. 2010;304:1173–80.
43. Nedrow A, Stecker NA, Hardman J. Physician resilience and burnout: can you make the switch? Fam Pract Manag. 2013;20(1):25–30.
44. Doctors and Divorce. http://hms.harvard.edu/news/doctors-divorce. Accessed on 15 Sep, 2020.
45. Gawande A. "Why doctors hate their computers", published in the *new Yorker*. November. 2018;5
46. Collier R. Electronic health records contributing to physician burnout. CMAJ. 2017;189(45):E1405–6.
47. Friedberg MW, Chen PG, Van Busum KR, Aunon F, Pham C, et al. Factors Affecting Physician Professional Satisfaction and Their Implications for Patient Care, Health Systems, and Health Policy. Accessed at https://www.rand.org/pubs/research_reports/RR439.html on September 28, 2020.
48. Melnick ER, Dyrybe LN, Sinsky CA, Trockel M, West CP, et al. The association between perceived electronic health record usability and professional burnout among US physicians. Mayo Clin Proc. 2020 Mar;95(3):476–87.
49. Young RA, Burge SK, Kumar KA, Wilson JM, Ortiz DF. A time-motion study of primary care physicians' work in the electronic health record. Fam Med. 2018;50(2):91–9.
50. Strongwater S, Lee TH. Are EMRs to blame for physician burnout? NEJM Catalyst, October. 2016;24
51. https://eventpilotadmin.com/web/page.php?page=Speaker&project=SAGES20&id=3346. Accessed 7 Dec, 2020.
52. Buckingham M. The one thing you need to know: about great managing, great leading, and sustained individual success. New York: Free Press; 2005.
53. Romanelli J, Gee D, Mellinger JD, Alseidi A, Bittner JG, et al. The COVID-19 reset: lesson from the pandemic on burnout and the practice of surgery. Surg Endosc. 2020;34(12):5201–7.
54. Perlo J, Balik B, Swensen S, Kabcenell A, Landsman J, et al. IHI framework for improving joy in work. Cambridge, MA: Institute for Healthcare Improvement; 2017.

Chapter 39
The Disruptive Surgeon

M. Shane Dawson and Rebecca B. Kowalski

"The disruptive surgeon" is a phrase we have all heard. Most of us have experienced it firsthand: as a student, resident, or fellow being berated by an attending; witnessing inappropriate comments; observing a colleague decompensating; or any combination of these events. Writing this chapter was actually a struggle for the authors, as it brought up a lot of PTSD-like memories of some of the behaviors we have personally witnessed over the years. As a resident, one author watched an attending throw an instrument at the scrub tech, which landed on the field and shattered, spraying pieces all over the patient which then had to be located. Both authors have witnessed attendings making inappropriate comments in the operating room, when no one felt comfortable saying something to stop the comments. During their first year as an attending, one author had a surgeon from another surgical subspecialty burst into the operating room while performing an emergency case on a weekend evening because the other

M. S. Dawson · R. B. Kowalski (✉)
Northwell Health at Lenox Hill Hospital, New York, NY, USA
e-mail: shane@shanedawson.com; rkowalski@northwell.edu

© The Author(s), under exclusive license to Springer Nature   757
Switzerland AG 2022
J. R. Romanelli et al. (eds.), *The SAGES Manual of Quality, Outcomes and Patient Safety*,
https://doi.org/10.1007/978-3-030-94610-4_39

attending was angry at the circulating nurse, start yelling, and then had to become the "disruptive surgeon" who yelled at the other attending to leave the operating room so the team could focus on the emergency case.

It is key to point out that disruptive behavior is not limited to physicians or surgeons. Nurses, scrub techs, patients, and family members are often guilty of disruptive behavior as well, all of which can have an equally negative impact on patient safety and quality of care. However, this chapter will focus on the disruptive surgeon.

Some of us may have been labeled as "a disruptive surgeon" ourselves. Whether it is unacceptable behavior such as anger or throwing instruments, inappropriate or derogatory language, or otherwise creating an environment that is not conducive to other members of the team speaking up, the disruptive surgeon is a definite threat to quality, outcomes, and safety in the operating room and beyond.

What Is Disruptive Behavior?

Disruptive behavior can be categorized into aggressive, passive, or passive-aggressive behaviors [1]. While the aggressive behaviors are "more disruptive" in the sense that they are usually more easily recognized, the passive or passive-aggressive behaviors can be harmful over the course of time as they will "build up" more to the point of breaking.

The behavior can be overt, as with the use of profane, disrespectful, insulting, demeaning, insensitive, or abusive language; negative comments about colleagues (either spoken or in the patient's chart); verbal intimidation; inappropriate arguments with patients, family members, or colleagues; rudeness; boundary violations; outbursts of anger; bullying behavior; throwing or breaking things; or the use of or the threat of unwarranted physical force with patients, family members, or colleagues [2].

Disruptive behavior can also be covert or passive, such as refusal to comply with known and generally accepted practice standards; repeated failure to respond or late response to calls or requests for information or assistance when expected to be available; not working collaboratively with others; and creating rigid or inflexible barriers to requests for assistance [2].

There are some key terms that will be used through the remainder of this chapter that need to be clearly defined. These terms include:

1. *Professional competence*: "The habitual and judicious use of communication, knowledge, technical skills, clinical reasoning, emotions, values and reflection in daily practice for the benefit of the individual and community being served" [3]. The Accreditation Council for Graduate Medical Education (ACGME) and the American Board of Medical Specialties (ABMS) have divided competence into "competencies" in specific domains, including those that apply to all physicians and those that are unique to each specialty [3]. A deficiency in any of these domains can be referred to as a "dyscompetency," which can be a helpful term because no one is totally incompetent [3].

2. *Mental and behavioral problems*: Include depression, anxiety, substance abuse, personality disorders, and disruptive behavior with colleagues, patients, and subordinates [3].

3. *Disruptive physician*: A physician who exhibits abusive behavior that "interferes with patient care or could reasonably be expected to interfere with the process of delivering quality care" [3]. Examples include profane or disrespectful language, demeaning behavior, sexual comments or innuendo, outbursts of anger, throwing instruments or charts, criticizing hospital staff in front of patients or other staff, negative comments about another physician's care, boundary violations with staff or patients, inappropriate chart notes (e.g., criticizing the treatment provided by other caregivers), or unethical or dishonest behavior [3].

4. *Impaired physician*: Defined by the American Medical Association as a disability resulting from psychiatric illness, alcoholism, or drug dependence.

5. *Performance problems*: All types of deficiencies, regardless of cause [3].

Although surgeons have been the specialty most commonly identified as "disruptive physicians" [4], a disruptive physician in any field is an obvious source of concern in the patient care environment. The fact that surgeons have been most commonly identified as disruptive may be related to the higher stress environment of the operating room or the perceived high-stakes nature of surgical care.

Disruptive behavior in the healthcare environment is not new, but in the past, the disruptive behavior has been ignored, tolerated, reinforced, or not reported [5]. We have all heard some version of the phrase "the squeaky wheel gets the oil," which is one way the behavior has been reinforced: surgeons who make a scene when they do not get what they want get things their way because the staff does not want to deal with the fallout if they don't get what they want, which reinforces the disruptive behavior. Conversely, surgeons who do not exhibit the disruptive behavior often get negative reinforcement of their good behavior because the staff knows they will not "erupt" and therefore will choose to give the disruptive surgeon what they want over the nondisruptive surgeon. Over time, this can lead to the nondisruptive surgeon becoming disruptive, and lead to a general decline in operating room staff morale.

In 2018 when the American College of Surgeons (ACS) conducted their annual survey, one of the topics addressed was the disruptive or impaired surgeon, and the Board of Governors then published feedback related to the disruptive or impaired surgeon. "Disruptive behavior by a physician, often called abusive behavior, generally refers to a style of interaction by physicians with others - including hospital personnel, patients, and family members - that interferes with patient care or adversely affects the health care team's ability to work effectively. It encompasses behavior that adversely affects morale, focus and concentration, collaboration, and communication and information transfer - all of which can lead to substandard patient care" [6].

What Are the Underlying Causes of Disruptive Behavior?

Disruptive behavior is driven by multiple factors. Staffing shortages, stress of the clinical environment, production pressures, financial constraints, increased governmental oversight with increasing managed care regulations, and greater liability risks have all been cited as factors that can increase pressure and may contribute to disruptive behavior.

Thinking of performance problems as *symptoms of underlying disorders* (rather than a disease in and of itself) can be helpful in understanding the underlying causes of performance problems and disruptive behavior. These can include mental and behavioral problems, including substance abuse or dependence (drugs or alcohol); physical illness, including age-related and disease-related cognitive impairment; a decline in surgeon wellness; and failure to maintain or acquire knowledge and skills [3].

Contributing to or compounding these underlying problems are fatigue, stress, isolation, and easy access to drugs [3]. The "normal stress" of medical practice has been exacerbated by increasing educational debt loads for graduating physicians, increasing malpractice premiums, decreasing reimbursement, and increasing pressure to see more patients in a shorter amount of time [3]. Stress can lead to isolation and maladaptive coping strategies such as alcohol or drug abuse [3]. By the time these issues appear in the workplace, the physician's relationships with significant others, family, friends, and community have typically been "impaired" for a long time [3]. A decline in wellness, with "burnout" being the end stage of the spectrum, is another underlying cause of performance problems, and subsequent disruptive behavior. This is discussed further in Chap. 38, Surgeon Wellness.

What Is the Extent of the Problem?

According to data provided by the Federation of State Medical Boards of the United States, 4081 physicians were disciplined by state medical boards in 2017 [7]. This number has remained relatively stable over the past decade. These figures are difficult to interpret within the realm of the disruptive physician, as there are a variety of reasons physicians may be disciplined by a state medical board.

With regard to mental illness, there were an estimated 17.3 million adults (aged 18 or older) in 2017 diagnosed with a major depressive episode, which represents 7.1% of all adults in the United States [8]. The prevalence may be higher in physicians, as rates of suicide are noted to be higher in physicians than in the general population: male physicians have suicide rates as much as 40% higher than the general population, and female doctors up to 130% higher than the general population [9]. Substance abuse or dependence rates may also be higher in physicians than in the general public, with female physicians in particular having a higher rate of alcoholism than women in the general population [10].

Despite a lack of data, it is estimated that 3–5% of physicians exhibit disruptive behavior [2, 3], although the negative effects are disproportionately felt [2].

Physical illness specifically in physicians has not been studied, but an estimated 10% of physicians must restrict their practice for several months or more during their career because of a disabling physical illness [3]. Although physicians are subject to age-related cognitive decline just like nonphysicians, cognitive decline in physicians has not been quantified [3].

Knowledge and skill dyscompetencies are also difficult to estimate as there is limited data such as failure rates on recertification examinations. An estimated 10% of physicians will demonstrate significant deficiencies in knowledge or skills at some point in their career [3].

When all these conditions are taken into account, **at least one-third of physicians** will experience a period during which they have a condition that impairs their ability to practice medicine safely at some point in their career [3]. This translates into an average of 1–2 physicians per year in a hospital with a staff of 100 physicians. Referral rates to state physician health programs suggest that few practitioners get help, and even serious problems are often poorly handled at the hospital or practice level [3].

The impaired physician is in some ways easier to recognize and address, because there are defined metrics and pathways: substance tests, blood alcohol levels, and psychiatric evaluations. Most states have defined pathways for treatment for these issues, and there are delineated measurements and protocols for returning the impaired surgeon to clinical work.

The disruptive physician is more challenging in many ways. While recognizing the disruptive behavior may be easier, there are not standard pathways to manage the disruptive behavior or return the disruptive physician to clinical work. In addition, some surgeons have been labeled as "disruptive" for disagreeing with policies or changes. While many physicians labeled as disruptive have truly needed help, the ACS Board of Governors survey also revealed that more than one-third of Governors were aware of physicians being labeled as disruptive when they disagreed with policies at a hospital or system and/or disagreed with proposed changes [6]. Medical staff policies, procedures, and bylaws must be in place to protect due process. For those surgeons who exhibit disruptive behavior, we as colleagues need to provide them with assistance and training to address the disruptive behavior.

The best treatment for disruptive behavior is to prevent its development. Prevention can occur through a number of strategies, such as participation in an ongoing wellness program, improving surgeons' emotional intelligence, intervention from a colleague, or stress reduction activities. Establishing transparent rules for behavior, as well as the ramifications if the rules are breached, is a helpful adjunct. These actions can help improve morale and stave off conflict resulting from disruptive behavior [6].

Sadly, it is the case that physicians who generate high revenues for hospitals receive more favorable treatment when they are disruptive. Physician disruptive behavior is frequently ignored or tolerated, in part because those responsible for addressing the behavior find it to be a difficult and unpleasant task and because even when they undertake to do so, organizational mechanisms often prove inadequate to solve the problem [3]. Indeed, disruptive physicians are frequently "indulged," as healthcare managers give in to their demands simply to stop the disruptive behavior. This, in effect, rewards the disruptive behavior and has led to "normalization of deviance," with disruptive behavior becoming an accepted way of doing business for some physicians, and even for nonphysicians who imitate the behavior [11].

How Does Disruptive Behavior Impact Patient Safety?

The Joint Commission has reported in its root cause analysis of sentinel events that nearly 70% of the events can be traced back to a problem with communication [4]. Communication failures are the leading causes of inadvertent patient harm [12]. The Joint Commission also stated that "intimidating and disruptive behaviors" can result in medical errors that affect patient care and safety, which include "overt actions such as verbal outburst and physical threats, as well as passive activities such as refusing to perform assigned tasks or quietly exhibiting uncooperative attitudes," "reluctance or refusal to answer questions, return phone calls or pages, condescending language or voice intonation, and impatience with questions" [1]. All of these overt and passive actions can easily lead to a breakdown in communication, which can negatively impact patient safety.

Disruptive behavior can cause significant psychologic and behavioral disturbances that can have a critical effect on focus, concentration, collaboration, communication, and information transfer, which can lead to potentially preventable adverse events, errors, compromises in safety and quality, and patient mortality [4]. These adverse events or patient mortality can lead to a decline in physician wellness, which can worsen the cycle of disruptive behavior.

There are multiple ways that disruptive behavior impacts patient safety. Disruptive behaviors can directly affect patient satisfaction, hospital reputation, and, in some cases, quality ratings [5], which can all financially impact a hospital and indirectly impact patient safety. Disruptive behavior can also lead to a decrease in job satisfaction with staff, leading to a higher rate of turnover, which can adversely impact the functioning of the team in the operating room.

Disruptive behavior undermines teamwork and collegiality, which can lead to medical errors. Staff experience tension around a disruptive clinician will hesitate to ask for help or clarification when unsure about orders or withhold useful suggestions for patient care due to fear of criticism or intimidation [2]. The creation of a tense or "hostile" environment due to fear of criticism can prevent someone pointing out a potential issue before it occurs. Instead of the "if you see something, say something" attitude that should be encouraged, a student, resident, or staff member might recognize a potential problem but not mention it so as to avoid causing an outburst from the surgeon. One author witnessed this firsthand as a third year medical student: a sponge was left inside a patient during a Cesarean section, because the attending surgeon at one point unclamped the clamp holding the sponge; during the count, the surgeon insisted a sponge could not be left inside the patient and closed the abdomen despite the sponge count being incorrect. The patient ultimately stayed in the operating room while getting an X-ray and was then opened again to retrieve the sponge that was retained. Hierarchy frequently inhibits people from speaking up [12]. While surgery has a natural hierarchy that is unavoidable to some extent, as the surgeon must be the "captain of the ship," effective leaders flatten the hierarchy, which encourages team members to speak up and participate. Authoritarian leaders create unnecessary risk by reinforcing the hierarchy and creating an environment that does not feel "safe" to speak up [12]. These lessons have been introduced into the operative room environment by crew resource management techniques that were initially introduced in the United States Military.

When patients or families witness disruptive behavior, it undermines their confidence in the physician and the institution, as well as their willingness to participate in their own care [3]. They may not ask questions or admit they do not understand, so as to avoid having the disruptive behavior targeted toward themselves.

Outbursts or disruptive behavior from the surgeon causes a shift in the focus of those in the room from the care of the patient to managing the surgeon's behavior [13]. Rather than paying attention to the procedure or the patient or the safety of the patient, as well as the safety of the team, the members of the team become focused on de-escalating or pacifying the surgeon to try to prevent further outbursts [13]. There can also be a "snowball effect" of increasingly frequent errors, which may be due to impaired decision-making by team members, decreased efficacy of communication, or heightened anxiety in team members [3, 13].

The inherently stressful environment of the operating room becomes exponentially more stressful if the staff is worrying about the surgeon demonstrating disruptive behavior [13]. In addition, because of this, communication suffers as a result of members of the team being unwilling to speak up if they notice a problem. Repeated exposure to disruptive behavior can also lead to increased staff turnover due to the corrosive effect on morale [3], which can decrease the efficacy of the surgical team as a whole. These effects on quality, safety, and staff wellness can lead to large economic losses for healthcare institutions [5].

How Do we Identify the Disruptive Surgeon?

There are several issues surrounding the timely reporting of and intervention for disruptive behavior. One is that since the disruptive behavior is often exhibited by healthcare professionals in positions of power, healthcare workers are often concerned about retaliation [2]. There is also a pervasive culture of "medical *omertà*" (a code of silence) that makes healthcare workers reluctant to report performance problems in their colleagues [2].

The Joint Commission requires that hospitals have a code of conduct defining acceptable behavior and behavior that undermines a culture of safety, documenting behavioral standards and the repercussions of failure to comply, and establishing a process for managing disruptive behavior, but the extent to which these policies are enforced, compliance is tracked, or disruptive behavior is addressed is unknown [2]. Although hospitals are required to have credentialing and disciplinary processes, the details of implementing these processes are left up to the institutions [3]. There are few national or state standards of conduct or competence, or measures for monitoring performance [3]. This leads to widely varying institutional responses to disruptive behavior.

Hospitals, physician practices, and other healthcare institutions should not only have written standards and policies that set expectations for physician professional behavior but should also address unprofessional behavior in a strict but fair way, using an approach that escalates from coaching and counseling to punitive measures if the disruptive behavior persists after early interventions [2]. A recent study by Swiggart et al. indicates that many physicians who exhibit persistent patterns of disruptive behavior and undergo intensive programs can demonstrate improved behavior [1, 2].

Healthcare leaders and institutions must set expectations for professional behavior, enforce policies, and invest resources in programs to help distressed physicians [2]. The goal should always be remediation first, with appropriate escalation in severity as needed. Ideally, the goal would be to identify "at-risk" doctors before they become "problem" doctors and certainly before patient safety is affected. We need better metrics for identifying physicians who need help, and better programs for providing help to the physicians who need it [3]. The three essential characteristics of a system to identify these physicians are:

1. An *objective* system with a basis in data, as much of the criticism of the current methods is that they are based on subjective judgments of personality, motivation, or character instead of performance [3].
2. A *fair* system, where all physicians are evaluated on an annual basis according to the same measures in an open, unbiased, and labor-regulation-compliant manner [3].
3. A *responsive* system, with prompt intervention when a problem physician is identified [3].

The first step of developing this system is the creation of explicit performance standards of behavior and competence, which need to be developed at a national level and should address all aspects of professional behavior [3]. This would also remove the variability between institutions and would set professional standards across all levels.

The second step is that all physicians be required to acknowledge that they have read and understand the standards, have a responsibility to follow the standards, are aware that adherence will be monitored, and understand that persistent failure will lead to loss of privileges and dismissal [3]. This acknowledgment should be given in writing or as a part of annual web-based training as a condition of being granted clinical privileges [3]. This step would ensure that the policies are transparent to all involved.

The third step is monitoring for adherence to the explicitly stated standards by formal annual evaluations of all members of the staff using accepted and validated measures of competence and behavior, including confidential evaluations by colleagues and coworkers with analysis of complaints by patients or others [3]. It is important to have evaluations by colleagues and coworkers and not only supervisors as these disruptive behaviors are masked from supervisors until the physician is "past the point of no return." In order to identify "at-risk" physicians, early identification is crucial.

The fourth step is communication of the (de-identified) results to the individual. Identified deficiencies should prompt a response from the department chair, which could include evaluative testing, counseling, or referral for further assessment and treatment, or immediate action to limit practice during assessment and rehabilitation in the setting of cases that threaten patient welfare [3]. The de-identified results of evaluations are to protect the evaluators, but the communication of the results is critical for transparency. If the results are not shared with the physician, he or she will not be able to address the problems that are identified.

A system with these clearly delineated steps would serve several purposes: every person would understand their roles and responsibilities when a practitioner with performance issues has been identified, and there would be accountability on all levels, from the physician to the chair of the department to the hospital administration to the state boards [3]. Again, this would remove some of the variability from institution to institution. Once this standard system is in place, the next step is to develop a defined remediation pathway with clear metrics for evaluating the success of the remediation.

How Do we Remediate the Disruptive Surgeon?

A key aspect of managing the disruptive surgeon is the question of whether surgeons who exhibit disruptive behavior can be "trained" – can they be taught to behave more appropriately under stressful conditions, or do they need to be removed from the profession [13]? Remediation can include providing education and training to improve communication skills and professional interactions of physicians and medical students [1].

A program targeting the root causes of physician misbehavior (such as burnout, poor stress management, poor self-care, and inability to manage the demands of work and personal life) can help coach physicians to improve their behavior [1, 2]. As with any problem, getting to the root cause is one of the most important aspects of managing the issue. Programs like this can succeed when there is institutional commitment to physician professionalism and wellness, there are structured curricula, and there are quantitative metrics to assess improvement in behavior [1, 2].

One of the obstacles to developing strong remediation programs is a lack of expertise to oversee the programs. Few national programs exist, and hospital-level programs are often poorly organized [3]. In order to appropriately address this widespread issue, we should focus on developing a national quality program that will allow remediation. This would also address the issue of each individual hospital not having appropriately trained staff to help with remediation.

Another barrier is that often hospitals and physicians are reluctant to voluntarily guide, mentor, and supervise remediation activities, as department chairs and other leaders often lack the formal supervisory training or experience needed to effectively manage physicians with performance problems of any type [3]. Remediation will be ineffective if the program is not adequate, so the development of a national, standardized program is crucial. Following the COVID-19 pandemic, most meetings have been forced to be hosted virtually, and therefore it is possible that these remediation programs could be conducted virtually.

A separate but related barrier is the financial aspect: physicians may be unwilling to participate in the remediation programs due to financial burden, as they are already going to lose practice income during the programs and then are also responsible for paying for the cost of the program [3]. To ensure these programs are the most effective, the direct and indirect costs to the physician attending the program would need to be minimal, or covered in some other fashion.

Reimbursement for time spent at the remediation program would be challenging, but one option would be to schedule the program for alternative times or days that would not require the physician to lose income as a result of attending the program. One potential solution would be to offer some sort of incentive to all physicians who elected to preemptively attend these programs, similar to a new driver getting a lower insurance rate if they attended driver's education.

Documentation of evaluations, events, and interventions is an essential component of the remediation process. Clear communication also is critical in the prevention and management of disruptive behavior. As cases are reported, investigated, and adjudicated, differences of opinion can be part of the problem, and many stem from miscommunication. With prevention in mind, surgeons should be taught effective listening skills and work to improve their emotional intelligence to avoid conflict and escalating confrontations. Surgeons are natural problem solvers; given the appropriate tools and resources, they can handily deal with this challenge to improve their working environments [6]. Again, the focus on the "disruptive surgeon" should be at prevention rather than waiting to address the problem. As with many other wellness-related issues, we need to start these preventative measures earlier – most likely these measures should be started during medical school, but certainly during residency, if the ultimate goal is to prevent the behavior. Again, national standards would facilitate adopting the preventative measures.

Summary

Healthcare leaders and institutions must set expectations for professional behavior, enforce policies, and invest resources in programs to help distressed and disruptive physicians. The ideal solution would aim to prevent the disruptive behavior before it starts and focus on early identification and remediation. It is crucial to point out that while much of the literature focuses on the disruptive physician, disruptive behavior is not limited to physicians or surgeons. Disruptive behavior in other members of the healthcare team can equally impact patient safety and outcomes.

References

1. Swiggart WH, Bills JL, Penberthy JK, Dewey CM, Worley LLM. A professional development course improves unprofessional physician behavior. Jt Comm J Qual Patient Saf. 2020;46(2):64–71.
2. Gautham KS. Addressing disruptive and unprofessional physician behavior. Jt Comm J Qual Patient Saf. 2020;46(2):61–3.
3. Leape LL, Fromson JA. Problem doctors: is there a system-level solution? Ann Intern Med. 2006;144(2):107–15.
4. Rosenstein AH, O'Daniel M. A survey of the impact of disruptive behaviors and communication defects on patient safety. Jt Comm J Qual Patient Saf. 2008;34(8):464–71.
5. Rosenstein AH. The quality and economic impact of disruptive behaviors on clinical outcomes of patient care. Am J Med Qual. 2011;26(5):372–9.
6. Paramo JC, Welsh DJ, Kirby J, et al. ACS governors survey: the disruptive and impaired surgeon. 2018;2019.
7. Federation of State Medical Boards of the United States. U.S. Medical Regulatory Trends and Actions. 2018. Available at: https://www.fsmb.org/siteassets/advocacy/publications/us-medical-regulatory-trends-actions.pdf. Accessed Sep 24, 2020.
8. National Institute of Mental Health. Available at: https://www.nimh.nih.gov/health/statistics/mental-illness.shtml. Accessed Sep 24, 2020.
9. Kalmoe MC, Chapman MB, Gold JA, Giedinghagen AM. Physician suicide: a call to action. Mo Med. 2019;116(3):211–6.
10. Schernhammer E. Taking their own lives -- the high rate of physician suicide. N Engl J Med. 2005;352(24):2473–6.
11. Porto G, Lauve R. Disruptive clinician behavior: a persistent threat to patient safety. Patient Saf Qual Healthc. Available at: https://www.psqh.com/julaug06/disruptive.html. Accessed Sep 23, 2020.

12. Leonard M, Graham S, Bonacum D. The human factor: The critical importance of effective teamwork and communication in providing safe care. Qual Saf health care. 2004 Oct;13 Suppl 1(Suppl 1):i85–i90.
13. Cochran A, Elder WB. Effects of disruptive surgeon behavior in the operating room. Am J Surg. 2015;209(1):65–70.

Chapter 40
The Surgeon as Collateral Damage: The Second Victim Phenomenon

Rebecca Gates and Charles Paget

Introduction

> Virtually every practitioner knows the sickening realization of making a bad mistake. You feel singled out and exposed—seized by the instinct to see if anyone has noticed. You agonize about what to do, whether to tell anyone, what to say. Later, the event replays itself over and over in your mind. You question your competence but fear being discovered. You know you should confess, but dread the prospect of potential punishment and of the patient's anger. You may become overly attentive to the patient or family, lamenting the failure to do so earlier and, if you haven't told them, wondering if they know [1].

In 2000, Dr. Albert Wu, an internist at Johns Hopkins University, published an editorial calling for attention to the emotional needs of healthcare providers after a medical error or mistake. The terminology was "second victim syndrome" – the concept that medical error creates psychological distress in physicians, with unnecessary and unintended consequences [1]. This was the start of a culture change within the healthcare

R. Gates · C. Paget (✉)
Virginia Tech Carilion School of Medicine and Carilion Clinic, Roanoke, VA, USA
e-mail: rsgates@carilionclinic.org; cjpaget@carilionclinic.org

J. R. Romanelli et al. (eds.), *The SAGES Manual of Quality, Outcomes and Patient Safety*,
https://doi.org/10.1007/978-3-030-94610-4_40

field, with an impetus on caring for the caregiver. Surgeons, given the direct nature of our involvement, are particularly vulnerable.

Three quarters of all physicians and 83–91% of all surgeons will experience this phenomenon on at least one occasion throughout their career with more than 30% of surgeons experiencing an intraoperative adverse event within the past year [2]. It is postulated that 30% of all healthcare providers experience personal consequences (physical or psychological) related to an adverse event every year [3].

The Second Victim Phenomenon

To err is to be human, yet surgeons are inherently perfectionists and tend as a group to not look for excuses and to not consider ourselves as "victims." We want our operations to go smoothly, to fix discrete problems, and to have our patients recover well and leave the hospital better than the state in which they came. This doesn't always happen and our reaction to this determines the collateral damage. Medical error is the third leading cause of death in America [4]. Major complications or adverse events occur in up to 16% of all inpatient surgical procedures and can lead to permanent morbidity or mortality in almost 1% of cases [5]. Given the unique personal relationship between surgeons and their patients, complications or medical errors are often perceived as personal failures and can cause a cataclysm of negative emotions, which can result in anxiety, loss of confidence, insomnia, reduced job satisfaction, grief, shame, embarrassment, anger, sadness, indecision, and decreased efficacy [2, 6–11]. Over a career, these repetitive traumas may compound, leading to posttraumatic stress disorder, burnout, depression, suicidality, or career change, among others [6, 12, 13].

As described by Scott et al., the second victim experience is characterized by distinct stages. First, there is a period of "chaos and accident response" which generally occurs in the immediate period around the complication or event. This stage is characterized by confusion and/or decreased efficacy [7]. The second stage is one of "intrusive reflections," where the surgeon dwells on the event and it dominates the mindspace. This can lead to anger, frustration, distraction, and lack of confidence. Isolation may also be a part of this stage, especially if the adverse event has come to the attention of other surgeons, which may trigger the isolation as a result of guilt or shame. The third stage is "restoring personal integrity," where the surgeon begins to reintegrate into their normal daily activities [7]. In practice this frequently occurs, at least in part, over the ensuing hours when the surgeon must focus on the next case. The fourth stage is "enduring the inquisition," which can take multiple forms, from root cause analysis, peer review, or morbidity and mortality conference to legal action or disciplinary actions. The fifth stage is characterized by "emotional first aid," where the surgeon seeks peer support, family support, or perhaps even visits with their institution's Employee Assistance Program or a licensed counselor. Finally, the last stage is "moving on" [7]. As with former stages, this can look vastly different for different surgeons in different scenarios, from emotional healing and resumption of former duties to restricting clinical practice or even retiring. Similar to other models of grief, individuals do not always move through these stages linearly and may have difficulty achieving resolution of these feelings and "moving on" (Fig. 40.1).

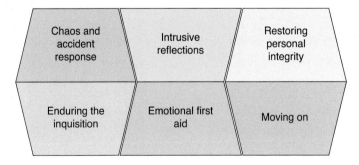

FIGURE 40.1 Six stages of second victim syndrome. (Adapted from Scott et al. 2009)

Risk Factors for Experiencing Second Victim Phenomenon

Empathy Overload

Empathy is treasured as a positive trait in physicians, and generally leads to fulfilling physician-patient relationships. It is natural to feel guilt after an adverse event given our common humanity and the relationships we have with our patients. Unfortunately, this "empathy-based guilt" can quickly transition to "pathogenic guilt," where the surgeon may misinterpret the event and inappropriately assign responsibility for the event, creating more guilt, shame, and feelings of failure [14]. This type of "pathogenic guilt" is found commonly in individuals suffering from psychiatric conditions such as posttraumatic stress disorder [14].

Perfectionism

Many surgeons identify as perfectionists. This trait drives the surgeon to succeed and to accomplish technical excellence. Many have heard the expression, "don't let perfect be the enemy of good" though heeding this advice is not straightforward. The very same attribute that drives many surgeons to success can also be at the heart of emotional distress after a clinical mistake or adverse event. The emotional impact of a mistake may be greater in physicians who demonstrate more perfectionistic traits, with lower confidence, more indecision, and higher levels of depression and thoughts of career change [8–10]. This maladaptive perfectionism may also increase the risk of suicide in response to the emotional turmoil associated with the second victim syndrome [9]. It is especially important to offer support to surgeons with perfectionistic traits after an adverse event.

Training

Second victim syndrome is not solely a problem of the independently practicing surgeon. In a 2017 article in the *New York Times*, Dr. Chen noted "you can't go through [residency] training without making an error unless you are not taking care of patients" [15]. Residents struggling for the first time with the emotions related to medical error may not have a strong framework for how to cope with these feelings, leading to development of second victim syndrome. Over time, this may lead to development of burnout or PTSD. In fact, in a national study, 22% of surgical residents screened positive for posttraumatic stress disorder, and an additional 52% were deemed "at-risk" based on their responses to survey questions [13]. In some programs, residents may be ashamed to admit their mistakes due to fear of judgment from other residents, fellows, or attendings. This is problematic, as [one of the most helpful strategies for residents struggling with the emotional consequences of a medical error is to discuss the errors with a peer or co-resident [16].

Female Gender

Some literature suggests that female surgeons may also be particularly vulnerable to the second victim experience [3, 17]. 49% of female physicians reported involvement in a medical mistake at some point in their medical career. Following this adverse event, 82% experienced guilt, 64% experienced loss of confidence, 53% experienced shame, 49% experienced sadness, and 1% reduced their clinical volume or left clinical practice [17].

Call to Action

Individuals experiencing the second victim phenomenon manifest many of the same outcomes as those with physician burnout, including substance abuse, depression, absenteeism, suicidality, and increased rates of medical error [18]. The vicious cycle of medical error begetting more medical error can be devastating to a physician's career and psyche.

On average, 39% of practicing physicians will experience depression, and 400 physicians will die by suicide yearly (National Academy of Medicine). Not only do these events have implications for the physicians' family, friends, and colleagues but also for the health system. Replacing a single physician lost to early retirement, a transition away from clinical practice, or suicide costs the healthcare system somewhere between $250,000 and 1,000,000 (National Academy of Medicine).

By creating a "just" culture and a safe space for surgeons to heal from the emotional consequences of medical error, future adverse events are decreased, and there is less physician turnover, which ultimately results in improved personal and financial gains for the surgeon and the healthcare system [2].

Recommendations for Practice at an Institutional or Department Level

Although a high proportion of surgeons will experience some degree of the second victim phenomenon, 90% of physicians report that they are not adequately supported in processing the emotional implications of an adverse event [6]. Creating a safe space for second victims to heal requires a multifaceted approach, including offering support/counseling, creating a space to analyze the mistake and learn from it, discussing mistakes with appropriate disclosure and apologies and system changes, focusing on wellness, and changing the overall culture at an institutional level [19].

Step 1: Create a Just Culture in your Department, Hospital, or Organization

Just culture is largely credited to an attorney by the name of David Marx, who described a system in which the response to workplace errors would depend on the behavior that led to the error [20]. He described three behaviors – human error, at-risk behavior, and reckless behavior – and recommended that the reaction to these behaviors should resemble consoling, coaching, and punishing/sanctioning, respectively [20]. Most errors that surgeons make are not related to at risk or reckless behavior. As such, they should be handled with a supportive environment rather than a punitive one. This is not the culture that many surgeons were trained in, but when adopted creates an environment that decreases the repercussions for individuals who report an adverse event related to human error. In sequence, workers are more likely to report errors [20] (Fig. 40.2).

In essence, creating a just culture leads to increased event reporting, which allows a healthcare system to address adverse events and near misses without penalizing an individual for being human and making a mistake. Having a just culture in which surgeons feel comfortable speaking up or sharing their negative experiences is essential to supporting

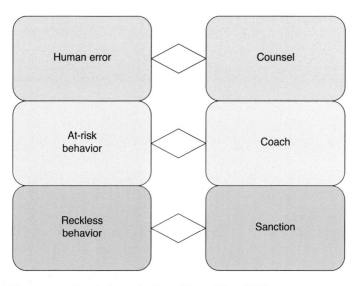

FIGURE 40.2 Just culture. (Adapted from Marx [20])

providers who have been personally affected by an adverse event.

In solidarity with a just culture, some institutions including the authors' institution have adopted a proactive response to both medical errors and the resulting risk to the healthcare profession. The TRUST team program began 6 years ago at Carilion Clinic to both proactively identify and give support to second victims, with a goal of providing just treatment and granting the individual in question with respect, understanding and compassion, supportive care, and transparency required to mitigate the damage [21]. As with just culture, this approach encourages disclosure of errors with a focus on learning from them and improving rather than placing blame on the physician and pursuing punitive action.

 Food for Thought How does your institution and your department handle near misses? If a surgeon overlooks significant hyperkalemia on morning labs and 12 hours go by before the nurse notifies him/her that the patient has EKG changes, what happens? If the surgeon's colleagues or the chair of the department find out about the incident, do they think "I cannot believe that Dr. X missed that?!", or do they think "thank goodness for the bedside nurse?" Are the near misses framed as near misses, or as "great catches"? Is there a way to reframe these events in a positive way? Can you help to create a culture that accepts human error, counsels the provider responsible for the error, and celebrates the individual who identified and corrected the mistake?

Step 2: Create a Network of Support and Aggregate Additional Resources

When creating a program to support colleagues struggling with an adverse event, it is important to consider the overall structure of the program first. It is important to establish whether the program will be primarily one of peer support or one of counselor/non-peer support. Each of these can be successful alone or can be combined for greater access. It is well-described in the literature that Employee Assistance Programs are historically underutilized by physicians, who primarily use peers as resources during stressful circumstances [22]. However, it should be noted that male and female surgeons differ in their assistance-seeking behaviors, with males generally seeking assistance from colleagues or friends and females more likely to seek assistance in the form of a professional counselor [23]. When creating a program, it is paramount to consider which type of program may be most successful in your institution or department. A short survey may be beneficial in determining which resources (peer or non-peer) would be most utilized by surgeons in your group.

Successful peer support programs have been described at multiple institutions [24–26] and may be easier to institute at a departmental level as they require fewer resources. Peer support programs mainly rely on self-identification or peer identification, which requires significant buy-in from providers. A well-functioning peer support program requires recruitment of a large number of peer coaches who represent the institution in terms of demographic characteristics such as specialty, age, gender, race, and years in practice. Oftentimes, these initial peer coaches are identified by surveying physicians in a department to determine which of their peers they would feel most comfortable talking to about an adverse event. It should be emphasized that the support should be about the emotional response. Often the tendency of two surgeons discussing a complication is to dissect out the technical and clinical issues. *These details should specifically be avoided.* For this reason, a peer from outside of the surgical discipline can often be helpful. These individuals should be trained on how to respond and provide nonjudgmental support to peers who are struggling, focusing on emotions rather than the technical components or clinical details of the case. Peer support programs are not protected by law, so if the adverse event ends in legal action, a peer supporter may be called on to testify about any discussion between themselves and the surgeon they are supporting. As such, it may be helpful to discuss a proposed peer support program with legal or risk management departments at your institution to mitigate these risks as much as possible [27]. Once peer supporters are trained, a notification system must be designed in which peer supporters are mobilized. A multifaceted approach with email, text, call, or survey options is likely most effective. For most efficient mobilization of resources, there should be an individual (surgeon or support staff) who acts as the initial point of contact and triages requests appropriately. In this type of system, there may be times that a peer supporter does not suffice, and the type of support must be escalated to a provider such as a licensed counselor or psychiatrist. In some cases, the struggling physician may even need to be referred to the emergency department. Peer supporters/coaches should be trained to identify signs of distress that may represent the need for a higher level of care.

An alternative approach is primarily referring struggling surgeons to non-peer counselors, often licensed professional counselors. This system functions much the same as a peer support program but can support a larger multidisciplinary system. Individuals (surgeons, nurses, pharmacy technicians, etc.) who are struggling with an adverse event are identified in much the same way as previously described, via self or peer identification. A central point of contact is notified and mobilizes a counselor to reach out to the specified individual. This is the method used at the authors' institution by the TRUST team, housed within the Employee Assistance Program. In addition to self-identification or peer identification, individuals who could potentially be in crisis are identified via a standard reporting system for adverse events. At our institution, "SafeWatch" reports are identifiable or anonymous reports of adverse events or events felt by the reporter to represent a "near miss." SafeWatch reports are routed to the TRUST team who uses the information to identify individuals who may be at risk for experiencing personal distress related to the event. This process of actively identifying at-risk individuals rather than relying on referrals has significantly increased the outreach of the TRUST team, with more individuals accepting support after these adverse experiences (Fig. 40.3).

Regardless of the system, it is paramount that surgeons in leadership roles validate the experiences of second victims and encourage colleagues to seek assistance if needed. After the support system is designed, it must be publicized and surgeons must feel comfortable utilizing it. The system should be frequently re-examined and improved, using participant feedback as a pillar of evaluation. In a peer support system, it is also important to ensure that the peer supporters are adequately supported themselves.

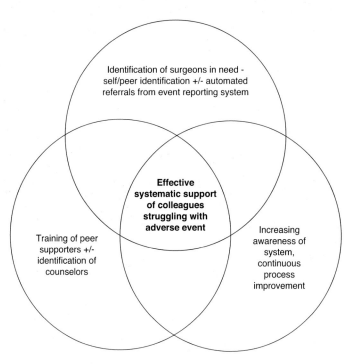

FIGURE 40.3 System design

Food for Thought What resources are available at your institution or within your department for individuals who are struggling on a personal level with a professional outcome? Are there any? If not, consider being the physician champion of this issue and recruit a group of other leaders to advocate for availability of peer support programs, counseling, etc. Be a voice for your surgical and medical colleagues who are struggling.

Recommendations for Practice at a Practice Group Level

Much more difficult than creating this at an institutional level is creating a stripped-down version for use at a local level. The same principles apply. The first step is creating a just culture within your practice group where human error is not punished but is supported. This requires that the group acknowledge that supporting one another is a vital function of the group – at least as important as the financial and call sharing aspects. The onus is on the partners within the group to be aware of complications and emotional reactions of others and to proactively address these with the affected surgeon. Secondary identification of resources that are available within your own community must also be part of this plan. The mantra that applies is "I am my brother's keeper," similar to the "no man left behind" mentality in the military. Unfortunately, this concept has been sorely missed in medicine. Utilizing a "strength in numbers" philosophy will allow the group to support its members and lessen the impact of poor patient outcomes on the provider.

Recommendations at a Personal Level

First, you must accept that as a surgeon, you and your fellow healthcare workers are at risk from the emotional collateral damage related to perceived medical mistakes. Second, you must commit to look for this in others and honestly attempt to help individuals in need. Finally, you must develop self-awareness to recognize when you are not "all right." This is not an easy task and is why the most successful assistance programs have looked for peers and others to recognize care-givers that have been affected. Despite the difficulty, a surgeon can remain introspective enough on multiple levels and realize that this fragility exists in all of us and that we are not invincible. The realization that experiencing emotional turmoil after an adverse event is a real risk and can be met in an affirmative manner can become an empowering and thoughtful way to remain mentally healthy for both our patients and our families.

Addressing Challenges

As with any intervention, programs are most successful when there is buy-in at a high level and a highly respected individual acknowledges the need for recognizing and supporting medical personnel affected by the second victim phenomenon. Our institution has been fortunate as our Chief Medical Officer is both an advocate and an expert with this issue. Furthermore, more locally within the Department of Surgery, both the Chair and the General Surgery Residency Program Director remain advocates of surgeon wellness. This can be duplicated elsewhere and in many different situations and institutions by seeking similar champions and enlisting existing departments such as Employee Assistance Programs. When encountering resistance or apathy, going back to the principles of just culture and improvement in provider wellness can be helpful. The association of provider wellness with improving retention, decreasing adverse outcomes and improving patient satisfaction are values that all within healthcare embrace.

Conclusions

The second victim phenomenon is a recently recognized and easily identified risk to medical providers. Surgeons are at particular risk given the type of care provided and the relatively frequent interaction with patients who have poor or less than ideal outcomes. Further, surgeons by their very nature assume ownership of their complications which can increase emotional turmoil after such an event. Recognition of the need to help the second victim to maximize provider wellness and subsequently improve patient care is an important concept of the new millennium. Successful programs at the institutional level that proactively identify and provide support are ideal, but the principles can be applied at more local levels as well. Part and parcel of successful support for the second victim is maintaining a just culture within the healthcare arena such that human error is not punished but rather the individuals involved in adverse events supported. Surgeons who are acknowledged leaders within their healthcare systems are ideally suited to champion this concept.

Special thanks are given to Dr. Patrice Weiss, internationally recognized in this area, for sharing her expertise and Neeley Connor, for her insight into creation of the TRUST team and its ongoing function at Carilion Clinic.

All images were created by the authors using ideas reflected in the sources credited in the figure title. The "food for thought" image was created using images listed as public domain (https://svgsilh.com/image/3246711.html; https://svgsilh.com/ms/3f51b5/image/310559.html).

References

1. Wu, A. W. (2000). Medical error: the second victim: the doctor who makes the mistake needs help too.
2. Han K, Bohnen JD, Peponis T, Martinez M, Nandan A, Yeh DD, et al. The surgeon as the second victim? Results of the Boston intraoperative adverse events surgeons' attitude (BISA) study. J Am Coll Surg. 2017;224(6):1048–56.
3. Seys D, Wu AW, Van Gerven E, Vleugels A, Euwema M, Panella M, Scott SD, Conway J, Sermeus W, Vanhaecht K. Health care professionals as second victims after adverse events: a systematic review. Eval Health Prof. 2013;36(2):135–62. https://doi.org/10.1177/0163278712458918. Epub 2012 Sep 12. PMID: 22976126.
4. Makary MA, Daniel M. Medical error—the third leading cause of death in the US. BMJ. 2016;353
5. Lives SSS. The second global patient safety challenge. World Health Organization; 2008.
6. Waterman AD, Garbutt J, Hazel E, Dunagan WC, Levinson W, Fraser VJ, Gallagher TH. The emotional impact of medical errors on practicing physicians in the United States and Canada. Jt Comm J Qual Patient Saf. 2007;33(8):467–76.
7. Scott SD, Hirschinger LE, Cox KR, McCoig M, Brandt J, Hall LW. The natural history of recovery for the healthcare provider "second victim" after adverse patient events. BMJ Quality & Safety. 2009;18(5):325–30.
8. Blatt SJ. The destructiveness of perfectionism: implications for the treatment of depression. Am Psychol. 1995;50(12):1003.
9. Kiamanesh P, Dieserud G, Dyregrov K, Haavind H. Maladaptive perfectionism: understanding the psychological vulnerability to suicide in terms of developmental history. OMEGA-J Death Dying. 2015;71(2):126–45.
10. Peters M, King J. 2012. Perfectionism in doctors. https://nam.edu/initiatives/clinician_resilience_and_well_being/.
11. Cabilan CJ, Kynoch K. Experiences of and support for nurses as second victims of adverse nursing errors: a qualitative systematic review. JBI Database System Rev Implement Rep. 2017;15(9):2333–64.

12. Shanafelt TD, Balch CM, Bechamps G, Russell T, Dyrbye L, Satele D, et al. Burnout and medical errors among American surgeons. Ann Surg. 2010;251(6):995–1000.

13. Jackson T, Zhou C, Khorgami Z, Jackson D, Agrawal V, Taubman K, et al. Traumatized residents—It's not surgery. It's medicine. J Surg Educ. 2019;76(6):e30–40.

14. O'Connor LE, Berry JW, Lewis TB, Stiver DJ. Empathy-based pathogenic guilt, pathological altruism, and psychopathology. Pathological Altruism. 2012:10–30.

15. Chen PW. Doctor and patient: when doctors make mistakes. New York Times; 2017.

16. West CP, Huschka MM, Novotny PJ, Sloan JA, Kolars JC, Habermann TM, Shanafelt TD. Association of perceived medical errors with resident distress and empathy: a prospective longitudinal study. JAMA. 2006;296(9):1071–8.

17. Gupta K, Lisker S, Rivadeneira N, Mangurian C, Linos E, Sarkar U. Save Dr Mom: second adverse event victim experiences: decisions and repercussions for mothers in medicine. In: Journal of general internal medicine (Vol. 33). 233 Spring ST, New York, NY 10013 USA: Springer; 2018. p. S334.

18. Shanafelt TD, Balch CM, Dyrbye L, Bechamps G, Russell T, Satele D, et al. Special report: suicidal ideation among American surgeons. Arch Surg. 2011;146(1):54–62.

19. Robertson JJ, Long B. Suffering in silence: medical error and its impact on health care providers. J Emerg Med. 2018;54(4):402–9.

20. Marx D. Patient safety and the "just culture": a primer for health care executives. New York (NY): Columbia University; 2001. p. 2001.

21. Denham CR. TRUST: the 5 rights of the second victim. J Patient Saf. 2007;3(2):107–19.

22. Hu YY, Fix ML, Hevelone ND, Lipsitz SR, Greenberg CC, Weissman JS, Shapiro J. Physicians' needs in coping with emotional stressors: the case for peer support. Arch Surg. 2012;147(3):212–7.

23. Sanfey H, Fromson J, Mellinger J, Rakinic J, Williams M, Williams B. Surgeons in difficulty: an exploration of differences in assistance-seeking behaviors between male and female surgeons. J Am Coll Surg. 2015;221(2):621–7.

24. El Hechi MW, Bohnen JD, Westfal M, Han K, Cauley C, Wright C, et al. Design and impact of a novel surgery-specific second victim peer support program. J Am Coll Surg. 2020;230(6):926–33.

25. Merandi J, Liao N, Lewe D, Morvay S, Stewart B, Catt C, Scott SD. Deployment of a second victim peer support program: a replication study. Pediatric Quality & Safety. 2017;2(4)
26. Edrees H, Connors C, Paine L, Norvell M, Taylor H, Wu AW. Implementing the RISE second victim support programme at the Johns Hopkins Hospital: a case study. BMJ Open. 2016;6(9)
27. Lane MA, Newman BM, Taylor MZ, O'Neill M, Ghetti C, Woltman RM, Waterman AD. Supporting clinicians after adverse events: development of a clinician peer support program. J Patient Saf. 2018;14(3):e56.

Chapter 41
The Surgeon in Decline: Can We Assess and Train a Surgeon as Their Skills Deteriorate?

Arthur Rawlings

Introduction

Ferdinand Sauerbruch (1875–1951) was held in high esteem in his lifetime as an outstanding surgeon. Internationally known, students and patients from far and wide traveled to Berlin to learn or receive care from his brilliant mind and gifted hands. Later in his career, colleagues voiced concern as they saw his demeanor change and his skills decline. At 74, he finally retired from the hospital (the alternative was the humiliation of a public dismissal), only to move his practice to his home with very unfavorable results [1].

Almost 70 years later, we are still wrestling with how to appropriately address a surgeon whose skills are in decline. With the aging of the US population, there is also an aging of the surgical workforce with 25% of surgeons above 65 years old in the United States, 19% in Australia and New Zealand, and 9% in the United Kingdom [2, 3]. Skills decline not only

A. Rawlings (✉)
General Surgery, University of Missouri, One Hospital Drive, Columbia, MO, USA

J. R. Romanelli et al. (eds.), *The SAGES Manual of Quality, Outcomes and Patient Safety*,
https://doi.org/10.1007/978-3-030-94610-4_41

as age increases but also from medical conditions. The majority of the following discussion focuses on the decline of skills with aging as every practicing surgeon will face this issue, unless they opt for early retirement.

What Skills Are Needed?

According to Astley Paston Cooper (1768–1841), the surgeon needs "an eagle's eye, a lady's hand, and a lion's heart" but, above all, a hard-fought knowledge of human anatomy [4]. The surgeon must have adequate visual-perceptual skills and fine motor skills to perform surgery safely, recall information (short-term and long-term memory) as well as apply both analytical and non-analytical reasoning to the surgical condition of the patient [5]. The passion and desire to help others is critical to success. The lack of heart will not be discussed in this chapter but is no less important than the hand or eye of the surgeon.

How Do We Know They Are Ready to Start?

No one is born a surgeon. A surgeon is made through prolonged personal dedication by an individual who desires to be a surgeon by submitting to training done mostly by those who are already surgeons. Looking at the development of a surgeon and the determination that a surgeon is ready to be released on the public may give some insight to addressing the surgeon in decline. Is it not reasonable that the bar should be the same for when one is able to enter into an independent practice as it is when one should end an independent practice?

Clinical Skills In and Out of the Operating Room

During residency, and for many followed by fellowship, a developing surgeon in the United States is assessed by practicing surgeons on a daily basis with informal feedback given periodically with at least one formal feedback session required by the Accreditation Council for Graduate Medical Education (ACGME) every 6 months. After successful completion of at least 5 years of Graduate Medical Education (GME), a trained individual could practice as a general surgeon. Other skills are required such as passing Advance Cardiac Life Support (ACLS), Advanced Trauma Life Support (ATLS), Fundamentals of Laparoscopic Surgery (FLS), and Fundamentals of Endoscopic Surgery (FES) before a program director can affirm that the resident is able to take the American Board of Surgery (ABS) Qualifying Exam, the penultimate assessment of knowledge. After passing the Qualifying Exam (QE), the ultimate assessment is the Certifying Exam (CE), which merits board certification if completed successfully. These two exams assess recall of information and clinical reasoning skills, the surgeon's head.

The developing surgeon's hands are assessed by FLS and FES, neither of which are sufficient in and of themselves for independent practice. More importantly, there is reliance upon a variety of faculty, each of which contribute to training, observing, and ultimately assessing the trainee, which truly determines when a trainee is ready for unsupervised practice. At the end of training, the program director verifies to the ABS that the skills observed – recall of knowledge, clinical reasoning, and operative ability – are sufficient for the individual to be eligible for board certification. Unlike assessing knowledge and reasoning skills with the QE and CE, there is no manual dexterity skills test to verify that a person can operate except that the person is observed to operate by faculty during training.

The Toll of Time

The presumption is that all residents who finish an ACGME training program are skilled enough in surgery to serve the general public and enter into an unsupervised practice. Board certification is not necessary to practice surgery in the United States, though it might be for credentialing in some locations. Those skills learned in training are expected to improve with time as graduates are now tackling cases independently and making clinical decisions for which they are solely accountable. The current ACGME General Surgery Milestones by which a resident's progress is reported are designed with the expectation that graduates will improve as level 5 of the Milestones "represents an expert resident whose achievements...are greater than the expectation" [5]. But what happens as more time passes? The question is whether skills continue to improve throughout one's career or there is a "U-shaped" performance curve.

Undoubtedly, there is a physical decline for everyone as the years advance. As a general characterization, vision and hearing decline with age. Visuospatial ability along with inductive reasoning and verbal memory all wane over time. One's stamina decreases as does fine-motor skills and the ability to tune out visual or auditory distractions [3, 6, 7]. The problem is that these declines vary from person to person with the variability in decline increasing with age [8, 9]. If this is true for the general population, how could a surgeon be exempt? [10]

Do Surgeons Decline?

When it comes to medical knowledge, decline with aging is easier to establish. Medical knowledge for board certification is tested with a written and oral examination. Prior to switching to the Maintenance of Certification process by the ABS, recertification to remain board certified required passing a written examination every 10 years. For the recertification examination, the failure rate for those at 10 years was 3.4%, at 20 years was 7.9%, at 30 years was 10.9%, and at 40 was 22% [11]. There may be confounding factors such as older surgeons having a narrower practice or have a less pressing need to do well because of dual board certification, yet the increasing failure rate should be noted. The Cognitive Changes and Retirement among Senior Surgeons (CCRASS) study demonstrated age-related cognitive decline in all areas studied, which were attention, reaction time, visual learning, and memory [12]. When it comes to decline in cognitive ability with age, surgeons are not exempt.

Operative skills, which would include performance in the operating room as well as clinical judgment before and after the operation, are more difficult to assess. There currently is no manual dexterity skills test that a practicing surgeon has to take on a periodic basis to establish retention of operative abilities after finishing training like there is for medical knowledge. So, there is nothing to directly examine like the recertification pass rate to establish operative decline. One surrogate approach is to look at outcomes of surgeries – death, morbidity, and readmissions – based on the age of the surgeon. There are mixed reports using this approach. On the one hand, there are studies that raise concern over declining outcomes in relation to a surgeon's age. In a review of 12,725 cases of a carotid endarterectomy from the 284 nonfederal Pennsylvania hospitals, years since licensure was associated with a greater mortality. There was no association of years since licensure and morbidity, though low patient volume was associated with an increased morbidity in the study [13]. When looking at the Medicare files of 461,000 patients undergoing 1 of 8 procedures and comparing the mortality of surgeons 40 years old and younger with those 41–50, 51–60, and over 60, mortality was only increased for pancreatectomy, coronary artery bypass grafting, and carotid enterectomy when done by surgeons over 60. This was mainly restricted for surgeons with low volumes and was not demonstrated in several other complex surgeries such as an esophagectomy [14].

On the other hand, there are studies that indicate that there is no difference in outcome based on surgeon age or that outcomes may even improve with age. In a study that compared new and experienced surgeons in 1221 US hospitals, the patients of new surgeons had significantly higher overall 30-day mortality, but when the patients were matched on the operation type, emergency admissions status, and complexity, the differences between new and experienced surgeons were practically erased [15]. More interestingly, one study that looked at 25 common surgical procedures in Canada from 2007 to 2015 of over 1 million patients treated by over 3000 surgeons from age 27 to 81 found that an increase in the surgeon's age was associated with a decrease in postoperative deaths, readmissions, and complications in almost a linear fashion when adjusting for patient, procedure, surgeon, and hospital factors [16]. The problem is that the study does not take into account the potential self-selection by surgeons for the cases they perform as they mature. In the CCRASS trial, for example, surgeons did report that they had a decrease in caseload and complexity over time [17]. No such statement was clearly made in the Canadian study. Identifying whether the decrease in postoperative problems in Canada was a result of the surgeon's experience or the surgeon's self-selection for cases cannot be determined. Finally, in a study of 1629 herniorrhaphies in a multicenter, randomized trial comparing open and laparoscopic repairs conducted at the Veterans Administration hospitals, 45-year-old and older inexperienced surgeons had a higher recurrence rate than inexperienced surgeons less than 45 years old [18]. Is this a result of age, experience, or both? So, there is mixed evidence on the question of the relationship between surgeon age and patient outcomes. In the end, the outcome is truly the only metric that matters. If patients receive appropriate care, the age of the surgeon does not matter.

As can be seen from the studies stated, there is a decline in cognitive skills and motor function as a surgeon ages, but the variability of the decline as one ages increases, making it practically impossible to develop a standard decline curve that applies to all individuals. There are always outliers. One person may suffer from a significant decline in eyesight while retaining manual dexterity, while another may retain eyesight yet suffer from dementia. Surgical outcomes, what truly matters to the patient, do not appear directly to decrease based upon age. It is difficult to convincingly say if outcomes improve, remain the same, or decline, based more on patient selection, case volume, and restrained practices the more a surgeon ages. In other words, there is just no standard decline curve of aging that can be superimposed on every single surgeon. The problem is that the decline is dependent on many factors such as genetics, general health, and self-care. Generalizations about decline can be made, but the direct application to an individual surgeon is not possible. This is why age-based decisions such as retirement are fraught with concern. Such a situation should not be a surprise. Many families in the United States are challenged with the transition of parents into dependent situations, such as the decision of letting them drive or not. The decision is rarely age based, but is made by considering a parent's eyesight, memory, reasoning skills, reaction time, mobility, etc. There is no decline curve based on age that determines when a person has to hand over the keys; similarly, there is not one for when a surgeon should hand over the scalpel. But, as has already been observed, "in many states it is more difficult to maintain one's driving privileges than one's surgical privileges" [19]. Such observation should give the surgical community pause.

Are Assessments Available?

As stated earlier, one enters into the public practice of surgery by passing a qualifying skills exam. The operative skills in a trainee are assessed by multiple observations by multiple surgeons. The determination of a practicing surgeon should likely be the same. There are two problems with such an assessment in a practicing surgeon. The first is making the observations in an unbiased fashion. The second is in deciding where the bar of performance should be located. This is true for deciding if one is ready to graduate from training. It is also true for those out in practice. The bottom line is that patients do not care how well you can perform in a trainer box but how well you do with their body.

Assessment of the Surgeon's Head

In an office setting, there are some quick tests that have been developed to screen for dementia. The prevalence of dementia for individuals over 65 is reported as between 3% and 11%. The Mini-Mental State Exam and Clock-Drawing Test may help detect cognitive impairment, but physicians, in general, can often mask early mild cognitive impairment because of their training and cognitive reserve making such tests less useful in that setting [20]. The Montreal Cognitive Assessment (MoCA) is another brief screening exam that measures verbal, numerical, and word recall. There is a visuospatial skills, clock-face, and naming component to it as well. Again, this is a screening tool and has not been validated to predict the safe performance of surgery [21].

MicroCog, which has become the more used tool, is a computer-based test that assesses processing speed and accuracy using questions. Some are simple math while others test the ability to recall information from a short story. This hour-long test examines the five domains of attention and mental control, memory, reasoning and calculation, spatial processing, and reaction time. This is only a screening test. MicroCog has a demonstrated sensitivity of 0.83 and a specificity of 0.96, which means there is a 17% false negative rate and a 4% false positive rate [22]; thus, poor performance on the MicroCog should only lead to further testing [23].

In assessing the surgeon, one factor that is critical is having the correct normative controls [24]. It has been shown, for example, that surgeons that underwent three tests selected from the Cambridge Neuropsychological Test Automated Battery (CANTAB) test – the Reaction Time test (RTI), the

Rapid Visual Information Processing (RVIP) test, and the Visual Paired Associates Learning (VPAL) test – did demonstrate a decline in performance when comparing medical students (age 20–35), midcareer surgeons (age 45–60), and senior practicing surgeons (age 61–75). However, surgeon group performance was significantly better when compared with age-matched normative controls [25]. Dr. Lauri Korinek, whose PhD dissertation is in the field, has indicated that even though the MicroCog is a well-normed test for the general public, there are no norms for physicians. And, should the norms for a practicing surgeon be linked with scores of surgeons of the same age, or should it be linked to norms determined appropriate for any surgeon to be in practice? Or as Dr. Blaiser has pointed out, "there has not been any showing that a good score on the MicroCog correlates with good performance of surgery or that a low score on the MicroCog correlates with incompetency or lack of skill" [23]. This raises the question of what should the norms be for such testing and how is that to be established.

Though not studied as well as the cognitive domain, motor skills of a surgeon need an appropriate norm as well if they are going to be evaluated. For example, the CCRASS study noted that there was an expected cognitive decline in all measures based on age, but the reaction time was notably better than age-appropriate norms [12]. When practicing senior surgeons in the study were compared with their younger counterparts, though, the majority of them performed at or near their younger peers on all cognitive tasks suggesting that older age does not assure cognitive deficiency [26].

In Sherwood and Bismark's qualitative study of expert opinion on assessing the performance of aging surgeons, 52 experts hailing from 4 countries spoke about the lack of validated tools for assessing surgical performance. The online appendix to their work has a table listing ten different assessment methods along with respective issues or concerns, strengths, and limitations of each one. For example, direct observation of procedural skills as an assessment method is useful for the technical domains of surgery. The strengths are that there can be a clear scoring criterion with targeted feedback and a quantifiable future reassessment. However, the approach suffers from potential Hawthorne effect and requires trained observers for quantifiable data. None are validated for assessing surgical performance making it necessary to continue to develop robust processes to assess performance [27].

Turning Back the Clock

As stated in the introduction, there are two areas to discuss when it comes to trying to turn back the clock on a surgeon's decline: cognition and operative skills. First, when a concern for a cognitive decline is raised, the decline needs to be investigated, and, if present, the source of that decline needs to be ascertained. There are impairments brought on by depression, substance abuse, alcoholism, and stressful life events that can be improved through proper treatment and attention. With appropriate intervention, any one of these can be time-limited allowing the surgeon to return to full function [20]. Dementia, on the other hand, is the erosion of cognitive ability that currently cannot be corrected. That is why the investigation of cognitive concerns is so critical. Correction could be as straightforward as developing a more humane call schedule [28]. It may mean resources to help with an addiction such as alcohol. Or, it could mean the beginning of the end of a career as in the case of dementia. The one area where the surgeon will need to accept the passage of time is the development of mild cognitive impairment. Unfortunately, this is a road that has no U-turn once one starts down it. The discovery of mild cognitive impairment through testing needs to be handled with grace, helping the surgeon transition out of practice with the dignity that everyone should be treated with when confronted with this diagnosis.

The second area is operative skills. If the deficiency is a lack of training on a new technique or procedure, then partnering with another surgeon to mentor one through the learning curve is appropriate. This is how one learned surgery during residency in the first place. If the deficiency is from an intrinsic source, then the regaining of an appropriate skill level maybe possible. Undoubtedly, some athletes have recovered from a horrendous life-altering disease or significant trauma to go on to inspire others with a world-class performance. But that is likely the exception and not the rule. It is possible that there are surgeons that have recovered skills once lost by an accident or a health-related event, but such recoveries are so individualized that using them as a model for the general practice of surgery seems impractical at best.

Suggestions for Practice Groups and Hospitals

For the near future, the aging of the American population and the surgical workforce is inevitable. There might be areas in the world where this topic is avoidable in the short term, but not in most developed countries that do not have a mandatory retirement age. Even in those countries, there are surgeons whose decline precedes the retirement age, and so the concern of the practicing surgeon in decline is unavoidable. The primary principle is that oversight and intervention of the surgeon in decline should happen before a patient gets hurt [20]. Unfortunately, sometimes an investigation is only triggered after there is a complaint or patient injury [29]. It would be valuable to detect and assist the surgeon in decline, prior to a patient safety issue [30].

Establishing a mandatory retirement for surgeons is tempting and would be a simple solution, but would be illegal, inappropriate, and unfair in the United States [31]. Though decline is inevitable, the variability of that decline based upon age and the variability of decline in specific areas of ability needed to provide good patient care preclude a blanket retirement policy based upon age. It would be unfair for surgeons whose abilities would allow them to practice competently beyond that age, and it would be unfair to patients who need those services. It would also be unfair to both parties as there would be surgeons whose decline preceded that retirement date and should be retired from practice earlier than mandated. With a mandatory retirement date not an option, what can practice groups or hospitals do to detect and help the surgeon in decline?

First, there must be an acknowledgement that there is a lack of validated tools for assessing a surgeon's performance. If such assessments were available, training programs would already be incorporating them into graduation requirements. The most commonly proposed assessments are multisource feedback, direct observation, analysis of data to discover outliers or changes over time, self-evaluation, and cognitive assessment. Each approach has its own strengths and weaknesses. All of them are adequate when evaluating surgeon performance that is significantly above or below what is acceptable. None has the ability in and of itself to declare with fine precision who should and who should not continue to operate when the surgeon is at the line where it could go either way. In other words, it is easy to determine who should continue to operate or stop when there is a catastrophic event like a stroke and retirement is obvious to all. It is not easy to determine when a surgeon falls below the line when there is a slow decline.

Second, institutions should be aware that decline with the passage of time is not readily recognized in oneself as a surgeon, nor are colleagues eager to report the impairment of a fellow colleague. The CCRASS study demonstrated that there was "no notable relationship, however, between subjective cognitive change and objective cognitive measures" [32]. Even though there was a measurable decline in cognitive skills, visual learning, and memory with age, retirement decisions based on subjective cognitive awareness may not accurately reflect objective cognitive abilities leading some to retire to early while encouraging others to practice longer than they should. Even though institutions may encourage surgeons to practice good self-care and volunteer reporting for testing when decline is self-perceived, institutions should not rely upon surgeons doing so [33]. For example, the American College of Surgeons recommends voluntary physical examination, eye examination, and online screening tests of cognition for surgeons between ages 65 and 70 [34]. Currently, this is not a mandate, and this does not mean that all surgeons in that age group will thus comply. Also, a national survey on professionalism suggested that, although the majority of those surveyed (96%) believed that an impaired colleague should be reported, 45% of those who knew of such a colleague had not reported the impairment [35]. That is why mechanisms other than self-reporting of decline need to be in place for institutions to protect patients and surgeons from untoward events because of decline.

Third, a decision does need to be made about mandatory testing. The options are a "whole of career" testing, an age-based trigger, and an incidence-based trigger. A whole of career testing approach does eliminate any concern over age-based discrimination but does seem less cost-effective for the institution. An age-based trigger could make testing more cost-effective, but this is a concern in the United States as at least two court cases have ruled against it based upon the Age Discrimination in Employment Act [36]. As of 2016, though, it was estimated that 5% of the US medical centers have developed age-based triggers for screening [6]. An incidence-based trigger should be a part of every institutional policy. There are many reasons to launch an investigation into a surgeon's practice besides chronology. The institution should have an established and adhered to routine of collecting data on practitioners such as outcomes, operative times, readmissions, infections, etc. Deviations from established norms in these categories should initiate a look into the reasons for them. This is also true for patient and staff complaints [21].

Fourth, there needs to be the establishment of local norms for practice. In the same way institutions establish norms for informed consent and preoperative antibiotics in the hospital, local norms for clinical practice can be established as well. What are the local institutional norms for wound infections, OR time for index cases, readmissions, etc.? If it is true that skills are "U-shaped" throughout one's career, it would be important for a surgeon to be assessed in competency with the beginning of one's career and not at the apex of the career. It is easy to say that a surgeon is not as good as the surgeon once was, but that does not mean that the surgeon is not safe enough to continue in practice. Establishing institutional norms, applicable to surgeons regardless of where they are in their career, would make the assessment of a surgeon in decline appropriate and fair.

Fifth, the development of a well-thought-out process for evaluation and determination of clinical privileges is needed. Regardless of the trigger for an assessment, the process should be as objective as possible, fair, and appropriately normed. For example, it is not appropriate to dismiss a surgeon just because of a decline in ability. The surgeon may not be as good as the surgeon once was, but the surgeon may still be better than any recent graduate. In other words, the bar to enter practice should be the same as the one to force a person to exit a practice. There are at least ten assessment centers that will offer testing [20]. Multidisciplinary, objective, and confidential evaluation of a surgeon's physical and cognitive function can be obtained through an independent agency, but such agencies only provide a report to the surgeon's hospital of the surgeon's performance of the evaluation. The decision to continue with full privileges or privileges with some forms of restriction is left up to the hospital medical staff.

Sixth, the evaluation process should end with a clear determination of the surgeon's future. Since decline is so individualized, the way forward for each surgeon is different as well. The options for the institution are a return to full practice, remediation, restriction, and retirement. It may not be possible to turn back the clock, but the clock can be slowed down by deferring on longer, more challenging cases, reducing amount or frequency of call and workload to a less stressful pace. Such alterations may keep a surgeon in practice for longer time but will need a supportive environment to implement these changes. This maybe more palatable if the seasoned surgeon is perceived as a mentor resource for the younger surgeons who desire to benefit from years of experience and wisdom.

Finally, each individual practice group and hospital should have a well-thought-out and documented policy to addressing this issue of the surgeon in decline. There should also be a retirement policy. The hospital or surgical group should collect the appropriate data of surgical activity and outcomes in order to track outcomes and make such data available to individual surgeons. Validated tools for assessment should be developed. Remediation or rehabilitation should be offered to those whom would benefit, or work patterns should be changed when necessary to support safe practices. And, at some time every surgeon will stop operating. Having a policy that details a pathway to retirement if the surgeon is in decline or not may be helpful for the surgeon and institution or practice group [37]. For example, the policy may have a provision that the surgeon is able to have no call the last year of practice. That would allow the surgeon to wind down the practice while also giving the institution or group a year's notice that a new surgeon will need to be hired. These policies should incorporate the above discussion and must be compliant with any local, state, and federal policies and laws.

Conclusion

There is no short and easy answer to evaluating and determining what to do with the surgeon in decline. It would be convenient if there were cognitive testing and manual dexterity testing that could determine if a person was safe to continue to be a surgeon. Residency programs would use these tools to launch a surgeon's career, and institutions and practice groups would use them to end a surgeon's career. When age or disease brings incremental decline, the decision to remove the scalpel from a surgeon's hand is complex, should be made by peers based on robust observations as well as input from independent assessment, and should be handled firmly yet with the grace deserved by a surgeon who has spent a career wielding the scalpel for the betterment of the patients the surgeon served.

References

1. Cherian S, Nicks R, Lord R. Ernst Ferdinand Sauerbuch: rise and fall of the pioneer of thoracic surgery. World J Surg. 2001;25(8):1012–20.
2. Kurek N, Darzi A. The ageing surgeon. BMJ Qual Saf. 2020;29(2):95–7.
3. Schenarts P, Cemaj S. The aging surgeon implications for the workforce, the surgeon, and the patient. Surg Clin N Am. 2016;96(1):129–38.
4. Bell A. The anatomy of Astley. Lancet. 2007;369(9572):1510.
5. ACGME Surgery Milestones, Second Revision: January 2019. Accessed on Mar 14, 2021 at https://www.acgme.org/Portals/0/PDFs/Milestones/SurgeryMilestones.pdf?ver=2020-09-01-152718-110.
6. Kaups K. Competency not age determines ability to practice: ethical considerations about sensorimotor agility, dexterity, and cognitive capacity. AMA J Ethics. 2016;18(10):1017–24.
7. Mani T, Bedwell J, Miller L. Age-related decrements in performance on a brief continuous performance test. Arch Clin Neuropsychol. 2005;20(5):575–86.
8. Dellinger E, Pellegrini C, Gallagher T. The aging physician and the medical profession: a review. JAMA Surg. 2017;152(10):967–71.
9. Durning S, Artino A, Holmboe E, Beckman T, van der Vleuten C, Schuwirth L. Aging and cognitive performance: challenges and implications for physicians practicing in the 21st century. J Contin Educ Health Prof. 2010;30(3):153–60.
10. Beekman A. Aging affects us all: aging physicians and screening for impaired professional proficiency. Am J Geriatr Psychiatry. 2018;26(6):641–2.
11. Buyske J. Forks in the road: the assessment of surgeons from the American Board of Surgery perspective. Surg Clin N Am. 2016;96(1):139–46.

12. Bieliauskas L, Langenecker S, Graver C, Jin Lee H, O'Neill J, Greenfield L. Cognitive changes and retirement among senior surgeons (CRASS): results from the CRASS study. J Am Coll Surg. 2008;207(1):69–78.
13. O'Neill L, Lanska D, Hartz A. Surgeon characteristics associated with mortality and morbidity following carotid endarteredtomy. Neurology. 2000;55(6):773–81.
14. Waljee J, Greenfield J, Dimick J, Birkmeyer J. Surgeon age and operative mortality in the United States. Ann Surg. 2006;244(3):353–62.
15. Kelz R, Sellers M, Niknam B, Sharpe J, Rosenbaum P, Hill A, Zhou H, Hochman L, Bilimoria K, Itani K, Romano P, Silber J. A national comparison of operative outcomes of new and experienced surgeons. Ann Surg. 2021;273(2):280–8.
16. Satkunasivam R, Klaassen Z, Bheeshma R, Kai-Hoi F, Menser T, Kash B, Miles B, Bass B, Detsky A, Wallis C. Relation between surgeon age and postoperative outcomes: a population-based cohort study. CMAJ. 2020;192(15):385–92.
17. Jin Lee H, Drag L, Bieliauskas L, Langenecker S, Graver C, O'Neill J, Greenfield L. Results from the cognitive changes and retirement among senior surgeons self-report survey. J Am Coll Surg. 2009;209(5):668–71.
18. Neumayer L, Gawande A, Wang J, Giobbie-Hurder A, Itani K, Fitzgibbons R, Reda D, Jonasson O. Proficiency of surgeons in inguinal hernia repair effect of experience and age. Ann Surg. 2005;242(3):344–51.
19. Katlic M, Coleman J. The aging surgeon. Adv Surg. 2016;50(1):93–103.
20. LoboPrabhu S, Molinari V, Hamilton J, Lomax J. The aging physician with cognitive impairment: approaches to oversight, prevention, and remediation. Am J Geriatr Psychiatry. 2009;17(6):445–54.
21. Hickson G, Peabody T, Hopkinson W, Reiter C. Cognitive skills assessment for the aging orthopaedic surgeon. J Bone Joint Surg Am. 2019;101(2):1–5.
22. Korinek L. Neuropsychological differences between physicians referred for competency evaluations and a control group of physicians. Unpublished dissertation. 2005. p. 86. Accessed on 14 Mar 2021 at https://assets.documentcloud.org/documents/5980346/Lauri-Korinek-Dissertation.pdf.

23. Blasier R. The problem of the aging surgeon: When surgeon age becomes a surgical risk factor. Clin Orthop Relat Res. 2009;467(2):402–11.

24. Williams B, Flanders P, Grace E, Korinek E, Welindt D, Williams M. Assessment of fitness for duty of underperforming physicians: the importance of using appropriate norms. PLoS One. 2017;12(10):e0186902. https://doi.org/10.1371/journal.pone.0186902.

25. Boom-Saad Z, Langenecker S, Bieliauskas L, Graver C, O'Neill J, Caveney A, Greenfield L, Minter R. Surgeons outperformed normative controls on neuropsychologic tests, but age-related decay of skills persists. Am J Surg. 2008;195(2):205–9.

26. Drag L, Bieliauskas L, Langenecker S, Greenfield L. Cognitive functioning, retirement status, and age: results from the cognitive changes and retirement among senior surgeons study. J Am Coll Surg. 2010;211(3):303–7.

27. Sherwood R, Bismark M. The ageing surgeon: a qualitative study of expert opinions on assuring performance and supporting safe career transitions among older surgeons. BMJ Qual Saf. 2020;29(2):113–21.

28. Wesnes K, Walker M, Walker L, Heys S, Warren R, Eremin O. Cognitive performance and mood after a weekend on call in a surgical unit. Br J Surg. 1997;84(4):493–5.

29. Williams B. The prevalence and special educational requirements of dyscompetent physicians. J Contin Educ Health Prof. 2006;26(3):173–91.

30. Soonsawat A, Tanaka G, Lammando M, Ahmed I, Ellison J. Cognitively impaired physicians: how do we detect them? How do we assist them? Am J Geriatr Psychiatry. 2018;26(6):631–40.

31. Katlic M, Coleman J, Russell M. Assessing the performance of aging surgeons. JAMA. 2019;321(5):449–50.

32. Bieliauskas L, Langenecker S, Graver C, Jin Lee H, O'Neil J, Greenfield L. Cognitive changes and retirement among senior surgeons (CCRASS): results from the CRASS study. J Am Coll Surg. 2008;207(1):69–78.

33. Davis D, Mazmanian P, Fordis M, Harrison R, Thorpe K, Perrier L. Accuracy of physician self-assessment compared with observed measures of competence: a systematic review. JAMA. 2006;296(9):1094–102.

34. American College of Surgeons (ACS). Statement on the aging surgeon. ACS website. Published Jan 1, 2016. Accessed 9 Dec 2020.

35. Campbell E, Regan S, Gruen R, Ferris T, Rao S, Cleary P, Blumenthal D. Professionalism in medicine: results of a national survey of physicians. Ann Intern Med. 2007;147(11):795–802.
36. Grandjean B, Grell C. Why no mandatory retirement age exists for physicians: important lessons for employers. Mo Med. 2019;116(5):357–60.
37. Bhatt N, Morris M, O'Neil A, Gillis A, Ridgway P. When should surgeons retire? Br J Surg. 2016;103(1):35–42.

Chapter 42
Fatigue in Surgery: Managing an Unrealistic Work Burden

V. Prasad Poola, Adam Reid, and John D. Mellinger

Introduction

The condition of chronic fatigue, burnout, or "burnout syndrome" is defined as a state of depersonalization (loss of empathy), emotional exhaustion, and a sense of reduced personal accomplishment (competence and achievement). Since Herbert Freudenberger first described symptoms including exhaustion, headaches, and irritability among volunteers at a free drug clinic in 1974, as "burnout," [1] it has grown to epidemic proportions, especially among healthcare workers [2]. The recent literature suggests worsening work-life balance and increasing burnout across all specialties, and surgery is no exception [3]. In fact, it is noted that surgeons and surgical trainees are more prone to burnout compared to their peers in other specialties due to long work hours, stressful work environments, and lack of schedule control during their prolonged training and beyond. The increasing exhaustion

V. P. Poola · A. Reid · J. D. Mellinger (✉)
Southern Illinois University School of Medicine, Department of Surgery, Springfield, IL, USA
e-mail: ppoola@siumed.edu; areid@siumed.edu; jmellinger@siumed.edu

© The Author(s), under exclusive license to Springer Nature Switzerland AG 2022
J. R. Romanelli et al. (eds.), *The SAGES Manual of Quality, Outcomes and Patient Safety*,
https://doi.org/10.1007/978-3-030-94610-4_42

813

and depersonalization components in particular are fostering substance abuse [4], broken relationships, depression [5], and suicide [6] at a personal level and correlate with increasing medical errors [3], decreasing quality of care and patient satisfaction [7], and decreasing clinical and scholarly productivity as well [8].

Surgeons have historically and appropriately taken pride in their noble and privileged vocation and have labored to improve the quality of surgical care they deliver. Simultaneously, the single-minded focus on patient care and quality of life appears to have fostered an unintended jeopardy for surgeons themselves, related to the physical and emotional toll of an unrealistic work burden. Current burnout prevalence has reached a level that threatens the profession and the institutions it serves. If the current trajectory continues, it is apparent there will be significant consequences in attracting young talent into the discipline [9], as well as in retaining and effectively utilizing the skills of current surgical providers to their full career potential.

In this chapter, we discuss the factors that have contributed to burnout among surgeons over the years, review tools for measuring burnout, and outline evidence-based interventions that can help prevent and mitigate its consequences.

Etiology and Risk Factors for Burnout

Understanding the etiology and risk factors that contribute to surgeons' fatigue is essential prior to considering interventions that are aimed at prevention and treatment. Burnout is a global crisis and seems to affect physicians from developed countries disproportionately in comparison to physicians from low-income and middle-income countries, partly due to the unique individual and societal expectations in such settings, coupled with the work environment [10]. The etiology described in this chapter is mostly pertinent to the developed world and multifactorial, which is categorized into personal and workplace or system-related factors.

Personal/Demographic Risk Factors

There are several personal and demographic factors that correlate with susceptibility for burnout. In the study by Campbell et al., an inverse correlation between age and burnout among surgeons was noted, contrary to the authors' hypothesis that older surgeons would be more likely to experience burnout as a function of the longer periods of exposure to instigating pressures and factors in comparison to younger colleagues [11]. In the same study, they also found a strong association between burnout and a desire to retire among young surgeons. In a study on gender variations in work-life balance and burnout by Dyrbye et al., it was noted that even though the factors contributing to burnout were remarkably similar for female and male surgeons, women were more likely to experience work-home conflict than men, which correlated with higher levels of burnout among women surgeons [12]. Lindeman et al. studied the emotional intelligence and personality features of surgery residents and their association with burnout [13]. In that study, while burnout was generally noted to be high among surgery residents, residents with high emotional intelligence and positive work experiences were noted to be of lower risk.

Workplace-/System-Related Factors

There are a number of well-intended system developments that have taken place in the last several decades which have significantly impacted healthcare training and delivery. All of these changes were deemed necessary and well thought out at the time they were instituted, and many of them continue to serve the purpose for which they were intended to the present day. However, if one considers the collective or holistic impact, these adjustments have had the unintended or unconsidered consequence of imposing an unrealistic burden of change and added work on surgical providers in a short and compressed amount of time. We describe some of these significant changes which have contributed to "job creep" and workflow pressure in what follows.

1. *The Quality Movement*

   Quality improvement in healthcare is not a new concept; however, public reporting of quality and tying it to the payment structure is a novel and recent trend [14]. The Institute of Medicine (IOM) report "To Err is Human" was published in 1999 and served to energize the public conversation on the quality of healthcare and ways and means to improve it [15]. Since then, several national organizations, both public and private, along with surgical societies, have implemented well-designed quality improvement processes. As a result, the quality of care delivered to patients has significantly improved across many aspects of medicine. In the process, a number of regulatory, reporting, and compliance mechanisms were put in place to facilitate measurement and monitoring of quality, including patient satisfaction scores and cost accounting measures, among others.

2. *Electronic Medical Records (EMRs)*

   Transition to EMRs was inevitable, given challenges posed by the ever-increasing complexities in medical care in the present information age, so as to improve the portability, transparency, quality [16], and value of medical records. The Health Information Technology for Economic and Clinical Health (HITECH) Act authorized incentive payments through Medicare and Medicaid to clinicians and hospitals to promote EMR adoption and implementation, and they became ubiquitous.

   Since the current-generation EMR is billing and quality metric capture-driven, it engenders a culture oriented to checking boxes, cut-and-paste formatting, and information bloating of records with unnecessary information; the related time expenditure involves "desktop medicine" rather than patient contact for physicians. In the place of bedside care and compassion, we have gradually moved in the direction of efficiency and metric documentation, entailing in the eyes of many providers an inherent compromise of priorities in the patient-doctor relationship [17].

More thoughts about EMRs and how they contribute to burnout are elucidated in Chap. 38.

3. *Ergonomics in the Operating Room*

With the advent of minimally invasive surgery, the man-machine interface became increasingly common and important in the operating room. In the initial phase of widespread adoption of laparoscopy, the equipment and training of laparoscopic surgeons did not incorporate principles of ergonomic science including equipment design, workplace environment layout, operating team, as well as patient safety and environment-related productivity. This neglect resulted in prolonged operations and significant physical strain for surgeons [18]. The recent trend toward increasing use of robotic surgery with improved ergonomic design, including attention to the machine interface with both patient and provider, may help in addressing this challenge [19]. More thoughts about ergonomics and injury prevention to maintain surgical wellness are discussed in detail in Chap. 45.

4. *Information Overload*

In the present information age, it only takes about 18 months to double medical knowledge, as opposed to 100 years prior to World War I. As we rapidly accumulate and adapt knowledge for the betterment of humankind, it is easy to underestimate the cognitive pressures entailed, which can lead to feelings of inadequacy on the part of providers. Surgical societies and specialty boards employ continuing medical education (CME) programs to help assure their membership and the public that they are up-to-date in their knowledge. Documentation of engagement with such programs are among the requirements for continued certification, which 81% of physicians believed was a burden as reflected in a nationwide cross-specialty survey [20]. The growing necessity of multispecialty algorithms of care, incorporating innovations in genetics, pharmacotherapy, and both diagnostic and therapeutic technology, has added to the challenges of contemporary delivery of optimal patient care.

5. *Changes in Surgical Education*

The duty hour restrictions and supervision requirements for trainees instituted by the Accreditation Council of Graduate Medical Education (ACGME) have represented a significant and positive development for the learning environment; however, they have entailed a "seniorization" of clinical work, with resulting heightened pressure on faculty and post-training care providers [21]. These changes, again promoted by a safety-oriented culture, have gradually pushed responsibility for the care of patients toward those with higher levels of experience and contributed to diminished levels of autonomy and concerns regarding adequacy of training both in the operating room and beyond for surgery residents. This is now a major concern, as graduating surgery residents felt not well prepared for either fellowship training or independent practice [22].

6. *Moral Insult*

Moral insult in medicine is described as "the challenge of simultaneously knowing what care patients need but being unable to provide it due to constraints that are beyond our control." Experiences of such moral insults are far too common and start unfortunately in a medical student [23]. Surgeons may be particularly prone to such challenges, as complications and the technical and resource challenges entailed in their management are unavoidable in one's career [24]. In a guest editorial by Dean et al., they propose a change of nomenclature from "burnout" to "moral insult," as the former suggests the problem resides within the individual, disregarding the presence of circumstances beyond his or her control [25]. In the same article, they suggested inviting administrators to join in clinical rounds, making physician satisfaction a financial priority, and establishing a sense of community among clinicians, among other interventions, as a part of a strategy to prevent or share the burden of moral insult. This is also elaborated on further in Chap. 38.

7. *Medicolegal Issues*

Malpractice risk is inherent for surgeons [26], and malpractice stress syndrome has significant psychological and physical effects on physicians that include isolation, negative self-image, and feelings of hopelessness and depression [27]. The risk of malpractice continues to rise as healthcare becomes more and more complex. The practice of defensive medicine is more prevalent in specialties at high risk for malpractice, including emergency medicine, general surgery, orthopedic surgery, neurosurgery, obstetrics and gynecology, and radiology. Interestingly, rates of burnout seem to correlate with the same specialties in which the risk of malpractice litigation is high [28].

8. *Economics*

The average medical student debt in 2011 was $170,000, and it increased to $190,000 by 2017 in the United States [29]. It is projected that if this trend continues, about 50% of physician salary will be consumed by monthly repayments of student loans in the years to come [30]. Student loan debt has significant influence on surgery resident career and lifestyle decision-making [31]. During the time the student loan debt has continued to increase, physician payments and salaries have gradually declined. Most physicians and surgeons over the past two to three decades have become employees of larger healthcare systems rather than independent practitioners, with an attendant decrease in autonomy in decision-making and other aspects of patient care.

Measuring Burnout/Fatigue

It is important to understand how the profession can meaningfully assess and measure burnout before considering the potential means of intervention. Both quantitative and qualitative elements are important in this discussion. There are many assessment tools available for this purpose, and a few of those commonly used are outlined in Table 42.1. Among

TABLE 42.1 Common burnout measurement tools

Name of the inventory	Description	Cost
Maslach Burnout Inventory-Health Services Survey (MBI-HSS)	22 items and 3 subscales: 1. Emotional exhaustion 2. Depersonalization 3. Diminished personal accomplishment	Yes
Single-item measures of emotional exhaustion and depersonalization	Consists of only two questions of the full 22-item MBI-HSS: 1. I feel burned out from my work 2. I have become more callous toward people since I took this job	Free
Copenhagen Burnout Inventory (CBI)	Consists of 19 items in 3 sub-dimensions: personal burnout, work-related burnout, and client-related burnout	Free
Utrecht Work Engagement Scale (UWES)	Consisting of 17 items. "Work engagement" is considered to be the antipole of burnout. This scale measures work engagement and arises from the research in positive psychology	Free
Jefferson Scale of Empathy-Health Professions (JSE-HP)	Consists of 20 items and measures empathy in healthcare providers and students	Yes

them, the Maslach Burnout Inventory-Health Sciences Survey (MBI-HSS) is the most reliable, validated, and commonly used for both clinical and research purposes [32, 33]. Even though MBI-HSS is considered the gold standard test for measure burnout, it is not without limitations. These would include its cost and lack of query in regard to nonprofessional confounders such as child care demands, the schedule and support of a spouse or partner, other significant life events, and financial concerns [34]. To mitigate the cost of MBI-HSS, West et al. proposed a single-item measure of both emotional exhaustion and depersonalization, which has been shown to provide meaningful information on burnout among medical professionals [35]. Tools that measure depression and anxiety distinct from burnout can and should also be considered in select situations in which burnout is highly prevalent. By measuring and monitoring burnout, organizations can demonstrate care for the well-being of their employees, which is a critical systemic first step toward providing a solution.

Strategies to Address and Prevent Burnout/Fatigue

Once burnout is identified, measured, and studied, it is possible to recognize and categorize the realities of unrealistic and unsustainable work burden at both the individual and institutional levels. Even though most of the factors that have contributed to "job creep" for surgeons will stay, there are strategies that can be employed to minimize the burden arising from contemporary pressures, while professionals and institutions continue to adapt. Most mitigation interventions are aimed at preventing the negative aspects of burnout (emotional exhaustion and depersonalization). While this is not inappropriate, a special emphasis should be given to strategies that enhance the sense of personal accomplishment, alongside efforts mitigating the negative domains, in order to achieve an overall sense of well-being. These strategies can be generalized or tailored to the etiology or to the circumstances once the source of burnout is identified and measured through a standardized tool. Interventions may be focused on the individual, on structural or organizational solutions, or ideally and optimally on both. The literature indicates that both individual and system-based interventions will result in meaningful reduction in physician burnout, if selected and executed appropriately. A systematic review and meta-analysis of available studies on intervention to prevent physician burnout showed a reduction in overall burnout rates from 54% to 44%, with improvement of both emotional exhaustion and depersonalization scores [36].

Improving a sense of personal accomplishment or job satisfaction is again as important as mitigating emotional exhaustion and depersonalization. Strategies to improve the sense of personal accomplishment are often rooted in the principles of positive psychology and personal well-being and include strategies promoting alignment of intrinsic and extrinsic motivation factors to primary work outcomes.

Several strategies or solutions will be provided in what follows, which have been proven useful in mitigating the negative elements of burnout, as well as in improving a sense of personal accomplishment. Some of these strategies can be executed at an individual level and also reinforced and supported at the institutional level. It is often both the commitment from the individual physician or employee, coupled with organizational changes that foster the culture of well-being by providing adequate resources, which can drive sustainable and desirable outcomes.

1. *Self-care/Interventions at the Individual Level*

Self-care strategies are at the center of all the measures that aim to prevent burnout and promote well-being. These include concepts such as self-calibration, stress management, mindfulness, meditation, exercise/fitness programs, sleep management, dietary recommendations, personal finance, access to relationship assessment and counseling services, and various approaches to work life integration.

In a prior study, brief self-care workshops of 2-month duration were offered to physicians, which resulted in an improvement in depersonalization; however the overall level of burnout remained the same [37]. Physical activity has been shown to improve both physical and mental health; hence the Center for Disease Control and Prevention recommends regular physical activity for all Americans [38]. Physicians, especially during their training period, tend to be more sedentary, and team-based, institutionally incentivized exercise programs are one way to improve physical activity and quality of life [39].

A mental skills curriculum implemented for novice learners in surgical training has been shown to reduce stress and enhance performance [40]. Mindfulness-based approaches address work-related stress by teaching the quality of awareness skill, including the ability to pay attention in a particular way: on purpose or intentional, in the present moment, and nonjudgmental [41]. Krasner et al. offered a CME course on mindfulness as an intervention to physicians which included didactics, formal mindfulness meditation, and narrative and appreciative inquiry exercises followed by discussions. In that study, they demonstrated the participants had improved personal well-being, decreased burnout, improved mood (including overall, depression, vigor, tension, anger, and fatigue elements), and also experienced positive changes in empathy and psychosocial beliefs [42].

Targeted communications skills training, especially where moral insults are likely, such as when dealing with difficult end of life situations and oncology care, has been shown to improve physician confidence and reduce subsequent burnout [43, 44]. A simple intervention such as organizing a "debriefing" meeting, where participants meet their peers, share their experiences, and support each other to create a sense of community and belonging, can be very valuable in reducing stress and burnout [45].

2. *Institutional/Organizational Interventions*

Institutional/organizational support is extremely important for a sustainable change in culture to be achieved, oriented enduringly to workforce well-being. This means providing adequate resources where necessary and at times making required changes in policies and guidelines geared toward balancing productivity and provider well-being. Self-care alone is often not sustainable without support from leadership and complementary organizational structure. Besides providing resources and support for self-care, evidence-based organizational interventions are categorized or centered around the themes which follow.

(a) *Balancing Productivity vs. Well-Being*

As outlined in the section on the etiology of burnout, physician or surgeon productivity and the related economics for healthcare organizations can promote unhealthy competition at both individual and organizational levels. Highlighting physician well-being as a quality metric at the institutional level, alongside patient-related quality indicators, may help create awareness and vet provider well-being as an indicator or quality of care as well as an organizational value. Such approaches also have the potential to impact institutional financial performance favorably by enhancing physician recruitment and retention. Given the economic reality where return on investment (ROI) drives organizational change and policy, a case for investment in surgeons' well-being has according fiscal merit and hence can be leveraged at the institutional and organizational level [46]. Increasing the productivity and income equation for surgeons has been shown to be associated with a degree of increased career satisfaction, as most surgeons at present graduate from training with significant financial debt [47]. For academic surgeons in particular with significant non-revenue-generating job expectations including teaching, administration, and scholarship, having "clinical academic service contracts" has been shown to increase satisfaction with professional activities and should be considered in situations where it is feasible [48].

(b) *Providing Structured Mentorship/Coaching*

Providing structured mentorship from a senior faculty member or through a designated program implemented at an institutional level has been shown to mitigate fatigue by improving the sense of boundary setting as well as prioritization, self-compassion, self-care, and self-awareness [49]. Role modeling by a senior faculty member, division chair, or department chair, alongside mentoring and coaching activities, can be very impactful at both professional and personal levels. Many institutions at present have a "Chief Wellness Officer" (CWO), who is primarily focused on improving their organizations' work environment and culture, complementing individual-level interventions [50]. CWOs can impact the organizational culture through helping to promote a positive work and learning environment and by guiding the organization in reducing administrative burden and aligning both workforce and leadership in achieving a sustainable balance of productivity and well-being.

(c) *Autonomy*

Autonomy at clinical work has been shown to directly correlate with surgeons' work satisfaction at the individual level [51]. That being noted, it remains controversial as to whether increasing departmental autonomy in the choice of quality and productivity metrics facilitates a higher quality of care, or otherwise [52]. Career satisfaction is highly dependent on work-life balance, and control over schedule and work hours is an important aspect thereof [53]. Creating an opportunity for autonomy and flexibility as surgeons create their own work schedule should be considered in policy changes and may be particularly important in allowing for major life events such as having children and parenting. Fostering or adapting to the "servant leadership model" as proposed by Greenleaf in 1970 might be one effective strategy in bridging the gap between the physicians and other frontline providers and institutional leadership through deliberate and cultivated listening.

(d) *Motivation*

Self-determination theory is a broad framework for understanding psychological well-being in the context of both intrinsic and extrinsic motivation [54]. While the meaning of work, autonomy, and mastery still remains deep rooted and intrinsic motivations for most surgeons, extrinsic motivation factors and rewards such as compensation and other recognitions for productivity are highly tangible and are often perceived as being crucial to the alignment of individual and organizational goals and priorities. Khullar et al. demonstrated that institutional payment models with higher reimbursement tied to performance, rather than productivity per se, may empower physicians to be not just aligned agents, but change agents [55]. Where the productivity model is well-suited and/or difficult to change, changing or augmenting the reward structure by including non-monetary currencies such as more scheduling flexibility, or more time to pursue activities such as teaching, research, and other mission-oriented work, can enable physicians to accomplish both professional and personal fulfillment as distinct from a raise in pay [56, 57].

(e) *Positive Psychology*

One of the criticisms of the present evidence as well as interventions on burnout is that it is aimed heavily toward reducing and mitigating on the negative side of the equation and achieving absence of burnout rather than pursuing a positive sense of well-being [34]. Although mitigating the negative effects of burnout or fatigue is extremely important, certainly a complementary and likely even more important concept would be applying principles such as those of positive psychology. This emphasizes strength, happiness, growth, and resilience and which in turn focuses on the ability to thrive rather than just cope and survive. If we could better understand when and how to apply the principles of positive psychology, many of which are ancient and well-attested in spiritual and other traditions, redirecting some of our research and scientific efforts on the theme of well-being and fulfillment in the context of surgeons' lives, we might save a significant amount of stress or fatigue to ourselves going forward. Indeed, focusing only on resilience strategies and amelioration of the negatively framed side of the burnout equation tends to promote a survival and victim orientation that limits generative and aspirational thinking critical to creative problem-solving. Institutional resources and efforts should be gradually redirected or shifted toward improving the well-being of their workforce as a means to not only achieve a lower prevalence of burnout but also to improve work satisfaction.

(f) *Human and Organization Potential*

Leveraging and enhancing human and organizational potential by deliberate efforts that are executed at the institutional level so as to mitigate burnout and enhance the well-being of physicians can make a significant difference [58]. The Center for Human and Organizational Potential (cHOP) at Southern Illinois University School of Medicine (Editors' note: this is the authors' home institution) is a current example of an entity created to do just that, providing faculty, staff, and learners with the tools to achieve professional growth and satisfaction by offering resources in professional development, leadership and excellence, and wellness [59].

Conclusion

Fatigue/burnout is a well-recognized occupational hazard, which has the potential to affect all healthcare personnel including surgeons. The etiology of burnout is multifactorial, an unintentional consequence of a constellation of well-intended measures. Measuring burnout and devoting effort to identifying the source at both the individual and institutional level are important. There are several evidence-based remedies that can be tailored to prevent or mitigate the negative effects of burnout. Efforts that improve a positive sense of well-being are equally important, if not more important, to creating and sustaining a joyful workforce.

References

1. Freudenberger HJ. Staff burn-out. J Soc Issues. 1974;30(1):159–65.
2. Shanafelt TD, et al. Burnout among physicians compared with individuals with a professional or doctoral degree in a field outside of medicine. Mayo Clin Proc. 2019;94(3):549–51.. Elsevier.
3. Shanafelt TD, et al. Burnout and medical errors among American surgeons. Ann Surg. 2010;251(6):995–1000.
4. Oreskovich MR, et al. Prevalence of alcohol use disorders among American surgeons. Arch Surg. 2012;147(2):168–74.
5. Bianchi R, Schonfeld IS, Laurent E. Burnout–depression overlap: a review. Clin Psychol Rev. 2015;36:28–41.
6. Shanafelt TD, et al. Special report: suicidal ideation among American surgeons. Arch Surg. 2011;146(1):54–62.
7. Anagnostopoulos F, et al. Physician burnout and patient satisfaction with consultation in primary health care settings: evidence of relationships from a one-with-many design. J Clin Psychol Med Settings. 2012;19(4):401–10.
8. Turner TB, et al. The impact of physician burnout on clinical and academic productivity of gynecologic oncologists: a decision analysis. Gynecol Oncol. 2017;146(3):642–6.
9. Are C, et al. A multinational perspective on "lifestyle" and other perceptions of contemporary medical students about general surgery. Ann Surg. 2012;256(2):378–86.
10. https://www.thelancet.com/journals/lancet/article/PIIS0140-6736(19)31573-9/fulltext.
11. Campbell DA Jr, et al. Burnout among American surgeons. Surgery. 2001;130(4):696–705.
12. Dyrbye LN, et al. Relationship between work-home conflicts and burnout among American surgeons: a comparison by sex. Arch Surg. 2011;146(2):211–7.
13. Lindeman B, et al. Association of burnout with emotional intelligence and personality in surgical residents: can we predict who is most at risk? J Surg Educ. 2017;74(6):e22–30.
14. • No Authors Listed. Rule emphasizes quality and cost savings. Hosp Case Manag. 2011;19:148–9. Summary of The Centers for Medicare and Medicaid Services (CMS) 2012 final rule on the Inpatient Prospective Payment System (IPPS). Rule establishes that hospitals will receive a net 1% increase in reimbursement, also proposes to add a measure of Medicare spending per beneficiary to the Hospital Inpatient Quality Reporting program and

the Value Based Purchasing program in effort to reduce costs by rewarding efficient care rather than volume. Finally in an effort to reduce preventable healthcare associated infections HAIs, the rule introduces new quality measures to be implemented in 2014 and 2015.

15. Kohn L, Corrigan J, Donaldson M, editors. To err is human: building a safer health system. Washington, DC: National Academy Press; 1999.
16. Bates DW, et al. Effect of computerized physician order entry and a team intervention on prevention of serious medication errors. JAMA. 1998;280(15):1311–6.
17. Zulman DM, Shah NH, Verghese A. Evolutionary pressures on the electronic health record: caring for complexity. JAMA. 2016;316(9):923–4.
18. Berguer R, Forkey DL, Smith WD. The effect of laparoscopic instrument working angle on surgeons' upper extremity workload. Surg Endosc. 2001;15(9):1027–9.
19. van der Schatte Olivier RH, et al. Ergonomics, user comfort, and performance in standard and robot-assisted laparoscopic surgery. Surg Endosc. 2009;23(6):1365.
20. Cook DA, et al. Physician attitudes about maintenance of certification: a cross-specialty national survey. Mayo Clin Proc. 2016;91(10):1336–45. Elsevier.
21. Dacey RG, Nasca TJ. Seniorization of tasks in the academic medical center: a worrisome trend. J Am Coll Surg. 2019;228(3):299–302.
22. Mattar SG, et al. General surgery residency inadequately prepares trainees for fellowship: results of a survey of fellowship program directors. Ann Surg. 2013;258(3):440–9.
23. Wiggleton C, et al. Medical students' experiences of moral distress: development of a web-based survey. Acad Med. 2010;85(1):111–7.
24. Munch S, de Kryger L. Moral wounds: complicated complications. JAMA. 2001;285(9):1131–2.
25. Dean W, Dean A, Talbot S. Reframing clinician distress: moral injury not burnout. Fed Pract. 2019;36(9):400.
26. Jena AB, et al. Malpractice risk according to physician specialty. N Engl J Med. 2011;365(7):629–36.
27. Maroon JC. Catastrophic cardiovascular complications from medical malpractice stress syndrome. J Neurosurg. 2019;130(6):2081–5.

28. Martini S, et al. Burnout comparison among residents in different medical specialties. Acad Psychiatry. 2004;28(3):240–2.
29. PAYE, IBR. Medical student education: debt, costs, and loan repayment fact card. 2013.
30. Youngclaus J, Fresne JA. Physician education debt and the cost to attend medical school: 2012 update. Association of American Medical Colleges; 2013.
31. Gray K, et al. Influence of student loan debt on general surgery resident career and lifestyle decision-making. J Am Coll Surg. 2020;230(2):173–81.
32. Maslach C, et al. Maslach burnout inventory, vol. 21. Palo Alto: Consulting Psychologists Press; 1986.
33. Maslach C, Jackson SE. The measurement of experienced burnout. J Organ Behav. 1981;2(2):99–113.
34. Eckleberry-Hunt J, Kirkpatrick H, Barbera T. The problems with burnout research. Acad Med. 2018;93(3):367–70.
35. West CP, et al. Single item measures of emotional exhaustion and depersonalization are useful for assessing burnout in medical professionals. J Gen Intern Med. 2009;24(12):1318.
36. West CP, et al. Interventions to prevent and reduce physician burnout: a systematic review and meta-analysis. Lancet. 2016;388(10057):2272–81.
37. Martins AE, et al. Impact of a brief intervention on the burnout levels of pediatric residents. J Pediatr. 2011;87(6):493–8.
38. https://health.gov/sites/default/files/2019-09/Physical_Activity_Guidelines_2nd_edition.pdf.
39. Weight CJ, et al. Physical activity, quality of life, and burnout among physician trainees: the effect of a team-based, incentivized exercise program. Mayo Clin Proc. 2013;88(12):1435–42. Elsevier.
40. Anton NE, et al. Effectiveness of a mental skills curriculum to reduce novices' stress. J Surg Res. 2016;206(1):199–205.
41. Kabat-Zinn J. Wherever you go, there you are: mindfulness meditation in everyday life. Hachette Books; New York, 2009.
42. Krasner MS, et al. Association of an educational program in mindful communication with burnout, empathy, and attitudes among primary care physicians. JAMA. 2009;302(12):1284–93.
43. Clayton JM, et al. Evaluation of a novel individualised communication-skills training intervention to improve doctors' confidence and skills in end-of-life communication. Palliat Med. 2013;27(3):236–43.

44. Bragard I, et al. Insight on variables leading to burnout in cancer physicians. J Cancer Educ. 2010;25(1):109–15.
45. Gunasingam N, et al. Reducing stress and burnout in junior doctors: the impact of debriefing sessions. Postgrad Med J. 2015;91(1074):182–7.
46. Shanafelt T, Goh J, Sinsky C. The business case for investing in physician well-being. JAMA Intern Med. 2017;177(12):1826–32.
47. Leigh JP, et al. Physician career satisfaction across specialties. Arch Intern Med. 2002;162(14):1577–84.
48. Clifton J, et al. The effect of clinical academic service contracts on surgeon satisfaction. Can J Surg. 2007;50(3):175.
49. Schneider S, Kingsolver K, Rosdahl J. Physician coaching to enhance well-being: a qualitative analysis of a pilot intervention. Explore (NY). 2014;10(6):372–9.
50. Ripp J, Shanafelt T. The health care chief wellness officer: what the role is and is not. Acad Med. 2020;95(9):1354–8.
51. Raptis DA, et al. Job satisfaction among young board-certified surgeons at academic centers in Europe and North America. Ann Surg. 2012;256(5):796–805.
52. Larsen KN, Kristensen SR, Søgaard R. Autonomy to health care professionals as a vehicle for value-based health care? Results of a quasi-experiment in hospital governance. Soc Sci Med. 2018;196:37–46.
53. Keeton K, et al. Predictors of physician career satisfaction, work–life balance, and burnout. Obstet Gynecol. 2007;109(4):949–55.
54. Ryan RM, Deci EL. Self-determination theory: basic psychological needs in motivation, development, and wellness. Guilford Publications; New York, 2017.
55. Khullar D, et al. How 10 leading health systems pay their doctors. Healthc (Amst). 2015;3(2):60–2. Elsevier.
56. Berwick DM. The toxicity of pay for performance. Qual Manag Health Care. 1995;4:27–33.
57. Shanafelt TD, et al. Career fit and burnout among academic faculty. Arch Intern Med. 2009;169(10):990–5.
58. Shanafelt TD, et al. Changes in burnout and satisfaction with work-life balance in physicians and the general US working population between 2011 and 2014. Mayo Clin Proc. 2015;90(12):1600–13. Elsevier.
59. https://www.siumed.edu/chop/chop.html.

Chapter 43
Training New Surgeons: Maintaining Quality in the Era of Work Hour Regulations

Ingrid S. Schmiederer and James R. Korndorffer Jr

Quality training requires efficient, guided learning for trainees that includes required operative time, appropriate evaluations, and reliable testing. In the current climate of surgical training, there are many factors that impact this quality of training. These factors include safety initiatives, new systems of documentation, higher case complexities with new techniques, and duty-hour restrictions. One might argue that these factors, especially work hour regulations, could be obstacles to quality; however, review of operative experience and resident wellness within duty-hour regulations shows that the perceived obstacles may actually be opportunities to improve mentorship and entrustment of residents.

_____

I. S. Schmiederer · J. R. Korndorffer Jr (✉)
Department of Surgery, Stanford University School of Medicine, Stanford, CA, USA
e-mail: ischmied@stanford.edu; korndorffer@stanford.edu

© The Author(s), under exclusive license to Springer Nature   833
Switzerland AG 2022
J. R. Romanelli et al. (eds.), *The SAGES Manual of Quality, Outcomes and Patient Safety*,
https://doi.org/10.1007/978-3-030-94610-4_43

Restrictions to limit the time residents spend on hospital-related activities were implemented in 2003, when the Accreditation Council for Graduate Medical Education (ACGME) set mandatory limitations on resident work hours to mitigate the potential effect of resident fatigue on patient safety. These rules limited residents to working 80 h per week in the hospital with strict guidelines for on-call schedules and rest periods in between shifts. In 2011, the ACGME further restricted maximum shift lengths for interns and increased the rest time after overnight on-call shifts for residents, and this was ultimately adjusted a third time for more leeway. The current iterations of duty hours have been studied in multiple contexts over the last 10+ years. Through systematic investigations of the resident workplace and work time, stakeholders have agreed that regulations are important, but wide variability has been evident in the benefits of duty-hour restrictions within the contexts of patient safety, resident education/experience, or resident wellness. For instance, most studies have shown no significant difference in patient health outcomes. One of the most widely cited studies, Bilmoria's Flexibility in Duty Hour Requirements for Surgical Trainees (FIRST) Trial during the 2014–2015 academic year, showed no significant differences or negative effects in patient outcomes when there were less restrictions to duty hours [1].

Operative volume is needed for the quality development of a surgical training graduate, but the change in volume cannot be directly attributed to restricted resident time. In 2010, Fairfax et al. noted a marked decrease in cases in the era of work duty restrictions after review of ACGME case log data from 1999 to 2008. According to comparison of "pre" duty hours and "post" duty hours, notable declines occurred in endoscopy (91 ± 3 vs 82 ± 2, $P < 0.001$) and vascular surgery (164 ± 29 vs 126 ± 5, $P < 0.01$) [2]. With broadening focus on increasingly diverse general surgical approaches at the same time that hours are restricted, sub-specialty cases could understandably fall out of focus, especially when vascular surgery has concomitantly developed integrated residency programs and endoscopy typically overlaps with gastroenterology trainees. This broadened focus on general surgery might also be predictable as the development and refinement of laparoscopic and robotic surgery techniques has expanded the scope of general surgical training. Further analysis of physical case load and operative experience for residents through operative logs and data reviews confirms that there is increased focus on general surgery procedures and decreased experience of subspecialty domains in the last 10–20 years of general surgery residency training [3].

When looking strictly at the amount of time in the physical learning environment (the hospital), the work hour restrictions still allow for proficiency and expertise – traits needed for quality outcomes – to develop. According to Anders Ericsson, psychologist and expert in the practice of learning, so-called expertise requires at least 10,000 h of deliberate practice [4]. A surgery resident might be able to achieve this in the 19,200–20,000 h of a duty-hour restricted surgical residency (80 h per week, 48 weeks, 5–7 years). With this argument, the approach to quality surgical training might be better suited when time-based training is de-emphasized. Competency-based education is structured on learner-centered environment and ability, as well as patient need [5].

Therefore, while the change in hours may not have shown an effect on patient outcomes, the improvement of the learning environment within the duty hours may ultimately lead to enhanced quality of training and graduate skill. In addition to patient care outcomes, the FIRST Trial looked at resident perceptions of their own training and education within duty-hour restrictions. There were no significant differences in overall resident satisfaction with education, between strict duty hours and flexible resident duty hours in cluster-randomized programs, but results did suggest that residents found some improvements in certain aspects of resident education (e.g., ability to stay for a late operative case) with flexible duty-hour policies. There was also the acknowledgment that flexible policies seem to affect time for personal activities and certain aspects of well-being outside of work [1]. The effect on education, then, may be felt in crucial influencers of resident learning and wellness – like fatigue and burnout. A systematic review by Ahmed et al. reported improvement in resident fatigue and burnout with the implementation of the 80-h workweek in 2003 [6]. Limited fatigue and burnout may lead to improved overall quality of the educational result, but to compare resident wellness since 2011 or since 2003 to resident self-assessment before duty-hour restrictions is inadequate and arguably unfair, as close study of the resident experience before 2003, or even 2011, is lacking.

There is ultimately not enough evidence to argue that work hour regulations have directly affected the quality of resident learning positively or negatively since 2003. The differences may lie in residents' perspectives within duty-hour training, as several surveys since 2013 indicate that general surgery residents actually feel prepared and confident entering practice or fellowship, despite the 2012 concerns expressed in a national survey of sub-specialty fellowship program directors about ill-preparedness of residency graduates [7–9]. This disconnect in perceptions – between trainees and trainers in resident self-efficacy – adds to the misconceptions about effects of duty hours on the quality of education of learners.

Direct effects of work hour restrictions on education quality or patient care quality have not been demonstrated clearly, though indirect effects may exist. A relationship with faculty, based on familiarity and entrustment, is crucial for trainee development. In this way, one could argue that work hour restrictions could hinder the growth of mentorship relationships between resident and faculty and, perhaps, this is where the quality of education has the most potential to fall behind. Torbeck found this concept of mentorship to be emphasized in an academic institution where senior residents identified faculty who allowed for the most and least independence in their trainees and then identified behaviors or teaching techniques of those faculty members in how they relate to residents. They found that independence depends on a trusting relationship between faculty and trainee that might only happen when time is given for trust to mature.

Entrustment and independence of the trainee allow for improved preoperative preparedness, improved skill based with modeling and repetition of technique, and more meaningful postoperative debriefing [10].

To maintain quality education and to prevent the potential negative effect of duty-hour restrictions, program directors must be proactive in finding ways to establish meaningful mentor-mentee relationships between faculty and trainees within time constraints earlier in training. The first step is the acknowledgment of the importance of mentorship within the program. Establishment of a mentorship-focused culture promotes resident integration into the general workplace culture earlier and leads to collaborations more quickly. This model may address the perception that graduates are unprepared by instilling skills, as well as confidence, more effectively and earlier in residency training. Within training time constraints, mentors can ensure that mentees achieve academic milestones and demonstrate competencies in a timely fashion. Faculty can correct a trainee's course more readily as they are most familiar with them. A good mentor creates a supportive environment and enforces confidence through entrustment and provides essential, regular feedback [11]. This also requires an effort on the part of the program, and a clear framework, to enable and enhance the process of feedback and entrustment between faculty and trainees.

Entrustable Professional Activities (EPAs) are a potential way for educational objectives and training outcomes to be linked to healthcare and patient safety within surgical residency. These are objectives that can be assessed but also discussed as developmental checkpoints. Instead of using nonspecific or reductionist statements such as numbers or grades (e.g., A–F, or outstanding to failing), the focus with EPAs shifts to statements about required supervision and prompts further discussion. Faculty are able to discuss residents progress in terms that are generalizable among surgeons (e.g., "Can I leave the room when this resident is operating?" or "Can the trainee manage the preop/postop patient without proactive assistance?") [12]. EPAs translate these general and understandable assessments into levels of supervision required for the trainee to execute a task:

1. Deficient execution by the trainee, even with direct supervision
2. Execution with proactive supervision
3. Execution with supervision as needed/requested
4. Supervision at a distance if at all
5. Supervision provided by the trainee to more junior colleagues

In these clear terms, the goal for the resident is "supervision at a distance" before independent practice (Level 4 of the EPA scale) [13]. The activities deemed necessary for independent general surgery practice are listed into attainable and concrete skills within the five different EPAs listed below, which are still developing and being integrated into the assessment of general surgery trainees:

1. Evaluation and management of a patient with an inguinal hernia.
2. Evaluate and manage a patient with right lower quadrant pain.
3. Evaluate and manage a patient with gallbladder disease.
4. Evaluation and initial management of a patient presenting with blunt or penetrating trauma.
5. Provide general surgical consultation to other healthcare providers.

Within the confines of duty-hour restrictions and busy clinical environments, perhaps shifting the focus from hours to competency-based education, which relies on abilities rather than time logs, might ensure and enrich quality training. Both trainees and supervisors may be supported by EPAs to optimize shared information that is discussed within one-on-one trainee meetings, as well as competency or promotion committees. For mentors or faculty, the smaller pieces of information or tangible experiences about a trainee are collected in understandable and concrete terms to convey where the trainee stands more clearly, earlier, and more efficiently. Focusing on competency-based, concrete activities and required levels of supervision can help frame discussion and feedback while maintaining quality training.

Suggested Reading

1. Bilimoria KY, Chung JW, Hedges LV, et al. National cluster-randomized trial of duty-hour flexibility in surgical training. N Engl J Med. 2016;374(8):713–27. https://doi.org/10.1056/NEJMoa1515724.
2. Fairfax LM, Christmas AB, Green JM, Miles WS, Sing RF. Operative experience in the era of duty hour restrictions: is broad-based general surgery training coming to an end? Am Surg. 2010;76(6):578–82. https://doi.org/10.1177/000313481007600619.
3. Kassam A-F, Lynch CA, Cortez AR, Vaysburg D, Potts JR III, Quillin RC III. Where has all the complexity gone? An analysis of the modern surgical resident operative experience. J Surg Educ. Published online 2020. https://doi.org/10.1016/j.jsurg.2020.06.016.
4. Hirschl RB. The making of a surgeon: 10,000hours? J Pediatr Surg. 2015;50(5):699–706. https://doi.org/10.1016/j.jpedsurg.2015.02.061.
5. Frank JR, Mungroo R, Ahmad Y, Wang M, DeRossi S, Horsley T, Rossi SDE. Toward a definition of competency-based education in medicine: a systematic review of published definitions. Med Teach. 2010;32(8):631–7.
6. Ahmed N, Devitt KS, Keshet I, et al. A systematic review of the effects of resident duty hour restrictions in surgery: impact on resident wellness, training, and patient outcomes. Ann Surg. 2014;259(6):1041–53. https://doi.org/10.1097/SLA.0000000000000595.
7. Rasmussen JM, Najarian MM, Ties JS, Borgert AJ, Kallies KJ, Jarman BT. Career satisfaction, gender bias, and work-life balance: a contemporary assessment of general surgeons. J Surg Educ. Published online 2020. https://doi.org/10.1016/j.jsurg.2020.06.012.
8. Friedell ML, VanderMeer TJ, Cheatham ML, et al. Perceptions of graduating general surgery chief residents: are they confident in their training? J Am Coll Surg. 2014;218(4):695–703. https://doi.org/10.1016/j.jamcollsurg.2013.12.022.

9. Mattar SG, Alseidi AA, Jones DB, et al. General surgery residency inadequately prepares trainees for fellowship: results of a survey of fellowship program directors. Ann Surg. 2013;258(3):440–9. https://doi.org/10.1097/SLA.0b013e3182a191ca.

10. Torbeck L, Wilson A, Choi J, Dunnington GL. Identification of behaviors and techniques for promoting autonomy in the operating room. Surgery. 2015;158(4):1102–12. https://doi.org/10.1016/j.surg.2015.05.030.

11. Sanfey H, Hollands C, Gantt NL. Strategies for building an effective mentoring relationship. Am J Surg. 2013;206(5):714–8. https://doi.org/10.1016/j.amjsurg.2013.08.001.

12. Wagner JP, Lewis CE, Tillou A, et al. Use of entrustable professional activities in the assessment of surgical resident competency. JAMA Surg. 2018;153(4):335–43. https://doi.org/10.1001/jamasurg.2017.4547.

13. Brasel KJ, Klingensmith ME, Englander R, et al. Entrustable professional activities in general surgery: development and implementation. J Surg Educ. 2019;76(5):1174–86. https://doi.org/10.1016/j.jsurg.2019.04.003.

14. Sandhu G, Magas CP, Robinson AB, Scally CP, Minter RM. Progressive entrustment to achieve resident autonomy in the operating room: a national qualitative study with general surgery faculty and residents. Ann Surg. 2017;265(6):1134–40. https://doi.org/10.1097/SLA.0000000000001782.

15. Ulmer C, Wolman DM, Johns MME. Resident duty hours: enhancing sleep, supervision, and safety. National Academies Press; 2009. https://search-ebscohost-com.laneproxy.stanford.edu/login.aspx?direct=true&db=nlebk&AN=280408&site=ehost-live. Accessed 9 Sept 2020.

Chapter 44
Maintaining Surgical Quality in the Setting of a Crisis

John R. Romanelli

With the recent COVID-19 pandemic, it is certainly reasonable to reflect upon the maintenance of surgical quality in the setting of a crisis situation. Given what has transpired – and in fact is still ongoing at the time of this writing – there are certainly lessons that are applicable to future events that can be learned from how we treated surgical patients during the crisis situation. This chapter will delve into the following topics: hospital resources and the impact on surgical scheduling; cessation of elective surgery and ramifications for patient care; scarce resource allocation during the crisis; redeployment of surgical workforce during a crisis; delays in care delivery of routine problems due to the crisis; and the re-emergence back into elective surgical care following a crisis. The challenges in maintaining surgical quality during this crisis are illustrated, while the solutions highlight principles that are foundational in quality systems.

J. R. Romanelli (✉)
Department of Surgery, University of Massachusetts Chan Medical School - Baystate Medical Center, Springfield, MA, USA
e-mail: John.Romanelli@baystatehealth.org

© The Author(s), under exclusive license to Springer Nature Switzerland AG 2022
J. R. Romanelli et al. (eds.), *The SAGES Manual of Quality, Outcomes and Patient Safety*,
https://doi.org/10.1007/978-3-030-94610-4_44

Hospital Resources During Crisis Situations

Most hospitals have an administrative structure that springs into action once a crisis situation unfolds. While the pandemic is fresh on our minds, this could also result from other crisis states such as a bed crunch caused by influenza; other infectious agents, much like the Ebola scare in the last decade; mass casualty incidents such as multiple traumas in blunt or penetrating situations; or other crises that cause normal hospital functions to cease or be altered significantly.

Typically, hospitals start with an incident command team. This should be structured to include key administrators, department chairs or other designated leaders, the emergency department, supply chain, nursing, bed control, and other important stakeholders, some of which may be unique to the crisis at hand. Many healthcare systems have a disaster plan of some type, and this should be activated as soon as it is apparent that the hospital's function has to shift to new priorities. Early priorities of the incident command team should be to assess what critical resources are needed immediately and what shortcomings they believe the healthcare system or hospital has or will have and to establish a timeline of need. They must begin to assess the capability of an expanded number of beds (and where to house the surge of patients) and an expanded number of critical care beds (and again, where to house those units). They must also decide whether or not the cause of the crisis will lead to unique needs (e.g., in the case of an infectious pandemic, if isolation beds will be needed and negative airflow rooms are available or could be created). Communication systems have to be tested and implemented.

An important aspect of a crisis affecting healthcare delivery is the impact of this crisis on the local or regional area. If the crisis affects many centers, such as the COVID-19 crisis, regular communication between leadership of local hospitals – even if from competing systems – is critical to understand the regional impact of both the problem itself and the altering of other healthcare deliveries. Further, if the crisis is broader in scope, then communication between hospital leadership (with representation on the incident command team) and local, state, and federal government officials is also important. These conversations must be bidirectional: the governmental authorities need to learn about the scope of the problem, and the hospital systems need to be informed about decision-making that impacts delivery of care. One such example during the COVID-19 crisis was the edict that elective surgery cease in most states. While societies such as the American College of Surgeons (ACS) and SAGES published communication suggesting the need to stop performing elective surgery, state governments and their Departments of Health made the call for this to be implemented by hospitals.

A critical step in early crisis management is to gain an understanding how much "say" the healthcare providers might have. In this example of the shutdown of elective surgery, most states left it to surgeons to determine what cases were truly elective and what cases were of an urgent or emergent nature. While certainly some surgeons could abuse this distinction, and still perform relatively elective cases (by calling them "urgent"), it is incumbent upon operating room leadership or department chairs to monitor for this activity and stop it if necessary. Nonetheless, the decision-making power should never be taken away from doctors and their patients to make surgical decisions, and at least in this most recent crisis, that decision was urged to stay between the providers and patients by both surgical societies and most states governments.

One of the most important tasks of the incident command group is to have a committee or subgroup that monitors bed availability. In surge conditions, they must continually plan for new units to be created, staffed by appropriate nursing and ancillary support, and to have these units equipped with all of the necessary medical and computing equipment. As the surge begins to ease, understanding how many beds per day become available will be a necessary step before lifting a prohibition on elective surgery. The same holds true for interventional radiology and interventional cardiology or vascular procedures, which may require bed usage post-procedure.

Central to quality in disaster management are data, transparency, and continuous analysis. Hospital systems are able to learn and adapt to various resource constraints using these important principles. As regards data, critical to an institutional response is the acceptance of information from all staff and, uniquely for COVID, from around the world. The data should be distilled and actionable such as the use of PaO_2/FiO_2 ratio in determining which patient requires prone positioning or D-Dimer levels in determining which patients require therapeutic anticoagulation. For transparency, daily briefings within specific units and about overall hospital operations reduce staff anxiety about resource constraints and encourage collective solutions. Data transparency is important at all levels from individual patients to regional trends. Lastly, in learning, eventually, a generative approach can be employed to anticipate and adapt; protocols are collected, updated, and shared continuously based on data and evidence. A mature operational team continuously reviews performance and can plan for a progressively better response.

Cessation of Elective Surgery and Ramifications for Patient Care

The decision to cease elective surgery is a difficult one for hospitals as it is a major source of revenue. It is typically a last step that happens once a crisis situation unfolds. In the case of COVID-19, this difficult decision was made by both societies and state governments, and it was one of the first times that this has ever occurred on a mass scale, at least in the United States.

Once elective surgery stops, two situations must be monitored. The first is that the clinical staff supporting surgeons must be in contact with patients who are displaced off of the schedule to ensure that their disease processes do not worsen, moving them into the "urgent" category. If so, they need to be re-scheduled and have their surgeries performed. The second is that medical offices must keep "bumped patient lists" so that re-scheduling can occur in a timely and orderly fashion once the cessation of elective surgery is lifted.

Another question that can be raised by the cessation of elective surgical work is how to manage patients with unfolding clinical needs. For example, a patient with right upper quadrant pain might still be able to receive an ultrasound to diagnose cholelithiasis. If that is negative, a nuclear medicine study might be needed to diagnose biliary dyskinesia. But what if that is unavailable? Would upper endoscopy be available, or were the endoscopy units also limited to emergent and urgent cases only? And then how that patient would be managed without surgical intervention?

Separating patients into acuity levels is a potential helpful exercise to help determine what patients should not be delayed in receiving surgical care. The ACS published a very helpful document [1] called COVID-19: Guidance for Triage of Non-Emergent Surgical Procedures. In this document, they described the Elective Surgery Acuity Scale, which separates patients into three tiers based on low, intermediate, or high acuity and then subdivides those tiers into healthy and unhealthy patients. In this example, Tier 1 patients (low acuity) are recommended for postponement of having the cases be performed at an ambulatory surgery center (ASC); Tier 2 are recommended for postponement "if possible" or consideration of being moved to an ASC; and Tier 3 are recommended to not be postponed and should only be performed at a hospital setting. Obviously, there is room for clinical decision-making by the surgeon and patient in this regard.

Cancer patients present a unique and interesting dilemma regarding the timing of surgical intervention. SAGES published very useful documents [2–4] offering recommendations on how to treat cancer patients in the setting of the COVID-19 crisis, but these recommendations could be broadly applied.

Another consideration is that operating room personnel are now a resource that could be redeployed into other critical need situations throughout the healthcare system. The operating room nurses could assist with triage, help in other critical care units, or work toward screening patients, in the case of infectious disease. Post-anesthesia care units could be re-purposed as critical care beds if needed. Hospital supply chain personnel could be tasked with managing the needs dictated by the crisis and as such could be diverted from operating room tasks.

Scarce Resource Allocation During a Medical Crisis

One of the more frightening aspects of a crisis is the dwindling of resources to an amount insufficient to meet the needs of patients. One can argue that the inability to perform elective surgery amounts to a scarce resource situation. This concept delves into ethical decision-making in choosing which patients received what is deemed as limited in supply. An early consideration for hospitals during, for example, a pandemic, is to form a scarce resource team led by an institutional bioethicist (if one is available). The idea is that such a team would comprise of clinicians that are not charged with taking care of a particular patient facing a need of an item in scarce supply at the given time. The formation of a team like this would be directed by the incident command team.

During the early part of the COVID-19 pandemic, a central concern was the availability of ventilators. Confronting the difficult concept of having to choose between two patients for one available ventilator is a terrifying prospect for physicians who took an oath to "Do no harm." Having guidance as to how to choose which patient is awarded the scarce resource is impossible as the clinician charged with care delivery to multiple patients that may drain said resources. Given that we all serve as advocates for those we care for, it would be a conflict to advocate for the same ventilator for two different patients. Alas, the concept of a scarce resource team, divorced from direct care delivery, can help choose where to allocate ventilators when there remains an insufficient number.

This concept is not limited to ventilators during an infectious pandemic. Dialysis could become available on a limited basis if many patients were going into acute renal failure. And of course, many care givers were troubled by a lack of appropriate personal protective equipment during the recent pandemic. Even operating room availability in a mass casualty event should be considered a scarce resource.

There are medical resources to guide scarce allocation teams in decision-making. The Massachusetts Department of Public Health issued this guide [5] to advocate for the formation of teams such as described herein and to help clinicians make these difficult decisions. Typically, one must factor survivability as an initial criterion. Triaging patients into low, intermediate, and high chance of survival can help to direct resources appropriately. This concept originated in battlefield and military medicine but can certainly be applied in a civilian crisis. Next a score such as SOFA (Sequential Organ Failure Assessment) could be employed to help make such a determination. The elements of SOFA [6] include PaO_2/FiO_2 ratio, platelet count, total bilirubin, blood pressure, Glasgow Coma Scale, and creatinine, thus quantifying dysfunction of the respiratory, coagulation, hepatic, cardiovascular, neurologic, and renal systems. This score could be combined with an analysis of major comorbidities and indicators of 1-year morbidity to objectively predict which patient has a better chance for survival and thus would be more appropriate to direct a resource toward.

Trauma systems apply these lessons of scarce resource allocation by using two principles: reduction of uncertainty through risk stratification (triage) and staged interventions that achieve the most in a minimal time. Quality, in a classic mass casualty event, means that arriving patients should be quickly risk stratified based on their apparent injury and vital signs, imaging studies kept to a minimum, and interventions be limited to 30–60 min per patient. This allows for rescue first, followed by recovery and restoration. Arguably, the nature of the COVID-19 pandemic cannot achieve this type of quality, as scientists have not identified a means to rapidly limit the extent of illness on presentation, while risk stratification requires time and extensive testing. The best achievable quality for this current mass casualty event is in the prevention of errors, that is, good quality might be defined by teams adept at early identification of escalating severity. Good quality might be defined by rapid intervention teams that are organized around specific interventions such as intubation, proning, invasive lines, or clinical trial enrollment.

Surgeons bring unique skills in this scarce resource allocation situation. Surgeons could and should be added to allocation teams, especially if time is freed with the shutdown of elective surgery, such as in COVID-19. Given that general surgeons have to be conscientious of all organ systems, they, along with internists, can take a generalized look at patients without the bias of being a single-organ system-based specialist. Further, surgeons might be forced into making these difficult choices if operating rooms become scarce (like a mass casualty situation) or if post-anesthesia care unit or critical care beds are limited by a patient surge. Lastly, surgeons may have to decide upon the relative urgency of a disease process to decide if patients need to have their operations performed in a more timely fashion, as previously described, and some of these tools could be employed to help in that decision-making analysis (e.g., choosing which urgent patient to operate on first).

Redeployment of the Surgical Workforce During a Crisis

In some critical situations, surgeons may be forced to redeploy to other areas of the hospital to augment the existing, if not exhausted, workforce. This might mean seeing patients in the emergency department; it might mean working in intensive or critical care units; or it might mean covering other areas of general surgery such as trauma or emergency general surgery. As stated in the SAGES publication, the Primer for Taking Care of Yourself During and After the COVID-19

Crisis [7], while being forced into unplanned clinical situations may provoke feelings of fear and anxiety, "what we do know is that regardless of our current specialty and regardless of the time since we practiced general medicine, that our contribution in fighting this medical nightmare is a unique and noble one. Our surgical training and heritage will support us. The role we may serve during the present need eclipses and stretches our normal patterns of practice, but not beyond the depth of our training backgrounds." Certainly needing to cover trauma admissions may seem uncomfortable and outright daunting after not performing trauma surgery for years – decades? – but our training will indeed begin to guide us, and our colleagues deployed to critical care units for pandemic needs can certainly assist us in decision-making. Materials such as those published as a part of ATLS can also serve as a reminder of basic core principles to help the redeployed surgeon.

Further, the surgical workforce comprises of more than just the attending surgeons. Trainees or advanced practice providers may also need to cover different areas of the hospital, leaving surgical teams short of their normal coverage. OR nurses or PACU nurses may be asked to work in other areas of the healthcare system to help handle surge or crisis needs, or they may be uprooted from an ambulatory OR to an inpatient OR. This may force urgent surgical procedures to be conducted with an unfamiliar team, which can hamper outcomes, slow operative times, and lead to frustration on the part of the surgeon or the team. Thus it becomes incumbent to prepare diligently for these cases, foster good communication in the room (and with the anesthesia team), and anticipate delays that would otherwise be atypical. Similarly, anesthesia staff will likely be asked to help in the critical care units in the setting of a pandemic or mass casualty, reducing the complement of available anesthetists that can work in the operating room. Lastly, hospital systems may have to divert resources away from community hospital settings toward the tertiary care centers as they may need an increase in help to combat the crisis. This may adversely impact the ability for surgeons to be able to care for their patients at the community hospital.

The ultimate concern for surgeons is to be placed into a situation where they have to urgently operate on a disease process or patient with a clinical situation far outside the norm of their practice. While there is no "one size fits all" solution to this issue, open discussion with surgical leaders at your institution about your concerns, communication with colleagues with more experience in treating the problem, and utilizing best clinical judgment and learning developed after rigorous and thorough surgical training and experience should, at a minimum, produce an outcome that is acceptable given the difficulties and obstacles created by the crisis. "Damage control" methodology might serve as a base to deliver the patient to an acceptable state until more experienced help can be lent to aid in the definitive surgical procedure to address an emergent problem. Also, some clinical decisions might need to be altered given the limitations in resources; for example, if the institution has no critical care beds available, then leaving the patient intubated with an open abdomen and wound vac may not be preferable in a patient with an acute abdominal catastrophe. In that case, temporary closure of the abdomen and extubation may be a preferable alternative.

Delays in Care Delivery of Routine Problems Due to the Crisis

One of the unexpected issues that may arise during or after a crisis situation, especially if prolonged, is the delay in treating clinical problems. This may lead to disease processes that worsen over the interval of time that operating rooms are not functioning at peak capacity. This has the potential to be a hidden issue as patients may avoid coming to the hospital for a period of time even after the crisis eases. One can foresee that, in an infectious disease crisis, patients may be afraid to present with clinical problems for fear of catching the illness and then in turn putting their families at risk.

There are two aspects to this delay in care. The first is obvious – clinical problems such as biliary colic, diverticulitis, or paraesophageal hernia with volvulus that may not be emergent, and may not even be urgent, so they are delayed during the period of reduced operating room availability. While these patients can potentially wait to receive surgery, they also are not purely elective cases (e.g., bariatric or cosmetic surgery). It is incumbent on surgeons and their outpatient staff to remain in communication with patients, who may become urgent should their disease and symptoms worsen. One can surmise that these patients could easily be overlooked as the emphasis on care delivery is crisis-related, but this could lead to worsened outcomes if the operation is then performed under less-than-ideal circumstances.

The second aspect to care delays is patient-driven. During the COVID-19 crisis, there were anecdotal reports of an increase in the number of amputations from limbs that were not salvaged by vascular surgery due to patients remaining at home for fear of contracting the virus. There were similar reports of patients presenting in a delayed fashion with long bone fractures, who presented with DVT and/or pulmonary emboli that may not have occurred had the orthopedic repairs taken place shortly after injury. One could foresee diverticulitis turning into an urgent Hartmann's procedure rather than a planned minimally invasive diverticular resection due to the disease smoldering at home without timely intervention. Although surgeons could not have prevented these complications, it is important to consider how messaging is done by healthcare systems about the safety of having medical procedures performed in the setting of an infectious pandemic. Similarly, in the urban mass casualty setting, indicating that the area around the hospital is safe for patients to arrive and receive care can help prevent unnecessary delays in treating urgent problems, which could then lead to poorer outcomes.

Re-emergence Back into Elective Surgical Care Following a Crisis

How to reschedule surgery must be coordinated with the operating room as block availability may not immediately be repatriated. At the hospital level, decisions have to be made as to what types of surgery to prioritize. For example, the hospitals may want to begin with purely outpatient procedures at low risk for needing an inpatient bed when overall bed availability may be strained. In hospital systems that blend employed and private practice surgeons, there might be consideration of giving the private surgeons earlier or more access to operating rooms as they were likely financially impacted by the crisis in a more severe manner. Certainly, acuity should be considered in the rescheduling of cases. One must also consider the impact on cancer patients that might have been delayed; these cases may have some priority although one could argue that some of the patients were likely given different care plans (chemotherapy, radiation therapy, etc.) to initiate some form of treatment while waiting for surgery to become an option. The remaining cancers likely were tumors with slow growth (e.g., papillary thyroid, prostate), such that the delay likely would not have impacted the outcome. Nonetheless, it is likely that surgical oncologists would want some type of priority prior to initiating a re-emergence plan. SAGES has released an excellent document with recommendations as to how to manage cancer patients during the COVID-19 crisis [7], but how to integrate the delayed patients back into the operating room schedule is a concept made more complex by the interim care decisions that were implemented during the delay.

An obvious factor in developing such a re-emergence plan is the total number of operating rooms available. Was some of the PACU space re-allocated to critical care beds? If so, this can limit how much surgery – elective or not – can be completed safely. When governmental agencies lift the restrictions on elective surgeries, will the hospitals have the full suite of rooms available? Will redeployed staff now be repatriated to the operating room? Will the anesthesia staff be completely available for the operating room schedule? Can outlying community hospitals in healthcare systems be utilized as an alternative source of operating room real estate – and can the same level of surgical quality be delivered there? Are there staff losses from people who left healthcare jobs later in the pandemic that now impact the number of operating rooms that can be safely utilized?

Furthermore, some thought has to be given to what occurred with patients during the delay created by the crisis. For instance, what happens if bariatric patients gained weight during the period of delay – should that now further delay their ability to undergo elective bariatric surgery? What happens if patients who had stable medical conditions have worsened while at home and isolated – do they now need more extensive preoperative medical clearance (which, in turn, will delay them further)? Do patients need to be seen again by surgeons, either in the office or via video or telehealth, prior to rescheduling their operations?

The recovery of normal operations across the United States and globally is dependent on local epidemiology, but the quality metrics remain the same. CMS has suspended penalties understanding that quality metrics will be necessarily be worse under the pandemic; however, at least a few regions that have achieved low infection levels have returned to normal levels of surgical volume with normalized quality. Length of stay, mortality, thromboembolic events, respiratory failure, and renal failure were measurably worse for surgical patients requiring urgent and emergent care but have improved to baseline during the period of recovery. Unwinding the redeployed surgical workforce and their operating environment requires attention to our quality systems and metrics. They serve as a guide to safe restoration. If quality remains compromised during recovery, we as surgeons must use our measurement systems to understand why and course correct.

While during a crisis the return to "normal" is a highly desirable achievement, arriving there in a safe and orderly fashion actually represents a complex series of decisions, both by providers and hospitals, to ensure maximum efficiency, safe surgical outcomes, and the ability to service all of those who were inconvenienced by the crisis itself.

Conclusion

A crisis such as a pandemic or mass casualty creates a ripple effect across a healthcare system; surgery is one of the most affected areas. Hospital resources often have to be commandeered quickly to provide for the needs of the crisis. The cessation of elective surgical care wreaks havoc with schedules and inconveniences of many patients but is often a necessary step to prepare for a surge of admitted patients. Scarce resources need to be allocated and addressed in a thoughtful, yet ethical manner. The surgeons and their teams may have to be redeployed to other areas of critical need. Delays in care may have clinical ramifications for patients that have to be dealt with and may worsen their ultimate outcomes. Emergence from the crisis and gravitating back to normal involves critical discussions with key stakeholders in a fair attempt to provide the best care to the most patients in as timely a fashion as possible.

References

1. https://www.facs.org/covid-19/clinical-guidance/triage.
2. https://www.sages.org/recommendations-surgical-management-colorectal-cancer-covid-19/.
3. https://www.sages.org/sages-recommendations-surgical-management-gastric-cancer-covid-19-crisis/.
4. https://www.sages.org/sages-ahpba-recommendations-surgical-management-of-hpb-cancer-covid-19/.

5. https://www.mass.gov/doc/crisis-standards-of-care-draft-planning-guidance-for-public-comment-october-6-2020/download.
6. https://www.mdcalc.com/sequential-organ-failure-assessment-sofa-score.
7. Dort J, Romanelli J, Choudhury N, et al. SAGES primer for taking care of yourself during and after the COVID-19 crisis. Surg Endosc. 2020;34(7):2856–62.

Chapter 45
Ergonomic Considerations for Surgeon Physical Wellness

Marinda Scrushy and Diana L. Diesen

Introduction

Why Does Ergonomics Matter?

Work-related injuries in healthcare are common: OSHA reports hospital workers have a higher risk of injury or illness requiring time away from work than construction workers or manufacturing sector workers [1], and hospitals have a worker injury rate three times that of professionals in other traditional professional or business services. Greater than 64% of hospital worker injuries are musculoskeletal (MSK) in nature, involving injury to muscles, nerves, tendons, joints, cartilage, or spinal discs. When these injuries are sustained due to the work environment, prolonged working time, or the performance of specific work, they are referred to as work-related MSK disorders (WR-MSKD) [2]. Costs associated with these injuries, which include medical cost, lost wages,

M. Scrushy · D. L. Diesen (✉)
Department of Surgery, University of Texas Southwestern Medical Center, Dallas, TX, USA
e-mail: MARINDA.SCRUSHY@phhs.org

© The Author(s), under exclusive license to Springer Nature Switzerland AG 2022
J. R. Romanelli et al. (eds.), *The SAGES Manual of Quality, Outcomes and Patient Safety*,
https://doi.org/10.1007/978-3-030-94610-4_45

857

decreased productivity, sick time, turnover, and decreased quality of life are estimated at $200 billion annually based on workers' compensation losses [3]. Unfortunately, work-related injuries are vastly underreported particularly in the surgical specialties.

WR-MSKD are due to a combination of repetitive activities, prolonged static positions, extreme body positions, and vibrating tools, all of which are common during surgery, putting surgeons at particularly high risk for work-related MSK disorders. The incidence of work-related MSK injuries in surgeons is remarkably high, with rates of 72–87.5% in open surgeons [4–8],78–100% for laparoscopic surgeons [9, 10], and 28–45% for robotic surgeons [11, 12].

The most common sites for pain or injury were back, neck, arms, and shoulders. These injuries are found across surgical specialties [2].

The physical environment, the surgical tools/equipment, the physical demands, and the overall culture of surgery put surgeons at increased risk for injury. Healthcare is often seen as a selfless profession, with healthcare workers often ignoring their own health or being injured as they put the patient's well-being above their own. Furthermore, the surgical culture of efficiency, strong work ethic, and grit puts surgeons at even higher risk. An institutional survey found that 65% of surgeons never sought help or reported their injuries to occupational health [5].

The consequences of surgeon injury are far-reaching, impacting not only the surgeon but also the healthcare system and patients. Surgeon injury leads to missed days of work, fewer operations, and even early retirement [3] and can lead to a decline in surgeon wellness by increasing fatigue, affecting personal relationships, decreasing sleep, and increasing fear of surgical error while operating [15]. Surgeon discomfort while operating may influence surgical approach, with up to 30% of surgeons in one survey reporting that they took their own physical symptoms into account when recommending a surgical approach to the patient [13]. The burden on the healthcare system includes costs of injury treatment, increased utilization of resources, decreased operating room efficiency, and increased missed days of work.

This chapter focuses on the ergonomic challenges specific to surgeons and optimal ergonomic strategies to mitigate these challenges. Attention to these strategies can improve the mental and physical well-being of the surgeon, the outcomes of the patients, and efficacy of our healthcare system.

Ergonomic Challenges in the Operating Room

Posture and Operative Fatigue

Activities in the operating room are prone to repetitive movements and awkward body positioning including extreme trunk rotation, arm movements, and significant force on the neck, spine, and upper extremities. Furthermore, static positions while operating can lead to a maladaptive posture that increases compressive force on surrounding tissues over time [16]. The type of surgical procedure, instruments, equipment, and duration of operation are also significant contributors to MSK pain. Studies have used electromyography (EMG) to measure muscle fatigue and stress while operating. Changes on EMG can be correlated to indicate muscle fatigue as well as measure the contraction force of the muscle [17], with muscle fatigue noted to increase as operative time increases [18].

Instruments and Equipment

Some of the factors in the operating room that contribute to MSK pain are specialized equipment such as loupes and headlamps, surgical instruments, operating table height, and monitor height.

Loupes and headlamps contribute to cervical spine symptoms due to increased weight on the head and neck, which

alters the surgeon's posture and causes an increase in neck
flexion and forward head position. Positions that require
neck flexion greater than 15° are more likely to cause cervical
spine pain and increase cervical loading up to 40% [19].
Similarly, microscopic surgery causes the neck to be in
extreme flexion or laterally deviated for prolonged periods of
time [16]. Improper table height has been cited as the most
common cause of pain following surgery, and inappropriate
monitor positioning during laparoscopic surgery can lead to
awkward trunk and neck rotation [5].

Poor positioning of the operating table and monitors during minimally invasive surgery (MIS) can lead to static or
abnormal positioning of head, neck, and back. The use of the
laparoscope also leads to uncomfortable arm positioning in
order to achieve appropriate camera view [20]. The level of
upper extremity muscle strain as measured by EMG is significantly higher while performing laparoscopic surgery when
compared to other surgical modalities [21]. Laparoscopic
instrument design may contribute to increased muscle strain
and fatigue, as these instruments are designed with a long
shaft requiring excessive force and pressure in order to
manipulate the tools [22]. Poor instrument handle design also
contributes to MSK pain and fatigue of the wrist and hands
by altering upper extremity posture [2, 21]. When compared
to robotic surgery, traditional laparoscopic surgery has shown
higher muscle activation and strain. Muscle fatigue is the
highest in the upper extremities including biceps, triceps, and
deltoid muscles [23, 24]. In addition, robotic instruments have
better ergonomic outcomes for surgeons due to improvement
in hand posture [25].

Implications of Poor Ergonomics

The risk of poor ergonomics for the surgeon is risk of physical
injury, fatigue, frustration, burnout, disability, and even the
need for early retirement. When examined over a 12-month
period, the estimates for WR-MSK pain were of the 65%

neck, 52% shoulder, 59% back, and 39% upper extremity [26]. These rates are comparable with manual labor occupations such as construction workers. This pain has been found to interfere with personal relationships, impair sleep, increase time away from work, increase need for medication and physical therapy, and reduce technical performance [27]. This physical pain combined with impaired relationships, decreased sleep, and limitations on one's practice surgery can ultimately led to burnout and/or early retirement [28].

Less is known about the direct effect of poor ergonomics and work-related injuries experienced during surgery on patient outcomes. Previous research looking at nurses has shown an increase in medication errors and infections related to caregiver fatigue, injury, and stress [1]. Lower patient satisfaction scores are associated with higher rates of job dissatisfaction, burnout, and frustration among the nursing staff [29].

The direct impact of WR-MSKD on patients is difficult to assess, as the only data available to date is retrospective self-reporting from surgeons who stated they took their own discomfort into account when deciding on an approach to a patient or reporting their pain affected their surgical care [13]. Other surveys have shown that 55% surgeons said their injuries had impact on surgical performance, with 13% reporting moderate to severe impact on surgical performance [3]. These numbers assume surgeon self-awareness of the impact of their injuries and thus are likely an underestimation of the true impact on patient care. This area needs focused attention and research.

When surgeons are injured, there is a much larger cost to the overall healthcare system. Substantial investment is made in the medical education and training of surgeons. When a surgeon is unable to fully work due to injury or illness, his/her position cannot be quickly filled given that it takes 5–10 years after medical school to train a surgeon. If a significant proportion of surgeons are experiencing chronic, repetitive injuries, the potential workforce impact and cost on society are considerable.

The direct, immediate cost of MSKD is the most obvious. These costs include cost of medical treatment, but there are other implications to the health system including absenteeism, reduced workload, early retirement, delays in patient care, and decreased team morale. Work-related injuries caused 22–27% of surgeons to take time off from work [3]. Those surgeons at highest risk included those aged >55 years, with more than 20 years of practice, and with an increasing number of procedures per year [30]. Fifty-three percent reported their injuries resulted in minimal or moderate effects on performance in OR [3]. Of surgeons who experienced an injury, 35% of surgeons had to cut back on operations during recovery [3]. For example, 27% of orthopedic surgeons reported an incidence of cervical radiculopathy, with 10.7% requiring surgery and 19% requiring time off work/early retirement [31]. Sivak-Callcott et al. found that 31% of surgeons had symptomatic bulging or herniated spinal discs. Of those surgeons with injuries, 2% had to modify their practice, 7.6% had to undergo surgery, and 9.2% had to retire due to injury [7].

MSKD are the number one cause of long-term disability claims and 20% of short-term disability pain, with acute back pain being the most common cause. Specifically, one in five short-term disability claims is caused by some form of MSK disorder [32]. Nearly 20% of surgeons in the UK and the USA and 15% of surgeons surveyed in Germany think they may need to retire early due to physical impact of conducting laparoscopic surgery [14]. While these rates of injuries are surprisingly high, only 19% of surgeons reported their injuries to their institution; the implication of these injuries may be grossly underestimated by the institution [3].

Strategies for Optimal Ergonomic Approach

The surgical community's awareness and appreciation of the ergonomic challenges in the operating room has increased, and with this increasing knowledge comes innovation and research to attempt to mitigate the consequences. Studies have focused on four specific areas in order to decrease the incidence of surgeon pain: First, increasing surgeon awareness of their own ergonomics and how they can design their operating room to accommodate these needs. Second, institutions have trialed developing ergonomics education programs that focus on increasing physician knowledge of ergonomics, how to avoid pitfalls, and an emphasis on institutional resources. Third, an emphasis on microbreaks, or small intra-operative pauses, to avoid or improve poor posture has also been provided. Last, development of specialized instruments and equipment has been suggested as a potential solution.

Surgeon Awareness of Their Environment [20]

It is imperative for surgeons to be aware of their environment and be proactive in designing an operating room that appeals to their individual ergonomic needs. This includes operating room setup as well as awareness of their own posture to make necessary adjustments to decrease their risk of injury. Studies have found that poor personal postural awareness and lack of attention to ergonomic design of the operating room are some of the most common causes of MSK injuries [19]. The need for proper room setup is specifically important in laparoscopic surgery where multiple different types of equipment are required to perform a case. Important variables in room setup include monitor positioning, choosing specialized instruments, optimal operating table height, and foot pedal placement. The implementation of an operating room checklists designed by each surgeon prior to the start of the case is one solution. Surgeons should also be aware of their own individual ideal table height, calculated to be 21 cm lower than the elbow height of the surgeon [33].

Setting Up the Operating Room for Success

During the performance of surgery, awkward body positioning is required at times, so it is important for surgeons to
maintain a neutral body position throughout as much of the
case as possible. The bed height should be positioned for the
tallest surgeon, with steps provided for other team members
to ensure every member of the team has optimal positioning.
The bed height is calculated to be 21 cm lower than the elbow
height of the tallest surgeon [33]. The bed height should be
such that the upper arms are perpendicular to the floor and
90° to the forearms with the shoulder at <30 degrees of
abduction. The forearms should be parallel to the floor and
neither supinated nor pronated with the elbows between 90°
and 120° (Fig. 45.1, Table 45.1). The back and trunk should be
positioned perpendicular to the floor with the feet hip's width
apart with weight distributed evenly between both feet.
Twisting or flexing the pelvic girdle should be avoided when
possible.

Monitors should be positioned 10–30° below eye level
(Fig. 45.1). Every degree of extension above the horizon
increases cervical load, which is exacerbated if wearing
loupes or a headlight [34–36]. Repeated sustained increases
in cervical load with or without shearing forces are thought to
exacerbate or accelerate development of degenerative disc
disease.

Elbows should rest at the surgeon's side with horizontal
forearms. This neutral position allows for a greater range of
motion when operating laparoscopically by allowing instruments to be comfortably moved up and down in the laparoscopic ports [33]. Studies have implemented the use of arm
rests during laparoscopic surgery to keep a neutral arm and
shoulder position, which improved discomfort in test subjects while they performed prolonged laparoscopic skills
tasks [37].

It is important to maintain a neutral position when seated.
A neutral seated position is sitting upright with a small lumbar lordosis (natural curve in the small of the back) and the

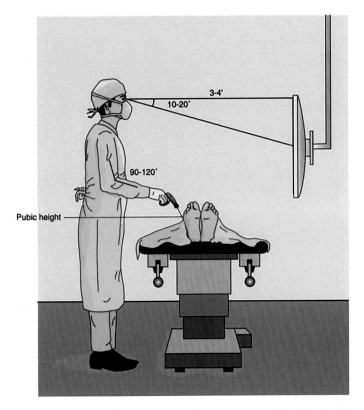

FIGURE 45.1 Ergonomic laparoscopic arrangement. (Reprinted with permission from Ronstrom et al. [54])

shoulders back. The feet should rest on the ground with the knees at least a 90-degree angle or greater [38]. When performing robotic surgery, the feet should be positioned so that no more than 25 degrees of movement is needed to activate the foot pedal [39].

Education

A survey of physicians showed that 100% of them thought that ergonomics were important, although 89% had poor

TABLE 45.1 Published surgical ergonomics recommendations, listed by applicable body site or equipment

Body part/ equipment	Recommendation	Studies— first author, year(s)
Shoulder/ upper arm	Upper arm should remain perpendicular to floor	Craven 2013
	Shoulders should be dropped and hands relaxed. Intraoperative stretching with arm raises recommended	Rosenblatt 2013
	Shoulder abduction should be <30°. Arms should be slightly abducted and rotated inward	Xiao 2012
	Assistants should rotate responsibility for retraction to avoid prolonged strain for any individual	Hullfish 2009
	In laparoscopic and vaginal surgery, assistants and surgeons should consider rotating sides to balance upper extremity strain	
Forearm/ elbow	Angle between forearm and upper arm should be 90°	Craven 2013
	To avoid excessive elbow flexion/ extension, forearm should be held in horizontal position, parallel to the floor. To avoid excessive torque, forearm should be held in neutral position between supination and pronation	Matern 2009
	Elbows should be held between 90-and 120-degree flexion	Xiao 2012
Wrist	Wrist should be held in slight extension with fingers bent slightly	Matern 2009

TABLE 45.1 (continued)

Body part/ equipment	Recommendation	Studies— first author, year(s)
	Avoid wrist deviations beyond 20-degree extension, 40-degree flexion, 15-degree radial deviation, and 25-degree ulnar deviation. Extreme wrist excursions should not occupy >30% of operating time	Van Veelen 2004
Hand/fingers	Instruments should not require more force than 15 N to completely close	Van Veelen 2004
Neck	Neck flexion should be about 20°. In robotic surgery, forehead should rest only lightly on the headrest	Craven 2013
	Surgeons should avoid excessive "head forward" posture, as this increases degenerative changes in the cervical spine	Rosenblatt 2013
	Prolonged static positioning of the neck, particularly if in excessive flexion, should be avoided	Szeto 2012
	Neck should be flexed at an angle between 10 and 30°. Excessive twisting should be avoided; surgeons should limit axial rotation to less than 15°	Van Det 2008
Back/trunk	Avoid pelvic girdle asymmetry by keeping feel hip's width apart with weight evenly distributed	Rosenblatt 2013

(continued)

TABLE 45.1 (continued)

Body part/ equipment	Recommendation	Studies— first author, year(s)
	Do not lock knees. Engage deep muscles of trunk and pelvis to maintain neutral position. Perform postural "resets" and intraoperative stretching with squats	
	Prolonged static positioning should be avoided	Szeto 2012
Lower extremity	In robotic surgery, excessive knee flexion should be avoided. Feel should rest on ground in front of pedals at angle ≥90°	Craven 2013
	Dorsal flexion of the fool should be <25° when controlling foot switch	Van Veelen 2004
	Consider antifatigue mats in the operating room to decrease lower extremity fatigue. Surgeons should also consider supportive hose if prolonged standing is required	Hullfish 2009
Monitor position	Laparoscopic monitors should be between 10 and 30° below eye level	Van Det 2009
	Image should be 15–45° below eye level	Van Veelen 2004
	Screen height of 160 cm is recommended	Zehetner 2006
Table height	Table heights in general should be adjusted to the height of the tallest surgeon with step stools used for other team members	Hullfish 2009

TABLE 45.1 (continued)

Body part/ equipment	Recommendation	Studies— first author, year(s)
	In vaginal surgery, surgeons should be seated whenever possible with table and stool heights adjusted so primary surgeon is looking straight ahead	Hullfish 2009
	To prevent extreme upper extremity excursions during laparoscopic surgery, the operating table should be between a factor 0.7 and 0.8 of surgeons' elbow height so instruments can rotate around elbow level	Berquer 2002
Standing support	Standing support adjustable between 780 and 1020 mm may help prevent prolonged static standing posture	Van Veelen 2004
Instrument manipulation	Working angle between instruments when stitching and knotting should be 60°. This will keep arms in comfortable, slightly inwardly rotated, position	Matern 2009
	Instrument intracorporeal to extracorporeal ratio should be >1	Xiao 2012
Arm boards	To avoid trunk twisting, surgeons should tuck patient's arms whenever possible	Rosenblatt 2013
Foot pedal position	Surgeons should be able to reach pedals without balancing on one foot	Matern 2009

(continued)

TABLE 45.1 (continued)

Body part/ equipment	Recommendation	Studies— first author, year(s)
	Foot pedals should be placed next to foot in line with target instruments toward the target quadrant	Rosenblatt 2013
Postsurgery interventions	Perform neck, hamstring, and back stretches immediately after breaking scrub. Surgeons should incorporate stretching/flexibility modules into their exercise programs (e.g., yoga, pilates) and engage in regular massage	Hullfish 2009

Reprinted with permission from Catanzarite et al. [2]

understanding of the ergonomic recommendations and resources at their own institutions [13]. This lack of training is strikingly high as studies have shown clear benefit from providing physicians with formal ergonomic training and physical tools to improve posture and decrease their pain [40]. Ergonomics training for surgical residents has shown particular benefits including overall decrease in pain and improvement in posture with targeted instruction by physical therapist targeting common areas of fatigue and pain [41]. Integration of ergonomic training early (medical school/residency) has the greatest potential to prevent these MSK injuries improving quality of life for the surgeon, extending years of practice, improving patient care, reducing burnout, and decreasing overall healthcare costs.

Steps to Alleviate Strain

Maintaining static body positions for extended lengths of time can lead to muscle fatigue and strain. There are steps available to mitigate the stress on the body during prolonged cases. For example, movement or rotation of the muscle groups responsible for retracting, changing position of the hands while retracting if possible, alternating hands [39], and intraoperative stretching with the arms raised [42] can all help mitigate prolonged strain on the muscles.

Neck flexion should be limited to approximately 20° to limit the strain on the neck [43]. Axial rotation should be limited to 15°, and excessive twisting or straining of the neck from a neutral position should be avoided [35].

Cervical stretches, specifically extension exercises, can help mitigate the strain on the neck. These stretches are shown in Fig. 45.2, Panel 1, and are performed by starting with the head displaced anteriorly and then pulling the head

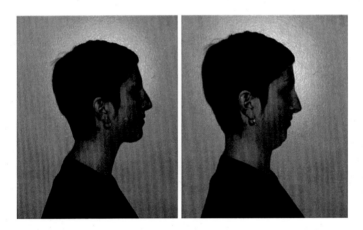

Figure 45.2 Stretches to address highest risk areas – before, during, and/or after surgery. Panel 1 Cervical retraction to counterbalance the excessive cervical load caused by flexion with or without headlights and loupes during the procedure. One may also perform cervical lateral flexion for cases with particular neck strain. Panel 2 Lumbar extension to counterbalance the excessive lumbar flexion during the case. Panel 3 Shoulders and upper back. Postural reset is performed by raising arm up above your head with the thumbs facing forward and then bringing arms straight down to your sides while pressing scapula together. (Reprinted with permission from Hullfish et al. [39])

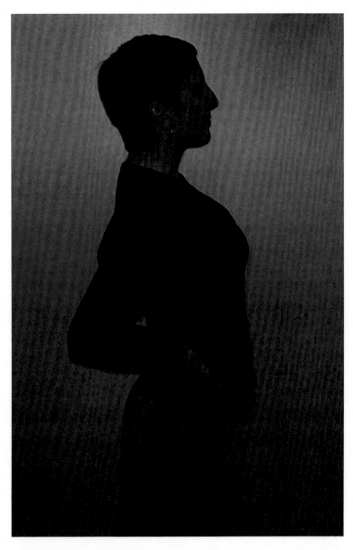

FIGURE 45.2 (continued)

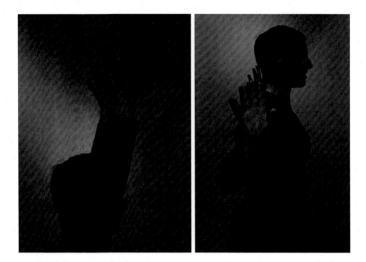

Figure 45.2 (continued)

back into an exaggerated posterior position. These cervical stretches are particularly helpful if the head is in an abnormal position for an extended period or if the surgeon is wearing loupes or a headlamp. Other exercises including stretching exercises focusing on the trapezius, sternocleidomastoid, and levator scapulae have been shown to improve cervical spine pain and reduce forward head positioning by strengthening the muscles responsible for deep cervical flexion [44] (Fig. 45.3).

Core strength is key to alleviating strain on the back and trunk. Engagement of the deep muscles of the trunk is needed to maintain neutral positioning. Regular postural resets and intraoperative stretching with squats and lumbar extensions (as shown in Fig. 45.2, Panel 2) can mitigate the flexion often needed during surgical procedures. Postural reset is performed by raising the arms up above the head with the thumbs facing forward and then bringing the arms straight down to the sides of the body while pressing the scapulae together (Fig. 45.2, Panel 3). These exercises can be

Neck & Head forward/flexion Exercises
1. Wall Chin Tucks (2 sets 30-40 secs)
2. Supine Neck Flexion (2 sets 30-40secs)
3. Lacrosse Ball Upper Trap Release
4. True Lateral Neck Flexion with Depressed Shoulders (2 sets x 5-8 reps)

Shoulders & Internal Rotation Exercises
1. Y 's, T 's, W's (3 sets, 5-10 reps with 3 second hold)
2. Wall Slide (3 sets: 30 second hold at 90, then 10 slides overhead)
3. Doorway Pectoralis Stretch (2-3 sets, 30-60 sec hold)
4. Pectoralis Minor Release with Lacrosse Ball (1x 1-2min)
5. Latissimus Dorsi Release with Lacrosse Ball (1x 1-2min)
6. Doorway stretch (2-3 sets, 30-60 sec hold)

Thoracic Spine Mobility
1. Prone Ws, Ys, Ts Extensions (2 sets x 8-10 reps, hold 3 secs)
2. Foam Roller Extensions (2-3 sets x 30 secs)
3. Puppy Dog Stretch (2-3 sets x 30 secs)
4. Cat-Cow Yoga (2 sets x 5 reps, hold 3 seconds at each position)

Lumbar Spine, Pelvic Tilt & Lower Extremity
1. Waiters Bow with Flat T-Spine (1-2 sets x 5 reps hold for 3-5 seconds)
2. Supine Bent Knee Hip Extension (2 sets x 5-8 reps, hold 3 seconds at top)
3. Prone Single Leg Hip Extension (2 sets x 5-8 reps, hold 3-5 seconds at top)
4. Wall Calf Stretch Varied Angles of Foot (2 sets, 20-30 second hold each angle)
5. Body Weight Squat Flat Footed (3 sets x 10 reps)

FIGURE 45.3 Strength and stretching exercises for problematic areas. (Reprinted with permission from Winters et al. [19])

performed prior to the case, during a longer case, or after the case is completed.

Avoiding excessive flexion of the knees or feet helps to mitigate strain on the lower extremities. The foot pedal should be positioned such that the surgeon does not have to balance on one foot to activate the instruments. Avoid locking the knees or twisting the pelvic girdle, which in addition to causing strain on the back can also cause strain on the leg experiencing the increased load [34, 38]. Lower extremity stretching, specifically squats and calf stretches, can also mitigate lower extremity pain and fatigue [2, 19].

Training sessions can also focus on increasing the surgeon's proprioception through techniques like the Alexander method, which focuses on the relationship with the head, neck, and spine and the individual's awareness of the body as a whole during each movement. This technique has been shown to improve overall posture by participants [40].

Participating in regular exercise at least 3 days per week (or 5 hours per week) also directly reduces MSK pain [41]. Exercise is the only intervention that has consistently been shown to decrease self-reported back problems [45], examples of which are included in Fig. 45.3.

Microbreaks

Microbreaks have been found to decrease surgeon discomfort without increasing operative time. Microbreaks are frequent but quick pauses during a case. These breaks are meant to be both mental and physical pauses, with three main goals: stress relief, posture correction, and reduction in tissue tension [46]. The overall goal is to reduce mental and physical fatigue through physical activities including posture realignment and stretching. When surgeons implemented short quick exercises or targeted stretching during these breaks, they were more likely to self-report improvement not only in pain and performance but in mental focus as well [27]. The idea is to perform these activities in a 1-min (or less) break without disrupting sterility. The body movements are meant to target multiple body segments and muscles at one time, which allows for effective and efficient improvement [46] (Fig. 45.2, Panel 2). Counterarguments against the implementation of microbreaks include concerns about increasing operating time or disrupting workflow, although microbreaks have not been found to increase operating time [41]. They can also be performed during natural breaks in workflow including scrub tech or nurse change over, instrument counting, or other communications with operating room staff.

Specialized Tools

Surgical Instruments

Due to the high volume of use, tools that allow for ideal ergonomic body positioning and enforce the proper technique for continued repetitive movements are essential. Surgical tool handle design has been shown to affect surgeons' upper extremity posture and is a significant contributor to discomfort, muscle fatigue, and even paresthesias [21, 22].

When looking at the root cause of discomfort, the method of gripping the tool was found to be the most important factor due to increased flexion and extension of the wrist, which increases ulnar deviation. Education on the proper gripping method of tools can reduce this hyperflexed positioning [22]. Laparoscopic tools are particularly problematic as the tool activation often requires extreme ulnar deviation and wrist flexion. This is caused by tool tips requiring pinching the thumb and three most medial fingers together while simultaneously rotating the tool head with the index finger, which increases the muscle force exerted by the surgeon in order to perform the desired movement while actually reducing the potential forces that can be exerted by the tool operatively [21]. Potential solutions include designing laparoscopic tools with a pistol grip to reduce stress on the hands and fingers. Studies implementing this design found that it leads to more neutral wrist posture and reduced hand discomfort, tremor, and fatigue in participants [21]. Robotic instruments have also been shown to provide better operative ergonomics by improving surgeon hand posture when compared to traditional laparoscopic instruments [25].

Laparoscopic tools are a "one size fits all" design. The handles on the laparoscopic instruments, cameras, and staplers are uniform and set for a size 7.5 glove size. Female surgeons average a glove size of 6.5, as compared to their male counterparts' average size of 7.5 [47]. Doctors with a larger glove size tend to describe these instruments as easy to use, while those with a smaller glove size tend to describe these instruments as awkward. Surgeons with a smaller glove size are more likely to need two hands to operate a reported "one-handed device" [47]. Other studies have found female gender and those with smaller glove size were more likely to report MSK symptoms related to instrument handle [48]. Given the rising number of female surgeons, this should serve as a clarion call to develop a line of laparoscopic instruments geared toward smaller hands.

Loupes and Headlamps

Any increased weight increases the strain on the neck due to increased cervical loading. Loupes and headlamps must be properly fitted to the surgeon. The two most important aspects of fit are the working distance of the lens and the declination angle. The design of these features contributes to the surgeon's line of sight during the case and, if not aligned properly, can increase forward head positioning. The declination angle is important to decrease forward head posture. Loupes should require less than a 20-degree downward head tilt to avoid neck and shoulder pain [2].

The weight of the headlamp and loupes should be considered when purchasing these items. Consider if loupes or a headlamp is needed for each case. If a headlamp is needed, ensure it is appropriately adjusted to allow the head to remain in a neutral position.

Lead Shields

The weight of lead shields worn to decrease radiation exposure caused discomfort in the neck, shoulder, and back which has been reported by surgeons/residents 42% of the time, anesthesiologists 36% of the time, and surgical nurses 49% of the time. This weight increases the axial load on the back and lower legs and has been associated with increased

MSK disorders over time. Some considerations for lead shields include the design, the amount of radiation protection (weight), and alternatives. A two-piece wrap distributes some weight over the hips and some weight onto the shoulders which may be more comfortable than a one-piece wrap, which distributes all of the weight over the shoulders. While traditional lead shields are 0.5 mm in thickness, recent data suggests lighter 0.3 mm shields provide sufficient protection. Another alternative is to use a floor standing barrier. The use of this barrier limits the surgeon's ability to move, as the surgeon must always stand behind the barrier, and is therefore only useful when fluoroscopy is needed for a short period of time requiring minimal active manipulation by the surgeon [49].

Footwear

Prolonged standing at work has been well established in multiple professions to lead to adverse health outcomes such as MSK pain in the lower back, lower extremities, shoulder, and neck as well as fatigue, chronic venous insufficiency, and preterm birth [39, 50]. These symptoms are worsened if the surgeon is wearing lead aprons. Interventions to mitigate these outcomes have included floor mats, sit-stand work stations, shoes, shoe inserts, foot stools, and supportive hose [51]. Shoe inserts or anti-fatigue mats are well known to be useful for decreasing lower extremity fatigue and lower back pain in multiple professions [52, 53]. Studies are mixed on which provides the best reduction on MSK discomfort [53]. Compression stockings have been shown to decrease leg swelling [51] for those who are required to stand for long periods of time [39]. While these interventions and ergonomic best practices are widely accepted in many other fields of industry, these principles have been largely ignored in the field of surgery.

Office Ergonomics Should Not Be Ignored

Once the surgeon leaves the operating room, a significant amount of time is spent in the office performing administrative tasks. The ergonomic setup of the surgeon's desk is shown in Fig. 45.4.

Additional steps that can be considered are to contact human resources to determine if there is an ergonomics consultant available to assist in ensuring optimal workspace ergonomics; checking/changing the position and height of the desk; considering a standing desk with an anti-fatigue mat; checking the height and angle of the computer monitor; considering glare protection on the computer screens; ensuring

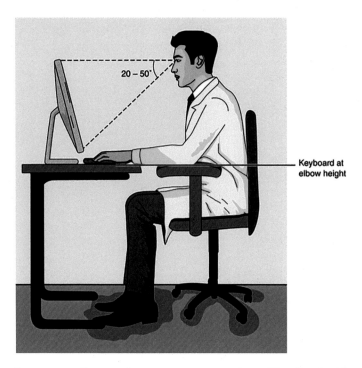

FIGURE 45.4 Ergonomic computer arrangement. (Reprinted with permission from Ronstrom et al. [54])

the desk chair height relative to the floor and desk is correct and has adequate lumbar support and arm rests; and ensuring the keyboard and mouse shapes and heights are appropriate.

Conclusion

Attention to the working environment and use of optimal ergonomic strategies can improve the well-being of the surgeon, the outcomes of patients, and the cost of healthcare. Surgery is far behind other industries in recognizing the impact of ergonomics. The best practices defined by other industries should be embraced and modified for the unique work environment of surgeons. When MSK discomfort does occur during surgery, it should be recognized and immediately mitigated prior to causing an acute injury. This is needed to protect surgeons, healthcare teams, patients, and the healthcare system as a whole.

References

1. OSHA. Secondary. https://www.osha.gov/sites/default/files/1.1_Data_highlights_508.pdf.
2. Catanzarite T, Tan-Kim J, Whitcomb EL, Menefee S. Ergonomics in surgery: a review. Female Pelvic Med Reconstr Surg. 2018;24(1):1–12. https://doi.org/10.1097/spv.0000000000000456. [published Online First: Epub Date]|.
3. Davis WT, Fletcher SA, Guillamondegui OD. Musculoskeletal occupational injury among surgeons: effects for patients, providers, and institutions. J Surg Res. 2014;189(2):207–12.e6. https://doi.org/10.1016/j.jss.2014.03.013. [published Online First: Epub Date]|.
4. Tan K, Kwek E. Musculoskeletal occupational injuries in orthopaedic surgeons and residents. Malays Orthop J. 2020;14(1):24–7. https://doi.org/10.5704/MOJ.2003.004. [published Online First: Epub Date]|.
5. Soueid A, Oudit D, Thiagarajah S, Laitung G. The pain of surgery: pain experienced by surgeons while operating. Int J Surg. 2010;8(2):118–20. https://doi.org/10.1016/j.ijsu.2009.11.008. [published Online First: Epub Date]|.

6. Babar-Craig H, Banfield G, Knight J. Prevalence of back and neck pain amongst ENT consultants: national survey. J Laryngol Otol. 2003;117(12):979–82. https://doi.org/10.1258/002221503322683885. [published Online First: Epub Date]|.

7. Sivak-Callcott JA, Diaz SR, Ducatman AM, Rosen CL, Nimbarte AD, Sedgeman JA. A survey study of occupational pain and injury in ophthalmic plastic surgeons. Ophthalmic Plast Reconstr Surg. 2011;27(1):28–32. https://doi.org/10.1097/IOP.0b013e3181e99cc8. [published Online First: Epub Date]|.

8. Szeto GP, Ho P, Ting AC, Poon JT, Cheng SW, Tsang RC. Work-related musculoskeletal symptoms in surgeons. J Occup Rehabil. 2009;19(2):175–84. https://doi.org/10.1007/s10926-009-9176-1. [published Online First: Epub Date]|.

9. Esposito C, El Ghoneimi A, Yamataka A, et al. Work-related upper limb musculoskeletal disorders in paediatric laparoscopic surgery. A multicenter survey. J Pediatr Surg. 2013;48(8):1750–6. https://doi.org/10.1016/j.jpedsurg.2013.01.054. [published Online First: Epub Date]|.

10. Miller K, Benden M, Pickens A, Shipp E, Zheng Q. Ergonomics principles associated with laparoscopic surgeon injury/illness. Hum Factors. 2012;54(6):1087–92. https://doi.org/10.1177/0018720812451046. [published Online First: Epub Date]|.

11. Santos-Carreras L, Hagen M, Gassert R, Bleuler H. Survey on surgical instrument handle design: ergonomics and acceptance. Surg Innov. 2012;19(1):50–9. https://doi.org/10.1177/1553350611413611. [published Online First: Epub Date]|.

12. Franasiak J, Craven R, Mosaly P, Gehrig PA. Feasibility and acceptance of a robotic surgery ergonomic training program. JSLS. 2014;18(4) https://doi.org/10.4293/JSLS.2014.00166. [published Online First: Epub Date]|.

13. Stucky CH, Cromwell KD, Voss RK, et al. Surgeon symptoms, strain, and selections: systematic review and meta-analysis of surgical ergonomics. Ann Med Surg (Lond). 2018;27:1–8. https://doi.org/10.1016/j.amsu.2017.12.013. [published Online First: Epub Date]|.

14. Secondary. https://cmrsurgical.com/news/one-in-five-surgeons-set-to-retire-early-due-to-physical-toll.

15. Koshy K, Syed H, Luckiewicz A, Alsoof D, Koshy G, Harry L. Interventions to improve ergonomics in the operating theatre: a systematic review of ergonomics training and intra-operative

microbreaks. Ann Med Surg (Lond). 2020;55:135–42. https://doi. org/10.1016/j.amsu.2020.02.008. [published Online First: Epub Date]|.

16. Lakhiani C, Fisher SM, Janhofer DE, Song DH. Ergonomics in microsurgery. J Surg Oncol. 2018;118(5):840–4. https://doi. org/10.1002/jso.25197. [published Online First: Epub Date]|.

17. Luttmann A. Detection of muscle fatigue with electromyography. Wien Med Wochenschr. 1996;146(13–14):374–6.

18. Slack PS, Coulson CJ, Ma X, Webster K, Proops DW. The effect of operating time on surgeons' muscular fatigue. Ann R Coll Surg Engl. 2008;90(8):651–7. https://doi.org/10.1308/003588 408x321710. [published Online First: Epub Date]|.

19. Winters JN, Sommer NZ, Romanelli MR, Marschik C, Hulcher L, Cutler BJ. Stretching and strength training to improve postural ergonomics and endurance in the operating room. Plast Reconstr Surg Glob Open. 2020;8(5):e2810. https://doi. org/10.1097/gox.0000000000002810. [published Online First: Epub Date]|.

20. Janki S, Mulder E, JNM IJ, Tran TCK. Ergonomics in the operating room. Surg Endosc. 2017;31(6):2457–66. https://doi. org/10.1007/s00464-016-5247-5. [published Online First: Epub Date]|.

21. Tung KD, Shorti RM, Downey EC, Bloswick DS, Merryweather AS. The effect of ergonomic laparoscopic tool handle design on performance and efficiency. Surg Endosc. 2015;29(9):2500–5. https://doi.org/10.1007/s00464-014-4005-9. [published Online First: Epub Date]|.   22.   Trejo A, Jung MC, Oleynikov D, Hallbeck MS. Effect of handle design and target location on insertion and aim with a laparoscopic surgical tool. Appl Ergon. 2007;38(6):745–53. https://doi.org/10.1016/j.apergo.2006.12.004. [published Online First: Epub Date]|.

23. Zihni AM, Ohu I, Cavallo JA, Cho S, Awad MM. Ergonomic analysis of robot-assisted and traditional laparoscopic procedures. Surg Endosc. 2014;28(12):3379–84. https://doi.org/10.1007/ s00464-014-3604-9. [published Online First: Epub Date]|.

24. Hislop J, Tirosh O, McCormick J, Nagarajah R, Hensman C, Isaksson M. Muscle activation during traditional laparoscopic surgery compared with robot-assisted laparoscopic surgery: a meta-analysis. Surg Endosc. 2020;34(1):31–8. https://doi. org/10.1007/s00464-019-07161-7. [published Online First: Epub Date]|.

25. Sánchez-Margallo JA, Sánchez-Margallo FM. Initial experience using a robotic-driven laparoscopic needle holder with ergonomic handle: assessment of surgeons' task performance and ergonomics. Int J Comput Assist Radiol Surg. 2017;12(12):2069–77. https://doi.org/10.1007/s11548-017-1636-z. [published Online First: Epub Date]|.

26. Epstein S, Sparer EH, Tran BN, et al. Prevalence of work-related musculoskeletal disorders among surgeons and Interventionalists: a systematic review and meta-analysis. JAMA Surg. 2018;153(2):e174947. https://doi.org/10.1001/jamasurg.2017.4947. [published Online First: Epub Date]|.

27. Hallbeck MS, Lowndes BR, Bingener J, et al. The impact of intraoperative microbreaks with exercises on surgeons: a multicenter cohort study. Appl Ergon. 2017;60:334–41. https://doi.org/10.1016/j.apergo.2016.12.006. [published Online First: Epub Date]|.

28. Kristin Chrouser M, Fran Foley, Mitchell Goldenberg, Joseph Hyder, Fernando J. Kim, Jodi Maranchie, James M. Moore, Michelle J. Semins, CDR Sean Stroup, Glenda B. Wilkinson. Optimizing outcomes in urologic surgery: intraoperative considerations. Guidelines 2018. https://www.auanet.org/guidelines/optimizing-outcomes-in-urologic-surgery-intraoperative-considerations.

29. McHugh MD, Kutney-Lee A, Cimiotti JP, Sloane DM, Aiken LH. Nurses' widespread job dissatisfaction, burnout, and frustration with health benefits signal problems for patient care. Health Aff (Millwood). 2011;30(2):202–10. https://doi.org/10.1377/hlthaff.2010.0100. [published Online First: Epub Date]|.

30. Alqahtani SM, Alzahrani MM, Tanzer M. Adult reconstructive surgery: a high-risk profession for work-related injuries. J Arthroplast. 2016;31(6):1194–8. https://doi.org/10.1016/j.arth.2015.12.025. [published Online First: Epub Date]|.

31. Auerbach JD, Weidner ZD, Milby AH, Diab M, Lonner BS. Musculoskeletal disorders among spine surgeons: results of a survey of the Scoliosis Research Society membership. Spine (Phila Pa 1976). 2011;36(26):E1715–21. https://doi.org/10.1097/BRS.0b013e31821cd140. [published Online First: Epub Date]|.

32. Alzahrani MM, Alqahtani SM, Tanzer M, Hamdy RC. Musculoskeletal disorders among orthopedic pediatric surgeons: an overlooked entity. J Child Orthop. 2016;10(5):461–6.

https://doi.org/10.1007/s11832-016-0767-z. [published Online First: Epub Date]|.

33. Lenoir C, Steinbrecher H. Ergonomics, surgeon comfort, and theater checklists in pediatric laparoscopy. J Laparoendosc Adv Surg Tech A. 2010;20(3):281–91. https://doi.org/10.1089/lap.2009.0226. [published Online First: Epub Date]|.

34. van Veelen MA, Kazemier G, Koopman J, Goossens RH, Meijer DW. Assessment of the ergonomically optimal operating surface height for laparoscopic surgery. J Laparoendosc Adv Surg Tech A. 2002;12(1):47–52. https://doi.org/10.1089/109264202753486920. [published Online First: Epub Date]|.

35. van Det MJ, Meijerink WJ, Hoff C, Totte ER, Pierie JP. Optimal ergonomics for laparoscopic surgery in minimally invasive surgery suites: a review and guidelines. Surg Endosc. 2009;23(6):1279–85. https://doi.org/10.1007/s00464-008-0148-x. [published Online First: Epub Date]|.

36. van Det MJ, Meijerink WJ, Hoff C, Pierie JP. Interoperative efficiency in minimally invasive surgery suites. Surg Endosc. 2009;23(10):2332–7. https://doi.org/10.1007/s00464-009-0335-4. [published Online First: Epub Date]|.

37. Galleano R, Carter F, Brown S, Frank T, Cuschieri A. Can armrests improve comfort and task performance in laparoscopic surgery? Ann Surg. 2006;243(3):329–33. https://doi.org/10.1097/01.sla.0000201481.08336.dc. [published Online First: Epub Date]|.

38. Craven R, Franasiak J, Mosaly P, Gehrig PA. Ergonomic deficits in robotic gynecologic oncology surgery: a need for intervention. J Minim Invasive Gynecol. 2013;20(5):648–55. https://doi.org/10.1016/j.jmig.2013.04.008. [published Online First: Epub Date]|.

39. Hullfish K, Trowbridge E, Bodine G. Ergonomics and gynecologic surgery: "surgeon protect thyself." J Pelvic Med Surg. 2009;15(6):435–9. https://doi.org/10.1097/SPV.0b013e3181bb89e5. [published Online First: Epub Date]|.

40. Reddy PP, Reddy TP, Roig-Francoli J, et al. The impact of the alexander technique on improving posture and surgical ergonomics during minimally invasive surgery: pilot study. J Urol. 2011;186(4 Suppl):1658–62. https://doi.org/10.1016/j.juro.2011.04.013. [published Online First: Epub Date]|.

41. Allespach H, Sussman M, Bolanos J, Atri E, Schulman CI. Practice longer and stronger: maximizing the physical well-being of surgical residents with targeted ergonomics train-

ing. J Surg Educ. 2020;77(5):1024–7. https://doi.org/10.1016/j.
jsurg.2020.04.001. [published Online First: Epub Date]|.

42. Park AE, Zahiri HR, Hallbeck MS, et al. Intraoperative
"micro breaks" with targeted stretching enhance surgeon
physical function and mental focus: a multicenter cohort
study. Ann Surg. 2017;265(2):340–6. https://doi.org/10.1097/
SLA.0000000000001665. [published Online First: Epub Date]|.

43. Rosenblatt PL, McKinney J, Adams SR. Ergonomics in the operating room: protecting the surgeon. J Minim Invasive Gynecol.
2013;20(6):744. https://doi.org/10.1016/j.jmig.2013.07.006. [pub-
lished Online First: Epub Date]|.

44. Lynch SS, Thigpen CA, Mihalik JP, Prentice WE, Padua D. The
effects of an exercise intervention on forward head and
rounded shoulder postures in elite swimmers. Br J Sports Med.
2010;44(5):376–81. https://doi.org/10.1136/bjsm.2009.066837.
[published Online First: Epub Date]|.

45. Bigos SJ, Holland J, Holland C, Webster JS, Battie M, Malmgren
JA. High-quality controlled trials on preventing episodes of
back problems: systematic literature review in working-age
adults. Spine J. 2009;9(2):147–68. https://doi.org/10.1016/j.
spinee.2008.11.001. [published Online First: Epub Date]|.

46. Coleman Wood KA, Lowndes BR, Buus RJ, Hallbeck
MS. Evidence-based intraoperative microbreak activities for
reducing musculoskeletal injuries in the operating room. Work.
2018;60(4):649–59. https://doi.org/10.3233/wor-182772. [pub-
lished Online First: Epub Date]|.

47. Adams DM, Fenton SJ, Schirmer BD, Mahvi DM, Horvath K,
Nichol P. One size does not fit all: current disposable laparoscopic devices do not fit the needs of female laparoscopic surgeons. Surg Endosc. 2008;22(10):2310–3. https://doi.org/10.1007/
s00464-008-9986-9. [published Online First: Epub Date]|.

48. Shepherd JM, Harilingam MR, Hamade A. Ergonomics in
laparoscopic surgery – a survey of symptoms and contributing
factors. Surg Laparosc Endosc Percutan Tech. 2016;26(1):72–7.
https://doi.org/10.1097/SLE.0000000000000231. [published
Online First: Epub Date]|.

49. Dixon RG, Khiatani V, Statler JD, et al. Society of interventional
radiology: occupational back and neck pain and the interventional radiologist. J Vasc Interv Radiol. 2017;28(2):195–9. https://
doi.org/10.1016/j.jvir.2016.10.017. [published Online First: Epub
Date]|.

50. Waters TR, Dick RB. Evidence of health risks associated with prolonged standing at work and intervention effectiveness. Rehabil Nurs. 2015;40(3):148–65. https://doi.org/10.1002/rnj.166. [published Online First: Epub Date]|.

51. Kraemer WJ, Volek JS, Bush JA, et al. Influence of compression hosiery on physiological responses to standing fatigue in women. Med Sci Sports Exerc. 2000;32(11):1849–58. https://doi.org/10.1097/00005768-200011000-00006. [published Online First: Epub Date]|.

52. Aghazadeh J, Ghaderi M, Azghani MR, Khalkhali HR, Allahyari T, Mohebbi I. Anti-fatigue mats, low back pain, and electromyography: an interventional study. Int J Occup Med Environ Health. 2015;28(2):347–56. https://doi.org/10.13075/ijomeh.1896.00311. [published Online First: Epub Date]|.

53. Speed G, Harris K, Keegel T. The effect of cushioning materials on musculoskeletal discomfort and fatigue during prolonged standing at work: a systematic review. Appl Ergon. 2018;70:300–14. https://doi.org/10.1016/j.apergo.2018.02.021. [published Online First: Epub Date]|.

54. Ronstrom C HS, Lowndes B, Chrouser K. Surgical ergonomics. In: Springer, editor. Surgeons as educators; 2017. p. 387–417.

Part VI
Surgical Controversies That Impact Quality

Chapter 46
Hernia Repair: Robot or No Robot?

Matthew Madion and Rana M. Higgins

Introduction

The utilization of minimally invasive techniques to repair hernias has continued to rise, and with the increasing use of the *da Vinci* robotic surgical system in general surgery, new methods have begun to emerge to repair abdominal wall hernias robotically. The touted benefits of utilizing the robot for hernia repairs can be subdivided into three aspects: clinical benefits, technical enhancement, and ergonomic improvement. Clinical benefits include decreased postoperative pain, earlier return to work, and shorter length of stay while also maintaining the advantages of traditional laparoscopy over open repairs, particularly with decreased wound complications. Technically, in particular repairs, there is an added ability to approximate fascia without conversion to an open operation as well as an ability to perform certain myofascial dissections not possible via simple laparoscopy and previously requiring an open repair. Possible ergonomic benefits include greater three-dimensional visualization, wristed instrumentation to

M. Madion · R. M. Higgins (✉)
Medical College of Wisconsin, Milwaukee, WI, USA
e-mail: mmadion@mcw.edu; rhiggins@mcw.edu

© The Author(s), under exclusive license to Springer Nature   889
Switzerland AG 2022
J. R. Romanelli et al. (eds.), *The SAGES Manual of Quality, Outcomes and Patient Safety*,
https://doi.org/10.1007/978-3-030-94610-4_46

facilitate intracorporeal suturing, and improved surgeon positioning.

Clinical benefits in the literature for robotic hernia repair thus far are limited to primarily single-institution case series, with a handful of national database reviews, and minimal randomized controlled trials. Despite the aforementioned benefits, early critiques of the robotic system include the added initial cost of the device and the continued cost of the disposable instruments. Furthermore, the need for surgeons to learn to use the new tool requires a learning curve, which leads to prolonged operative times. This chapter will examine the current published results, including discussion on utilization techniques, outcomes, and cost of robotic inguinal and ventral hernia repairs.

Robotic Inguinal Hernia Repair

The robotic transabdominal pre-peritoneal (rTAPP) has been established as another minimally invasive technique to repair inguinal hernias. Indications for rTAPP are similar to those for laparoscopic inguinal hernia repair, including any inguinal or femoral hernia that is symptomatic and recurrent inguinal hernias previously repaired with an open technique. rTAPP has been cited to be advantageous in inguinal hernias in patients with a prior surgical history of prostatectomy or lower pelvic surgery and large incarcerated or complicated hernias where optimal visualization and fine dissection are needed [1]. The touted benefits of rTAPP over a traditional laparoscopic repair are decreased postoperative pain, likely related to the avoidance of placing tacks during mesh fixation, and an improved ergonomic environment for the operating surgeon [2].

Although rTAPP continues to be adopted in centers that have robotic capabilities, most data indicates that this is done with increased cost and additional drawbacks including longer operative times. A recent multicenter randomized controlled study of 102 patients comparing traditional laparoscopic TAPP to rTAPP showed that rTAPP had a median cost of $3258 versus $1421 ($p < 0.001$) [2]. This difference is consistent with prior cost-analysis studies. A Vizient database review of 3547 patients showed that robotic repairs had the highest average cost at $9431 compared to $8837 in the open group and $6502 in the laparoscopic group ($p < 0.001$) [3]. Abdelmoaty et al. reported a cost difference of $5517 in their robotic inguinal repair group versus $3269 in the laparoscopic group ($p < 0.001$) and with longer average in-room, skin to skin, and recovery room times in the robotic group [4]. A single-institution retrospective review of 321 patients reported a mean operative time of 116 min and average hospital cost of $9993 in their robotic group versus 95 minutes and $5994 in their laparoscopic group ($p < 0.01$) [5].

In addition to higher cost and longer operative times, studies have looked at levels of frustration during robotic inguinal hernias. The NASA Task Load Index (NASA-TLX) Scale gauges on a scale of 1–100 the cognitive workload of a task through five distinct categories, namely, demand, performance, effort, frustration, and workload. Lower scores indicate lower cognitive workload. In the aforementioned randomized controlled trial by Prabhu et al., NASA-TLX scores demonstrated significantly higher overall surgeon reported frustration in the robotic group (32.7 versus 20.1, $p = 0.004$) as well as increased effort (36.7 versus 27.4, $p = 0.05$) [2].

Despite the current high cost of rTAPP, there is a growing body of evidence that it can be done feasibly and with comparable or improved clinical outcomes to laparoscopic and open inguinal hernia repairs. A recent systematic review and meta-analysis of 12 studies comprised of 1645 patients showed that rTAPP had comparable postoperative urinary retention (4.1%), seroma/hematoma (3.5%), overall complication (7.5%), and recurrence rates (0.18%) to laparoscopic TAPP and total extraperitoneal (TEP) repairs [6]. Additionally, early results from the Prospective Hernia Study indicate that patients undergoing rTAPP required fewer prescription pain medications than both open and laparoscopic repair groups and had a quicker return to work compared to patients who underwent open inguinal repair, all with comparable complication rates [7].

Other studies demonstrate improved clinical outcomes in robotic inguinal hernia repairs. The previously mentioned Vizient national database review of 3547 patients showed that robotic inguinal hernia repairs had the lowest overall 30-day complication rate (0.67%) compared to laparoscopic (4.44%) and open (3.85%) ($p < 0.05$). With respect to 30-day postoperative infection rates, robotic inguinal hernia repairs had no infections, compared to 0.56% in laparoscopic repairs and 8.33% in open repairs ($p < 0.05$) [8].

Overall, utilization of robotics to repair inguinal hernias can be performed safely and with comparable or improved clinical outcomes to laparoscopic and open repair techniques, but with significantly increased cost and likely initial increased operative time that may decline with surgeon experience. rTAPP may have a role in situations where a TEP repair is not feasible given prior anatomic violation of the space and the surgeon is not facile with laparoscopic TAPP. However, the exact role of rTAPP compared to laparoscopic TAPP and TEP has yet to be determined.

Robotic Ventral Hernia Repair

The variability and complexity of ventral hernias is reflected in the breadth of repair techniques utilized. Among robotic ventral hernia repairs performed, they can be distinguished into four approaches: robotic intraperitoneal onlay mesh (IPOM), robotic pre-peritoneal, robotic retrorectus and transversus abdominis release (TAR), and robotic extended total extraperitoneal (eTEP).

Robotic Intraperitoneal Onlay Mesh (rIPOM)

Intraperitoneal placement of coated mesh to cover the hernia defect has been a popular technique to laparoscopically repair ventral hernias, which has now also taken hold as a popular robotic approach. When compared with open repairs, laparoscopic repairs have been shown to have decreased length of stay and postoperative pain, fewer surgical site infections, but with typically longer mean operative times [9]. However, closing the fascial defect laparoscopically can be challenging and is not consistently accomplished when undergoing a laparoscopic IPOM.

The rIPOM offers a similar minimally invasive benefit profile as the laparoscopic approach, with an increased ability to re-approximate the fascia prior to placing the mesh given the wristed instrumentation to facilitate intracorporeal suturing. Fascial closure provides the added benefit of decreasing the incidence of postoperative seroma by compressing or excising the hernia sac and incorporating it into the closure. A retrospective 1:1 case-matched comparison of laparoscopic hernia repair with transcutaneous fascial closure versus standard laparoscopic repair without fascial closure showed a seroma difference from 27.8% in the non-closure group to 5.6% in the fascial closure group ($p = 0.02$) [10]. Another review of studies comparing fascial closure versus non-closure in laparoscopic hernia repairs showed a range of hernia recurrence of 4.8–16.7% in the non-closure groups versus 0.0–5.7% in the closure groups [11]. The ease of closing the fascia is a crucial technical aspect of the robotic IPOM and other robotic hernia repair techniques, but more studies need to be performed to elucidate the benefit of more consistent re-approximation of the fascia when placing mesh in an onlay fashion. Additionally, although not proven in the literature, given the circumferential fascial fixation of the mesh in rIPOM, transfascial mesh fixation can be avoided, potentially decreasing anecdotally reported post-operative pain.

Most data regarding clinical outcomes in rIPOM has been limited to single-institution studies and retrospective data. Results have shown that rIPOM can be accomplished with complication rates equivalent to traditional laparoscopy and with recurrence rates similar to those previously reported for both open and laparoscopic techniques [9, 12, 13]. A review by the Americas Hernia Society Quality Collaborative (AHSQC) of 631 patients comparing laparoscopic IPOM with robotic IPOM found that laparoscopic IPOM was associated with a higher surgical site occurrence rate (14.5% versus 5%, $p < 0.001$) and increased median length of stay (1 versus 0 days, $p < 0.001$) with robotic IPOM having a higher rate of fascial closures (93% versus 56%, $p < 0.001$) [14]. Gonzalez et al. compared a single-institution cohort of patients undergoing robotic IPOM with fascial closure to laparoscopic IPOM without fascial closure and found that the robotic group trended toward decreased recurrence rate (1.5% versus 7.5% $p = 0.095$ with median follow-up of 9.5 months in rIPOM and 12.1 months in laparoscopic IPOM) and fewer complications (3% versus 10.4%, $p = 0.084$) but without statistical significance [9]. A recent multicenter review of 215 patients comparing robotic and laparoscopic IPOM repairs showed that robotic hernia repairs were associated with comparable incidence of recurrence (7.7% versus 6.8%, $p = 1.0$), increased incidence of fascial closure rates (71% versus 54%, $p = 0.05$), and decreased surgical site occurrence (0.0% versus 6.8%, $p < 0.01$) with a propensity score matching indicating a decreased risk of recurrence (2.1% versus 4.2%, $p < 0.01$) when mean follow-up was 4.9 weeks for robotic repair and 6.0 weeks for laparoscopic repairs [15].

Prolonged operative time is a primary limitation of rIPOM compared to the laparoscopic approach. Currently, most studies identify an increased operative time with rIPOM compared to laparoscopic. Specifically, one retrospective review demonstrated average operative times of 127 minutes in robotic versus 67 minutes in laparoscopic ($p < 0.001$) [16]. Gonzalez et al. reported mean operative time of 107.6 minutes in their robotic group versus 87.9 minutes in their laparoscopic group ($p = 0.012$) [9]. A meta-analysis calculated a 52-minute longer operative time in robotic repairs versus laparoscopic repairs ($p = 0.04$) [13]. The aforementioned AHSQC review showed that 46% of rIPOM cases had an OR time of greater than 2 hours versus only 30% in the laparoscopic IPOM group ($p < 0.001$) [14]. Walker et al.'s multicenter review of 215 patients calculated a mean case length of 116.9 minutes in the robotic group compared to 98.7 minutes in the laparoscopic group ($p = 0.03$) [15].

Robotic IPOM offers a more feasible method of re-approximating the fascia prior to placing an intraperitoneal mesh compared to the laparoscopic IPOM and, in some studies, has been shown to have lower rates of surgical site occurrences. Most studies show that robotic repair has a longer operative time, which can be compensated by a shorter length of stay. rIPOM can be considered in patients when laparoscopic onlay mesh placement is particularly difficult, such as in obese patients, where transfascial suture placement and perpendicular tack placement are more ergonomically challenging. Additionally rIPOM can be utilized to facilitate primary fascial closure, potentially decreasing the incidence of postoperative seroma.

Robotic Pre-peritoneal Ventral Hernia Repair

Pre-peritoneal placement of mesh for ventral hernias offers the advantage of a peritoneal covering over the mesh, therefore avoiding intra-abdominal mesh placement. This can potentially reduce concerns associated with IPOM placement, which includes adhesions, seroma formation, and possibly chronic pain associated with tack and transfascial suture placement, none of which have been delineated with significance in the literature. This peritoneal covering is accomplished in a similar technique to robotic inguinal hernia via a transabdominal pre-peritoneal (TAPP) approach by raising peritoneal flaps around the defect where mesh will be placed and subsequently suturing closed the peritoneal defect over the mesh. Compared to onlay mesh placement, widespread adoption of pre-peritoneal mesh placement via traditional laparoscopy has been limited due to the technical difficulty of dissecting the pre-peritoneal plane along the anterior abdominal wall [17]. The robotic platform allows for easier dissection and closure of the pre-peritoneal plane, as well as the continued ease in closure of the fascial defect, as previously discussed with the rIPOM technique.

Pre-peritoneal repair of ventral hernias has been shown to be a feasible and safe approach and, when compared to robotic IPOM techniques, has not added significant operating time in certain single-institution studies—one retrospective review showed an average operative time of 167 minutes for rIPOM versus 158 minutes for pre-peritoneal repair ($p = 0.57$) [17]. In a single-institution comparison of different robotic hernia repair techniques for primary ventral hernias, pre-peritoneal mesh placement compared to rIPOM had a lower rate of minor complications (2.8% versus 12.2%, $p = 0.028$) and offered a higher mesh to defect overlap ratio compared to rIPOM [18]. Furthermore, intraperitoneal placed mesh was a risk factor for any grade of Clavien-Dindo postoperative complication [18]. As in rIPOM, approximation of fascial defects can be more consistently accomplished robotically compared with laparoscopy alone while also continuing to have the added benefit of less wound complications and pain that the laparoscopic techniques offer over an open repair technique. In the largest single surgeon series of robotic pre-peritoneal ventral hernia repair, the fascia was closed in all 54 patients and with only two post-operative complications, a seroma and a rectus sheath hematoma [19].

Robotic pre-peritoneal hernia repairs can be accomplished with a similar side effect profile to previously discussed rIPOM, with a potentially added benefit of placing mesh in a space that is isolated from the visceral contents. A robotic pre-peritoneal hernia repair may be advantageous in similar patients that would benefit from a rIPOM, such as in obese patients, a demographic at high risk for wound complications and in whom even laparoscopic surgery can be ergonomically challenging. As in rIPOM, fascial defect closure is more feasible than in laparoscopic ventral hernia repair. A preperitoneal repair could be attempted over robotic IPOM if a pre-peritoneal dissection if feasible to avoid intraperitoneal mesh placement.

Robotic Retrorectus and Transversus Abdominus Release (TAR)

The most ideal use of robotics techniques in ventral hernia repairs is to accomplish successful and durable repairs in patients that would have previously required an open repair. Due to the technical difficulty of a traditional laparoscopic repair, retromuscular dissections with transversus abdominis release (TAR) have been mostly limited to open approaches. However, given the increased range of motion of the robotic instruments, these dissections can be more easily accomplished robotically compared to laparoscopically. Retromuscular dissections with TAR offer the added benefit of bringing fascial edges back to their normal anatomic position in hernias whose defects would otherwise not be able to be approximated due to tension or defect size. Furthermore, in similar fashion to the previously described pre-peritoneal technique, mesh is placed in a retromuscular/pre-peritoneal position, thus preventing intraperitoneal mesh placement.

Robotic TAR (rTAR) is a relatively new technique, so data has been mostly limited to single-institution series and retrospective series but shows promise in its ability to significantly reduce length of stay but typically with longer operative times compared to open TAR repairs. A recent analysis from the Americas Hernias Society Quality Collaborative comparing propensity matched open and robotic retrorectus hernia repairs demonstrated that robotic repairs had a significantly decreased length of stay compared to open repairs (2 days versus 3 days, $p < 0.001$) without any differences in intraoperative complications, surgical site infections, reoperation, or readmissions, but with longer overall operative times [20]. A double institution case-matched review of a total of 114 patients showed a decreased length of stay of 1.3 days in the rTAR group versus 6.0 days in the open group ($p < 0.001$), however with prolonged operative times of 299 minutes in the rTAR versus 211 minutes in the open group ($p < 0.001$) [21]. Another single-institution retrospective review of 102 patients also demonstrated a decreased length of stay of 3.8 days in the rTAR group versus 7.1 days in the open group ($p < 0.01$), but also with prolonged operative times of 365 minutes versus 287 minutes ($p < 0.01$) [22]. Overall, although there is an increased operative time to complete a rTAR compared to an open TAR, surgeon learning curve must be considered given the advanced nature of this case. Additionally, costs incurred from prolonged operative time can theoretically be compensated through a significantly decreased length of stay when compared to open repairs.

Although data is new and evolving, the robotic retrorectus repair with TAR offers the most promising current use for robotics in repairing ventral hernias in a cost-effective and clinically effective method. It can be performed in place of open repairs while having comparable clinical results and decreased length of stay while also maintaining the technical benefits over traditional laparoscopy including extraperitoneal mesh placement, fascial defect closure, and avoidance of transfascial sutures. However, retrorectus repair with possible TAR is a technically challenging operation and should only be attempted robotically by surgeons who have significant experience with both complex open hernia repairs and robotics.

Robotic Extended (or Enhanced-View) Total Extraperitoneal Ventral Hernia Repair (eTEP)

Robotic eTEP ventral hernia repair utilizes the technical principles initially described and currently widely utilized in TEP inguinal hernia repairs. Access to the pre-peritoneal or retrorectus space is gained via direct cutdown or optical trocar, and repair is accomplished without accessing the intra-peritoneal space. After access, the surgical dissection and hernia repairs in the total extraperitoneal space can utilize aforementioned techniques of both the pre-peritoneal and retrorectus with TAR including defect closure, extraperito-neal mesh placement, and component separation. Additional benefits of robotic eTEP include complete exclusion of mesh from the peritoneal cavity without the requirement of closing the peritoneum or posterior sheath as is required in the other techniques that avoid mesh exposure to visceral contents. Robotic eTEPs have been adopted by some institutions that are previously adept in performing laparoscopic eTEP for ventral hernias, and their data has mostly been limited to retrospective institutional reports. Lu et al. reviewed 206 patients undergoing robotic versus laparoscopic eTEP and showed longer average operative times of 174 minutes in the robotic eTEP versus 120 minutes in the laparoscopic group ($p < 0.05$) and comparable recurrence rates of 1.2% in the robotic group versus 1.7% in the laparoscopic group ($p = 0.771$) at an average follow-up of 5.5 months [23]. Belyansky et al. looked at 37 patients who underwent robotic eTEP and had no intraoperative complications, two seromas with one requiring drainage, and one readmission for poor oral intake. There were no recurrences when mean follow-up was 36 days [24]. Overall robotic eTEP is a hernia repair tech-nique that has not yet been fully established in the surgical community but offers yet another repair option that may find a footing as robotic hernia repairs become more widely adopted.

Cost of Robotic Ventral Hernia Repair

The challenge of analyzing costs related to robotic ventral hernia repairs is that choosing the correct comparison control group is difficult. A single-institution review of robotic versus laparoscopic ventral hernia repairs has shown similar direct hospital costs between the two groups, specifically $13,943 in the laparoscopic group versus $19,532 in the robotic group

(p = 0.07) with a decreased length of stay in the robotic group (1 day versus 2 days, p = 0.004) [25]. However, a systematic review of the literature and meta-analysis showed generally increased overall costs [13]. Most recently, a multicenter, blinded randomized control trial of robotic versus laparoscopic IPOM technique showed increased overall costs at 90 days of $15,865 in the robotic group versus $12,955 in the laparoscopic group (p = 0.004) [26]. Many comparisons are made between traditional laparoscopic hernia repairs; however, robotics offers a tool that may be able to successfully repair more complex hernias that would have previously been repaired in an open technique, thus offering the added benefit of decreased surgical site occurrences and decreased length of stay, both of which contribute to cost [13]. Overall, analysis of robotic ventral hernias continues to show a higher overall cost compared to a traditional laparoscopic repair, with that additional cost being slightly lower in centers that perform high-volume robotic surgeries [16, 27].

Recent reviews have concluded that it may be possible to achieve reduced costs; however that has not yet been consistently displayed in the literature [28]. Cost offset of robotic ventral hernia repairs can be accomplished in several ways including efficient robotic instrument utilization, decreased operative time, and reducing mesh costs. Utilization of a simple uncoated pre-peritoneal mesh can potentially reduce the overall material cost compared to a coated intraperitoneal mesh. Pursuing use of a robotic ventral hernia repair in cases where length of stay could be significantly reduced, as has been shown in robotic TARs, avoids the additional hospital costs of overnight stays.

Ergonomics of Robotic Hernia Repairs

One of the touted benefits of the *da Vinci* robotic surgical system over traditional laparoscopy has been the improved ergonomics in sitting at a console and being able to work with improved posture, wristed instrumentation, and three-dimensional visualization. Anecdotally, many surgeons report improved comfort while operating on the console; however, little objective data has been found to display improved ergonomics, particularly to a degree that improves outcomes or surgeon performance. Some of the lack of clarity on ergonomics may be due to the possibility that like operating, managing the ergonomics on the console also takes experience to master. A survey of 289 gynecologic oncology surgeons showed that of surgeons who performed more than 200 robotic cases per year, 34% reported symptoms including finger, neck, back, shoulder, wrist, and eye discomfort versus 60% in those performing 50 or fewer cases per year [29].

Ergonomics in robotic surgery has been examined using the Rapid Upper Limb Assessment (RULA), which is a tool that assesses posture and movements of the neck, upper back, and upper limbs to identify motions that may put the subject at risk for injury [30]. The RULA score was used to examine surgeons during the only randomized controlled trial comparing laparoscopic and robotic TAPP inguinal hernias and showed no differences in overall scores. Specifically, when examining the grand composite score, which includes posture, upper arms, and wrists on each side of the body, the mean left and right grand composite scores for laparoscopic were 9.8 and 10.1 compared to 10.3 and 10.2 robotic ($p = 0.31$ and $p = 0.94$), demonstrating no difference in ergonomics between laparoscopic and robotic inguinal hernia repair [2]. Data on ergonomic benefits in robotic cases with longer operative times, more complex dissection, and obese patients is limited in the literature. More evidence and studies on the ergonomic benefits in robotics are warranted.

Conclusion

The use of minimally invasive techniques to repair inguinal and ventral hernias will continue to rise. The use of the *da Vinci* robotic surgical system to repair inguinal hernias can achieve clinical results similar to traditional laparoscopy but with additional cost and operative time. A robotic inguinal hernia repair can be considered in situations where a laparoscopic transabdominal pre-peritoneal approach is necessary but prior surgeon experience with laparoscopic TAPP is limited. Robotic ventral hernia repair offers a wide variety of repair techniques, many of which have been previously accomplished via traditional laparoscopy. However the robotic equivalent techniques can typically accomplish increased fascial closure rates and avoiding transfascial sutures. More research need to be conducted on the clinical benefits of increased fascial closure rates, but some studies point to a possible reduction in recurrence rates. Currently, the most promising use of the robot in ventral hernias is with retrorectus and transversus abdominis release wherein the traditional laparoscopic repair is not achievable; therefore the clinical benefits of reduced wound morbidity, decreased postoperative pain, and reduced length-of-stay compared to the open technique are obtainable. Cost-effective practices in robotic hernia repairs have generally not been able to reach costs that compete with traditional laparoscopy or open-repair techniques; however cost savings can occur if robotic repair techniques are chosen in situations that utilize cheaper non-coated mesh while reducing length of stay. Although touted and anecdotally reported as having an ergonomic benefit compared to traditional laparoscopy, more studies are required to examine the true ergonomic benefits in utilizing the *da Vinci* robotic surgical system.

References

1. Podolsky D, Novitsky Y. Robotic inguinal hernia repair. Surg Clin N Am. 2020;100:409–15.
2. Prabhu AS, Carbonell A, Hope W, Warren J, Higgins R, Jacob B, Blatnik J, Haskins I, Alkhatib H, Tastaldi L, Fafaj A, Tu C, Rosen MJ. Robotic inguinal vs transabdominal laparoscopic inguinal hernia repair: the RIVAL randomized clinical trial. JAMA Surg. 2020;155:380.

3. Pokala B, Armijo PR, Flores L, Hennings D, Oleynikov D. Minimally invasive inguinal hernia repair is superior to open: a national database review. Hernia. 2019;23:593–9.
4. Abdelmoaty WF, Dunst CM, Neighorn C, Swanstrom LL, Hammill CW. Robotic-assisted versus laparoscopic unilateral inguinal hernia repair: a comprehensive cost analysis. Surg Endosc. 2019;33:3436–43.
5. Khoraki J, Gomez PP, Mazzini GS, Pessoa BM, Browning MG, Aquilina GR, Salluzzo JL, Wolfe LG, Campos GM. Perioperative outcomes and cost of robotic-assisted versus laparoscopic inguinal hernia repair. Surg Endosc. 2020;34:3496–507.
6. Aiolfi A, Cavalli M, Micheletto G, Bruni PG, Lombardo F, Perali C, Bonitta G, Bona D. Robotic inguinal hernia repair: is technology taking over? Systematic review and meta-analysis. Hernia. 2019;23:509–19.
7. The Prospective Hernia Study Group, LeBlanc K, Dickens E, Gonzalez A, Gamagami R, Pierce R, Balentine C, Voeller G. Prospective, multicenter, pairwise analysis of robotic-assisted inguinal hernia repair with open and laparoscopic inguinal hernia repair: early results from the Prospective Hernia Study. Hernia. 2020;
8. Pokala B, Armijo PR, Flores L, Hennings D, Oleynikov D. Minimally invasive inguinal hernia repair is superior to open: a national database review. Hernia. 2019;23:593–9.
9. Gonzalez A, Escobar E, Romero R, Walker G, Mejias J, Gallas M, Dickens E, Johnson CJ, Rabaza J, Kudsi OY. Robotic-assisted ventral hernia repair: a multicenter evaluation of clinical outcomes. Surg Endosc. 2017;31:1342–9.
10. Clapp ML, Hicks SC, Awad SS, Liang MK. Trans-cutaneous closure of central defects (TCCD) in laparoscopic ventral hernia repairs (LVHR). World J Surg. 2013;37:42–51.
11. Nguyen DH, Nguyen MT, Askenasy EP, Kao LS, Liang MK. Primary fascial closure with laparoscopic ventral hernia repair: systematic review. World J Surg. 2014;38:3097–104.
12. Fuenmayor P, Lujan HJ, Plasencia G, Karmaker A, Mata W, Vecin N. Robotic-assisted ventral and incisional hernia repair with hernia defect closure and intraperitoneal onlay mesh (IPOM) experience. J Robotic Surg. 2020;14(5):695–701.
13. Henriksen NA, Jensen KK, Muysoms F. Robot-assisted abdominal wall surgery: a systematic review of the literature and meta-analysis. Hernia. 2019;23:17–27.

14. Prabhu AS, Dickens EO, Copper CM, Mann JW, Yunis JP, Phillips S, Huang L-C, Poulose BK, Rosen MJ. Laparoscopic vs robotic intraperitoneal mesh repair for incisional hernia: an Americas Hernia Society Quality Collaborative Analysis. J Am Coll Surg. 2017;225:285–93.
15. Walker PA, May AC, Mo J, Cherla DV, Santillan MR, Kim S, Ryan H, Shah SK, Wilson EB, Tsuda S. Multicenter review of robotic versus laparoscopic ventral hernia repair: is there a role for robotics? Surg Endosc. 2018;32:1901–5.
16. Zayan NE, Meara MP, Schwartz JS, Narula VK. A direct comparison of robotic and laparoscopic hernia repair: patient-reported outcomes and cost analysis. Hernia. 2019;23:1115–21.
17. Kennedy M, Barrera K, Akelik A, Constable Y, Smith M, Chung P, Sugiyama G. Robotic TAPP ventral hernia repair: early lessons learned at an inner city safety net hospital. JSLS. 2018;22:e2017.00070.
18. Kudsi OY, Gokcal F. Lateral approach totally extraperitoneal (TEP) robotic retromuscular ventral hernia repair. Hernia. 2021;25(1):211–22.
19. Orthopoulos G, Kudsi OY. Feasibility of robotic-assisted transabdominal preperitoneal ventral hernia repair. J Laparoendoscop Adv Surg Tech. 2018;28:434–8.
20. Carbonell AM, Warren JA, Prabhu AS, Ballecer CD, Janczyk RJ, Herrera J, Huang L-C, Phillips S, Rosen MJ, Poulose BK. Reducing length of stay using a robotic-assisted approach for retromuscular ventral hernia repair: a comparative analysis from the Americas Hernia Society Quality Collaborative. Ann Surg. 2018;267:210–7.
21. Martin-del-Campo LA, Weltz AS, Belyansky I, Novitsky YW. Comparative analysis of perioperative outcomes of robotic versus open transversus abdominis release. Surg Endosc. 2018;32:840–5.
22. Bittner JG, Alrefai S, Vy M, Mabe M, Del Prado PAR, Clingempeel NL. Comparative analysis of open and robotic transversus abdominis release for ventral hernia repair. Surg Endosc. 2018;32:727–34.
23. Lu R, Addo A, Ewart Z, Broda A, Parlacoski S, Zahiri HR, Belyansky I. Comparative review of outcomes: laparoscopic and robotic enhanced-view totally extraperitoneal (eTEP) access retrorectus repairs. Surg Endosc. 2020;34:3597–605.
24. Belyansky I, Reza Zahiri H, Sanford Z, Weltz AS, Park A. Early operative outcomes of endoscopic (eTEP access) robotic-

assisted retromuscular abdominal wall hernia repair. Hernia. 2018;22:837–47.

25. Warren JA, Cobb WS, Ewing JA, Carbonell AM. Standard laparoscopic versus robotic retromuscular ventral hernia repair. Surg Endosc. 2017;31:324–32.

26. Olavarria OA, Bernardi K, Shah SK, Wilson TD, Wei S, Pedroza C, Avritscher EB, Loor MM, Ko TC, Kao LS, Liang MK. Robotic versus laparoscopic ventral hernia repair: multicenter, blinded randomized controlled trial. BMJ. 2020;370:m2457.

27. Khorgami Z, Li WT, Jackson TN, Howard CA, Sclabas GM. The cost of robotics: an analysis of the added costs of robotic-assisted versus laparoscopic surgery using the National Inpatient Sample. Surg Endosc. 2019;33:2217–21.

28. Nikolian VC, Coleman NL, Podolsky D, Novitsky YW. Robotic-assisted transabdominal preperitoneal ventral hernia repair. Surg Technol Int. 2020;36:95–7.

29. Lee MR, Lee GI. Does a robotic surgery approach offer optimal ergonomics to gynecologic surgeons?: a comprehensive ergonomics survey study in gynecologic robotic surgery. J Gynecol Oncol. 2017;28:e70.

30. McAtamney L, Nigel CE. RULA: a survey method for the investigation of work-related upper limb disorders. Appl Ergon. 1993;24(2):91–9.

Chapter 47
The Consistent Operating Room Team

Leena Khaitan and Joseph Youssef

Objectives

1. What are the measurable impacts of team consistency?
2. What are the pros and cons of team consistency vs cross-trained teams?

Introduction

A team is defined as a group of people who perform interdependent tasks to achieve a common objective. In healthcare, there are many types of teams. For example, they can vary from teams whose members work together often and are highly specialized, such as a team in a cardiac catheterization suite, to teams who sporadically come together for temporary measures, such as the stroke or trauma team. In the operating room, a typical team includes anesthesiologists and/or nurse anesthetists, surgeons, residents, nurses, physician assistants, and technicians.

L. Khaitan (✉) · J. Youssef
University Hospitals, Department of Surgery, Cleveland, OH, USA
e-mail: leena.khaitan@uhhospitals.org;
joseph.youssef@uhhospitals.org

© The Author(s), under exclusive license to Springer Nature   907
Switzerland AG 2022
J. R. Romanelli et al. (eds.), *The SAGES Manual of Quality,
Outcomes and Patient Safety*,
https://doi.org/10.1007/978-3-030-94610-4_47

Several studies have shown that team training in the operating room can improve efficiency and improve the culture of patient safety [1]. It is evident in this era of healthcare that teams need to be optimized to deliver the best performance in accomplishing care. To achieve optimization, emphasis has been placed on teamwork through effective communication between those team members and a culture of safety. Teams are structured within this paradigm and objectives can be met utilizing different formats. In this chapter, the importance and impact of team training and team interaction in the operating room environment will be reviewed. Methodologies to achieve these goals will also be discussed.

Types of Teams

Cross-Trained Team

One emerging team structure is the cross-trained team. There are several definitions for what a cross-trained team is—one of which is some or every team member has been trained to perform other job functions than their primary designated function. For example, a scrub technician may help transport the patient, or a post-anesthesia care unit (PACU) nurse may rotate into the operating room and assist the circulating nurse. Another definition, which will be the primary focus of this chapter, is that team members are trained to perform their respective duties in a wide variety of procedures and circumstances. In essence, each team member becomes a "Jack of all trades, master of none." An example of this is a scrub technician or a physician assistant who has been trained for a wide variety of specialty cases, such as a member of the orthopedic team assisting in a bariatric case.

Cross-trained teams are not a new phenomenon but rather something that has been advocated by other industries as well as sports and the military. For example, in sports, by mixing different exercises for players, coaches can prevent overuse injuries, balance development, and avoid monotony. In the military, operational success is dependent on each team member's understanding of each other's roles and tasks. This is primarily to ensure that if one member is unable to continue, others can replace them and accomplish the mission at hand. In industry, cross-trained teams of employees help increase productivity and mitigate risk and inefficiency.

Team members involved in cross-training programs become proficient at tasks outside the usual limitations of their job. Hence, they can anticipate and help with the needs of other team members. For their employers, this also provides more flexibility. It makes it easier for employers to seamlessly fill in certain employees for a variety of tasks. By ensuring that team members are trained for multiple roles, it is easier to respond to and troubleshoot problems and mitigate disasters.

By providing scheduling flexibility, cross-trained team members are better suited to meeting varied operating room demands. For example, in Geisinger Health System in Pennsylvania, two centers with different team paradigms were set up to deal with thrombectomies for stroke patients. Center A utilized a cross-trained team that was trained in both operating and neuroendovascular procedures, while Center B maintained a dedicated on-call neuroendovascular team. When comparing the effectiveness of both teams, successful reperfusion was achieved in 98% and 97% of cases in Centers A and B, respectively ($p = 0.79$), but door-to-puncture time differed significantly between 50 minutes in center A compared to 121 minutes in center B (58% reduction, $p < 0.02$) [2]. This is due to Center A relying on in-house staff members that are trained to fit in different roles whenever it is asked of them. Center B relied on a highly trained specialty-specific team. These teams are more experienced in their specific specialties but logistically require more time to mobilize.

Cross-trained teams can be more economical as members of the staff can fill different functions. Larger institutions with more financial resources are more adept at having multiple specialty-specific teams. The smaller surgical department, however, may only have a limited number of staff members. Thus, cross-training those few staff members becomes imperative to handle the wide variety of procedures that need to be performed.

Consistent Teams

On the other end of the spectrum of team models is a paradigm of consistency in team members and their functions, i.e., each member is tasked with certain functions that do not change. This type of team has been espoused by other fields as well. In sports, it is equivalent to special teams on an NFL professional team or the special tactical unit in the police force or military. For these teams, there are clear expectations for each team member's functions, responsibilities, and accountabilities. This helps to optimize the team's efficiency toward a concentrated goal. In the setting of an operating room, these teams are typically trained toward a particular surgery or set of surgeries and spend the majority of their time performing these procedures. Members of the team would function in their primary designated function but would work as such in a dedicated subspecialty.

Consistent teams affect multiple factors when it comes to the operating room. Communication, for example, is more effective in teams that have worked together longer and have familiarity with each other. This, in turn, causes increased efficiencies, as demonstrated by one study, in which there was an average of 5.1% time gain per similar case performed within the same day with the same team. This consistency builds trust among team members; thus, individual team members can rely on dependable working conditions, knowing the reliability and acumen of each team member through experience and consistent feedback [3]. The effects of this consistency can outlast just same-day similar surgeries. In another study, which examined 754 cases of bilateral reduction mammoplasty procedures over 12 years, there was a reduction of 16 minutes of operative time as the team members became familiarized with one another [4].

As surgical departments try to rein in spending and cut costs, they must find the optimal level of efficiency to take advantage of their infrastructure, equipment, and team setup. In one study, it was demonstrated that it is possible to increase operating room efficiency by changing the patient flow from patients linearly moving through their operative day to one of parallel processing. In this model, the team members are effectively able to work on two patients simultaneously. To achieve this, each member had a well-defined role, and the team acted as a unit. Therefore, by mandating consistent teams, there was a reduction of overall costs per case [5]. To achieve this model, additional personnel may be needed. However, cost-effectiveness analysis suggests that the additional costs incurred by higher staffing ratios are likely to be offset by increases in throughput [6]. To increase efficiency utilizing this team model, it is important to have a high volume of surgery. The more surgeries performed, the more opportunity teams have to work together and thus contribute to the team's overall effectiveness.

Factors Affected by Team Format

Communication

The concept of a culture of safety has been featured prominently in the literature on quality and outcomes. At the heart of the culture for safety is effective communication between team members. Operating room safety does not just happen organically, but rather it is largely a result of the behaviors and attitudes of the involved individuals and how well they communicate [7]. In the operating room, communicative events were found to be clustered around certain phases: patient preparation, the start of the procedure, moments where surgery is difficult, the conclusion of the procedure, and patient hand-off [8].

Team dynamics play a large role in how effective communication is. Team members' familiarity with one another and comfort level in addressing each other play a significant role in how effective the team is in maintaining the appropriate culture and addressing common concerns that arise in the operating room (Table 47.1). The consistent team members are aware of the equipment needed for the procedure and how to prepare the patient. They can get the patient on the table and have the room appropriately ready faster than their counterparts on cross-trained teams [9]. Thus, at least in the phases of communicative clusters, at the beginning and end of cases, it is more optimal to have a consistent team. The authors also made this observation when looking at the importance of team consistency in their own experience. They also noted that with consistent teams, the setup time and time after surgery out of the operating room were shorter with a consistent team [16].

Additionally, team members of a consistent team are more likely to know the goal of the operation and the procedure steps as compared to members of a cross-trained team [10]. This will give them more confidence in speaking up on safety issues as well as bring up concerns regarding steps in the procedure as they become more familiarized with the procedure [11].

TABLE 47.1 Common concerns in the operating room

Coordinating patient preparedness (room readiness, cancellation)

Resources (locating correct equipment, troubleshooting equipment)

Staffing (assign particular staff to cases, coordinating coverage during breaks)

Safety (timeout, operating room fire, instrument counts)

Error Reduction

In the operating room, situations can arise in which the team has to act quickly and decisively in response to changing conditions. This has to be achieved without necessarily being able to halt surgery to discuss the best plan of action. To be successful in the operating room, teams need to intuitively know what to do and how to do it together efficiently. To do this, they need a good shared mental model. A shared mental model is a "knowledge structure held by each member of a team that enables them to form accurate explanations and expectations…and in turn, to coordinate their actions and adapt their behavior to demands of the task and other team members" [12].

A shared mental model is the notion of being on the "same page." Team members who are part of consistent teams will, over time, develop a shared mental model through repetition of the procedure. This, in turn, allows for error reduction and the ability to meet challenges as they arise. This can be attributed to team members identifying errors or potential errors due to previous encounters of similar problems or due to knowing the capabilities and shortcomings of the team members at hand [13].

In one study, questionnaires were given to surgical teams performing video-assisted thoracoscopic surgery to assess their shared mental model [14]. The questions addressed three overall topics, namely, (1) risk assessment of the procedure, (2) familiarity with team members/perception of those team members' skills, and (3) recognition of challenges arising during the operation for different team members. As noted in Fig. 47.1, the team member who was most familiar with the team and who team members, in turn, felt most familiar with was the surgeon. This has important ramifications regarding leadership and guidance of the procedure to a resolution safely. More importantly though were the final results of the questionnaire: it noted that only one-third of perceived problems were identified by other team members, as outlined in Table 47.2.

The data suggests that despite some level of familiarity, perceptions of other team members' challenges may not be recognized by other team members. This study also suggests that as teams become more familiar, they demonstrate a greater degree of concordance for each other's perceived skill levels as well as recognizing other member's challenges. Furthermore, this mutual understanding also improves adaptive coordination within teams which is essential for overall performance. As teams became more consistent, there was an improvement in recognizing challenges. For cross-trained teams, it is important to have explicit coordination strategies to obtain shared mental models that can help compensate for lack of familiarity [15].

It is also important to note that consistent teams may also have limitations. Team members who have the same mental

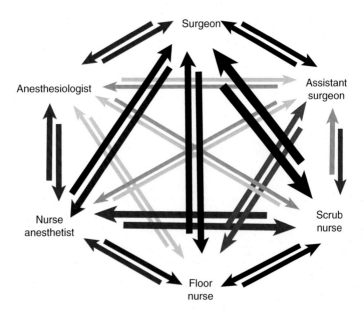

FIGURE 47.1 Familiarity within the team. Each arrow represents the mean familiarity of one team member toward another team member; darker and thicker arrows represent higher familiarity. (Reproduced from Gjeraa et al. [14])

TABLE 47.2 Team members' awareness of other team members' challenges or problems, as percentage of self-identified problems and challenges

| Awareness of challenges/ problems | Problems of | | | | | | Team member's awareness (average) |
	Surgeon	AS	SN	FN	Anesth	NA	
Surgeon	...	44	22	27	65	60	44
Assistant surgeon	48	...	0	27	58	50	37
Scrub nurse	27	47	...	27	49	35	37
Floor nurse	24	44	25	...	17	15	25
Anesthesiologist	35	31	33	40	...	32	34
Nurse anesthetist	27	31	22	30	47	...	32
Rest of team (average)	32	39	21	30	47	38	35

Reproduced from Gjeraa et al. [14]
Anesth anesthesiologist, *AS* assistant surgeon, *FN* floor nurse, *NA* nurse anesthetist, *SN* scrub nurse

model may also hinder the goal of the team through "group think." This term refers to a situation in which team members all have a consensus of a mental model, but the mental model is incorrect. Also, familiar teams are less innovative when faced with new problems. This is an area where cross-trained team members may be more advantageous. They can provide a different lens by which the challenge can be met and can bring experience from other specialties to use in dealing with the procedure at hand.

Team members possessing a common understanding of the case at hand, including its major steps and points at which challenges are most likely to be encountered, do better than teams that do not. However, one way to mitigate this is through creating specialty-specific preoperative briefings [16]. This will help decrease surgical flow disruptions as well as improve patient safety [17].

OR Efficiency

The operating room is a complex dynamic work environment. It requires multiple professionals to interact with each other as well as with complicated technologies seamlessly. This must be done with safe and effective patient care as the primary goal, but it is also important for it to be efficient. As discussed earlier, in large hospital settings, it is common that during the day, personnel are utilized across many different ORs and different types of surgeries. Although the staff members may be adequately prepared for some of these surgeries through prior experience, it is possible that some members will not be familiar with the procedures or surgeon at all. For staff who have been part of the team during previous surgeries, it is also possible for them to require a period of familiarization time at the beginning of the surgical procedure or during it. This can form an obstacle for smooth workflow and reduce efficiency.

In one study in the Netherlands, scheduling similar consecutive cases and performing them with a consistent team resulted in faster case time and lower turnover and preparation time. The study focused on two procedures: an open inguinal hernia repair and a laparoscopic cholecystectomy. The procedure time of the inguinal hernia repair decreased significantly and had practical scheduling implications. Surgeons were able to increase the number of cases they perform per day due to an increase in efficiency. For the more complex operation, laparoscopic cholecystectomy, there was no significant effect on procedure time, but there was a decrease in turnover time [18].

In our institution, we observed similar results. Operating room data was obtained for 180 cases of laparoscopic Roux-en-Y bypasses performed at two hospitals. One hospital had a highly consistent operating room team (eight circulating and scrub nurses, four anesthetists, three anesthesiologists), and the other had much greater variability of staff (39 circulating nurses, 57 scrub nurses/technicians, 59 anesthetists or anesthesia residents, 24 anesthesiologists).

There was no statistical difference between the total mean OR time. However, the preparation and turnover time for cases were shorter in the hospital with a consistent operating room team [19].

Training

Multiple modalities exist for training, including on-the-job training, apprenticeship, as well as simulation models. On-the-job training is an explicit type of training where team members are instructed via targeted information and observed as they perform their duties. This is followed up by feedback based on observed performance. An example of this is when a new surgical assistant is placed with the surgeon, and instructions with feedback are continuously given throughout the operation. In an apprenticeship model, new team members are paired with coworkers who have more experience. The older team members mentor and advise on how to succeed in that particular team role. The newer team members observe, learn, and assimilate the different responsibilities of their role. For example, a new scrub technician may shadow a more experienced scrub technician to learn the steps and responsibilities of a particular surgery before attempting them on their own. In the simulation model, the goal is to replace real experiences with guided and immersive replicas. Team members are immersed in surgical settings that evoke or replicate what they may encounter during surgery.

The goal of any training should be to ensure patient safety while providing an optimal training environment. Another goal is to increase productivity and efficiency. Simulation-based training can be the answer to foster those goals regardless of the team configuration. Simulations can be used to expose the team members to the steps and conditions of the surgery. It allows for knowledge sharing and feedback to be done in a setting without the possibility of patient harm. This gives team members access to valuable information not just on the steps needed to get the job done but also on the skills and capabilities of other team members. The feedback on potential errors, which might otherwise be missed during the usual clinical setting, can be exposed during the simulation and prevented [20]. A simulated environment allows the team members to grow, learn, and be challenged. Additionally, simulation scenarios can be created from basic common experiences or atypical experiences that the team may encounter, thus preparing the team for a myriad of possibilities. This can be particularly effective when preparing to perform a new procedure for the first time in the operating room.

Team members with proper training have improved efficiency and productivity. There is less wasting of time and resources. Training also improves morale as team members are more likely to feel confident if they feel more prepared for the surgeries. This causes less team turnover. Most importantly, fewer mistakes occur if team members do not lack the knowledge and skills required for the job. The more proficient each team member becomes, the less likely an error will occur.

Conclusion

The reality of most operating room teams is perhaps a hybrid between the consistent team and the cross-trained team models. Operating rooms utilize nurses, technicians, anesthesiologists, and physician assistants in their functional capacity but in an ever-shuffling mix as per the demands of the operating schedule as well as logistical and staffing issues. Additionally, as to be expected in emergency surgery, most operating room teams form ad hoc for the procedure. Thus, it is commonplace for the surgeon to have a team consisting of different members for different procedures throughout the operative day. This is most evident as the institutions become larger as they can employ dozens to hundreds of operating room staff.

Ultimately, having a large operating room staff that is not organized into teams results in team members working loosely together and never developing the same cohesiveness as a pure, consistent team should. It is for this reason that team training in surgery is paramount to having a safe and efficient operating room that communicates effectively with mutual respect among all members of the team. The surgeon, regardless of the team format, must first be a team player but also a leader. They must establish a clear vision for the case, provide the knowledge and method by which that goal can be achieved, and coordinate/balance the conflicting interests of all team members—avoiding the hierarchical model and realizing that every member in the operating room is equally important in achieving the best patient care results in a better "team" environment. As leaders, they must demonstrate that leadership by taking all concerns into account in a safe manner and providing an environment whereby team members are encouraged to speak about their concerns and feel that their concerns matter to everyone on the team, all in the name of patient safety.

Through team training, improvements in operating room efficiency, quality of care, operating time, turnover time, and overall team morale can all be improved and optimized.

References

1. Armour Forse R, Bramble JD, McQuillan R. Team training can improve operating room performance. Surgery. 2011;150(4):771–8. https://doi.org/10.1016/j.surg.2011.07.076.
2. Callahan AM, et al. Abstract TP239: cross-training in-hospital operating staff significantly improves door-to-puncture time in thrombectomy patients. Stroke. 12 Feb. 2020. www.ahajounals.org/doi/abs/10.1161/str.51.suppl_1.TP239. Accessed 18 Feb 2021.
3. Stepaniak PS, Heij C, Buise MP, Mannaerts GHH, Smulders JF, Nienhuijs SW. Bariatric surgery with operating room teams that stayed fixed during the day. Anesth Analg. 2012;115(6):1384–92. https://doi.org/10.1213/ANE.0b013e31826c7fa6.
4. Xu RAB, Carty MJ, Orgill DP, Lipsitz SR, Duclos A. The teaming curve. Ann Surg. 2013;258(6):953–7. https://doi.org/10.1097/SLA.0b013e3182864ffe.

5. Friedman DM, Sokal SM, Chang Y, Berger DL. Increasing operating room efficiency through parallel processing. Ann Surg. 2006;243(1):10–4. https://doi.org/10.1097/01. sla.0000193600.97748.b1.

6. Stahl JE, Sandberg WS, Daily B, Wiklund R, Egan MT, Goldman JM, Isaacson KB, Gazelle S, Rattner DW. Reorganizing patient care and workflow in the operating room: a cost-effectiveness study. Surgery. 2006;139(6):717–28. https://doi.org/10.1016/j. surg.2005.12.006. PMID: 16782425.

7. Yates GR, Hochman RF, Sayles SM, et al. Sentara Norfolk General Hospital: accelerating improvement by focusing on building a culture of safety. Jt Comm J Qual Saf. 2004;30(10):534–42.

8. Lingard L, Reznick R, Espin S, Regehr G, DeVito I. Team communications in the operating room: talk patterns, sites of tension, and implications for novices. Acad Med. 2002;77(3):232–7. https:// doi.org/10.1097/00001888-200203000-00013. PMID: 11891163.

9. Cendán JC, Good M. Interdisciplinary workflow assessment and redesign decreases operating room turnover time and allows for additional caseload. Arch Surg. 2006;141(1):65–9. https://doi. org/10.1001/archsurg.141.1.65; discussion 70. PMID: 16415413.

10. Haig KM, Sutton S, Whittington J. SBAR: a shared mental model for improving communication between clinicians. Jt Comm J Qual Patient Saf. 2006;32(3):167–75.

11. Fagin CM. Collaboration between nurses and physicians. Academic Med. 1992;67(5):295–303.

12. Cannon-Bowers JA, Salas E, Converse SA. Shared mental models in expert team decision-making. In: Castellan Jr NJ, editor. Current issues in individual and group decision making. Hillsdale, NJ: Erlbaum; 1993. p. 221–46.

13. Gjeraa K, Dieckmann P, Spanager L, Petersen RH, Østergaard D, Park YS, Konge L. Exploring shared mental models of surgical teams in video-assisted Thoracoscopic surgery lobectomy. Ann Thorac Surg. 2019;107(3):954–61. https://doi.org/10.1016/j. athoracsur.2018.08.010. Epub 2018 Oct 4. PMID: 30292841.

14. Gjeraa K, et al. Exploring shared mental models of surgical teams in video-assisted thoracoscopic surgery lobectomy. Ann Thorac Surg. 2019;107(3):954–61.

15. Burtscher MJ, Kolbe M, Wacker J, Manser T. Interactions of team mental models and monitoring behaviors predict team performance in simulated anesthesia inductions. J Exp Psychol Appl. 2011;17:257–26.

16. Henrickson SE, Wadhera RK, Elbardissi AW, Wiegmann DA, Sundt TM 3rd. Development and pilot evaluation of a preoperative briefing protocol for cardiovascular surgery. J Am Coll Surg. 2009;208(6):1115–23. https://doi.org/10.1016/j.jamcollsurg.2009.01.037. Epub 2009 Apr 17. PMID: 19476900; PMCID: PMC4282162.
17. Nundy S, Mukherjee A, Sexton JB, et al. Impact of preoperative briefings on operating room delays: a preliminary report. Arch Surg. 2008;143(11):68–72.
18. Stepaniak PS, Vrijland WW, de Quelerij M, de Vries G, Heij C. Working with a fixed operating room team on consecutive similar cases and the effect on case duration and turnover time. Arch Surg. 2010;145(12):1165–70. https://doi.org/10.1001/archsurg.2010.255. PMID: 21173290.
19. Lam W, Kim GY, Petro C, Alhaj Saleh A, Khaitan L. Bariatric efficiency at an academic tertiary care center. Surg Endosc. 2020;34(6):2567–71. https://doi.org/10.1007/s00464-020-07507-6. Epub 2020 Mar 27. Erratum in: Surg Endosc. 2020 Apr 16;: PMID: 32221751.
20. Grogan EL, Stiles RA, France DJ, et al. The impact of aviation-based teamwork training on the attitudes of health-care professionals. J Am Coll Surg. 2004;199:843–8.

Chapter 48
Prevention of Common Bile Duct Injury: What Are we as Surgeons Doing to Prevent Injury

Nabajit Choudhury, Manoj Kumar Choudhury, and Rebecca B. Kowalski

History of Common Bile Duct Injury

Anatomical knowledge of the biliary tree has been traced back as far as 2000 BC [1]. Gallstone disease was found in a mummy from Egypt from around 1500 BC [1]. In contrast, the history of gallbladder surgery is relatively brief. The first

N. Choudhury (✉)
The University of Tennessee Health Science Center,
Memphis, TN, USA
e-mail: nchoudh2@uthsc.edu

M. K. Choudhury
Senior Consultant, GI and MIS, Nemcare Superspecialty Hospital,
Assam, India

R. B. Kowalski
Northwell Health at Lenox Hill Hospital, New York, NY, USA
e-mail: RKowalski@northwell.edu

© The Author(s), under exclusive license to Springer Nature   923
Switzerland AG 2022
J. R. Romanelli et al. (eds.), *The SAGES Manual of Quality,
Outcomes and Patient Safety*,
https://doi.org/10.1007/978-3-030-94610-4_48

surgical interventions on the biliary tree were removal of gallstones by Fabricus in 1618 [1] and creation of a cholecystostomy by Bobbs in 1867 [1]. The creation of a cholecystostomy provided temporary relief but led to other issues, namely, persistent pain and fistulas [2]. This was the standard treatment for biliary disease until Carl Langenbuch performed the first cholecystectomy in 1882 [1, 2]. By 1897, over 100 cholecystectomies had been performed [2]. Courvoisier performed the first choledochotomy in 1890 [1]. The first iatrogenic bile duct injury was described by Sprengel in 1891 [1], and the first choledochoduodenostomy was also performed by Sprengel in a patient whose distal common bile duct (CBD) was unable to be cleared of stones following a cholecystectomy [1]. The first intraoperative cholangiogram was performed by Mirizzi in 1931 [3]. In 1985, Erich Mühe performed the first laparoscopic cholecystectomy, and the surgical treatment of biliary disease was transformed. Unfortunately, one of the unexpected consequences of the rapid adaptation of the new surgical technique of laparoscopic cholecystectomy was a two- to fourfold increase in the rate of bile duct injury compared to open cholecystectomy: the rate of bile duct injury (BDI) is estimated to be approximately 0.2% by Roslyn et al. in an analysis of 42,474 patients undergoing open cholecystectomy [4] and up to 0.5% in an analysis of 40 series by MacFayden et al. in 114,005 patients undergoing laparoscopic cholecystectomy [5]. Unfortunately, despite the many advantages of laparoscopic cholecystectomy, the rate of bile duct injury remains higher in laparoscopic cholecystectomy than in open cholecystectomy. There is significant morbidity associated with bile duct injury [6–9] and a significant alteration in the patient's life after this devastating complication.

Multiple studies have been done to try to identify bile duct injury prevention strategies during laparoscopic cholecystectomy. Since the overall incidence is low, definitive studies to compare the techniques will likely never be performed [10]. However, these studies have identified factors that are related to an increased risk of bile duct injury, including timing of the procedure and patient selection [11–15]. Two of the most frequently used techniques are clear identification of the Critical View of Safety, which was first described by Strasberg et al. over 25 years ago [11, 16], and intraoperative cholangiography.

SAGES Safe Cholecystectomy Task Force

The SAGES Safe Cholecystectomy Task Force was launched in 2014 to tackle the issue of educating residents, fellows, and practicing surgeons about technical steps to prevent bile duct injury, such as the Critical View of Safety and intraoperative biliary imaging [17]. There are six steps recommended by the Safe Cholecystectomy Task Force to help reduce the incidence of BDI [10]:

1. Use the Critical View of Safety (CVS) method of identification of the cystic duct and cystic artery during laparoscopic cholecystectomy. Three criteria are required to achieve the CVS:

    (a) The hepatocystic triangle is cleared of fat and fibrous tissue. The hepatocystic triangle is defined as the triangle formed by the cystic duct, the common hepatic duct, and inferior edge of the liver. The common bile duct and common hepatic duct do not have to be exposed.

    (b) The lower one third of the gallbladder is separated from the liver to expose the cystic plate. The cystic plate is also known as liver bed of the gallbladder and lies in the gallbladder fossa.

    (c) Two and only two structures should be seen entering the gallbladder (see Fig. 48.1a and b).

2. Understand the potential for aberrant anatomy in all cases.

    (a) Aberrant anatomy may include a short cystic duct, aberrant hepatic ducts, or a right hepatic artery that

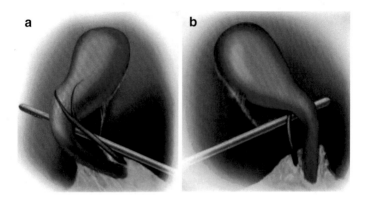

FIGURE 48.1 (**a**). The critical view of safety: anterior view [10]. (**b**) The critical view of safety: posterior view [10]

crosses anterior to the common bile duct. These are some but not all common variants.

3. Make liberal use of cholangiography or other methods to image the biliary tree intraoperatively.

   (a) Cholangiography may be especially important in difficult cases or unclear anatomy.
   (b) Several studies have found that cholangiography reduces the incidence and extent of bile duct injury but controversy remains on this subject.

4. Consider an intraoperative momentary pause during laparoscopic cholecystectomy prior to clipping, cutting, or transecting any ductal structures.

   (a) The intraoperative momentary pause should consist of a stop point in the operation to confirm that the CVS has been achieved utilizing the doublet view.

5. Recognize when the dissection is approaching a zone of significant risk and halt the dissection before entering the zone. Finish the operation by a safe method other than cholecystectomy if conditions around the gallbladder are too dangerous.

(a) In situations in which there is severe inflammation in the porta hepatis and neck of the gallbladder, the CVS can be difficult to achieve. The sole fact that achieving a CVS appears not feasible is a key benefit of the method since it alerts the surgeon to possible danger of injury.

(b) The surgical judgment that a zone of significant risk is being approached can be made when there is failure to obtain adequate exposure of the anatomy of the hepatocystic triangle or when the dissection is not progressing due to bleeding, inflammation, or fibrosis.

(c) Consider laparoscopic subtotal cholecystectomy or cholecystostomy tube placement and/or conversion to an open procedure based on the judgment of the attending surgeon.

6. Get help from another surgeon when the dissection or conditions are difficult.

(a) When it is practical to obtain, the advice of a second surgeon is often very helpful under conditions in which the dissection is stalled or the anatomy is unclear or under other conditions deemed "difficult" by the surgeon.

Intraoperative Cholangiography

In addition to achieving the CVS, intraoperative cholangiography (IOC) is a critical tool during laparoscopic or open cholecystectomy to identify anatomical abnormalities or unclear biliary anatomy. There has been significant debate about routine versus selective cholangiography [7, 17–23]. While IOC may help in early identification of bile duct injuries, it does not in and of itself prevent bile duct injuries [17].

Indications for IOC include abnormal liver function tests, suspicion of CBD stone on preoperative imaging, CBD diameter more than 6 mm, history of jaundice, history of pancreatitis or cholangitis without preoperative ERCP, presence of unclear biliary anatomy due to congenital anomalies, distorted anatomy due to pathological process of the gallbladder, identification of bile duct injury, determination of the severity of bile duct injury, or detection of bile leakage.

Other intraoperative techniques such as choledochoscopy or common bile duct exploration (CBDE) can be similarly helpful in the management of choledocholithiasis and its complications. Additional intraoperative techniques and tools include a variety of dissection techniques such as "top-down" dissection if the infundibulum of the gallbladder is difficult; landmark techniques such as Rouvière's sulcus, which indicates the plane of the main bile duct, where any dissection below this point is avoided in order to eliminate any danger to the bile duct during surgery [24]; intraoperative ultrasound; and intraoperative fluorescence cholangiography.

In the future, ultrasound and intraoperative fluorescence cholangiography may help to reduce bile duct injury without requiring IOC. In this respect, near-infrared fluorescence cholangiography (NIRFC) was developed [25–27], and a multicenter randomized controlled trial is currently recruiting to compare NIRFC-assisted laparoscopic cholecystectomy with conventional laparoscopic cholecystectomy (FALCON trial) [28]. To use NIRFC, indocyanine green (ICG) is injected intravenously, and an NIR light-emitting xenon-based light source and a camera that can detect NIR fluorescence emitted by indocyanine green-dyed bile are used to visualize the biliary anatomy [25–29]. Neither the dye (at normal doses) nor the equipment is dangerous (no irradiation) for the patient or surgeon [11]. NIRFC has been shown to be quicker to perform and to cost less when compared with IOC [30]. Increased safety has yet to be proven [11]. Theoretically, it should be possible to perform NIRFC in all cases versus a 93% rate for IOC due to difficulty with cannulation of the cystic duct [11, 31–33]. The one clinical situation in which ICG may not be able to be administered is in the pregnant patient, as it is considered a Category C medication with unknown affects to the fetus and has not been studied or tested in pregnant women [34]. The other factor is that in order to be able to be used efficiently, it needs to be given at least 20 minutes before attempts to visualize the NIRFC to allow uptake of the ICG into the liver and excretion into the bile. Therefore, it would need to be administered prior to the incision and would be less useful if the anatomy was unclear in the middle of the cholecystectomy.

Summary

The rate of bile duct injury increased with the introduction of laparoscopic cholecystectomy, and while the rate during laparoscopic cholecystectomy has decreased, it remains higher than during open cholecystectomy. Routine cholangiography has not been demonstrated to reduce the rate of bile duct injury, although it can help identify an injury. The SAGES Safe Cholecystectomy Task Force has six steps that have been identified to help prevent bile duct injuries. Indocyanine green and intraoperative ultrasound are potential future tools that may be helpful in preventing bile duct injuries, although further studies are needed to demonstrate a decrease in the rate of bile duct injury. The SAGES Safe Cholecystectomy Task Force endeavored to standardize best practices for the elimination of BDI, a rare complication of one of the most common general surgical procedures. These efforts should serve as a template for organizing and presenting evidence-based standards for reducing complication rates of other common general surgical procedures. These society-led efforts to improve quality care and patient outcomes in focused clinical areas are at the heart of the purpose of their existence.

References

1. Jabłońska B, Lampe P. Iatrogenic bile duct injuries: etiology, diagnosis and management. World J Gastroenterol. 2009;15(33):4097–104. https://doi.org/10.3748/wjg.15.4097.
2. The History of Medicine: The Galling Gallbladder. https://columbiasurgery.org/news/2015/06/11/history-medicine-galling-gallbladder.

3. Litynski GS. Erich Mühe and the rejection of laparoscopic cholecystectomy (1985): a surgeon ahead of his time. JSLS. 1998;2(4):341–6.

4. Roslyn JJ, Binns GS, Hughes EF, Saunders-Kirkwood K, Zinner MJ, Cates JA. Open cholecystectomy. A contemporary analysis of 42,474 patients. Ann Surg. 1993;218(2):129–37.

5. MacFadyen BV Jr, Vecchio R, Ricardo AE, Mathis CR. Bile duct injury after laparoscopic cholecystectomy. The United States experience Surgical Endoscopy. 1998;12:315–21.

6. Keus F, de Jong JAF, Gooszen HG, Van Laarhoven CJHM. Laparoscopic versus open cholecystectomy for patients with symptomatic cholecystolithiasis. Cochrane Database Syst Rev. 2006:CD006231.

7. Buddingh KT, Weersma RK, Savenije RA, van Dam GM, Nieuwenhuijs VB. Lower rate of major bile duct injury and increased intraoperative management of common bile duct stones after implementation of routine intraoperative cholangiography. J Am Coll Surg. 2011;213:267–74.

8. Kern KA. Malpractice litigation involving laparoscopic cholecystectomy. Cost, cause, and consequences. Arch Surg. 1997;132:392–7; discussion 7-8.

9. Flum DR, Flowers C, Veenstra DL. A cost-effectiveness analysis of intraoperative cholangiography in the prevention of bile duct injury during laparoscopic cholecystectomy. J Am Coll Surg. 2003;196:385–93.

10. The SAGES Safe Cholecystectomy Program. Strategies for Minimizing Bile Duct Injuries: Adopting a Universal Culture of Safety in Cholecystectomy. https://www.sages.org/safe-cholecystectomy-program/. Accessed December 10 2020.

11. Renz BW, Bösch F, Angele MK. Bile duct injury after cholecystectomy: surgical therapy. Visc Med. 2017;33(3):184–90.

12. de Mestral C, Rotstein OD, Laupacis A, et al. Comparative operative outcomes of early and delayed cholecystectomy for acute cholecystitis: a population-based propensity score analysis. Ann Surg. 2014;259:10–5.

13. Blohm M, Österberg J, Sandblom G, Lundell L, Hedberg M, Enochsson L. The sooner, the better? The importance of optimal timing of cholecystectomy in acute cholecystitis: data from the national Swedish registry for gallstone surgery. GallRiks J Gastrointest Surg. 2017;21:33–40.

14. da Costa DW, Dijksman LM, Bouwense SA, et al. Cost-effectiveness of same-admission versus interval cholecystectomy

after mild gallstone pancreatitis in the PONCHO trial. Brit J Surg. 2016;103:1695–703.

15. Tan JKH, Goh JCI, Lim JWL, Shridhar IG, Madhavan K, Kow AWC. Same admission laparoscopic cholecystectomy for acute cholecystitis: is the 'golden 72 hours' rule still relevant? HPB (Oxford). 2017;19:47–51.

16. Strasberg SM, Hertl M, Soper NJ. An analysis of the problem of biliary injury during laparoscopic cholecystectomy. J Am Coll Surg. 1995;180:101–25.

17. Brunt LM, Deziel DJ, Telem DA, Strasberg SM, Aggarwal R, Asbun H, et al. Safe cholecystectomy multi-society practice guideline and state of the art consensus conference on prevention of bile duct injury during cholecystectomy. Ann Surg. 2020;272(1):3–23.

18. Fletcher DR, Hobbs MS, Tan P, et al. Complications of cholecystectomy: risks of the laparoscopic approach and protective effects of operative cholangiography: a population-based study. Ann Surg. 1999;229:449–57.

19. Alvarez FA, de Santibañes M, Palavecino M, et al. Impact of routine intraoperative cholangiography during laparoscopic cholecystectomy on bile duct injury. Brit J Surg. 2014;101:677–84.

20. Buddingh KT, Nieuwenhuijs VB, van Buuren L, Hulscher JBF, de Jong JS, van Dam GM. Intraoperative assessment of biliary anatomy for prevention of bile duct injury: a review of current and future patient safety interventions. Surg Endosc. 2011;25:2449–61.

21. Hugh TB, Kelly MD, Mekisic A. Rouvière's sulcus: a useful landmark in laparoscopic cholecystectomy. Br J Surg. 1997;84:1253–4.

22. Ferzli G, Timoney M, Nazir S, Swedler D, Fingerhut A. Importance of the node of Calot in gallbladder neck dissection: an important landmark in the standardized approach to the laparoscopic cholecystectomy. J Laparoendosc Adv Surg Tech. 2015;25:28–32.

23. Pucher PH, Brunt LM, Fanelli RD, Asbun HJ, Aggarwal R. SAGES expert Delphi consensus: critical factors for safe surgical practice in laparoscopic cholecystectomy. Surg Endosc. 2015;29:3074–85.

24. Singh M, Prasad N. The anatomy of Rouviere's sulcus as seen during laparoscopic cholecystectomy: a proposed classification. J Minim Access Surg. 2017;13(2):89–95.

25. Daskalaki D, Fernandes E, Wang X, et al. Indocyanine green (ICG) fluorescent cholangiography during robotic cholecystec-

tomy: results of 184 consecutive cases in a single institution. Surg Innov. 2014;21:615–21.

26. Ashitate Y, Stockdale A, Choi HS, Laurence RG, Frangioni JV. Real-time simultaneous near-infrared fluorescence imaging of bile duct and arterial anatomy. J Surg Res. 2012;176:7–13.

27. Ankersmit M, van Dam DA, van Rijswijk A-S, van den Heuvel B, Tuynman JB, Meijerink WJHJ. Fluorescent imaging with indocyanine green during laparoscopic cholecystectomy in patients at increased risk of bile duct injury. Surg Innov. 2017; https://doi.org/10.1177/1553350617690309.

28. van den Bos J, Schols RM, Luyer MD, et al. Near-infrared fluorescence cholangiography assisted laparoscopic cholecystectomy versus conventional laparoscopic cholecystectomy (FALCON trial): study protocol for a multicentre randomised controlled trial. BMJ Open. 2016;6:e011668.

29. Boni L, David G, Mangano A, et al. Clinical applications of indocyanine green (ICG) enhanced fluorescence in laparoscopic surgery. Surg Endosc. 2015;29:2046–55.

30. Dip FD, Asbun D, Rosales-Velderrain A, et al. Cost analysis and effectiveness comparing the routine use of intraoperative fluorescent cholangiography with fluoroscopic cholangiogram in patients undergoing laparoscopic cholecystectomy. Surg Endosc. 2014;28:1838–43.

31. Ishizawa T, Bandai Y, Hasegawa K, Kokudo N. Fluorescent cholangiography during laparoscopic cholecystectomy: indocyanine green or new fluorescent agents? World J Surg. 2010;34:2505–6.

32. Livingston EH, Miller JAG, Coan B, Rege RV. Costs and utilization of intraoperative cholangiography. J Gastrointest Surg. 2007;11:1162–7.

33. Ambe PC, Plambeck J, Fernandez-Jesberg V, et al. The role of indocyanine green fluoroscopy for intraoperative bile duct visualization during laparoscopic cholecystectomy: an observational cohort study in 70 patients. Patient Saf Surg. 2019;13:2.

34. https://www.accessdata.fda.gov/drugsatfda_docs/label/2006/011525s017lbl.pdf

Chapter 49
OR Attire: Does it Impact Quality?

Yasmin Essaji, Kelly Mahuron, and Adnan Alseidi

"Quality is never an accident; it is always the results of high intention, sincere effort, intelligent direction and skillful execution; it represents the wise choice of many alternatives." - William A. Foster.

Introduction

Operating room (OR) attire has come a long way since the days of Dr. William Grant performing what is believed to be the first successful appendectomy in the USA in 1885, in Iowa. ORs in the nineteenth century were structured as stages with rows of seats for students to watch, and surgeons either wore their business suits or donned their favorite coat, which some used to wipe their bloody scalpels between cases. Surgical

Y. Essaji
Division of HPB Surgery, Virginia Mason Medical Center,
Seattle, WA, USA

K. Mahuron · A. Alseidi (✉)
Department of Surgery, University of California San Francisco,
San Francisco, CA, USA
e-mail: Adnan.alseidi@ucsf.edu

© The Author(s), under exclusive license to Springer Nature   933
Switzerland AG 2022
J. R. Romanelli et al. (eds.), *The SAGES Manual of Quality,
Outcomes and Patient Safety*,
https://doi.org/10.1007/978-3-030-94610-4_49

attire began to evolve with the widespread acceptance of germ theory in the late nineteenth century. Evaluation of photographs from early surgical operations shows the general implementation of surgical gowns in 1863, while caps, gloves, and masks followed between 1900 and 1916 [1]. Through the years, it has by and large been accepted that surgical gowns, gloves, caps, and masks protect both the surgeon and the patient and decrease surgical site infection (SSI) rates. SSIs are the most common hospital-acquired infection and contribute to increased length of stay and risk of mortality. The idea that OR attire is linked to increased SSIs has been further explored in several retrospective studies and meta-analyses, for example, glove perforation being associated with increased SSI rates and that changing gloves before closure during colorectal surgery reduces SSI rates. Studies dating back to 1976 by Noble and colleagues demonstrated that the human body and inanimate surfaces in the OR contribute to microbial contamination, and this has been extrapolated to contribute to increased SSI rates. However, few randomized control trials (RCTs) exist evaluating this surgical dogma. One RCT from England showed no difference in SSIs when non-scrubbed OR personnel wore face masks or not. Despite the lack of strong evidence, many guidelines have been established in attempts to reduce SSI rates given the clinical impact they have on patients. One of the principles of Hippocrates is to treat the ill to the best of one's abilities, and most surgeons would agree that everything must be done to one's best ability to protect the patient from harm, including SSIs. However, guidelines made without any evidence are equivalent to opinion. Dr. Guyatt first introduced the concept of evidence-based medicine in 1992 as critical appraisal and judicial application of the evidence [2]. It has served as a guiding principle of medicine in the modern era by which judicial evaluation of guidelines and practices is performed. Margaret McCartney from the Cochrane Colloquium Edinburgh said: "Ignoring evidence leads to avoidable harm, and failing to admit our uncertainties means we don't get better evidence." This further highlights the frustration which can come from imposed guidelines in perioperative safety, especially as it pertains to

OR attire and personal freedoms. This chapter will serve as a review of the previous guidelines, current evidence, and implications for future practice.

Types of Surgical Attire

Surgical attire revolves around the dichotomy of reusable and disposable [3]. Most facilities have moved to reusable cloth scrubs which are changed daily and laundered by the respective institution. Surgical jackets, as seen in Fig. 49.1, are typically reusable and laundered by the institution. Individual

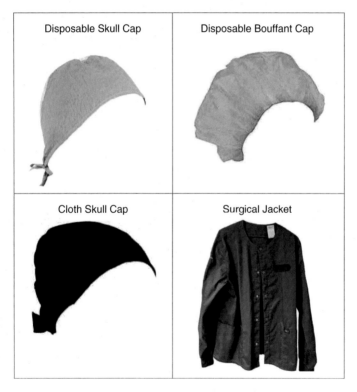

Disposable Skull Cap

Disposable Bouffant Cap

Cloth Skull Cap

Surgical Jacket

FIGURE 49.1 Types of surgical attire illustrating both disposable and cloth skull cap, disposable bouffant cap, and surgical jacket

healthcare workers have purchased reusable cloth hats; however, this is dependent on institutions laundering each individual's hat and returning it to them which can be an arduous process. Many guidelines have dissuaded against healthcare workers laundering any perioperative clothing in their private homes given the potential risk of contamination with bloodborne pathogens to themself and, as well, concern that there would not be standardized adherence to necessary laundering protocols. Many centers have adopted and mandated disposable surgical caps. Typically, the skull cap would be specific for short-haired individuals and the bouffant hat would be for those with longer hair, ponytails, or buns in order to cover it adequately.

Current Guidelines

AORN 2015 (Updated Publication in January 2020)

A critical paradigm shift occurred in 2015 with the publication of the revised Guideline for Surgical Attire by the Association of periOperative Registered Nurses (AORN). These guidelines, written by perioperative registered nurses, were challenged on many fronts and were felt to be based upon weak evidence. Additionally, the OR team comprises many different healthcare disciplines including nurses, scrub technicians, surgeons, anesthesiologists, and custodians, among others. The AORN guidelines were criticized for only involving a single discipline's input.

Many state health organizations and accreditation bodies utilize AORN's Guidelines for Perioperative Practice for continued evaluation that a center is upholding current perioperative practices. AORN guidelines are also the only evidence-based guidelines for perioperative nurses approved by the National Guideline Clearinghouse which is run by the Agency for Healthcare Research and Quality. AORN guidelines published in 2015 were updated in January 2020; however, the 2015 version is currently in practice in most centers.

The 2015 guidelines sparked an onslaught of research regarding the impact of OR attire and revolutionized how perioperative guidelines are created and implemented. Some perioperative healthcare workers saw these guidelines as an attack on personal liberties thinly veiled in weak or no evidence. In particular, recommendation III endorsed surgical head attire with complete coverage of the scalp, hair, nape of the neck, and ears. As the AORN guidelines were considered the standard for measuring patient safety, many hospitals received citations for noncompliance and subsequently banned skull caps. The American College of Surgeons (ACS) responded by publishing their first dress code in 2016, based upon "professionalism, common, sense, decorum, and the available evidence [4]." Other organizations, including the Centers for Disease Control and Prevention (CDC) and the World Health Organization (WHO), followed suit and published their updated guidelines. Several collaborative summits occurred, most notably the Operating Room Attire Summit of 2018. This summit contained members from ACS, the American Society of Anesthesiologists, AORN, the Association for Professionals in Infection Control and Epidemiology, the Association of Surgical Technologist, the Council on Surgical and Perioperative Safety, and The Joint Commission. The organizations reviewed the available evidence relating to OR attire recommendations, specifically focusing on the recommendations related to ear and hair covering. They concluded that (1) evidence-based recommendations on OR attire should be developed with a multidisciplinary team, (2) current evidence is not sufficient to require ear coverage or associate the type of hat or extent of hair coverage with SSI rates, and (3) other areas of surgical attire need further evaluation.

AORN subsequently published revisions to their Guidelines for Perioperative Practice in July 2019 that were aligned with the summit, and these revisions were officially updated in January 2020 after review by AORN members. Notable changes included retraction of their previous surgical headwear recommendation stating "no recommendation can be made for the type of head covers worn in semi-restricted and restricted areas" with retained recommendation to "cover the scalp and hair when entering the semi-restricted and restricted areas." The type of surgical head cover may be determined by the individual healthcare facility, but they expanded their recommendations to include the covering of beards when entering the restricted areas and while preparing and packaging items in the clean assembly section of the sterile processing area. Additionally, they noted that no recommendation could be made regarding arm coverage other than when performing preoperative patient skin antisepsis. There is a conditional recommendation to cover the arms while performing skin antisepsis referring to one semi-experimental study published in *American Journal of Infection Control* in 2018 which showed decreased bacterial shedding when arms were covered by the healthcare worker who was sterile prepping the surgical site.

The most recent AORN guidelines point to a stronger support for double-gloving citing a systematic review that showed a reduced risk of sharps injury. This is further supported by a Cochrane Review published in 2006 which showed that double-gloving reduced perforations to the innermost glove; however, the study had insufficient power to determine any effect on SSIs. A further Cochrane Review in 2014 concluded that there is moderate-quality evidence that double-gloving reduces blood stains on skin which may translate to lower risk of contracting serious blood-borne viral infections.

The AORN guideline revisions made notable changes to the use and classification of evidence for each guideline and now provide summary tables ranking the evidence. These revisions were developed around evidence-based practices, and they reflect the collaborative efforts of a multidisciplinary team.

ACS 2017

Probably the most practical and pragmatic guidelines were published by ACS in 2017. Appropriate OR attire is regarded by ACS as a reflection of professionalism as it can help to establish and maintain a patient-physician relationship as well as reduce healthcare-associated infections and improve patient safety by reducing SSIs. ACS guidelines for surgical attire are based on professionalism as well as a degree of common sense availing to the limited high-quality evidence available. AORN disagreed with this approach as the guidelines were not solely based upon evidence. ACS guidelines on surgical attire are summarized in Table 49.1.

TABLE 49.1 ACS statement on operating room attire

ACS statement on OR attire 2016
Soiled scrubs and/or hats should be changed as soon as feasible and certainly prior to speaking with family members after a surgical procedure
Scrubs and hats worn during dirty or contaminated cases should be changed prior to subsequent cases even if not visibly soiled
Masks should not be worn dangling at any tim
OR scrubs should not be worn in the hospital facility outside of the OR area without a clean lab coat or appropriate cover up over them
OR scrubs should not be worn at any time outside of the hospital perimeter
OR scrubs should be changed at least daily
During invasive procedures, the mouth, nose, and hair (skull and face) should be covered to avoid potential wound contamination. Large sideburns and ponytails should be covered or contained. There is no evidence that leaving ears, a limited amount of hair on the nape of the neck or a modest sideburn uncovered contributes to wound infections
Earrings and jewelry worn on the head or neck where they might fall into or contaminate the sterile field should all be removed or appropriately covered during procedures
The ACS encourages clean appropriate professional attire (not scrubs) to be worn during all patient encounters outside of the OR

Reproduced with permission from [4]

ACS additionally wrote that "the skullcap is symbolic of the surgical profession." They emphasized patient quality and safety and established that as stewards of the healthcare profession, surgeons much retain emphasis on key principles of their culture and uphold the public perception of surgeons as highly trustworthy, attentive, professional, and compassionate.

CDC 2017

The CDC's Guideline for the Prevention of Surgical Site Infection, 2017, consists of broad and overarching guidelines regarding topics such as perioperative antibiotics, glycemic control, and normothermia. Due to the paucity of evidence, the CDC only published one statement regarding OR attire:

- Available evidence suggested uncertain trade-offs between the benefits and harms of orthopedic space suits or the healthcare personnel who should wear them for the prevention of SSI in prosthetic joint arthroplasty (no recommendation/unresolved issue).

Although the CDC guidelines are based on higher-quality evidence, they highlight the need for individual institutional review of guidelines prior to implementation.

WHO 2018

The WHO's Global Guidelines for the Prevention of Surgical Site Infection, originally published in 2016 [5] and updated in 2018, has several guidelines on reducing major contributors to SSIs including preoperative measures and skin preparation, nutritional maintenance, prevention of hypothermia, and antibiotic prophylaxis. These guidelines are based on global practices which can be varied based on a country's economic standing and healthcare access. The WHO provides one recommendation regarding OR attire:

- The panel suggests that either sterile, disposable, non-woven or sterile, reusable woven drapes and surgical gowns can be used during surgical operations for the purposes of preventing SSI (conditional recommendation, moderate to very low quality of evidence).

The WHO acknowledges the research gaps in the field of OR attire, especially in lower-resource countries, and they continue to support well-designed RCTs for the evaluation of further guidelines.

Evidenced-Based Practices

Since the publication of the revised Guidelines for Surgical Attire by AORN in 2015, there has been an outpouring of research on this topic to help better understand the implication of surgical attire on SSI rates. Most researchers understand the limitations of semi-experimental bacterial-based research findings and how these wrestle with the difficulties of implementing pragmatic OR attire guideline changes. As well, some researchers express difficulties in conducting higher-level studies such as RCTs due to reluctance in altering already imposed guidelines. This culminates in the majority of the body of research being retrospective reviews which do help to show associations, however remain of lower-quality evidence in the pyramid of evidence-based medicine. The National Academy of Medicine's Standards for Developing Trustworthy Clinical Practice Guidelines addresses the limitations of evaluating the available evidence. They provide standards for the development of medical guidelines and as well provide a model for formulating recommendations as shown in Figs. 49.2 and 49.3.

Surgical Head Coverings

The 2015 AORN recommendation that skull caps be replaced with disposable bouffant hats led to multiple studies compar-

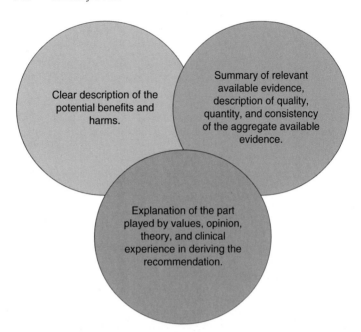

FIGURE 49.2 National Academy of Medicine's Standards for Developing Trustworthy Clinical Practice Guidelines. Establishing evidence

ing the associated SSI rates between the two. A study published in *Hernia* in 2017 by Haskins and colleagues sent a survey to surgeons who submitted at least 10 patients with 30-day follow-up in the Americas Hernia Society Quality Collaborative database [6]. From this survey, 6210 cases were identified, and the authors found no association between reported surgical hat type and wound events at a 30-day follow-up after ventral hernia repair. Another study, published in *Neurosurgery* in 2018 by Shallwani and colleagues, was a single-center retrospective review that included over 15,000 clean neurosurgical cases spanning 13 months before and 13 months after the ban of surgical skull caps [7]. This study showed a 0.07% increase in overall infections, a 0.03% increase in infections in spinal procedures, and a 0.2% decrease in infections in

Standards:
I. Establish transparency
II. Management of conflict of interest
III. Guideline development group composition
IV. Clinical practice guideline-systematic review intersection
V. Establishing evidence foundations for and rating strength of recommendations
VI. Articulation of recommendations
VII. External review
VIII. Updating

FIGURE 49.3 National Academy of Medicine's Standards for Developing Trustworthy Clinical Practice Guidelines

craniotomy/craniectomy cases after the switch from skull caps to bouffant hats. None of the outcomes reached statistical significance, and the authors concluded that banning skull caps did not significantly reduce infection rates. A third study, published in the *Journal of the American College of Surgeons* in 2018 by Kothari and colleagues, was a retrospective review of 1543 patients undergoing general surgery and abdominal surgeries [8]. Similar to the other studies discussed, no correlation was found between the use of skull caps versus bouffant hats and SSI rates. The authors of these studies therefore concluded that there is no clear evidence that the type of surgical hat impacts the rate of SSIs.

However, there was one study that suggested a possible advantage of skull caps over bouffant hats. Markel and colleagues evaluated the passive and active microbial shed from different head gear in a simulated sterile OR environment [9]. Their results were published in the *Journal of the American College of Surgeons* in 2017. They found that although there was no significant difference in particle or actively sampled microbial contamination between the head wear types, there was a higher passive microbial shed among disposable bouffant hats than disposable skull caps ($p < 0.05$). Additionally, disposable bouffant hats exhibited significantly higher particle size and passive microbial shed than cloth skull caps. The study did not include cloth bouffant hats. The authors concluded that disposable bouffant hats had greater permeability, penetration, and passive microbial shed than disposable or cloth skull caps. This study supports the revisions made to the AORN guidelines, which no longer recommend the avoidance of skull caps. Currently there is no clear benefit to support one type of surgical head covering over another for the reduction of SSI rates, and further research is needed before evidence-based recommendations can be made.

Surgical Masks

A systematic review by Lipp and colleagues in the *Canadian Operating Room Nursing Journal* published in 2005 evaluated two RCTs involving 1453 patients undergoing clean surgery and showed a trend toward masks being associated with fewer infections in one trial; however, in neither trial was this significant [10]. This is further supported with the 2016 updated Cochrane review evaluating trials involving 2106 patients in which they found no significant difference in infection rates between masked and unmasked groups undergoing clean surgery [11]. The question of whether all OR personnel should wear masks versus only scrubbed surgical personnel was also evaluated in a 2010 RCT by Webster and colleagues which showed no difference in SSI rate when nonscrubbed personnel did not wear a face mask [12]. An additional Cochrane review published in 2018 also looked at the question of masks versus no masks and did not find a signficant difference in surgical site infections [13]. Surgical masks provide benefit to scrubbed surgical personnel from blood-borne pathogens and should be worn by scrubbed OR personnel for their own protection even if no direct benefit to patients can be shown in terms of reduced SSI rates.

OR Jackets and Bare Below the Elbows

AORN guidelines from 2015 quoted moderate evidence for all non-scrubbed personnel completely covering their arms with a long-sleeved scrub top or jacket when in restricted areas. An observational study from 2016 at the University of Minnesota compared SSI rates 12 months prior to the implementation of surgical jackets in their facility and 12 months following implementation of the AORN guidelines. They found no statistically significant difference in SSI rates. AORN quotes one study which did show increased bacterial shedding from uncovered arms only related to the individual prepping the surgical site and, therefore, recommends arm coverage for personnel performing skin antisepsis. The 2020 AORN guidelines were amended with no recommendation for covering arms outside of during skin prep.

The bare below the elbows (BBE) policy adopted by the National Health Service (NHS) in the UK has also been a source of controversy. It is published as a position statement by the NHS; however, direct implementation is referred back to individual health centers. The BBE policy states that arms must be bare below the elbows which restricts the use of watches and jewelry as well as white coats. There is limited evidence for its implementation, and further practical studies have not shown a difference. This has raised troublesome implementations with a cross-sectional study published in the *British Journal of Medicine* in 2019 which found that Muslim women reported experiencing challenges when wearing headscarves in ORs and, as well, adopting the BBE policy [14]. They found that in many instances, these guidelines infringed on their religious requirements and some respondents were dissuaded from entering surgical specialties preferring to specialize as a general practitioner due to dress code matters. This highlights a greater need for evidence-based guidelines especially when there is a risk of religious right and personal freedom infringement and a reflexive impact on reduction in workforce diversity.

Facial Hair: Clean Shaven and Bearded

A quasi-experimental study published in 2016 by Parry and colleagues evaluated bacterial shedding between ten clean-shaven and ten bearded male OR personnel [15]. They evaluated the subjects conducting several facial expressions while wearing a mask, unmasked, or wearing a hood. They found that while wearing a mask, there was no difference in bacterial shed between bearded and clean-shaven personnel. They also found that disposable hoods did not decrease the amount of shedding compared with masks alone. A cross-sectional study to evaluate the presence of bacteria between clean-shaven and bearded males with 408 subjects published in 2014 by Wakeam and colleagues found that bacterial shed rates among both groups were comparable, with the clean-shaven group having higher colonization rates for *Staphylococcus aureus* and methicillin-resistant *Staphylococcus aureus* [16]. A quasi-experimental study in 2000 by McLure and colleagues further complicated the limited available evidence as they compared ten clean-shaven men, ten bearded men, and ten women [17]. They found that wiggling the mask significantly increased the bacterial shedding among women and bearded men; however, this was not the case in the clean-shaven men. They suggest that bearded men could consider removing their beards; however, this does not address the surprising results that women had comparable bacterial shed to bearded men.

Cost

The matter of replacement of OR attire for every case also contributes to the overall cost of surgery and caring for a patient. Any cost to the healthcare system as a whole should be evaluated and efforts made to reduce this where possible. A retrospective review by Elmously and colleagues published in the *Journal of the American College of Surgeons* in 2018 evaluated data from the National Health Safety Network and included 30,493 general surgery, cardiac, neurosurgery, ortho-pedic, and gynecology procedures from January 2014 to November 2017, before and after implementation of the man-dated bouffant hats [18]. They showed no difference in rate of SSIs between groups. The cost of attire for one person enter-ing the OR increased from $0.07–0.12 before policy change to $1.11–1.38 after policy change which encompassed not only disposable surgical hat implementation but also mandated OR jackets. This was estimated to translate to an increase of $540 million per year for all US hospitals. Given the high cost of these implementations, their benefit must be evaluated in a cost-effectiveness review.

Environmental Waste

The growing impact of global warming has shone a light on the urgency for reduction of environmental waste. The healthcare system is the second largest contributor of trash in the USA with one-third of the four billion pounds of waste produced by ORs every year [19]. The waste from ORs has also been shown to translate to increased costs from not only waste elimination but also the associated increased cost of disposable materials; one such study showed $100,000 annual savings with the use of reusable gowns in their surgical center [20]. A survey conducted by AORN evaluated perioperative staff preference and demonstrated that the majority of sur-geons and surgical technologists actually preferred the reus-able products and they felt this would translate to a 65% decrease in regulated medical waste generated in the OR and reduce the cost of waste disposal [21].

Older studies had suggested that reusable gowns were inferior to disposable; however, they were using materials which are now considered obsolete, and more recent studies on newer materials in use show equivalence in safety. In simulated OR analysis, disposable bouffant hats were shown to have greater permeability and microbial shed than dispos-able skull caps and cloth skull caps. AORN has released a statement that donning cloth caps should be determined at the facility level. These factors taken together suggest that consideration for system-based assessment of reduction strategies for medical waste may decrease costs while not impacting safety or surgeon preference.

COVID-19 Impact

The COVID-19 pandemic and its uncertainty have resulted in significant perioperative changes that are constantly in flux as our understanding of the virus expands. These changes extend to OR attire as there is increased emphasis on improved protection for healthcare providers to minimize transmission of COVID-19. Furthermore, PPE shortages have created additional constraints on the US healthcare system, and institutions have had to develop new resource strategies to meet PPE demands.

As aerosolization and respiratory droplets are considered the primary mechanism of transmission for the COVID-19 virus, the use of N95 respirators has been recommended in addition to standard OR PPE and attire. The ACS and the CDC have recommended that N95 respirators should be worn while operating and during aerosol-generating procedures such as intubation for COVID-19 suspected and confirmed patients. Many institutions also encourage the use of N95 respirators during intubation regardless of a patient's COVID-19 status due the significance of false-negative test results.

PPE recommendations are challenging to follow due to national and international shortages. Hospitals have responded to these shortages with strategies that reduce the use of disposable PPE and reuse PPE when appropriate. Many institutions now encourage and even provide cloth scrub hats and non-disposable eye protection. SAGES has published a rotation and reuse strategy for N95 respirators to extend their use, and decontamination methods are being investigated. As OR PPE guidelines continue to evolve, it is critical that institutions find innovative ways to protect their healthcare providers while still maintaining a high level of care for their patients.

Correlation of Current Guidelines with Evidence

Since the publication of the controversial AORN Guidelines for Perioperative Practice in 2015, further revisions have been made and updated guidelines were published in January 2020. Considerable changes were made in regard to evidence appraisal and multidisciplinary input, both key factors that have been identified as important to successful guideline creation and implementation. AORN revised their model for evidence appraisal and rating which they published in their own journal in 2016. They also published the evidence table they created and used to support their guidelines. This aids in transparency and building trustworthy guidelines for implementation among multidisciplinary healthcare services. One notable update in their 2020 guidelines is that some policy decisions need to be determined at the facility level such as donning cloth caps and what form of head covers are needed. They continue to recommend that the scalp and hair are covered in restricted or semi-restricted areas. They acknowledge that the evidence does not show any association between type of head cover worn or extent of hair coverage and SSI rates. As well, they repeal the recommendation for covering arms other than when performing preoperative patient skin antisepsis.

When assessing the guidelines from an evidentiary basis, there are few guidelines that can be strongly recommended. Pragmatically, wearing a surgical gown and mask for scrubbed personnel is recommended for prevention of transmission of blood-borne pathogens to the surgical team. As well, there is building evidence for double-gloving, a recommendation from the AORN 2020 guidelines.

Further research is needed to determine optimal guidelines for protecting patients and reducing SSI rates. Medicine and in particular ORs already have many regulatory practices. It is important that efforts are focused on what will make the greatest impact on patient safety. If recommendations are made without evidentiary basis and without input from multidisciplinary teams, they can contribute to the overburdening of healthcare workers and physician burnout. Lack of input or control for physicians with respect to issues affecting their work lives has been shown to contribute to physician burnout. Transparency and physician input both help to reduce these negative effects in regard to guideline formation. A systematic review and meta-analysis published in *Medicine* in 2019 by Garcia and colleagues showed a correlation between high physician burnout and worse patient safety [22]. They also suggest that organized workflows that promote health professionals' autonomy help to improve patient safety practices. Another systematic review from England published in 2016 showed that higher levels of physician burnout correlated with increased medical errors [23]. The largest meta-analysis to date published in 2017 by Salyers and colleagues included over 210,000 healthcare providers over 82 studies [24]. They again showed consistent negative relationships between physician burnout and perceived quality including patient satisfaction and the perception of safety. Regulatory guidelines that include efforts to reduce healthcare worker burnout by being transparent and involving all involved disciplines, as outlined in the National Academy of Medicine's Standards for Developing Trustworthy Clinical Practice Guidelines summarized in Figs. 49.2 and 49.3, are essential as they produce benefits for patients as well as healthcare workers.

Summary

OR attire offers both protection for healthcare workers from blood-borne pathogens and infections and protection for patients from the most common, costly, and morbid hospital-acquired infection, SSIs. Expert evidenced-based guidelines are important in OR attire to maintain and uphold professionalism within the healthcare team. The ACS states that this also assists in establishing and maintaining the patient-physician relationship and upholds the perception of surgeons as highly trustworthy, attentive, professional, and compassionate. Establishment of guidelines should be made with a thorough evaluation of the available evidence and with input from all healthcare team members to ensure collegiality and adequate uptake. The AORN 2020 guidelines were created with multi-disciplinary input and a revised format for review of evidence. It will take time for uptake of these guidelines as many health-care facilities made significant changes to adopt the 2015 guidelines and the recommendations will need to be reviewed at the individual institution level. As well, the COVID-19 pandemic has ratified PPE use in the healthcare community and will have lasting and far-reaching repercussions. Clarity and engagement are paramount to establishing guidelines. Current guidelines are based on a combination of very few RCTs and mostly quasi-experimental microbial contamination studies as well as retrospective clinical studies. Many other factors also contribute to SSIs other than the minimal component of a small amount of hair exposed on the nape of the neck; there-fore, optimization of those factors (preoperative antibiotics, normothermia, postoperative wound care, and dressing choice) should take precedence. Current surgical attire prac-tices should also evaluate interventions in the context of their economic and environmental impact. Lastly, within our multi-cultural society, guidelines should be reviewed to address any infringement on religious practices or personal freedoms, especially when there is lack of proof of benefit. This may help also reduce the toll on physician and healthcare worker burn-out in a highly stressful workplace.

References

1. Adams LW, Aschenbrenner CA, Houle TT, et al. Uncovering the history of operating room attire through photographs. Anesthesiology. 2016;124(1):19–24.

2. Evidenced-Based Medicine Working Group. Evidence-based medicine: a new approach to teaching the practice of medicine. JAMA. 1992;268(17):2420–5.

3. Overcash M. A comparison of reusable and disposable perioperative textiles: sustainability state-of-the-art 2012. Anesth Analg. 2012;114(5):1055–66.

4. American College of Surgeons task force on operating room attire. Statement on Operating Room Attire. Bulletin of the American College of Surgeons website. October 1, 2016. Accessed Oct 10, 2020. https://bulletin.facs.org/2016/10/statement-on-operating-room-attire/

5. Allegranz B, Zayed B, Bischoff P, et al. WHO guidelines development group. New WHO recommendations on intraoperative and postoperative measures for surgical site infection prevention: an evidence-based global perspective. Lancet Infect Dis. 2016;16(12):e288–303.

6. Haskins IN, Prabhu AS, Krpata DM, et al. Is there an association between surgeon hat type and 30-day wound events following ventral hernia repair? Hernia. 2017;21(4):495–503.

7. Shallwani H, Shakir HJ, Aldridge AM, et al. Mandatory change from surgical skull caps to bouffant caps among operating room personnel does not reduce surgical site infections in class I surgical cases: a single-center experience with more than 15 000 patients. Neurosurgery. 2018;82(4):548–54.

8. Kothari SN, Anderson MJ, Borgert AJ, et al. Bouffant vs skull cap and impact on surgical site infection: does operating room headwear really matter? J Am Coll Surg. 2018;227(2):198–202.

9. Markel TA, Gormley T, Greeley D, et al. Hats off: a study of different operating room headgear assessed by environmental quality indicators. J Am Coll Surg. 2017;225(5):573–81.

10. Lipp A, Edwards P. Disposable surgical face masks: a systematic review. Can Oper Room Nurs J. 2005;23(3):20. -1, 24-5, 33-8

11. Vincent M, Edwards P. Disposable surgical face masks for preventing surgical wound infection in clean surgery. Cochrane Database Syst Rev. 2016;4(4):CD002929.

12. Webster J, Croger S, Lister C, et al. Use of face masks by non-scrubbed operating room staff: a randomized controlled trial. ANZ J Surg. 2010;80(3):169–73.

13. Liu Z, Dumville JC, Norman G, et al. Intraoperative interventions for preventing surgical site infection: an overview of Cochrane reviews. Cochrane Database Syst Rev. 2018;2(2):CD012653.
14. Malik A, Qureshi H, Abdul-Razakq H, et al. 'I decided not to go into surgery due to dress code': a cross-sectional study within the UK investigating experiences of female Muslim medical health professionals on bare below the elbows (BBE) policy and wearing headscarves (hijabs) in theatre. BMJ Open. 2019;9(3):e019954.
15. Parry JA, Karau MJ, Aho JM, et al. To beard or not to beard? Bacterial Shedding Among Surgeons Orthopedics. 2016;39(2):e290–4.
16. Wakeam E, Hernandez RA, Rivera Morales D, et al. Bacterial ecology of hospital workers' facial hair: a cross-sectional study. J Hosp Infect. 2014;87(1):63–7.
17. McLure HA, Mannam M, Talboys CA, et al. The effect of facial hair and sex on the dispersal of bacteria below a masked subject. Anesthesia. 2000;55(2):173–6.
18. Elmously A, Gray KD, Michelassi F, et al. Operating room attire policy and healthcare cost: favoring evidence over action for prevention of surgical site infections. J Am Coll Surg. 2019;228(1):98–106.
19. Wormer BA, Augenstein VA, Carpenter CL, et al. The green operating room: simple changes to reduce cost and our carbon footprint. Am Surg. 2013;79(7):666–71.
20. DiGiacomo JC, Odom JW, Ritota PC, et al. Cost containment in the operating room: use of reusable versus disposable clothing. Am Surg. 1992;58(10):654–6.
21. Conrardy J, Hillanbrand M, Myers S, et al. Reducing medical waste. AORN J. 2010;91(6):711–21.
22. Garcia C, de Abreu LC, Ramos JL, et al. Influence of burnout on patient safety: systematic review and meta-analysis. Medicina. 2019;55(9):553.
23. Hall LH, Johnson J, Watt I, et al. Healthcare staff wellbeing, burnout, and patient safety: a systematic review. PLoS One. 2016;11(7):e0159015.
24. Salyers MP, Bonfils KA, Luther L, et al. The relationship between professional burnout and quality and safety in health-care: a meta-analysis. J Gen Intern Med. 2017;32(4):475–82.

Selected Readings

Ban KA, Minei JP, Laronga C, Harbrecht BG, et al. American College of Surgeons and Surgical Infection Society: Surgical Site Infection Guidelines, 2016 Update. J Am Coll Surg. 2017;224(1):59–74.

Guideline for surgical attire. Guidelines for Perioperative Practice. Denver, CO: AORN, Inc.; 2020. p. 989–1006.

Liu Z, Dumville JC, Norman G, et al. Intraoperative interventions for preventing surgical site infection: an overview of Cochrane Reviews. Cochrane Database Syst Rev. 2018;2(2):CD012653.

Moalem J, Markel TA, Plagenhoef J, et al. Proceedings and Recommendations from the OR Attire Summit: A Collaborative Model for Guideline Development. Bulletin of the American College of Surgeons website. May 1, 2019. Accessed Oct 10, 2020. https://bulletin.facs.org/2019/05/proceedings-and-recommendations-from-the-or-attire-summit-a-collaborative-model-for-guideline-development/.

Nash D, Reifsnyder J, Fabius R, et al. Population Health: Creating a Culture of Wellness. 3rd ed. Jones & Bartlett Learning. 2010

Spruce L, Van Wicklin SA, Wood A. AORN's Revised Model for Evidence Appraisal and Rating. AORN J. 2016;103(1):60–72.

Chapter 50
Learning When Not to Operate: From Patient Selection to Withdraw of Care

Carolyn Judge, Kim Gerling, and Tiffany C. Cox

Objectives

1. Define consideration of appropriate patient selection and when to wait to operate.
2. What are the outcome measures supporting these concepts for surgical frailty?
3. Define the problem of care near the end of life.
4. Setting goals of care: who is right?
5. What is medical futility? Is it quantifiable?

C. Judge · K. Gerling · T. C. Cox (✉)
Department of Surgery, Uniformed Services University of Health Sciences & Walter Reed National Military Medical Center, Bethesda, MD, USA
e-mail: Carolyn.g.judge.mil@mail.mil;
Kimberly.a.gerling3.mil@mail.mil; tiffany.cox@usuhs.edu

© The Author(s), under exclusive license to Springer Nature Switzerland AG 2022
J. R. Romanelli et al. (eds.), *The SAGES Manual of Quality, Outcomes and Patient Safety*,
https://doi.org/10.1007/978-3-030-94610-4_50

Introduction

Fundamental adages for surgery that still apply today are timeless in their expression of the innate nature of our profession. "Residency is to learn how to operate, not do an operation." "Junior residents learn when to operate, Chief residents learn when NOT to operate." These concepts have not changed. Similar to other notions in surgery wherein you improve your technique over time, learning when not to operate is a skill. This skill is a responsibility of every mentor to bestow on their trainees so it can be instilled during training yet is mastered over years of practice. The tendency is to want to save everyone with an operation. Unfortunately, knowing when an operation isn't the best answer is much harder to discern. Included herein are considerations of when we need to rethink if an operation is the next appropriate step, from selection of patients and appropriate delay in timing of an operation. Whether for intentions of improved outcomes when delayed or never performed at all such as when to enact the provision of less care, this chapter will discuss when not operating is ultimately the more appropriate choice.

Patient Selection: *When to Wait First, Operate Later*

There are many dynamic patient characteristics that have a significant impact on surgical risk and prognosis. These factors include, but are not limited to, smoking, diabetes, and obesity, all of which have been linked to increased postoperative morbidity and mortality. Preoperative optimization of these factors can not only decrease complications but also decrease hospital charges secondary to minimizing rates of readmission and reoperation. Surgeons must also consider women of childbearing age in their patient selection for elective surgery. Hernia surgery is one of the best evidence-based examples to prove the case of consideration of delay of surgery until optimization of high-risk comorbidities.

Smoking

Tobacco use carries a 2.49 relative risk of wound complications [1]. Tobacco use increases the risk of surgical site infections [2] and specifically mesh infections following hernia repair [3]. It is also associated with increased readmission and reoperation rates [4]. The pathophysiologic relationship between smoking and poor wound healing is complex and remains to be fully elucidated. It has been shown, however, that decreased cutaneous blood flow to the wound bed causes tissue hypoxia [5, 6], reducing the migration of fibroblasts and the response of inflammatory cells leading to decreased wound healing [2]. Cessation is effective in reducing postoperative complications [7] even in just 4 weeks [8–10]; improved tissue oxygenation and reduced inflammatory cell response can be seen within a month of quitting smoking [2]. It is recommended to postpone surgery until cessation can be achieved. It should be considered to not perform elective surgery on actively smoking patients should the potential morbidity make the procedure maleficent to the patient and the patient is unwilling to cease tobacco use. If there is any doubt regarding compliance with smoking cessation, a urine test is available which detects cotinine, a metabolite of nicotine, suggesting tobacco use within 40 hours prior [11].

Obesity

The prevalence of obesity in the United States was 42.4% from 2017 to 2018 and has increased annually as has the prevalence of obesity-related type II diabetes [12]. Hernia recurrence increases for patients with obesity [13–15] which is higher risk as the BMI increases [16–20]. This recurrence may be precipitated by surgical site infection (SSI) which are known to be more common in the obese population. A stepwise increase in SSI with increasing BMI beginning at a threshold of 24.2 kg/m^2 has been observed [21]. Minimizing SSI is paramount to avoiding the "vicious cycle" of hernia repair, complication, recurrence, and reoperation [22]. A BMI ≥40 is an independent risk factor for readmission [4], increased risk of SSI [21], as well as hernia recurrence [15]. The etiology of SSI in patients with obesity may be due to increased intra-abdominal pressure [23] or decreased vascularity of adipose tissue [24]. Surgeons are advised to avoid elective repair in patients with a BMI 50 kg/m^2 or greater [25] in the elective setting. Preoperative BMI optimization may help decrease complications leading to recurrence for hernias or necessitating reoperation and ultimately greatly increasing hospital costs.

Diabetes

Patients with diabetes have increased postoperative morbidity and mortality during elective surgery [18, 26–30]. Increasing severity of disease has been correlated with increased risk of complications, increased length of stay, and greater inpatient charges overall [31]. Current data suggest a HbA1c ≤7.2 significantly decreased postoperative morbidity [18]. Diabetics are 7.25 times more likely to develop an SSI than nondiabetic patients, and uncontrolled diabetic patients are 3.25 times more likely to develop an SSI than patients with controlled diabetes [26]. This may be due to increased blood glucose level impairing blood flow through the small vessels and compromising mobilization and phagocytic activity of leukocytes, thereby increasing risk of infection [32]. In a study of the effect of varying severity of diabetes on open ventral hernia repair outcomes, it was shown that diabetics (both insulin dependent and non-insulin dependent) had increased complications as compared to nondiabetic patients [31]. Diabetic patients should be counseled to improve disease control as reflected by a lower hemoglobin A1c level as this has been shown to directly impact their postoperative course.

Multiple Comorbidities and Cost

Patients with comorbidities including diabetes, smoking, and obesity are more likely to have postoperative complications and generate higher hospital charges than those without [18, 33]. This effect is directly correlated with an increasing number of these comorbidities [33]. According to the American Society of Metabolic and Bariatric Surgeons, the combination of morbid obesity and smoking is linked to an increased risk of postoperative marginal ulceration and pneumonia [34]. Similarly, morbidly obese patients have an increased postoperative sepsis rate of 1% increased risk per pack-year of smoking [35].

Hospital charges, which need to be considered as part of patient counseling for an elective procedure, have also been shown to be higher in patients with multiple comorbidities [33]. In fact, patients with these aforementioned comorbidities but without complications still have higher hospital charges than patients without comorbidities who do not have a complication after surgery [33]. This has been seen in other studies as well, increasing the cost with readmission for actively smoking patients with obesity resulting in a rate of 25% readmission following elective hernia repair [4].

In the elective setting, patient selection and surgical timing should reflect the efficacy of preoperative optimization from associated high-risk comorbidities for these quality outcome concerns. It is prudent to delay surgical intervention otherwise.

Women of Child-Bearing Age

There is limited data on the operative management of hernias in pregnancy and 30-day outcomes. This void is compounded by the fact that what data there is within the American College of Surgeons National Surgical Quality Improvement Program (ACS-NSQIP) database does not include gestational age and trimester. Primary ventral hernia repair in women occurs with a bimodal distribution peaking at age 5 and again at 35–40 [36], and femoral hernia incidence increases after age of 30 [37]. Pregnancy itself has been proven to be a risk factor for hernia recurrence [38, 39]. The relative incidence of hernia presentation during pregnancy is quite low as was demonstrated in a study of 20,714 pregnant patients, of which 17 (0.08%) and 25 (0.12%) have primary ventral and groin hernias, respectively; none of the patients underwent elective or emergent repair during pregnancy and all had uncomplicated childbirth [40]. Watchful waiting for reducible hernias in pregnancy is recommended [40] with plan to proceed to surgical repair in the postpartum period should symptoms develop or persist. The presence of a hernia does not appear to negatively affect the pregnancy, labor, or delivery, and there exists the possibility for misdiagnosis of round ligament varicosities as a hernia [41]. The decision to proceed to surgery must be made after consideration of the risk of progression to bowel incarceration and strangulation weighed against the risk of maternal and fetal physiologic stress and teratogenic exposures [42]. It is important to ensure that elective surgical repair is performed at a hospital with neonatal capabilities as the risk of preterm labor in the pregnant surgical patient is 4% [43]. Additionally, it is recommended to postpone surgery until the second trimester and to use local or regional anesthesia if possible [44]. The consideration of waiting for surgery after childbearing age for elective hernia cases is well supported for improved quality outcomes.

End-of-Life Care: First, Do no Harm

While delaying an operation can be difficult, deciding not to operate on a patient is even more challenging. This decision is further complicated when we realize that this will ultimately lead to the patient's demise. Often, surgeons are used to working in the "black and white"; there is a sense that our technical skills can sustain life. Early in a surgeon's career, the end result may lead to a sense of guilt or failure. However, there will be a time when surgery is futile and may result in more harm than good. How do we decide where to draw that line? How do we tell patients and their families that we cannot offer a surgical intervention? How do we train future surgeons to know how and when to have that conversation? The ability to communicate risks and benefits of surgery to patients is becoming increasingly more important, as almost a third of Americans over the age of 65 undergo a surgical procedure in the last year of life, with a majority of those procedures in the last month of life [45]. This highlights the need to be able to master communicating options within the context of a critically ill or dying patients and the consideration of how to communicate when the choice not to operate is what is best for their care.

In order to communicate these options clearly, it is important to address why end-of-life care is difficult to discuss. Even in the most ideal situations, patient-physician communication is fraught with potential barriers, and end-of-life discussions are no different. Counseling patients on the dying process is inherently complex because it is more often than not a high-stress, emotionally charged event. Patients and their caregivers or families may feel a sense of unfinished business or finality, or they may have expectations of how their death should occur, even if these expectations are not aligned with the reality of what medical care can offer. Patient and caregiver concerns include a lack of understanding of the true complexities of their medical illness, possibly related to low health literacy or prior medical experiences. Sometimes patients anchor on their prior experiences and think that their current situation is the same as all of their other hospitalizations, even though they may be much more ill than during previous presentations. Their barriers of communication can include the patient's incapacity, absence of advanced directives, and failure to assign a surrogate for decision-making [46]. These concerns are further hindered by factors inherent to the surgeon, including prognostic uncertainty, inexperience with palliative care, time constraints, or their personal bias [46]. Additionally, system-based barriers such as limited availability of experts in palliation, fragmented information across multiple healthcare systems, and clinical inexperience at various institutions may also play a role [47]. All of these factors may confound the decision to operate and the ability to clearly communicate when an operation is not the answer.

Eliminating these barriers completely is not possible; however, we can improve communication techniques to benefit both the patient and the physician. Physicians should not always think of end-of-life discussions as a singular occurrence [48]. In an ideal world, discussions of possible outcomes and scenarios related to end-of-life care would occur in an outpatient setting. This allows for multiple conversations which could consider situations such as social support at home and earlier involvement of palliative care. Unfortunately, given the nature of many surgical interventions, these conversations tend to occur in an expedited manner without preamble or prior relationships. Time to develop relationships and establish the intimate familiarity is a luxury not often afforded to the surgeon on call. If at all possible, it's important to separate the "breaking of bad news" discussion from the "goals of care" discussion, as this allows the patient and their family time to process the context in which a decision regarding end-of-life care will be made [49]. This includes both the acute illness and change in status within the context of the patient's underlying medical conditions. This is often an overlooked step with many surgeons avoiding statements asserting poor prognosis with or without an intervention [49].

The patient's wishes are critical input to a discussion about treatment options near the end of life. Failure of goal-concordant care is considered in the palliative care literature as a medical error, and high-quality communication is the highest priority to achieve this goal [50]. For patients with chronic illness or a protracted clinical course, this conversation would occur in a more consistent setting with a physician that has developed rapport with the patient and their family. This is not often the case, and in the surgical community in times of critical care, this key component of goal concordance is lost without high-quality communication in situations of provision of less care or withdraw of care [50].

As a medical community, we assign significant weight to patient autonomy as it pertains to medical decision-making. In this context, this allows the patient to make an informed decision that further surgical treatment no longer meets their overarching goals. It also allows the patient to make decisions where the expected benefits from invasive surgical intervention no longer outweigh the potential harms and the emphasis of importance that the patient can come to this decision autonomously with proper counseling. Sometimes, this option not to intervene aligns with the physician's consensus. When it does not, surgeons cannot lean into the "rescue credo" that frameworks the conversation with the worst outcome equaling death [47]. It is imperative that surgeons express to patients and families that selection of nonoperative management does not equate to *giving up*. Furthermore, it is critical to convey that recommending nonoperative management does not mean that the physician team is abandoning the patient or their family [48]. This concern can be mitigated via consideration of follow-up with the patient even after the decision has been made to not undergo further surgical treatment and establishment of ongoing psychosocial care by connecting the patient with the appropriate teams, most significantly palliative care.

Even when death is inevitable and surgical intervention is futile, what we can do is continue to advocate for the patient. Early consultation of palliative care has been shown to improve patient's quality of life [51]. There is perception among surgical residents, and likely their mentors, that the palliative team does not need to be consulted until death is imminent or there are no more options for cure [52]. This is an incorrect assumption which is harmful to patients at the time in which they need medical counseling the most. The fact that metastatic cancer patients are four times more likely to have a fatal outcome from their admission than cohort matched cases excluding the cancer diagnosis [53] demonstrates we are subjecting patients to end of life within the confines of the hospital and late palliation is not sufficient. Many patients and physicians alike fear a sense of betrayal with consultation of a palliative team. There is a belief that consultation is equivalent to hospice care or, even worse, that this signifies end-of-care. In fact, patients who receive palliative care consultation perceive their end-of-life care more favorably than those who did not [54]. Despite the likely benefit to palliative care consultation, even among patients undergoing high-risk surgeries, only 3.5% received consultation [54]. Surgical practices should consider routine involvement of palliative care consultation where early engagement of the palliative team normalizes their involvement for patients prior to critical decision points.

Conclusion

When not to operate is a critical skill mastered at the crossroads of the art and science of medicine. Physicians have a responsibility to their patients to elicit their values in an ongoing dialogue of shared decision-making with proper counseling of their risks. As we move the needle from understanding to mastery, it is our responsibility to make the harder recommendation regarding when an operation should be delayed or not performed at all. When considering what we know about quality outcomes for patients with multiple comorbidities or impacting patient factors, we should consider preoperative optimization and delay surgical intervention in the elective setting. Patients must be appropriately risk stratified with awareness of the risk for increased morbidity, mortality, and healthcare costs on an individual basis. It is paramount that physicians continue actively engaging patients who are not yet surgical candidates or should not undergo surgery at all in situations requiring provision of less care so that they do not feel abandoned. Education in palliative care and ready integration of these services into surgical practice is essential in understanding how to manage patients necessitating withdraw of care.

The implicit trust patients place in their physicians must be ethically employed to balance our recommendations and patient autonomy such that patients feel supported and empowered to make informed decisions. Patients need to understand when not operating may be better aligned with their care goals. It is upon us to counsel patients in this manner and train the future of surgery to do the same.

Disclosure The views and opinions expressed herein are that of the authors and do not represent the opinions of the US Army, US Navy, or that of the DOD.

References

1. Gronkjaer M, Eliasen M, Skov-Ettrup LS, et al. Preoperative smoking status and postoperative complications: a systematic review and meta-analysis. Ann Surg. 2014;259(1):52–71.
2. Sorensen LT. Wound healing and infection in surgery: the pathophysiological impact of smoking, smoking cessation, and nicotine replacement therapy: a systematic review. Ann Surg. 2012;255(6):1069–79.
3. Novitsky YW, Porter JR, Rucho ZC, et al. Open preperitoneal retrofascial mesh repair for multiply recurrent ventral incisional hernias. J Am Coll Surg. 2006;203(3):283–9.
4. Henriksen NA, Bisgaard T, Helgstrand F. Smoking and obesity are associated with increased readmission after elective repair of small primary ventral hernias: a nationwide database study. Surgery. 2020;168(3):527–31.
5. Monfrecola G, Riccio G, Savarese C, Posteraro G, Procaccini EM. The acute effect of smoking on cutaneous microcirculation blood flow in habitual smokers and nonsmokers. Dermatology. 1998;197(2):115–8.
6. Arnold DL, Williams MA, Miller RS, Qiu C, Sorensen TK. Iron deficiency anemia, cigarette smoking and risk of abruptio placentae. J Obstet Gynaecol Res. 2009;35(3):446–52.
7. Rosen MJ, Krpata DM, Ermlich B, Blatnik JA. A 5-year clinical experience with single-staged repairs of infected and contami-

nated abdominal wall defects utilizing biologic mesh. Ann Surg. 2013;257(6):991–6.

8. Finan KR, Vick CC, Kiefe CI, Neumayer L, Hawn MT. Predictors of wound infection in ventral hernia repair. Am J Surg. 2005;190(5):676–81.

9. Lindstrom D, Sadr Azodi O, Wladis A, et al. Effects of a perioperative smoking cessation intervention on postoperative complications: a randomized trial. Ann Surg. 2008;248(5):739–45.

10. Sorensen LT, Karlsmark T, Gottrup F. Abstinence from smoking reduces incisional wound infection: a randomized controlled trial. Ann Surg. 2003;238(1):1–5.

11. Cooke F, Bullen C, Whittaker R, McRobbie H, Chen MH, Walker N. Diagnostic accuracy of NicAlert cotinine test strips in saliva for verifying smoking status. Nicotine Tob Res. 2008;10(4):607–12.

12. CDC. Obesity is a Common, Serious, and Costly Disease. https://www.cdc.gov/obesity/data/adult.html. Last Accessed 1JAN2021. 29 JUNE 2020.

13. Schumacher OP, Peiper C, Lorken M, Schumpelick V. Long-term results after Spitzy's umbilical hernia repair. Chirurg. 2003;74(1):50–4.

14. Venclauskas L, Silanskaite J, Kiudelis M. Umbilical hernia: factors indicative of recurrence. Medicina (Kaunas). 2008;44(11):855–9.

15. Stey AM, Russell MM, Sugar CA, et al. Extending the value of the National Surgical Quality Improvement Program claims dataset to study long-term outcomes: rate of repeat ventral hernia repair. Surgery. 2015;157(6):1157–65.

16. Tsereteli Z, Pryor BA, Heniford BT, Park A, Voeller G, Ramshaw BJ. Laparoscopic ventral hernia repair (LVHR) in morbidly obese patients. Hernia : the Journal of Hernias and Abdominal Wall Surgery. 2008;12(3):233–8.

17. Ko JH, Wang EC, Salvay DM, Paul BC, Dumanian GA. Abdominal wall reconstruction: lessons learned from 200 "components separation" procedures. Arch Surg. 2009;144(11):1047–55.

18. Colavita P, Zemlyak A, Burton P, et al. The expansive cost of wound complications after ventral hernia repair. Washington DC: Am College Surg Meeting; 2013.

19. Desai KA, Razavi SA, Hart AM, Thompson PW, Losken A. The effect of BMI on outcomes following complex Abdominal Wall reconstructions. Ann Plast Surg. 2016;76(Suppl 4):S295–7.

20. Sauerland S, Korenkov M, Kleinen T, Arndt M, Paul A. Obesity is a risk factor for recurrence after incisional hernia repair.

Hernia: The Journal of Hernias and Abdominal Wall Surgery. 2004;8(1):42–6.

21. Park H, de Virgilio C, Kim DY, Shover AL, Moazzez A. Effects of smoking and different BMI cutoff points on surgical site infection after elective open ventral hernia repair. Hernia: The Journal of Hernias and Abdominal Wall Surgery. 2020.

22. Holihan JL, Alawadi Z, Martindale RG, et al. Adverse events after ventral hernia repair: the vicious cycle of complications. J Am Coll Surg. 2015;221(2):478–85.

23. Sugerman H, Windsor A, Bessos M, Wolfe L. Intra-abdominal pressure, sagittal abdominal diameter and obesity comorbidity. J Intern Med. 1997;241(1):71–9.

24. Pierpont YN, Dinh TP, Salas RE, et al. Obesity and surgical wound healing: a current review. ISRN Obes. 2014;2014:638936.

25. MK, Liang JLH, Itani K, et al. Ventral hernia management: expert consensus guided by systematic review. Annals Surg. 2016(Published online 15MAR2016).

26. Novitsky YW, Orenstein SB. Effect of patient and hospital characteristics on outcomes of elective ventral hernia repair in the United States. Hernia: The Journal of Hernias and Abdominal Wall Surgery. 2013;17(5):639–45.

27. Hornby ST, McDermott FD, Coleman M, et al. Female gender and diabetes mellitus increase the risk of recurrence after laparoscopic incisional hernia repair. Ann R Coll Surg Engl. 2015;97(2):115–9.

28. Shah BR, Hux JE. Quantifying the risk of infectious diseases for people with diabetes. Diabetes Care. 2003;26(2):510–3.

29. Fischer JP, Wink JD, Tuggle CT, Nelson JA, Kovach SJ. Wound risk assessment in ventral hernia repair: generation and internal validation of a risk stratification system using the ACS-NSQIP. Hernia: The Journal of Hernias and Abdominal Wall Surgery. 2015;19(1):103–11.

30. Asolati M, Huerta S, Sarosi G, Harmon R, Bell C, Anthony T. Predictors of recurrence in veteran patients with umbilical hernia: single center experience. Am J Surg. 2006;192(5):627–30.

31. Huntington C, Gamble J, Blair L, et al. Quantification of the effect of diabetes mellitus on ventral hernia repair: results from two National Registries. Am Surg. 2016;82(8):661–71.

32. Casqueiro J, Casqueiro J, Alves C. Infections in patients with diabetes mellitus: a review of pathogenesis. Indian J Endocrinol Metab. 2012;16(Suppl 1):S27–36.

33. Cox TC, Blair LJ, Huntington CR, et al. The cost of preventable comorbidities on wound complications in open ventral hernia repair. J Surg Res. 2016;206(1):214–22.
34. Mechanick JI, Youdim A, Jones DB, et al. Clinical practice guidelines for the perioperative nutritional, metabolic, and nonsurgical support of the bariatric surgery patient--2013 update: cosponsored by American Association of Clinical Endocrinologists, The Obesity Society, and American Society for Metabolic & Bariatric Surgery. Obesity (Silver Spring, Md). 2013;21(Suppl 1):S1–27.
35. Blair LJ, Huntington CR, Cox TC, et al. Risk factors for postoperative sepsis in laparoscopic gastric bypass. Surg Endosc. 2016;30(4):1287–93.
36. Burcharth J, Pedersen MS, Pommergaard HC, Bisgaard T, Pedersen CB, Rosenberg J. The prevalence of umbilical and epigastric hernia repair: a nationwide epidemiologic study. Hernia: The Journal of Hernias and Abdominal Wall Surgery. 2015;19(5):815–9.
37. Burcharth J, Pedersen M, Bisgaard T, Pedersen C, Rosenberg J. Nationwide prevalence of groin hernia repair. PLoS One. 2013;8(1):e54367.
38. Lappen JR, Sheyn D, Hackney DN. Does pregnancy increase the risk of abdominal hernia recurrence after prepregnancy surgical repair? Am J Obstet Gynecol. 2016;215(3):390 e391–5.
39. Oma E, Jensen KK, Jorgensen LN. Increased risk of ventral hernia recurrence after pregnancy: a nationwide register-based study. Am J Surg. 2017;214(3):474–8.
40. Oma E, Bay-Nielsen M, Jensen KK, Jorgensen LN, Pinborg A, Bisgaard T. Primary ventral or groin hernia in pregnancy: a cohort study of 20,714 women. Hernia: The Journal of Hernias and Abdominal Wall Surgery. 2017;21(3):335–9.
41. Lechner M, Fortelny R, Ofner D, Mayer F. Suspected inguinal hernias in pregnancy--handle with care! Hernia: The Journal of Hernias and Abdominal Wall Surgery. 2014;18(3):375–9.
42. Buch KE, Tabrizian P, Divino CM. Management of hernias in pregnancy. J Am Coll Surg. 2008;207(4):539–42.
43. Cohen-Kerem R, Railton C, Oren D, Lishner M, Koren G. Pregnancy outcome following non-obstetric surgical intervention. Am J Surg. 2005;190(3):467–73.
44. Van De Velde M, De Buck F. Anesthesia for non-obstetric surgery in the pregnant patient. Minerva Anestesiol. 2007;73(4):235–40.

45. Kwok AC, Semel ME, Lipsitz SR, et al. The intensity and variation of surgical care at the end of life: a retrospective cohort study. Lancet (London, England). 2011;378(9800):1408–13.
46. Diaz MR. Barriers to high quality end of life Care in the Surgical Intensive Care Unit. Am J Hosp Palliat Care. 2020;1049909120969970
47. Cooper Z, Koritsanszky LA, Cauley CE, et al. Recommendations for best communication practices to facilitate goal-concordant Care for Seriously ill Older Patients with Emergency Surgical Conditions. Ann Surg. 2016;263(1):1–6.
48. Wancata LM, Hinshaw DB. Rethinking autonomy: decision making between patient and surgeon in advanced illnesses. Annals translat Med. 2016;4(4):77.
49. Taylor LJ, Johnson SK, Nabozny MJ, et al. Barriers to goal-concordant Care for Older Patients with Acute Surgical Illness: communication patterns extrinsic to decision aids. Ann Surg. 2018;267(4):677–82.
50. Sanders JJ, Curtis JR, Tulsky JA. Achieving goal-concordant care: a conceptual model and approach to measuring serious illness communication and its impact. J Palliat Med. 2018;21(S2):S17–27.
51. Kelley AS, Morrison RS. Palliative Care for the Seriously ill. N Engl J Med. 2015;373(8):747–55.
52. Suwanabol PA, Vitous CA, Perumalswami CR, et al. Surgery Residents' experiences with seriously-ill and dying patients: an opportunity to improve palliative and end-of-life care. J Surg Educ. 2020;77(3):582–97.
53. Majdinasab EJ, Puckett Y, Pei KY. Increased in-hospital mortality and emergent cases in patients with stage IV cancer. Supportive care in cancer : official journal of the Multinational Association of Supportive Care in Cancer. 2020.
54. Yefimova M, Aslakson RA, Yang L, et al. Palliative care and end-of-life outcomes following high-risk surgery. JAMA Surg. 2020;155(2):138–46.

Chapter 51
The Changing Paradigm in Acute Care Surgery: Who Is the Best to Offer the Care?

Freeman Condon and Robert Lim

Introduction

Emergency general surgery (EGS) patients constitute a particularly high-risk group of surgical candidates who suffer disproportionate morbidity and mortality rates compared to non-emergency patients undergoing similar procedures [1–3]. This may seem unsurprising as EGS patients tend to be older, sicker, and frailer than their elective counterparts [4, 5]. Nonetheless, EGS patients remain at increased risk of morbidity even after controlling for these factors [6, 7]. The data suggests emergency procedures convey increased risk of their own accord. As life expectancies extend and the population ages, an increased burden of emergency surgical care can be

F. Condon
Tripler Army Medical Center, Honolulu, HI, USA

R. Lim (✉)
University of Oklahoma School of Medicine Tulsa, Tulsa, OK, USA
e-mail: Robert-lim@ouhsc.edu

© The Author(s), under exclusive license to Springer Nature   971
Switzerland AG 2022
J. R. Romanelli et al. (eds.), *The SAGES Manual of Quality, Outcomes and Patient Safety*,
https://doi.org/10.1007/978-3-030-94610-4_51

anticipated. It is vital, therefore, to find ways to improve care of this vulnerable population.

What's in a Name?

In 2003, the American Association of the Surgery for Trauma (AAST) began to define acute care surgery (ACS). They envisioned an evolution of the subspecialty of trauma and surgical critical care (SCC) which would formally subsume expertise in EGS [8]. Specific ACS fellowships emerged in 2008. Some of these programs arose from existing SCC programs, while others were created de novo. There remains significant heterogeneity among the 1- or 2-year fellowships in SCC, trauma/SCC, and ACS; and the American Board of Medical Specialties does not recognize a specific subspecialty in ACS, or trauma surgery for that matter [9]. Proponents of an ACS model of care suggest that concentrating emergency surgical care into the hands of subject matter experts will allow for the development of expertise and improve outcomes. Additionally, the ACS surgeon who is on-call for that particular day generally has no other clinical obligations, like an elective OR schedule or clinic, which would take away their ability to see patients with emergent conditions. Further, the on-call ACS surgeon would be able to operate readily at all hours without fear of commitments the following day. These factors would make the ACS surgeon, and likely the operating room, more efficient. Since the establishment of ACS services in 2003, many centers have adopted such models for the care of trauma, EGS, and SCC patients.

The Existing Standards

While ACS models are gaining popularity in busy urban medical centers and academic hospitals, the traditional model of a general surgeon on-call (GSOC) remains the most common paradigm nationwide. A recent Joint Commission survey found that only 16% of hospitals with an emergency department and operating room utilize an ACS service [10]. Surgeons responsible for emergency care under the traditional GSOC model may be a blend of community general surgeons or academic fellowship-trained subspecialists. Surgeons in the traditional model tend to maintain an elective practice and frequently have pre-scheduled daytime obligations following a night on call. Criticism of this model focuses on the absence of required training in the care of critically ill surgical patients as well as the potential for acute care and elective practice patients competing for a surgeon's attention during a day on call and the day after call. GSOC systems frequently alternate clinical responsibility for ACS consults every 24-hour period. Formal ACS systems often utilize 12-hour shifts, 24-hour, or even weekly call responsibility during which the surgeon on call is responsible for ACS presentations and little if anything else. The scope of ACS teams is not standardized nationally, and there is variability as to whether the ACS team acts in conjunction with, alongside, or in addition to the trauma service.

Heartening Signs

Early data from institutions that have converted to an ACS model are encouraging. The implementation of ACS programs has been demonstrated to reduce complications and shorten hospital stays [11]. In one series, mortality was reduced by a staggering 31% under an ACS model versus the previous GSOC standard [12]. Costs overall have also been reduced, likely by way of shortened inpatient stays [13, 14]. Patients with appendicitis had shorter times from ED presentation to surgery and lower rates of perforation when care was provided by ACS surgeons [15]. Such trends suggest a tremendous potential for improvements in national EGS outcomes if ACS models were widely implemented.

Nonoperative Contributors to ACS Success

Specialty trained surgeons and operative care are vital components of the ACS model, but they are not the only piece of the equation. Outside of emergency operative expertise, one reason for improved outcomes in the ACS model may be familiarity with and formal training in critical care. EGS patients are more likely to require ICU-level care including mechanical ventilation and continuous renal replacement therapy than similar elective surgery patients [16]. Multiple recent studies have suggested that "closed" ICU management (i.e., care in which the critical care physician is the primary physician and the surgeon functions as a consultant) also results in superior outcomes [17–19]. Advocates for "open" ICUs argue that this model disrupts the continuity of the patient's care and may sideline the surgeon who has intimate knowledge of their patient's pathology. Formally trained ACS surgeons may, therefore, offer a "best of both worlds" scenario. An ACS surgeon with formal training in SCC may admit and operate on an EGS patient and continue to care for that patient as an intensivist in the postoperative period in a closed surgical ICU. Indeed, a national survey demonstrated that 93% of critically ill EGS patients were cared for in a surgical ICU in institutions with ACS models compared with 45% in those using a GSOC model.

Beyond the care of the operative surgeon, ACS models depend on robust non-physician staffing. The same national survey found that ACS hospitals are more likely to have overnight in-house scrub techs, OR nurses, and recovery room nurses [20]. A retrospective review of ACS outcomes found decreased mortality in EGS was associated not only with an in-house surgeon but also independently associated with in-house overnight recovery room nursing [21]. Drawing from the experiences of the surgical community, anesthesiology has experienced a similar recent push for specialists in "acute care anesthesia" [22, 23]. These trends suggest, unsurprisingly, that building effective ACS systems relies on multidisciplinary and institutional commitments to improving

EGS patients and not simply specializing the training of surgeons. Such a paradigm has proven effective in the care of trauma patients, for whom specialized team care has been accepted as a national standard in recent decades.

Obstacles to ACS Implementation

Despite the encouraging data, ACS models are a long way from being adopted as a national standard. This is likely due to multiple factors. The biggest obstacle to broad ACS adoption is a lack of surgeon availability. ACS models, as envisioned by the AAST, rely on a robust pool of surgeons with formal fellowship-level training in ACS. Currently, such a cohort of surgeons does not exist, and indeed a critical shortage of trauma and SCC surgeons is anticipated [24]. This shortage coincides with a larger shortage of surgeons in all subspecialties [25].

In addition to a surgeon shortage, many community hospitals only have three or four general surgeons, and there isn't enough case volume to justify adding more surgeons to only cover the ACS business. Indeed only 7% of ACS fellowship-trained surgeons work in a rural setting. The current portrait of ACS in the United States is a familiar map in which the coasts and urban centers have a relatively high proportion of ACS model institutions, but rural, poor, and less educated regions continue to operate under a traditional model [26].

Another potential hurdle to ACS adoption is a concern that ACS surgeons will take operative volume away from the non-ACS general surgeons. Such a diversion of cases has implications for experience and reimbursement. Fortunately, several studies examining this problem have found that emergency volume diverted from non-ACS general surgeons is quickly recouped with elective caseload [27, 28]. Moreover, increased productivity and job satisfaction have been seen with the ACS model [29]. These data suggest that coverage of EGS with an ACS model is a non-zero-sum game: ACS surgeons are not stealing pieces of a finite pie of surgical patients. In fact, there are an estimated 6.5 surgeons per 100,000 patients in settings where there are ACS surgeons, but 4.7 surgeons per 100,000 patients in rural settings. This would suggest that in an urban setting where there is no decrease in productivity with an ACS model, there would be an increase in productivity in underserved areas with an ACS model.

Who Is the Expert?

With the emergence of ACS as a specialty, the question has arisen asking if the ACS surgeon is a jack of all trades but a master of none. Detractors of the model argue that subspecialist surgeons will always remain the experts in their field, emergency or no. There is some data to support this concern. Surgeons with specific bariatric training, for example, when compared to those without, are more likely to utilize laparoscopy and have shorter length of stay in obese EGS patients [30]. Elsewhere, it has been demonstrated that emergent laparotomies are less morbid when performed by a surgeon with training that reflects that pathology in question [31]. In other words, laparotomies for perforated diverticulitis are best performed by colorectal surgeons, while those for perforated duodenal ulcers are best performed by foregut surgeons. Nonetheless, there is evidence that continues to support the role of ACS in these situations. In one series, the availability of an acute care surgeon decreased mortality in emergent colon surgery [32]. Indeed there is also data showing that patients who require emergent colectomy have similar outcomes when performed by ACS surgeons as compared to colleagues who routinely perform elective resections [33]. Again, it is not only the individual surgeon who improves the EGS patient's outcome but rather the system with a supportive administration, appropriate levels of nursing, and in-house 24-hour availability of a surgical team that improves the patient's chances of survival and decreased morbidity.

Alternative Means to ACS with Finite Resources

Given the disconnect between the need and availability of ACS surgeons to staff a national transition to an ACS model, two potential options have been proposed. The first is a system used widely in Canada, which in essence combines the surgical manpower of the GSOC model with the dedicated call time of ACS [34]. Under this system, general and subspecialty surgeons take 1 week of rotating ACS call during which they have no elective responsibilities, followed by a period of time in which they may focus on their elective practice with no concern for cases that require emergent attention. Although this system removes the potential for competing strains on a surgeon's attention, it fails to achieve the chief benefit espoused by advocates of ACS, namely, dedicated training and practice in surgical emergencies and critical care.

An alternative solution to ACS implementation nationally is the regionalization of EGS care to centers of excellence with expertise in surgical acute care. Proponents argue that trauma care has already been successfully regionalized to American College of Surgeons-designated trauma centers in much of the country and that EGS care could be similarly organized. Some early experiments with regionalization of EGS care to trauma centers report improved mortality and efficiency [35, 36]. Multiple authors have described superior outcomes for EGS patients who present directly to tertiary centers as opposed to those requiring interhospital transfer [37, 38]. This regionalization of EGS care would require the pre-hospital triage of EGS patients to an appropriate regional center.

Defining Quality and Standards with EGS

There are three well-defined national programs of accreditation that have seen improved surgical success and quality in surgery. They are the National Surgical Quality Improvement

Program (NSQIP), the Metabolic and Bariatric Surgery Accreditation and Quality Improvement Program (MBSAQIP), and the Trauma Quality Improvement Project (TQIP). The NSQIP evaluates a random 10% of a hospital's cases and compares their 30-day outcomes to equivalent hospitals and national averages. The MBSAQIP and the TQIP programs evaluate 100% of a hospital's cases in those specialties to establish national standards and expected outcomes in those patient populations. In the case of MBSAQIP, it has helped to standardize the practice of bariatric surgery and provide direction on what constitutes quality care in that specialty [39]. The success of the TQIP goes further, in that fewer deaths and fewer major complications in trauma patients are seen in hospitals that participate in the TQIP program [40].

There are no such definitions or metrics of success for the ACS surgeon. ACS has demonstrated a need for it as EGS continues to have a high surgical morbidity and mortality rate. For example, one study listed major morbidity and death after emergent colon resection to be around 40% [41]. Additionally, an increasing number of EGS pathologies are managed nonoperatively. A shortcoming of NSQIP is the failure to capture the *nonoperative* cases. Small bowel obstruction, diverticulitis, and appendicitis are being successfully managed nonoperatively at increasing rates [42–44]. Such management and their results must be analyzed if an honest comparison of EGS outcomes is to be made.

An EGS Quality Improvement Program (EGSQIP) would likely help define what skills a quality ACS provider would have and what resources a quality ACS hospital would have. In a model similar to regionalized trauma centers, institutions that do not have the appropriate ACS resources would be able to quickly transfer those patients to those that did. From the success of the aforementioned programs, there is every reason to believe that this would improve outcomes and quality in EGS surgery. Further, it is a system that under-resourced hospitals could use to get their sicker patients to the better-resourced hospital and fellowship-trained specialists.

Moreover, hospitals would have a mechanism for determining where their practice gaps lie and where they should seek improvement to provide better care for EGS patients.

Conclusion

In sum, it should come as no surprise that the fellowship-trained ACS surgeon working in an appropriately resourced and staffed facility is likely to see better patient outcomes in the field of EGS. Such improved outcomes are borne out of specialty training in the breadth and depth of surgical emergencies as well as familiarity with the complex care of an often very sick patient population in the intensive care unit. Unfortunately, there just aren't enough such surgeons to serve the entire US population; and in fact, most of the country is underserved in this regard. Surgeon workforce projections suggest this disparity is likely to worsen before it improves. Two concepts may be able to address this issue. The first is to develop an EGSQIP to help define skills, metrics, resources, and expected outcomes needed to provide quality care at different hospitals. The second is to regionalize ACS such that sicker patients who exceed the capabilities of a smaller hospital, to include individual physician skill, would have a mechanism for a more timely and more appropriate transfer.

References

1. Smith M, Hussain A, Xiao J, Scheidler W, Reddy H, Olugbade K Jr, Campbell D Jr. The importance of improving the quality of emergency surgery for a regional quality collaborative. Ann Surg. 2013;257(4):596.
2. Stoneham M, Murray D, Foss N. Emergency surgery: the big three–abdominal aortic aneurysm, laparotomy and hip fracture. Anaesthesia. 2014;69:70–80.

3. Sudarshan M, Feldman LS, Louis ES, Al-Habboubi M, Hassan MME, Fata P, Khwaja KA. Predictors of mortality and morbidity for acute care surgery patients. J Surg Res. 2015;193(2):868–73.
4. Farhat JS, Velanovich V, Falvo AJ, Horst HM, Swartz A, Patton JH Jr, Rubinfeld IS. Are the frail destined to fail? Frailty index as predictor of surgical morbidity and mortality in the elderly. J Trauma Acute Care Surg. 2012;72(6):1526–31.
5. St-Louis E, Sudarshan M, Al-Habboubi M, Hassan MEH, Deckelbaum DL, Razek TS, Khwaja K. The outcomes of the elderly in acute care general surgery. Eur J Trauma Emerg Surg. 2016;42(1):107–13.
6. Havens JM, Peetz AB, Do WS, Cooper Z, Kelly E, Askari R, Salim A. The excess morbidity and mortality of emergency general surgery. J Trauma Acute Care Surg. 2015;78(2):306–11.
7. Mullen MG, Michaels AD, Mehaffey JH, Guidry CA, Turrentine FE, Hedrick TL, Friel CM. Risk associated with complications and mortality after urgent surgery vs elective and emergency surgery: implications for defining "quality" and reporting outcomes for urgent surgery. JAMA Surg. 2017;152(8):768–74.
8. American Association of the Surgery for Trauma. Acute care surgery overview AAST. 2020, October 6. https://www.aast.org/acute-care-surgery-overview.
9. American Board of Medical Specialties. Specialty and subspecialty certificates ABMS. 2020, October 6. https://www.abms.org/member-boards/specialty-subspecialty-certificates/.
10. Daniel VT, Ingraham AM, Khubchandani JA, Ayturk D, Kiefe CI, Santry HP. Variations in the delivery of emergency general surgery care in the era of acute care surgery. Jt Comm J Qual Patient Saf. 2019;45(1):14–23.
11. Khalil M, Pandit V, Rhee P, Kulvatunyou N, Orouji T, Tang A, Joseph B. Certified acute care surgery programs improve outcomes in patients undergoing emergency surgery: a nationwide analysis. J Trauma Acute Care Surg. 2015;79(1):60–4.
12. To KB, Kamdar NS, Patil P, Collins SD, Seese E, Krapohl GL, et al. Acute care surgery model and outcomes in emergency general surgery. J Am Coll Surg. 2019;228(1):21–8.
13. Cubas RF, Gómez NR, Rodriguez S, Wanis M, Sivanandam A, Garberoglio CA. Outcomes in the management of appendicitis and cholecystitis in the setting of a new acute care surgery service model: impact on timing and cost. J Am Coll Surg. 2012;215(5):715–21.

14. Chana P, Burns EM, Arora S, Darzi AW, Faiz OD. A systematic review of the impact of dedicated emergency surgical services on patient outcomes. Ann Surg. 2016;263(1):20–7.

15. Earley AS, Pryor JP, Kim PK, Hedrick JH, Kurichi JE, Minogue AC, Schwab CW. An acute care surgery model improves outcomes in patients with appendicitis. Ann Surg. 2006;244(4):498.

16. Lissauer ME, Galvagno SM Jr, Rock P, Narayan M, Shah P, Spencer H, Diaz JJ. Increased ICU resource needs for an academic emergency general surgery service. Crit Care Med. 2014;42(4):910–7.

17. Ghorra S, Reinert SE, Cioffi W, Buczko G, Simms HH. Analysis of the effect of conversion from open to closed surgical intensive care unit. Ann Surg. 1999;229(2):163.

18. van der Sluis FJ, Slagt C, Liebman B, Beute J, Mulder JW, Engel AF. The impact of open versus closed format ICU admission practices on the outcome of high risk surgical patients: a cohort analysis. BMC Surg. 2011;11(1):18.

19. Klein AL, Brown CV, Aydelotte J, Ali S, Clark A, Coopwood B. Implementation of a surgical intensive care unit service is associated with improved outcomes for trauma patients. J Trauma Acute Care Surg. 2014;77(6):964–8.

20. Ricci KB, Rushing AP, Ingraham AM, Daniel VT, Paredes AZ, Diaz A, Santry HP. The association between self-declared acute care surgery services and operating room access: results from a national survey. J Trauma Acute Care Surg. 2019;87(4):898–906.

21. Daniel VT, Rushing AP, Ingraham AM, Ricci KB, Paredes AZ, Diaz A, et al. Association between operating room access and mortality for life-threatening general surgery emergencies. J Trauma Acute Care Surg. 2019;87(1):35.

22. McCunn M, Dutton RP, Dagal A, Varon AJ, Kaslow O, Kucik CJ, Grissom T. Trauma, critical care, and emergency care anesthesiology: a new paradigm for the "acute care" anesthesiologist? Anesth Analg. 2015;121(6):1668–73.

23. Conti B, Greco KM, McCunn M. The acute care anesthesiologist as resuscitationist. Int Anesthesiol Clin. 2017;55(3):109–16.

24. Cohn SM, Price MA, Villarreal CL. Trauma and surgical critical care workforce in the United States: a severe surgeon shortage appears imminent. J Am Coll Surg. 2009;209(4):446–52.

25. Williams TE Jr, Ellison EC. Population analysis predicts a future critical shortage of general surgeons. Surgery. 2008;144(4):548–56.

26. Khubchandani JA, Ingraham AM, Daniel VT, Ayturk D, Kiefe CI, Santry HP. Geographic diffusion and implementation of

acute care surgery: an uneven solution to the National emergency general surgery crisis. JAMA Surg. 2018;153(2):150–9.

27. Miller PR, Wildman EA, Chang MC, Meredith JW. Acute care surgery: impact on practice and economics of elective surgeons. J Am Coll Surg. 2012;214(4):531–5.

28. Austin MT, Diaz JJ Jr, Feurer ID, Miller RS, May AK, Guillamondegui OD, et al. Creating an emergency general surgery service enhances the productivity of trauma surgeons, general surgeons and the hospital. J Trauma Acute Care Surg. 2005;58(5):906–10.

29. Barnes SL, Cooper CJ, Coughenour JP, MacIntyre AD, Kessel JW. Impact of acute care surgery to departmental productivity. J Trauma Acute Care Surg. 2011;71(4):1027–34.

30. Pakula A, Skinner R. Do acute care surgeons need bariatric surgical training to ensure optimal outcomes in obese patients with nonbariatric emergencies? Surg Obes Relat Dis. 2018;14(3):339–41.

31. Boyd-Carson H, Doleman B, Herrod PJJ, Anderson ID, Williams JP, Lund JN, et al. Association between surgeon special interest and mortality after emergency laparotomy. Br J Surg. 2019;106(7):940–8.

32. Moore LJ, Turner KL, Jones SL, Fahy BN, Moore FA. Availability of acute care surgeons improves outcomes in patients requiring emergent colon surgery. Am J Surg. 2011;202(6):837–42.

33. Schuster KM, McGillicuddy EA, Maung AA, Kaplan LJ, Davis KA. Can acute care surgeons perform emergency colorectal procedures with good outcomes? J Trauma Acute Care Surg. 2011;71(1):94–101.

34. Ball CG, Hameed SM, Brenneman FD. Acute care surgery: a new strategy for the general surgery patients left behind. Can J Surg. 2010;53(2):84.

35. Diaz JJ Jr, Norris PR, Gunter OL, Collier BR, Riordan WP, Morris JA Jr. Does regionalization of acute care surgery decrease mortality? J Trauma Acute Care Surg. 2011;71(2):442–6.

36. Block EF, Rudloff B, Noon C, Behn B. Regionalization of surgical services in central Florida: the next step in acute care surgery. J Trauma Acute Care Surg. 2010;69(3):640–4.

37. Yelverton S, Rozario N, Matthews BD, Reinke CE. Interhospital transfer for emergency general surgery: an independent predictor of mortality. Am J Surg. 2018;216(4):787–92.

38. Santry HP, Janjua S, Chang Y, Petrovick L, Velmahos GC. Interhospital transfers of acute care surgery patients: should

care for nontraumatic surgical emergencies be regionalized? World J Surg. 2011;35(12):2660–7.

39. Dawson TH, Bhutiani N, Benns MV, Miller KR, Bozeman MC, Kehdy FJ, Motameni AT. Comparing patterns of care and outcomes after operative management of complications after bariatric surgery at MBSAQIP accredited bariatric centers and non-bariatric facilities. Surg Endosc. 2020:1–6.

40. Hemmila MR, Cain-Nielsen AH, Jakubus JL, Mikhail JN, Dimick JB. Association of hospital participation in a regional trauma quality improvement collaborative with patient outcomes. JAMA Surg. 2018;153(8):747–56.

41. Ingraham AM, Cohen ME, Bilimoria KY, Raval MV, Ko CY, Nathens AB, Hall BL. Comparison of 30-day outcomes after emergency general surgery procedures: potential for targeted improvement. Surgery. 2010;148(2):217–38.

42. Matsushima K, Sabour A, Park C, Strumwasser A, Inaba K, Demetriades D. Management of adhesive small bowel obstruction: a distinct paradigm shift in the United States. J Trauma Acute Care Surg. 2019;86(3):383–91.

43. Collaborative, C. O. D. A., Flum DR, Davidson GH, Monsell SE, Shapiro NI, Odom SR, et al. A randomized trial comparing antibiotics with appendectomy for appendicitis. N Engl J Med. 2020;383:1907–19.

44. Salem L, Anaya DA, Flum DR. Temporal changes in the management of diverticulitis. J Surg Res. 2005;124(2):318–23.

Chapter 52
Super-subspecialization of General Surgery: Is This Better for Patients?

Joseph A. Sujka and Christopher G. DuCoin

Objectives

1. Define the population impacts of care access in a specialized model.
2. Who owns the patient in a paradigm of specialists?
3. What is lost in super-specialization?

Specialization has been becoming more common in the world of general surgery. At the time of writing, the American Board of Medical Specialties has over 24 separate medical and surgical specialty boards. In a survey of US allopathic surgery residency graduates from 2009 to 2013, over 77% pursued a specialty [1], despite findings that long-term financial outcomes may not be improved [2]. Some suggest that this trend is motivated somewhat by mentorship and overall confidence when completing residency [1]. The trend toward specialization began around the World War II with the estab-

J. A. Sujka · C. G. DuCoin (✉)
Department of Surgery, University of South Florida Morsani
College of Medicine, Tampa, FL, USA
e-mail: josephsujka@usf.edu; cduoin@usf.edu

J. R. Romanelli et al. (eds.), *The SAGES Manual of Quality,
Outcomes and Patient Safety*,
https://doi.org/10.1007/978-3-030-94610-4_52

985

lishment of the British Association of Aesthetic Plastic Surgeons and has continued to change the world of general surgery since [3]. Many have written as detractors of this model and question whether or not subspecialization is truly better for the patient [4–6]. In this chapter, this question will be examined.

Clarification of the terms subspecialization and super-specialization is necessary: Subspecialization is when a surgeon is carrying out the broad practice of their specialty but develops an expertise in one area. Super-specialization is when a surgeon discontinues the broad practice of their specialty to concentrate on one particular area of surgery [7].

Population Impacts of Care Access in a Specialized Model

Healthcare disparities and access to care are important elements of social justice that must be considered in all aspects of healthcare delivery including access to specialists. Unfortunately, lower income, insurance status, race, and ethnicity have all been associated with limited surgical care access. Black and Hispanic patients have significantly higher rates of postoperative complications, blood transfusions, perioperative mortality, and longer hospital stays. On top of that, patients of color are less likely to receive a variety of oncologic and vascular procedures and are more likely to undergo open operations compared to white patients [8–10]. Access to procedures by specialists has been suggested to improve outcomes. One study examined access to colonoscopy from medical specialists and found colonoscopy was less likely to be performed by a specialist if the patient was non-white [11]. Due to these disparities, ongoing increases in surgical specialization may be indirectly worsening these inequities. Therefore, it is important that current disparities in patient care be examined and evaluated for ongoing areas of improvement.

Another important question alongside equitable access to care is this: Does subspecialization improve the quality of patient care and outcomes? At this time, there is no definitive answer to this question; however, it appears that specialization may improve patient care and outcomes. One study compared breast cancer outcome among patients in a cancer registry both before and after involving surgeons with surgical specialization. They found a significant improvement in disease-free survival and recurrence rates; however, the authors admit this may be due to an increase in the use of appropriate systemic therapy. It could be argued though that the increased education of a specialist leads to patients getting appropriate systemic therapy. There is also the possibility that this change was due to improvements in overall patient care and was independent of surgical specialization [12].

Colorectal surgery has also examined their outcomes in comparison to general surgery. One study examined 974 patients and found an overall higher 5-year survival in a group treated in a colorectal unit. Being treated in the specialized colorectal unit was found on survival regression analysis to be an independent predictor of survival. However, patients in the colorectal unit were also overall lower stage cancers, and the general surgery unit was heterogenous with ten total surgeons to the colorectal unit's one surgeon [13]. Another study retrospectively reviewed 196 consecutive patients who underwent emergent left-sided colonic resection. They compared outcomes of acute care and colorectal surgeons. Colorectal surgeons were found to have similar morbidity and mortality but lower overall stoma rates (40.4 versus 88.8%) and higher rates of primary anastomosis (85.5 versus 28.7%) both of which were statistically significant [14]. The authors do not go as far as to say that acute care surgeons should not perform these operations but suggest that acute care surgeons should receive sufficient experience to perform the technically more complex operation of a primary anastomosis.

It appears this improvement in patient outcomes may extend into the world of emergency surgery was well. A retrospective study examined 30-day operative mortality after emergency laparotomy and found lower mortality rates in patients who underwent emergency laparotomy by specialists with interest in the affected area of the GI tract (UGI or colorectal) [15].

Finally, a systematic review was performed focusing on surgeon volume and specialization in relation to patient outcomes. The 22 studies included contained 144,421 patients. Specialist surgeons had significantly better outcomes in 20 of the 22 studies in comparison to general surgeons. They also had lower mortality (11 of 12 studies), fewer complications (14 of 17 studies), and shorter hospital stays (5 of 5 studies). When examining specialization the majority of prospective and retrospective studies showed a beneficial effect for patients [16].

Based on the literature, it appears that a specialized patient care model may produce superior results, but in many studies the role of multidisciplinary conferences to discuss patients and specialized clinics is not evaluated as potential confounders.

Who Owns the Patient in a Paradigm of Specialists?

As the field of surgery becomes progressively more specialized, it can be frustrating and confusing to the patient on who is driving their care. Eugene Stead is quoted as saying, "what this patient needs is *a* doctor" [17]. This quote is particularly impactful now as one patient can have multiple treating physicians and not know whom to turn to for answers.

Some have opined that this fracturing of patient care and changes to resident training have led to a decrease in patient ownership, not only by residents but also by specialists caring for patients [18, 19]. Even the phrase "patient ownership" has been examined to see if its meaning has changed or requires redefining in this modern era of medicine [20, 21]. In many cases the admitting surgical or medical team takes the lead on overarching patient care issues, although the boundaries for whether consulting specialists may or may not adjust patient care is not standardized.

Sparse objective data exists on how much of a problem changes in patient ownership and care models may present; however, the cost of healthcare has been increasing along with the rise in specialists. This rise in cost has been implied by some to be indicative of an underlying problem with the specialist model [22]. In the simplest terms, having multiple specialists complicates planning of patient care, appears to increase cost, and separates a patient into multiple small parts based on their respective teams of care.

What Is Lost in Super-specialization?

Super-specialization, or when a surgeon discontinues the broad practice of their specialty to concentrate on one particular area of surgery, is a relatively new issue in the world of surgery. Minimal papers or opinion pieces have been written to discuss the potential pitfalls of this practice. Access to general surgeons remains a concern as the United States is projected to have a shortfall of general surgeons with some predicting a shortage of over 6,000 general surgeons by 2050 [23]. Even with ongoing specialization and changes seen in the field of surgery, a recent study found that general surgery still remains a heterogenous field with a strong need for a broad-based surgical education [24]. To extend this to super-specialization if the world of surgery was to be even further subdivided, this deficiency of general surgery and specializations would be further exacerbated potentially leading to difficulty finding care for patients outside of tertiary academic centers. Only time will tell if this practice becomes more widespread and what affect it may have on patient's care.

Where Do We Go from Here?

Specialization has become more common in the world of surgery for a variety of reasons. This has been in the background of disparities in medical care, which may be worsened by specialization. However, care from specialists does appear to improve patient outcomes if not patient ownership. We must be cautious that at-risk populations do not suffer from this increase in specialization and work diligently to improve their access to care. Specialization will not be eliminated as the knowledge and complexity of medicine increases, but it is our duty to make sure all patients receive the benefits of this increasing education.

Bibliography

1. Klingensmith ME, Cogbill TH, Luchette F, Biester T, Samonte K, Jones A, et al. Factors influencing the decision of surgery residency graduates to pursue general surgery practice versus fellowship. Ann Surg. 2015;262(3):449–55; discussion 454-455.
2. Baimas-George M, Fleischer B, Slakey D, Kandil E, Korndorffer JR, DuCoin C. Is it All About the Money? Not All Surgical Subspecialization Leads to Higher Lifetime Revenue when Compared to General Surgery. J Surg Educ. 2017;74(6):e62–6.
3. Burd DA. Super-specialization leads to higher surgical standards? Br J Plast Surg. 1990;43(1):112–5.
4. Silen W. Super-specialization fellowships in gastrointestinal surgery: an unrealistic dream. Surgery. 1992;111(4):479–80.
5. Black J. Has surgical subspecialization gone too far? Hosp Med Lond Engl. 1998. 1999;60(3):206–9.
6. Rajan P, Din NA. Sub-specialization in general surgery--the end of the "general" surgeon? Hosp Med Lond Engl 1998. 2005;66(3):185.
7. Milward TM. Sub-specialization or super-specialization. Br J Plast Surg. 1991;44(7):554.
8. Haider AH, Scott VK, Rehman KA, Velopulos C, Bentley JM, Cornwell EE, et al. Racial disparities in surgical care and outcomes in the United States: a comprehensive review of patient,

provider, and systemic factors. J Am Coll Surg. 2013;216(3):482–92.e12.

9. Kressin NR, Groeneveld PW. Race/Ethnicity and overuse of care: a systematic review. Milbank Q. 2015;93(1):112–38.

10. Ravi P, Sood A, Schmid M, Abdollah F, Sammon JD, Sun M, et al. Racial/Ethnic Disparities in Perioperative Outcomes of Major Procedures: Results From the National Surgical Quality Improvement Program. Ann Surg. 2015;262(6):955–64.

11. Josey MJ, Odahowski CL, Zahnd WE, Schootman M, Eberth JM. Disparities in Utilization of Medical Specialists for Colonoscopy. Health Equity. 2019;3(1):464–71.

12. Golledge J, Wiggins JE, Callam MJ. Effect of surgical subspecialization on breast cancer outcome. Br J Surg. 2000;87(10):1420–5.

13. Platell C, Lim D, Tajudeen N, Tan J-L, Wong K. Dose surgical sub-specialization influence survival in patients with colorectal cancer? World J Gastroenterol. 2003;9(5):961–4.

14. Gibbons G, Tan CJ, Bartolo DCC, Filgate R, Makin G, Barwood N, et al. Emergency left colonic resections on an acute surgical unit: does subspecialization improve outcomes? ANZ J Surg. 2015;85(10):739–43.

15. Brown LR, McLean RC, Perren D, O'Loughlin P, McCallum IJ. Evaluating the effects of surgical subspecialisation on patient outcomes following emergency laparotomy: A retrospective cohort study. Int J Surg Lond Engl. 2019;62:67–73.

16. Chowdhury MM, Dagash H, Pierro A. A systematic review of the impact of volume of surgery and specialization on patient outcome. Br J Surg. 2007;94(2):145–61.

17. Stead EA, Wagner GS, Cebe B, Rozear MP, Stead EA Jr. What this patient needs is a doctor. Durham, N.C: Carolina Academic Press; 1978. p. 244.

18. Conti CR. Some thoughts about patient ownership. Clin Cardiol. 2015;38(1):1.

19. Masters P. In our health system, who "owns" patients [Internet]. KevinMD. Available from: https://www.kevinmd.com/blog/2019/06/in-our-health-system-who-owns-patients.html

20. Kiger ME, Meyer HS, Hammond C, Miller KM, Dickey KJ, Hammond DV, et al. Whose patient is this? a scoping review of patient ownership. Acad Med J Assoc Am Med Coll. 2019;94(11S Association of American Medical Colleges Learn Serve Lead: Proceedings of the 58th Annual Research in Medical Education Sessions):S95–104.

21. Cowley DS, Markman JD, Best JA, Greenberg EL, Grodesky MJ, Murray SB, et al. Understanding ownership of patient care: A dual-site qualitative study of faculty and residents from medicine and psychiatry. Perspect Med Educ. 2017;6(6):405–12.
22. Jauhar S. https://doi.org/10.1002/clc.22348 [Internet]. Time. 2014. Available from: https://time.com/3138561/specialist-doctors-high-cost/.
23. Williams TE, Ellison EC. Population analysis predicts a future critical shortage of general surgeons. Surgery. 2008;144(4):548–54. discussion 554-556
24. Decker MR, Dodgion CM, Kwok AC, Hu Y-Y, Havlena JA, Jiang W, et al. Specialization and the current practices of general surgeons. J Am Coll Surg. 2014;218(1):8–15.

Chapter 53
What Is the Connection Between Physician Relationships with Industry and Patient Care?

Caroline E. Reinke, Peter M. Denk, Erin Schwarz, and Phillip P. Shadduck

All financial relationships between physicians and commercial interests should be disclosed. When financial relationships exist, the potential for bias can be mitigated by evaluating the relevance of the financial relationship to the educational/scientific content and peer reviewing the content for balance.

C. E. Reinke (✉)
Department of Surgery, Atrium Health, Charlotte, NC, USA
e-mail: Caroline.e.reinke@atriumhealth.org

P. M. Denk
GI Surgical Specialists, Fort Myers, FL, USA
e-mail: pmdenk@gisurgical.com

E. Schwarz
SAGES, Los Angeles, CA, USA
e-mail: erin@sages.org

P. P. Shadduck
Duke University, Durham, NC, USA

© The Author(s), under exclusive license to Springer Nature   993
Switzerland AG 2022
J. R. Romanelli et al. (eds.), *The SAGES Manual of Quality, Outcomes and Patient Safety*,
https://doi.org/10.1007/978-3-030-94610-4_53

994   C. E. Reinke et al.

Introduction

In society, government, and medicine, a tension exists between those who emphasize that physician relationships with healthcare companies have the potential to negatively impact patient care and those who emphasize that these relationships are necessary and beneficial to medical device and drug development. Both points of view are true. In rare instances, there have been examples of relationships between companies and physicians (or physician organizations) that have impacted educational programs and clinical initiatives in ways that were not in the best interest of the patient [1]. There have been reports of high-profile cases of financial kickbacks received by physicians in exchange for promoting various commercial products [2]. Such cases of professional misconduct undermine public trust. At the same time, relationships between physicians and industry are critical for the development of devices and procedures that improve clinical outcomes. Practicing physicians best understand the unmet clinical needs that should be addressed by new technologies. When engineers translate ideas and unmet needs into prototypes, direct feedback from physicians, to modify and advance medical devices and related procedures, is important to ensure the introduction of safe, effective, and cost-effective technologies and techniques [3–5]. Collaborations between stakeholders are also essential to ensure the safe adoption and implementation of novel techniques and instruments through education and large-scale hands-on training [3]. In this chapter, we will explore financial relationships with industry and potential conflicts of interest in medical education, conflicts that might directly or indirectly impact patient care, and we will detail the SAGES model for disclosing and managing relevant financial relationships.

For purposes of this chapter, we will utilize terms as defined by the Accreditation Council for Continuing Medical Education (ACCME). The ACCME is the organization that regulates accredited education (CME) to ensure that it is free of bias. In December 2020, the ACCME released its new guidance document, termed **Standards for Integrity and Independence (SII)**, which replaced its 2004 **Standards for Commercial Support (SCS)** [6, 7]. With the 2020 update came some new terminology and revised definitions. The terms "commercial interest," "industry," and "conflict of interest" were replaced by "ineligible company" and "relevant financial relationships." In the new SII, the ACCME defines an **ineligible company** as one "whose primary business is producing, marketing, selling, re-selling, or distributing healthcare products used by or on patients." The companies are called "ineligible" because they are not eligible to be accredited in the ACCME system. The ACCME SII requires that all the planning and implementation of accredited educational content must occur independently from any ACCME-defined ineligible companies. The ACCME states that "the accredited provider [of CME] is responsible for identifying **relevant financial relationships** between individuals in control of educational content and ineligible companies and managing these to ensure they do not introduce commercial bias into the education. Financial relationships *of any dollar amount* are defined as **relevant** if the educational content is related to the business lines or products of the ineligible company."

It is also worth noting that the terms "owner" and "employee" have been redefined in the December 2020 standards. "**Owners** are defined as individuals who have an ownership interest in a company, except for stockholders of publicly traded companies, or holders of shares through a pension or mutual fund. **Employees** are defined as individuals hired to work for another person or business (the employer) for compensation and who are subject to the employer's direction as to the details of how to perform the job" [6].

Relevant financial relationships, if not recognized and managed well, have the potential to bias not only CME but also the education of medical students and graduate trainees, drafting and promotion of clinical practice guidelines, funding of research, clinical study design and data analysis, scientific publication, and health system administration. Though financial relationships that influence patient safety and quality care can exist in many forms beyond the scope of CME, the ACCME provides the most broadly accepted and rigorous definitions around financial relationships. As a Professional Medical Association (PMA) steeped in surgical innovation, SAGES is an international leader in patient safety, quality, and outcomes through physician education. The ACCME standards have been the foundation for the SAGES work in this area.

Examples of Ways that Financial Relationships Can Impact Quality, Outcomes, and Patient Safety

In the late 1990s, there was a significant publicity surrounding more than 3000 lawsuits filed over cervical pedicle screws utilized in surgical operations for treatment of degenerative disc disease. In over 400 of these lawsuits, the litigants alleged that numerous specialty societies and several university centers had promoted, in medical education activities, the off-label use of the pedicle screw due to financial relationships between the organizations and the manufacturer. All of the lawsuits were eventually dismissed for lack of evidence [7]. The concerns raised by the patients in these cases, as well as many other pressures, contributed to the 2003 guidance issued by the Office of the Inspector General (OIG) of the US Department of Health and Human Services regarding commercial support of medical education activities. The OIG identifies educational grants as something that may place a company at high risk for violating FDA regulations and/or federal anti-kickback regulations [8]. It was in this environment, in 2004, that the ACCME dramatically revised the 1992 Standards for Commercial Support to clarify what was and was not allowable in CME programming [9].

There are, unfortunately, more recent examples of unrecognized/unmanaged relevant financial relationships that adversely impacted patient care. One recent example from academic medicine involved a prominent medical oncologist and chief medical officer at a world-renowned cancer center who "failed to disclose millions of dollars in payments from drug and health care companies in recent years, omitting his financial ties from dozens of research articles in prestigious publications like The New England Journal of Medicine and the Lancet." Also, "he put a positive spin on the results of two Roche-sponsored clinical trials that many others considered disappointments, without disclosing his relationship to the company. Since 2014, he has received more than $3 million from Roche..." It's difficult to know how widespread the negative impact on patient care was from this physician's biased research publications, academic presentations, society leadership influence, and medical center influence [10].

Research has demonstrated that there is a connection between payments received from commercial interests and both physician prescribing habits and research conclusions. ProPublica reported in 2016 that "the more money doctors receive from drug and medical device companies, the more brand-name drugs they tend to prescribe" [11]. Studies have also revealed that some authors with relevant financial relationships publish results that are more favorable toward industry [12, 13]. It is evident that improperly disclosed and managed relevant financial relationships with industry may impact quality, outcomes, and patient safety.

Unfortunately, a physician disclosure-alone approach, which had been allowed by the ACCME prior to 2004, has not proven to be effective at preventing bias [14, 15]. The 2004 ACCME Standards included the requirement that accredited CME providers must both identify and *manage* conflicts of interest in advance of educational activities. Voluntary physician disclosure of their financial relationships to the audience is a necessary but insufficient management mechanism. The 2020 ACCME SII requires that accredited education providers must (a) collect information from all individuals about their financial relationships, (b) exclude owners or employees of ineligible companies, (c) identify relevant financial relationships, (d) mitigate relevant financial relationships, and (e) disclose all relevant financial relationships to the learners [6].

SAGES Processes for Disclosure and Management of Relevant Financial Relationships

Recognizing the importance of internal oversight of potential and real conflicts of interest within its innovative membership, SAGES began developing conflict of interest (COI) review processes over a decade ago. In 2009, the SAGES Executive Committee established both an Industry Relations Task Force (IRTF) to study corporate-level financial relationships and a Conflict of Interest Task Force (CITF) to study physician-level financial relationships. These task forces were led by seasoned SAGES leaders, and they were charged with developing and implementing processes that accomplish two goals: (1) eliminate influence that financial relationships with industry might have upon educational content and (2) sustain innovation, research, education, and other worthy activities, including those performed collaboratively with pharmaceutical/device companies. The task forces produced several policies, procedures, and work products, including the SAGES 2010 Statement [16].

SAGES Statement on the Relationship Between Professional Medical Associations and Industry

In February 2010, the SAGES IRTF and Board published a "Statement on the Relationship between Professional Medical Associations and Industry" [16]. The statement affirms important differences between drug and device development. Early drug development is generally conducted by basic scientists, including chemists, immunologists, pharmacists, and others. Medical clinicians become more involved at the clinical trial stage of drug development. In contrast, surgeons are typically required throughout the development process for surgical devices including identifying unmet needs, defining device requirements, developing and testing device prototypes, performing preclinical research, and conducting clinical trials. Once new technologies and techniques are approved, surgeons are also necessary to guide their safe introduction into practice [16–18]. Surgeons and other specialists who perform invasive procedures (such as gastroenterologists, cardiologists, and interventional radiologists) require hands-on training for safe implementation of new technology. If regulatory changes regarding industry relationships exclude surgical innovators from safe device development and introduction, then negative clinical and economic repercussions would follow. Recognizing this, SAGES opined that with effective COI disclosure and management processes, Professional Medical Associations (PMAs) should be capable of providing educational activities that are scientifically and ethically sound, without eliminating all financial support from industry. Of course, with this position comes significant responsibility. The SAGES leadership understands and embraces that responsibility, and stringent internal policies and processes for the organization, leadership, and all educational activities have been developed accordingly.

Disclosure and Mitigation Process

SAGES endorses and complies with the newly released ACCME SII which requires that individuals who control CME content disclose all relevant financial relationships with ACCME-ineligible companies. The ACCME requires the accredited provider to identify and mitigate relevant financial relationships in advance of the activity. According to the ACCME, "financial relationships of any dollar amount are defined as relevant if the educational content is related to the business lines or products of the ineligible company" [19].

SAGES developed a comprehensive process for identifying and mitigating relevant financial relationships in 2009, prior to the CMSS Code, the Physician Payment Sunshine Act, and other developments. The SAGES process was refined over several years and published in 2014 [20, 21]. The process was also evaluated annually for its effectiveness during its first 3 years of implementation [21]. Notably stringent features of the SAGES disclosure and mitigation process include the following: (1) Reviews of disclosures are performed independently by at least three people—a CME staff member, one or more physicians (COI committee members and session chairs), and a final review by the COI committee chair, co-chairs, and staff; (2) for scientific abstract/video submissions, all authors (not just the presenting author) must disclose their financial relationships; (3) faculty who have SAGES-defined level 3 conflicts (relevant consulting relationships, Fig. 53.1) are required to submit their presentation for peer review prior to the presentation, with firm deadlines;

Level of Potential Conflict	Action by SAGES	Resulting Actions
Level 1: Nothing to disclose	Chairs to review for accuracy	Print disclosures in program
Level 2: Relationships with ineligible companies not relevant to content of session and/or lecture. *Example: Dr. X receives honorarium for consulting work for Company A. Company A manufactures hernia repair products. Dr. X is invited to speak on surgical management of acid reflux.*	Chairs to review for accuracy, confirm not relevant; secondary review by Conflict of Interest Committee (COIC) *Example: Dr. X's relationship is not relevant.*	Print disclosures in program
Level 3: Relationships with ineligible companies making products related to content. *Example: Dr. Y receives honorarium for consulting work for Company A. Company A manufactures hernia repair products. Dr. Y is invited to give a talk on complications following hernia repair*	Chairs to review relevance, confirm that faculty is best person to give lecture & adjust lecture subject if appropriate; secondary review by COIC; Determination of management technique (typically peer review) *Example: Dr. Y's presentation will be peer reviewed in advance of the meeting; all clinical care recommendations will be referenced; balance & impartiality will be obvious.*	Letter to faculty informing them of Commercial Support Policy, options for conflict management; Mitigation technique applied and documented in advance of activity; Print disclosures in program and include statement that "all relevant relationships were mitigated"

FIGURE 53.1 SAGES conflict management process

(4) faculty submitting their presentation after an initial deadline (10–21 days before the meeting) lose any PMA reimbursements or discounts being offered; (5) faculty submitting their presentation after a final deadline (3–5 days before the meeting) are removed from the program; and (6) the process is applied uniformly, regardless of speaker rank or role.

Less than five abstract submitters to each annual meeting are identified with a level 4 conflict (relevant ownership/employment relationship, Fig. 53.1), and they are not allowed to present. About 80–100 presentations (of the 500 or so presentations at each annual meeting) must be submitted to the COI committee for review, nearly all of the presentations requested by the COI committee are submitted before the posted deadlines, and about 10–15 presentations require modification before they can be delivered at the annual meeting. If any concerns remain (which is rare), then COI committee representatives attend the presentations. After each annual meeting, all attendee evaluations are reviewed by the COI committee, program committee, and executive committee. Any reports of perceived bias are evaluated per our policy established for this purpose (the SAGES COI Committee Procedures for Confidentially Evaluating Reports of Concerns).

The SAGES process is designed to be stringent, yet it does rely on physician self-disclosure. By intent, we have strict oversight of presentations. It was developed not only to meet regulatory requirements but primarily to accomplish the goal established by the SAGES Board in 2009: to provide educational activities that are both scientifically and ethically sound, without being required to achieve zero financial support from industry.

The SAGES experience with our mitigation process has demonstrated effectiveness at meeting the goals of transparent disclosure of COI when evaluated based on audience-perceived bias at our annual scientific meetings. In the first 3 years after its implementation, perceived bias as reported in attendee evaluations (1.2–2.2%) was one third of what it was in the 3 years prior to its implementation (4.4–6.2%). During this period, 14–42% of speakers at the annual meeting had financial relationships with industry [20]. Subsequent annual meetings have had similar low reports of perceived bias. Furthermore, post-meeting evaluations by the COI committee have revealed that most reports of perceived bias turn out not to be actual bias. Actual bias at the SAGES annual meetings appears to occur in less than 1% of presentations.

Conclusion

SAGES leadership carries on a decade-long tradition of embracing the importance of rigorous evaluation of financial relationships in education as a way to safeguard the safety and quality of patient care provided by SAGES members. The SAGES COI and executive committee leaders communicate regularly with the ACCME to continue refining definitions and policies, as the understanding of PMA and industry relationships evolves with time and technology advances.

References

1. Rothman DJ, McDonald WJ, Berkowitz CD, Chimonas SC, DeAngelis CD, Hale RW, et al. Professional medical associations and their relationships with industry: a proposal for controlling conflict of interest. JAMA. 2009;301(13):1367–72.
2. Advanced Medical Technology Association. Code of ethics 2020. Available from: https://www.advamed.org/issues/code-ethics/code-ethics.
3. Cervero RM, Gaines JK. Is there a relationship between commercial support and bias in continuing medical education activities? An updated literature review. Available from: https://www.accme.org/publications/there-relationship-between-commercial-support-and-bias-continuing-medical-education.
4. Ellison JA, Hennekens CH, Wang J, Lundberg GD, Sulkes D. Low rates of reporting commercial bias by physicians following online continuing medical education activities. Am J Med. 2009;122(9):875–8.

5. Kawczak S, Carey W, Lopez R, Jackman D. The effect of industry support on participants' perceptions of bias in continuing medical education. Acad Med. 2010;85(1):80–4.

6. Accreditation Council for Continuing Medical Education. Standards for integrity and independence in accredited continuing education standalone package. Available from: https://accme.org/publications/standards-for-integrity-and-independence-accredited-continuing-education-standalone.

7. Eisner W. Exorcising the "Ghost of Pedicle Screw Past". Orthopedics this week [Internet]. 2012 December 3, 2021. Available from: https://ryortho.com/2012/10/exorcising-the-ldquoghost-of-pedicle-screw-pastrdquo/#:~:text=Over%20 3%2C%20000%20lawsuits%20were,and%20SRS%20were%20 also%20sued.

8. Conflicts of Interest in Medical Education. In: Lo B, Field MJ, editors. Conflict of interest in medical research, education, and practice. Washington DC: National Academies Press; 2009.

9. Accreditation Council for Continuing Medical Education. ACCME standards for commercial support. Available from: https://www.accme.org/publications/accme-standards-for-commercial-support.

10. Ornstein C, Thomas K. Top cancer researcher fails to disclose corporate financial ties in major research journals. Sloan Kettering's Crisis [Internet]. 2018. Available from: https://www.propublica.org/article/doctor-jose-baselga-cancer-researcher-corporate-financial-ties.

11. Ornstein C, Tigas M, Grochowski R. Now there's proof: docs who get company cash tend to prescribe more brand-name meds. Dollars for Doctors [Internet]. 2016. Available from: https://www.propublica.org/article/doctors-who-take-company-cash-tend-to-prescribe-more-brand-name-drugs.

12. Cherla DV, Olavarria OA, Bernardi K, Viso CP, Moses ML, Holihan JL, et al. Investigation of financial conflict of interest among published ventral hernia research. J Am Coll Surg. 2018;226(3):230–4.

13. Turner EH, Matthews AM, Linardatos E, Tell RA, Rosenthal R. Selective publication of antidepressant trials and its influence on apparent efficacy. N Engl J Med. 2008;358(3):252–60.

14. Cain DM, Loewenstein G, Moore DA. When sunlight fails to disinfect: understanding the perverse effects of disclosing conflicts of interest. J Consum Res. 2011;37(5):836–57.

15. Loewenstein G, Sah S, Cain DM. The unintended consequences of conflict of interest disclosure. JAMA. 2012;307(7):669–70.

16. Society of American Gastrointestinal and Endoscopic Surgeons(SAGES)statement on the relationship between professional medical associations and industry. Surg Endosc. 2010;24(4):742–4.

17. Stain SC, Pryor AD, Shadduck PP. The SAGES manual ethics of surgical innovation. Springer; 2016.

18. Strong VE, Forde KA, MacFadyen BV, Mellinger JD, Crookes PF, Sillin LF, et al. Ethical considerations regarding the implementation of new technologies and techniques in surgery. Surg Endosc. 2014;28(8):2272–6.

19. Accreditation Council for Continuing Medical Education. Standard 3: identify, mitigate, and disclose relevant financial relationships. Available from: https://www.accme.org/accreditation-rules/standards-for-integrity-independence-accredited-ce/standard-3-identify-mitigate-and-disclose-relevant-financial-relationships.

20. Stain SC, Schwarz E, Shadduck PP, Shah PC, Ross SB, Hori Y, et al. A comprehensive process for disclosing and managing conflicts of interest on perceived bias at the SAGES annual meeting. Surg Endosc. 2015;29(6):1334–40.

21. Stain SC, Schwarz E, Shadduck PP, Shah PC, Ross SB, Hori Y, et al. A comprehensive process for identifying and managing conflicts of interest reduced perceived bias at a specialty society annual meeting. J Contin Educ Health Prof. 2015;35 Suppl 1:S33–5.

Index

J. R. Romanelli et al. (eds.), *The SAGES Manual of Quality, Outcomes and Patient Safety*,
https://doi.org/10.1007/978-3-030-94610-4